# Voluntary Food Intake and Diet Selection in Farm Animals

# Voluntary Food Intake and Diet Selection in Farm Animals

J.M. Forbes

*Professor*
*Department of Animal Physiology and Nutrition*
*University of Leeds*
*Leeds LS2 9JT*
*UK*

CAB INTERNATIONAL

CAB INTERNATIONAL
Wallingford
Oxon OX10 8DE
UK

Tel: +44 (0)1491 832111
Telex: 847964 (COMAGG G)
E-mail: cabi@cabi.org
Fax: +44 (0)1491 833508

A catalogue entry for this book is available from the
British Library.

ISBN 0 85198 908 X

Typeset by Solidus (Bristol) Limited
Printed and bound in the UK by Biddles Ltd, Guildford

# CONTENTS

# PREFACE

This book has its origins in *The Voluntary Food Intake of Farm Animals* published by Butterworths in 1986 since which time there has been steady development in our understanding of the control of voluntary food intake and there are plenty of new ideas and recent results to report, especially relating to diet selection. Although some of the material originates from the earlier book, the whole structure has been reorganized, with separate chapters on feeding behaviour, the role of the ruminant stomachs, learning, diet selection and specific appetites. All other sections have been revised, mainly by adding and reordering material, occasionally by omitting some information.

My approach throughout has been to provide examples to illustrate the principles of the subject and diagrams have been used wherever appropriate. I have given very many references to the literature. This is partly to justify the statements I have made but mainly as assistance to readers should they want to read in more detail about any aspect of the subject. By giving a list of contents at the beginning of each chapter it is hoped that the reader can, in conjunction with the index, quickly find any section in which (s)he might be interested.

J.M. Forbes

# 1 INTRODUCTION

- The significance of voluntary food intake
- Definitions
- Methods of measuring food intake
- Classical theories of intake control
- Problems and pitfalls
- Conclusion

The majority of farm animals are fed *ad libitum*; that is, they have food available almost all of the time. This is true whether they are kept intensively, the supply of food being under direct control of their keeper, or extensively, where the herbage available varies in quantity and quality according to the time of year, but is rarely completely unavailable. Despite this freedom of access to food there are many situations in which animals over- or under-eat and 'voluntary food intake' and the factors which control and influence it are of great importance to agriculturists across the world. The ramifications of the subject are so great that it is impossible to cover them all in one book and I have tried to give an even coverage of all aspects although, no doubt, some of my particular interests and prejudices will show through.

In the early chapters of the book, dealing with the physiological mechanisms of intake control, some reference is made to experimental work with laboratory animals, particularly the rat. This is necessary because many areas of study have been followed little or not at all with farm animals. However, the problem of balancing food intake with nutrient requirements has been with animals from an early stage in their evolution and it seems reasonable to assume that the mechanisms

1

are similar in all types of higher animal, unless this is proved otherwise. The later chapters deal with the more applied and agriculturally relevant aspects of the subject and here the coverage is restricted almost entirely to farm species.

This brief introductory chapter discusses in general terms why studies of the control of voluntary food intake in farm animals are important; the terminology is defined; a little of the history of the subject is described. The techniques used to measure food intake are briefly described while methods of monitoring feeding behaviour are dealt with in Chapter 2. The major features of domestic fowl and ruminants where they differ from the simple-stomached mammal are consigned to Appendix 1.

In a few places I have mentioned relevant findings with horses but have not dealt at all with fish. Recent reviews by Talbot (1993) and McCarthy *et al.* (1993) provide interesting reading and further reference on the latter.

## The Significance of Voluntary Food Intake

If voluntary intake is too low then the rate of production is likely to be depressed, making the requirements for maintenance become a very large proportion of the metabolizable energy in the food and so giving a poor efficiency of food conversion. If there is too high a level of intake then excessive fat deposition may occur, in some species at least. Thus the aim must be to match food consumption with the required level of production. This optimum level of production depends to a large extent on the relative costs of different types of feed and their nutrient values, and on the production response curve to changes to feed quantity and quality. For example, depending on the circumstances, it may be economically more efficient to feed a low rather than a high level of compound feed to a dairy cow, because forage intake increases and milk yield is not seriously depressed.

The quantitative importance of voluntary food intake is illustrated by the fact that poultry, which are invariably fed *ad libitum*, consume some 3.5 Mtonnes of food annually in the UK, accounting for some 70% of the total cost of poultry production.

Animals compete with man for food and there is a need to reduce the amount of grain-based feed especially with ruminants which are able to make use of grass, grass products and by-products of other agricultural and industrial activities; cereals can thus be saved for human consumption and for pigs and poultry which cannot digest cellulose, as can the ruminant. Because the bulk of a food as well as its nutritive value may limit intake, knowledge of the effects of changes in the type of food offered is essential.

The scientific study of voluntary food intake is important, there-fore, and demands a multidisciplinary approach. The nutritionist, the physiologist, the psychologist, the pharmacologist and, in the agricul-tural context, the animal and crop scientist all have to be involved to unravel the complexities of the subject.

## Problems of overeating

Whereas the problems of human obesity are obvious, those concerning farm animals are less so. That proverbial glutton, the pig, is often prevented from eating its fill by restricted feeding of a daily measured amount of food which is expensive in labour. Other species also become obese, however; cattle, sheep and broiler chickens fed *ad libitum* continue to deposit fat until they become grossly 'overweight' (Chapter 8). For example, Friesian dairy cows offered a feed low in roughage *ad libitum* and not remated were seen to increase in weight at the rate of about 1 kg per day and to show no sign of slowing down after 70 weeks, when they weighed 700 kg (Monteiro, 1972).

Do these animals get fat through overeating or because their energy output is too low? There has been much interest in the possibility that brown fat might 'burn off' excess energy intake (Stock and Rothwell, 1982; Hervey and Tobin, 1983) but brown fat appears to be absent in farm animals after the first few weeks of life. This then might be why cattle, sheep and pigs do not control their body fat content as well as the rat. Cattle, sheep, pigs and broilers seem to be more prone to obesity than other species, possibly as a result of selection by man for fast growth even if much of the rapid weight gain was in the form of fat.

Consumer preference has been to reduce the amounts of fat in meat over the last 50 years or so due, at least in part, to the general decrease in physical exertion of the human population. It is in the interests of the producer to reduce the amount of fat his animals deposit because of its low sale value and because the high energy content and low water content of adipose tissue make it very expensive to produce.

## Problems of undereating

Animals normally eat the amount of food which satisfies their energy requirements, including continued fat deposition in the adult. There are some circumstances, however, when insufficient is eaten, resulting in loss of body weight or a decrease in a productive process, such as growth or milk secretion (Chapter 9). Undereating can occur, in humans at least, even in the presence of adequate availability of food (e.g. the condition of anorexia nervosa). More commonly it occurs when there is a shortage of food (famine). In farm animals the problem of undereating is most often seen with ruminants where highly fibrous, bulky food is offered. This is digested slowly and its disappearance from the rumen sets a limit to the rate at which more food can be eaten; the mechanisms are dealt with in Chapters 4 and 10. This problem of undereating is at its most acute when other abdominal organs are competing for space (uterus, fat) or when the energy requirements are very high, as in early lactation. Food intake may be depressed also when the food is deficient in an essential component such as protein, a mineral, a vitamin or an amino acid (Chapter 11).

When the amount of herbage available for grazing is very sparse and each mouthful is small there may not be enough time in the day for the animal to eat enough to satisfy its nutrient demands. When snow, cold wind or hot weather prevent grazing there will again be inadequate food intake.

## Matching diet with appetite

Under natural conditions animals such as ruminants, pigs and poultry are 'general' feeders; that is, they eat from a wide range of foods. Initially they sample most potential foods but as they learn the nutritive (or toxic) properties of each type of material they become more selective. Although energy is probably the main controller of food intake there are other appetites, some innate, others learned, which influence the animal's choice of food and its total intake. The aim of the animal nutritionist is to match the quantity and quality of the diet with the nutrient requirements of the animal. If the diet is offered *ad libitum* this implies that the composition of the food should be such as to allow enough to be eaten to meet the animal's nutrient needs, but not to overconsume. In practice, this means offering a highly digestible nutrient-dense food (or foods) when high production is required (growth, late pregnancy, early lactation, egg production) but reducing the nutrient density of the feed at other times so as to prevent excessive fat deposition. This control of diet quality is often achieved with ruminants by varying the amount of a cereal-based compound food while allowing free access to a more fibrous forage. With pigs and poultry the greater degree of dilution with inert or poorly digestible 'fillers' which is necessary to depress intake of digestible nutrients usually renders this approach impractical and restriction of food must sometimes be practised (e.g. pregnant sows, broiler breeders).

With grazing animals (Chapter 16) intake is influenced by varying the stocking rate, herbage height or time available for grazing. The composition of the available herbage is not so amenable to manipulation and the changes in digestibility and composition which occur at different stages of the growing cycle must be understood if optimum use of grass is to be made. The formulation of diets has become increasingly sophisticated, especially for non-ruminants, so that they meet as closely as possible the requirements of the animals for which they are intended. Because requirements of an animal are for a given amount of a nutrient to be taken in a day, rather than per unit of feed, assessment of optimum levels of inclusion of nutrients depends on a knowledge or prediction of voluntary intake if it is intended that the feed should be given *ad libitum,* as is usually the case with poultry. It is unnecessary and impractical to control exactly the composition of ruminant feeds because they are going to be modified by rumen fermentation which precedes the normal processes of mammalian digestion (Appendix 1).

## Definitions

**Voluntary food intake** is the weight eaten by an animal or group of animals during a given period of time during which they have free access to food. In this book the word **food** describes the materials which animals eat whereas a **feed** is a portion of food offered to an animal, usually of a size and material determined by man.

Distinct eating periods which may include short breaks but which are separated by longer intervals are called **meals** and the short within-meal periods of eating are called **feeding bouts**. In analysing feeding behaviour a minimum **intermeal interval** is often adopted, meals separated by intervals of less than this value being considered as part of the same continuing meal. This critical intermeal interval, if it is to be applied, should not be selected arbitrarily but only after study of a frequency plot of intermeal intervals (Chapter 2). When an animal starts to eat it is said to do so because it is in a state of **hunger**; when it stops eating it does so because it is **satiated**. These two terms have no precise physiological meaning.

Given free access to food of good quality, individuals of many species may eat from ten to fifteen meals per day. Very often the distribution of meals through a 24 h period is not uniform, with more frequent, larger meals being taken during the photophase in those species, including the common farm animals, which are more active during that period.

Derived from measurements of meal size and intermeal interval are the **hunger ratio**, i.e. weight of meal divided by premeal interval, and the **satiety ratio**, i.e. weight of meal divided by postmeal interval. **Appetite** is used to describe a drive to eat a specific nutrient, rather than to eat food in general (Chapter 14). The word **palatability** has often been used to describe the overall sensory impression the animal receives from its food. However, there is no precise way of measuring palatability and ... 'there seems little point in using the term' (Lynch *et al.*, 1992).

The weight of food eaten per unit of time is the **rate of eating**. In this book the term refers to rate of eating during a meal rather than mean rate of eating over the whole day which is sometimes called **rate of intake**. In some cases it has been possible to measure instantaneous rates of eating at different times during a meal and to show, for example, that rate of eating declines as the meal progresses.

The total amount eaten during a given period of time (usually one day) is usually called the **voluntary intake**; this is often lower than the **potential intake** (the weight of food required to fulfil all of the animal's nutrient requirements) due to the physical or chemical constraints within the animal, or environmental limitations.

## Methods of Measuring Food Intake

In order to study factors affecting voluntary food intake and to develop methods of prediction (Chapter 17) we need to be able to measure intake in a variety of experimental and farm situations. Much of the more applied experimental work covered in later chapters has relied for measurement of voluntary food intake on single weighings of food at intervals of 24 h, but often shorter and occasionally longer periods. It is sometimes difficult to interpret data collected in this way because animals eat numerous meals during the day and a knowledge of the size and frequency of these meals is useful as will be seen in later chapters. The method of 24 h weighings is not applicable to the grazing situation, nor is it appropriate to the estimation of individual intakes of animals kept in a group and Chapter 2 describes methods for monitoring feeding behaviour.

When the fresh food is offered only once per day it is important to offer sufficient so that at least 15% remains; excessive allowance may, however, enable selection of the more preferred parts of feed mixtures which aggravates the difficulty of assessing the consumption of nutrients.

However, it is important to recognize that the ability of animals to select an optimum diet (Chapter 13) allows them to choose between different parts of the same plant and they can select a much more nutritious diet than the overall composition of the forage would provide, if given a sufficient excess of the food. For example, Brown *et al.* (1988) have shown that the digestibility of the herbage eaten increases with the amount on offer until this reaches about twice the dry matter eaten by the animals.

Sufficient time should be allowed for animals to become accustomed to new food before voluntary intake is recorded. For ruminants at least ten days is required because of the slow rate of passage and adaptation of the rumen micropopulation but prolonged standardization appears to be unnecessary (Heaney and Pigden, 1972). In view of the variability between individuals it is necessary to use a sufficient number of animals in order to get a reliable estimate of intake. Variability between animals in a group does not differ greatly between different feeds and is less when they are penned individually than when they are penned together (Heaney *et al.*, 1968). These authors observed that '... while intake is unquestionably an important index of forage value, high variability of estimates (coefficient of variation, 0.16) renders it not so useful as it might appear at first sight'. It has been suggested that the effects of between-animal variation in measurements of voluntary intake can be reduced by using the intake of a standard forage by each animal as a reference point (Abrams *et al.*, 1987) but this would be very difficult to apply over a long period of time with large numbers of animals.

## Classical Theories of Intake Control

This section briefly presents hypotheses of the way in which voluntary intake might be controlled. Various aspects are then covered in detail in subsequent chapters.

The history of studies of control of food intake is reviewed by Gallouin and Le Magnen (1987). Although there are many references to the subject before the beginning of the 20th century, it was not until around 1950 that much objective scientific study was directed to the problem. Having observed fluctuations in blood glucose concentration in synchrony with meals, and mindful of the central role of glucose in the metabolism of the rat, Mayer (1953) proposed the glucostatic theory in which he envisaged that the animal attempted to maintain a relatively constant level of glucose in the blood by a central nervous monitoring system. This has been modified in several ways, as described in Chapters 5 and 7, but the concept that it is the supply of energy to the body which the animal attempts to maintain by feeding is still very important. Whereas rats and other simple-stomached animals reduce their food intake when glucose is supplied, as would be expected, ruminant feeding is unaffected by glucose infusion. However, their intake is depressed by infusions of volatile fatty acids, the major products of rumen fermentation (Appendix 1), suggesting that their intake control depends on receptors for these acids.

It had long been suggested that the capacity of the digestive tract is an important limiting factor in feeding; this seems to be especially true for ruminants, in which fermenting bulky food remains in the rumen for very long periods. In the late 1950s the importance of gut fill had been demonstrated experimentally (Balch and Campling, 1962) and the positive relationship between the rate and extent of digestion of a forage and its level of voluntary food intake, which is so important in the utilization of forages, had been established and used as evidence for a 'physical' limit to intake. However, it is also generally accepted that ruminants can control their food intake to meet their nutrient requirements under quite a wide range of circumstances and there is evidence of sensitivity to the chemical and osmotic properties of the digesta which allow a 'metabolic' control of intake. It is likely that physical and metabolic controls of intake are not mutually exclusive, but additive.

Whereas short-term changes in energy supply and gut-fill can be seen to be involved in the control of meal size and frequency, it is unlikely that they would give a perfect balance between nutrient intake and nutrient requirements. A long-term imbalance must lead to an increase or decrease in body energy stores, particularly as fat, and it has been proposed that there is a route whereby the size of fat depots is relayed to the central nervous system (CNS) which uses this information in the control of intake: a lipostatic theory (Kennedy, 1953). This 'long-term' signal must be integrated with the various 'short-term' signals in order that the sum total of the food eaten at a series of meals is appropriate to the animal's long-term requirements.

When requirements change, intake should change in parallel. For example, lactation creates a massive increase in the requirements for energy, protein and other nutrients. Normally voluntary intake increases to match but sometimes, especially for ruminants offered forages, low voluntary intake limits milk yield and causes mobilization of body fat stores. Climatic changes also modify energy requirements and food intake normally responds appropriately (Chapter 15); the thermostatic theory of intake control (Brobeck, 1948) envisaged that animals eat to maintain a constant body temperature but this is now considered to be only a safety mechanism to avoid hyperthermia.

Because the unit of feeding is the meal, differences in meal size or intermeal interval must account for differences in food intake over any longer period from a few hours to a lifetime. If we can understand what causes an animal to start and stop eating then we can claim to understand the control of voluntary food intake. We do not yet have sufficient knowledge to be able to make such a claim; what we do know, however, is that several occurrences during a meal (stomach distension, accumulation and flow of products of digestion) are able to induce satiety when imposed experimentally, although it is often necessary to use levels which are greater than those encountered in the normal animal. These negative feedback signals will be considered further in Chapters 3 and 4 and the point will be made that it is likely to be the sum of these signals that controls not only satiety, but hunger also.

Nervous pathways from the viscera relay information to the brain concerning such parameters as stomach acidity, abdominal temperature and distension of various parts of the gastrointestinal tract. The lower part of the brain responds with changes in signals controlling metabolic hormones (including growth hormone, insulin and glucagon); it also activates the higher centres to initiate, continue or cease feeding. Information on the environment is relayed from the special senses influencing the basic control of feeding which is exerted by the lower centres. The identity of the parts of the brain which are involved is covered in Chapter 6. There are two major reasons for continuing to study the role of the brain in the control of food intake in farm animals: on the one hand there are the agricultural implications of the possibility of manipulating intake by pharmacological or other means to improve animal productivity and welfare. On the other hand there is the possibility of using these species, especially the pig, as a more adequate model than the rat, for gaining deeper understanding of basic feeding mechanisms which will improve chances of combating the human problems of obesity and anorexia.

## Problems and Pitfalls

In case this brief review gives the impression that we understand exactly how intake is controlled, it must be pointed out that there are numerous cases where different experiments and observations lead to contradictory conclusions. This situation can arise for many reasons. First, differences in experimental protocol such as the type of food offered or the duration of any period of food withdrawal before an experimental treatment or observation. Most studies of peripheral feedback signals either offer food *ad libitum* and add the infused substance to the contents already in the gut or precede feeding tests with fasts of many hours which put the animal in an abnormal state. The degree of stress to which animals are subjected might also influence the results of experiments on the control of intake.

Second, there are species differences. Hamsters do not increase their food intake after a period of food deprivation whereas rats invariably do (Silverman and Zucker, 1976). Would de Jong *et al.* (1981) have reached similar conclusions concerning the role of short-chain fatty acids in the control of feeding in goats if he had been working with sheep as did Anil and Forbes (1980a)?

Third, differences in interpretation occur. For example, Le Magnen and Tallon (1966) found a close correlation between the size of a meal and the postmeal interval, using an arbitrary minimum intermeal interval of 40 min, and proposed that the onset of feeding is determined largely by the rate of metabolic utilization of the products of the previous meal. Castonguay *et al.* (1986) have used an objective method, based on a sudden change in the frequency distribution of intermeal intervals, to determine the minimum intermeal interval and found it to be between 5 and 10 min. Applying this criterion they failed to obtain a significant relationship between size and postmeal interval and reached a different conclusion.

It is tempting to think that we can ultimately explain the control of food intake once we know about all the negative and positive feedbacks which pass information to the central nervous system (CNS). However, it is becoming increasingly clear that learning plays a vital role (Chapter 12). For example, animals learn the difference between two foods offered as a choice and base their relative intakes of the two on what they have learned. Why should the intake of a single feed not be subject to the same learning processes? That is, the metabolic consequences of previous meals of that food allow the animal to anticipate the likely consequences of the current meal and to adjust its size accordingly. Thus, the nutritional and metabolic history of the animal is as important in determining when and how much it eats as are the events which occur in the digestive tract, liver and CNS during the current meal.

## Conclusion

This brief introduction signposts areas covered in more detail in subsequent chapters. It will be clear that voluntary food intake and diet selection are complex subjects but that they are also important subjects, no less for farm animals than for human beings.

# 2 | FEEDING BEHAVIOUR

- Monitoring individual feeding behaviour
- Analysis of meal data
- Description of feeding
- Meal size and number
- Abnormal feeding-related behaviour
- Rate of eating
- Circadian rhythms
- Hunger and satiety ratios
- Food restriction and fasting
- Conclusions

In higher animals feeding occurs in discrete meals and, as indicated in Chapter 1, longer term changes in food intake can only occur by modification of the size of meals and/or the interval between them. Much effort, therefore, has gone into determining the factors which induce feeding to start and stop. In addition, many studies have described feeding behaviour without considering the underlying mechanisms. In any case, it is necessary to be able to monitor feeding behaviour and numerous methods have been devised to make this possible; once collected the copious amount of data needs to be reduced and analysed and appropriate methods for this have also been developed.

For further reading, the book of Fraser and Broom (1990) gives a useful introduction to behaviour, including feeding.

# Monitoring Individual Feeding Behaviour

This has traditionally been carried out by many hours of patient observation, noting at regular intervals whether or not each animal is eating, ruminating, standing, etc. Although there is no substitute for this in terms of learning about animal behaviour, and certain types of behaviour are not amenable to quantification in any other way, this method suffers from two major drawbacks: (a) it is very time-consuming (this can be overcome to some degree by video-recording and observing the play-back at a fast speed) and (b) it does not provide information on the weight of food eaten, but only on the timing of meals.

## Semi-automated systems

A more sophisticated system for recording the length of meals was developed by Wangsness *et al.* (1976) who used a light beam and photocell to detect when a sheep had its head in the feeder and employed this to move a new container of food into the feeding area automatically if at least 20 min had elapsed since the previous meal (i.e. a minimum intermeal interval defined as 20 min). This equipment, slightly modified, was also used to study the feeding behaviour of growing cattle (Chase *et al.*, 1976).

More comprehensive data can be collected by continuous automatic recording of the weight of the food container (e.g. Suzuki *et al.*, 1969). If the weight is static the animal is not eating. The duration of a meal is signalled by frequent oscillations in the weight of the container as it is disturbed by the animal's head; the weight of food eaten during that meal is the difference between the weights before and after the meal. It is often possible to obtain intermediate weights during a meal when the animal is not touching the container and thereby to determine the rate of eating at different stages during the meal.

V.R. Fowler (personal communication) adopted the simple expedient of suspending feed buckets for pigs from a spring balance whose face was continuously monitored by a video camera. A development of this principle has been described in which the weight of food is monitored by weighing on an electronic balance, the output of which is displayed at the bottom of a television picture of the animal (Baldwin *et al.*, 1983b). Such visual records must be scanned by eye and do not lend themselves to computerization.

For quail, Savory (1979) placed food on the pan of a balance and the weight was continuously recorded on a moving-paper recorder. The meals were so small, however, that their size was difficult to determine, although the occurrence and length of meals was easily ascertained. A more sophisticated system for chickens involved shielding the feed container from the bird once per hour to allow a stable weight to be recorded (Savory, 1976) but this did not give weights of individual meals, nor their timing.

## Fully automated systems

An automated system used at Leeds University for sheep, pigs and chickens is similar to that used by Suzuki *et al.* (1969). Although we used to make our own load beams and amplification system, more recently we have used proprietary balances with digital outputs, multiplexed to an IBM-compatible personal computer. Professional balances are robustly made and do not suffer from the drift which plagued our own set-up.

Each balance is programmed to transmit continuously the weight as a string of digits through the serial interface which is connected to the multiplexer, an electronically controlled switch. The PC instructs the multiplexer to connect a balance and reads in digits until it has got a meaningful weight; it then tells the multiplexer to connect to the next balance, and so on. Given that the length of each meal is at least several minutes, interrogating each balance at intervals of about 10 s is satisfactory and up to about 24 balances can be handled in that time. Each time a weight is obtained it is compared with the previous weight from that balance. If there has been no change then it is initially assumed that the animal is not eating; if previously the animal was eating then a potential end of meal is stored. However, in case this is just a pause in a meal, a series of stable weights over the period required for an intermeal interval is necessary to confirm that the meal has indeed ended.

If, on the other hand, there is a difference between two successive weights on the same balance then the animal is detected as eating; if this follows a period of stable, i.e. non-eating, weights, then the start of a meal is signalled. A simplified version of the program used is given in Appendix 2.

Each pen or cage can be provided with more than one weigher so that the intake of two or more different feeds and water can be monitored (e.g. sheep, Jones and Forbes, 1984; poultry, Shariatmadari and Forbes, 1992b).

## Operant conditioning

In the systems just described the animal has free access to the food; an alternative is to teach the animal to 'work' for a reward of food (reinforcement) by pressing a button (response), a technique known as

(a)

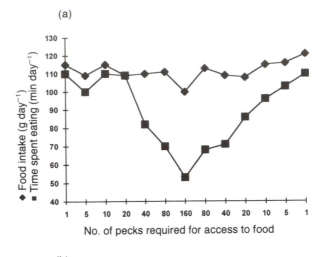

No. of pecks required for access to food

(b)

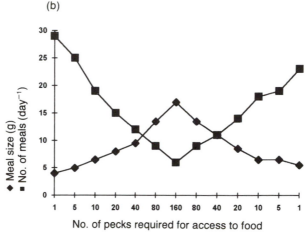

No. of pecks required for access to food

**Fig. 2.1.** The effect of the number of pecks (*y* axis) required for hens to obtain access to food on food intake and feeding behaviour (Savory, 1989). (a) Food intake (g day$^{-1}$) ◆; Time spent eating (min day$^{-1}$) ■. (b) Number of meals per day ■; Meal size (g) ◆.

**operant conditioning** (Baldwin, 1979, pigs and sheep; Clifton, 1979, chickens; Matthews and Kilgour, 1980, cattle). The number of responses the animal has to make before a reward is given (the **reinforcement schedule**) can be increased in order to see how strong is its desire for food, in relation to its other needs. The use of operant conditioning techniques ensures that the animal eats only when it has a definite urge to do so and not simply when it happens to find itself near to food. The apparatus used to control the reinforcement schedule can easily be adapted to keep a record of the timing of responses for subsequent analysis of meal occurrence.

Perhaps operant conditioning, in which the animal has to 'work' for food, might be a method of avoiding the social eating so often seen when animals are penned in sight of each other – one animal's eating often triggers that of another when the second would not have otherwise taken a meal at that time – thus confounding a strict 'physiological' experimental design. It must be recognized, however, that single confinement may induce abnormal behaviour. Savory (1989) has suggested that having to do a moderate amount of work for food avoids eating from boredom and gives more natural patterns of feeding under laboratory conditions. Figure 2.1 shows that, as the ratio of responses (pecks) to reinforcements (access to food) was increased, so the time spent eating and number of meals declined whereas the size of the meal and its rate of eating increased; daily food intake was unaffected.

## *Recording feeding behaviour in groups*

The relatively simple methods available for automatically recording the meals taken by individuals penned by themselves are not all suitable for monitoring the behaviour of individuals in a group. Observation, either direct or through the medium of video tape, is still possible for animals in groups when individuals can be identified by eye. In recent years electronic recognition has become available and it is now possible for a feed-dispensing system to recognize an animal's identity and to record the amount of food eaten by each individual. Such systems are available commercially for the recording and/or control of the concentrate allowance to individual dairy cows kept in groups (out-of-parlour dispensers; Broster *et al.*, 1982). Whereas this system is suitable for pelleted feeds it cannot be used to dispense long roughages.

If measurement of individual intakes of hay or silage is required and cattle cannot be fed individually then it is possible to use a marker dilution technique in which each animal is dosed by mouth with a known amount of an inert material. Chromic oxide has often been used, either given as a pellet or incorporated in a palatable feed. After several days to allow equilibrium to be reached faeces are collected from each animal, either by grab sampling from the rectum, or by collection of faeces identified by observation or by coloured plastic particles which can be given by mouth at the same time as the marker. From the content of the marker in the faeces, total faecal production can be calculated. It is then necessary to know the digestibility of the food in order to calculate the food intake; digestibility varies with level of intake so that ideally the individually penned animals used to determine the digestibility of the food should be of the same species, physiological state and level of intake as those whose intake is being estimated in the group. The cumulative errors involved in these procedures makes the result unreliable but useful for comparisons (see Chapter 16 for a discussion of these methods applied to grazing ruminants).

If the trough or bunker containing the forage could be weighed automatically and animals identified as they ate, then full details of meal patterns of individuals in a group would be available. This principle is embodied in the LUCIFIR system (Leeds University Cow Individual Feed Intake Recorder, Forbes *et al.*, 1987) in which cows wear collars with transponders of the type available commercially for identification in the milking parlour or at out-of-parlour concentrate dispensers. The food is placed in boxes mounted on top of load platforms which are capable of weighing to the nearest 0.1 kg. Both food weighing and identification systems are multiplexed to a PC which can be up to 1 km from the cattle yard. The software collects meal patterns at each weigher and also for each cow. Figure 2.2 shows part of the system. A further refinement is the provision of solenoid-controlled doors which allow certain animals to be prevented from eating from some or all of the feed boxes for some or all of the day. Thus, it is possible to have a group of animals, managed as a herd, in which different individuals have access to different feeds; it is also possible to restrict animals to eating within given periods of the day and/or to

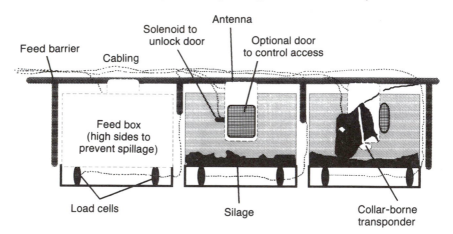

**Fig. 2.2.** Diagram of system to monitor feeding behaviour of several animals in a group, viewed from the side furthest from the animals. The left-hand feed station is shown with its feed box in place while the others are shown without boxes to enable the antennas and access control doors to be seen.

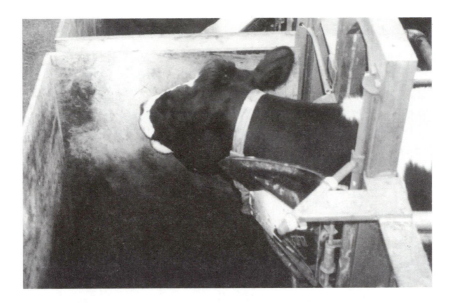

**Fig. 2.3.** The LUCIFIR system for monitoring feeding behaviour and feed intake of individual cattle kept in a group. Each cow wears a collar-borne transponder which allows it to be identified by the antenna loop through which she must put her head in order to eat. In this example feeding is controlled by computer-controlled doors which allows different animals to eat from different types of food (in this case grass silage).

predetermined weight of feed(s). Such a modification is shown in Fig. 2.3.

An example of a meal pattern of a cow obtained using this apparatus can be seen in Fig. 2.4 in which it can be seen that some 15 meals of silage varying in size from 1 to 7 kg of fresh matter were taken, with lengths from a few minutes to half an hour. Drinking occurred only three or four times per day, usually in close proximity to meals.

Systems such as this are expensive but yield a very large amount of detail about feeding behaviour; they also allow animals to be kept in groups and thus avoid the likely effects of individual confinement on intake. In addition to their use for research, they are being used by breeding companies in order to enable the intakes and thus efficiencies of individual animals to be used in the selection index. Thus, the largest cattle breeding organization in the UK is now using a LUCIFIR system in which the intakes of 70 heifers are monitored and a similar system is in use in Holland. Several pig breeding companies are also using automatic feed intake recorders to monitor daily intakes of individual pigs kept in a group (e.g. Brown and Henderson, 1989).

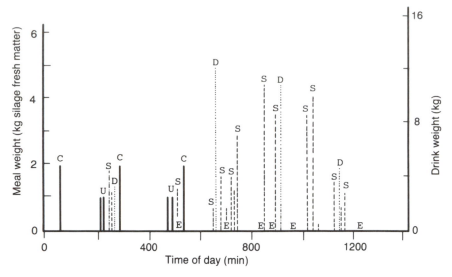

**Fig. 2.4.** An example of the meals of silage and concentrates and the drinks taken by a lactating dairy cow during a 24 h period using the LUCIFIR system (D.A. Jackson, J.M. Forbes and C.L. Johnson, unpublished results). S, meals of silage; D, drinks; C, meals of concentrates; U, visits to the concentrate dispenser which go unrewarded as the requisite time since last dispensation has not elapsed; E, visits to the concentrate dispenser which go unrewarded as the daily allowance has been exhausted.

## Analysis of Meal Data

*Reduction of meal data; calculation of intermeal interval*

Typically, the data generated by automatic recording systems are of the form:

> *Animal identity; serial number of feed station; times of start and end of meal; weights of start and end of meal*

each meal forming a record in a computer file. These data can be manipulated by statistical analysis programs, by purpose-written software or by means of a spreadsheet program. Calculation of total intake per day or during particular periods of the day is straight-forward, as is calculation of intermeal interval, rate of eating, hunger and satiety ratios. However, it is first necessary to consider 'When is a meal not a meal?' Animals invariably take short pauses during a meal and these must be differentiated from the longer gaps between separate meals. Sometimes an arbitrary period has been used (e.g.

20 min for sheep, Baile, 1975). However, examination of the frequency distribution of intermeal intervals often shows that these intervals form two distinct populations. In several species of bird, for example, intervals of more than a few minutes between feeding bouts are distributed in the form of negative exponentials, implying that there is a constant probability of a meal starting. However, the shortest intervals between meals do not follow this pattern and can be regarded as breaks in a meal, rather than true intervals between meals. Duncan *et al.* (1970) plotted the frequency distribution of intermeal intervals for domestic fowl and noted that there were far more intervals of 2 min or less than would be predicted from the negative exponential of the rest of the data and 2 min was therefore adopted as the minimum intermeal interval.

Metz (1975) derived survivorship curves for lengths of feeding bouts and interbout intervals for cows; bout length showed a distribution which is close to random. The bout-to-bout interval changes its frequency distribution at about 4 min, which is interpreted to mean that intervals of less than 4 min are within a meal. Metz also analysed rumination patterns in a similar manner and a thorough reading of his work is recommended to anyone who is planning to study feeding and ruminating behaviour.

For lactating cows fed grass silage at the Leeds University farm the critical intermeal interval was found to be close to 7 min (Forbes *et al.*, 1987) and this varied little between animals or with season or physiological state of the cows. However, it has not been possible to obtain such clear and consistent indications of the critical intermeal interval with cows at other sites.

Once the critical intermeal interval has been determined or estimated for the animal(s) in question, raw meal data can be merged into *true* meals. This is done by comparing the starting time of each meal in turn with the finishing time of the previous meal. If this interval is less that the chosen critical intermeal interval then the starting time and weight of the previous meal are assigned to the current meal and the previous meal is erased, thus merging the two.

## Statistical analysis of meal data

Various ways of analysing meal pattern data are discussed by Panksepp (1978). This section covers some of the more commonly used methods.

*Univariate analyses*

Methods such as *t*-test and analysis of variance have usually been used
to compare means of parameters such as daily intake, meal size and
rate of eating. However, because many feeding characteristics, such as
meal duration, meal size and intermeal intervals, are inter-correlated
the use of univariate tests for each variable is likely to yield some false
significant differences. It is, therefore, often advisable to use multivariate methods of analysis.

*Multivariate analyses*

These methods include multiple analysis of variance, discriminant
analysis and multiple regression analysis, in which more than one
meal-related variable can be included. This is a complex area of
statistical analysis (see Geiselman *et al.*, 1980 for examples applied to
rabbit data).

Sometimes, to reduce the huge amount of data collected by

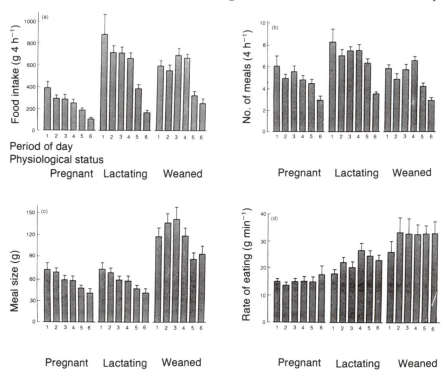

**Fig. 2.5.** Food intake (a), meal numbers (b), meal size (c), and rate of eating (d) by
pregnant, lactating, and weaned ewes fed hay during different periods of the day (Forbes
*et al.*, 1989)

automatic systems, calculations are made of mean meal size and intermeal interval. When done for whole days this disguises the fact that there is a circadian rhythm of feeding behaviour so the day can be divided into periods of, say 4 h and means calculated for each period (Forbes *et al.*, 1989). Figure 2.5 shows the number of meals, meal size, and rate of eating during the six 4-h periods of the day during late pregnancy, lactation and after weaning of ewes. The number of meals per 4 h declined from the time when fresh food was offered, as did meal size. However, rate of eating did not differ between different periods of the day. The increase in total food intake between pregnancy and lactation was due to an increase in meal numbers, whereas the slight fall in intake after weaning was due to fewer meals of larger size than in lactation, eaten at a faster rate.

Forbes *et al.* (1989) confirmed that feeding behaviour was markedly affected by physiological state using discriminant function analysis which showed that there was very little overlap between pregnancy, lactation and weaning in the characteristics of eating as described by total daily intake, rate of eating, meal weight, number of meals, satiety ratio and time spent eating.

Division of the day into arbitrary periods is an artificial procedure and methods which adopt a more continuous approach have been developed. Deswysen *et al.* (1989) used Fourier analysis to extract rhythms from meal patterns recorded from heifers offered maize silage. There were large and consistent cycles with phases of 24 h, 12 h and 8 h; the authors speculate about the physiological significance of these rhythms but only the 24 h cycle is clearly explicable as it is related to the solar cycle and the daily offering of fresh feed.

If in doubt, consult a statistician!

## Description of Feeding

It is not my intention to give an account of the minutiae of feeding but it is appropriate to describe briefly some of the main features.

### Poultry

For the first 2 days after hatching chicks are not dependent on eating food as they have sufficient reserves from the yolk sac. In the first few hours they eat little or nothing although they are exploring their environment and pecking at small round objects.

Chickens peck jerkily at food items, pick up the grain in their beak and then lift the head back before swallowing (see Appleby *et al.*, 1992a for a detailed description of feeding behaviour in poultry).

*Pigs*

Pigs grasp at food with their mouths and chew vigorously to mix it with saliva before swallowing the bolus. When kept outdoors they spend a lot of time rooting in the soil with their snouts. Stolba and Wood-Gush (1989) described the behaviour of domestic pigs in a seminatural environment. Concentrates were given at the normal time in normal quantities as the paddocks were not large enough to support the groups with natural food. Even so, on average, 31% of the time during the day was spent grazing and 21% rooting, i.e. over half the time was spent in ingestive activity. The animals turned turves over to get at worms and prized certain types of root, especially tree roots and those of sedge. Sterotypies and vices were absent.

*Cattle*

Dulphy *et al.* (1980) and Dulphy and Faverdin (1987) have reviewed the feeding behaviour of ruminants in detail. A characteristic of grazing cattle is that they wrap their tongue around herbage and pull rather than biting cleanly. They walk slowly forward, moving their head from side to side to take mouthfuls as they go.

The feed behaviour of housed cattle depends to a large extent on the ratio of animal numbers to length of trough. If there is sufficient space for all animals to eat at once then this they will do, especially when fresh food has been given or when they have just returned from milking. At other times a proportion will be eating leisurely. If, however, there is insufficient space for all animals to eat simultaneously then a great deal of manoeuvring takes place, dominant animals displacing timid ones, and meals tend to be a succession of brief episodes interspersed with movement to other feeding positions. Those cows lower in the social dominance order are forced to eat at less popular times of day, including late at night.

*Sheep*

Jaw movements start in the fetus about 40 days before birth, with evidence of swallowing; 'chewing' and 'sucking' occur during the last few days before birth (Harding *et al.*, 1984). Amniotic fluid and meconium (fetal faeces) are ingested, the latter occasionally causing death by choking at birth.

Lynch *et al.* (1992) describe teat-seeking and sucking activities of newborn lambs in detail. From two or three weeks of age lambs spend increasing amounts of time nibbling at food. After weaning they eat by prehending food with their lips and tongue, pulling it back into the mouth for extensive chewing.

Sheep can select well as they have a narrow bite. However, they have a blind area about 30 mm in front of the nose so they cannot see exactly what they are eating. Perhaps they use touch to decide exactly what to eat.

When they are selecting actively, e.g. green material from a predominantly dead sward, rate of eating is greatly reduced. The best way to monitor what sheep are selecting is to collect oesophageal extrusa from fistulated animals, although it is then difficult to identify the various parts of the plants. Lynch *et al.* (1992) give a detailed description of feeding behaviour in sheep.

# Meal Size and Number

*Poultry*

Isolated birds feed in frequent, brief bouts from which it is difficult to define a meal (Kaufman and Collier, 1983). However, when the cost of feeding is increased chickens exhibit similar patterns of feeding to mammals, and similar functional relations between foraging cost, meal frequency and meal size, i.e. meal frequency and, eventually daily intake, decline with increasing difficulty of obtaining food. The authors conclude that 'Meal patterns do not reflect momentary fluctuations in the internal environment; rather they appear to be a behavioural

**Table 2.1.** Comparison of feeding behaviour between growing chickens of broiler and layer strains (Masic *et al.*, 1974).

|  | Broilers | Layers | Significance |
|---|---|---|---|
| Age of birds (weeks) | 10.8 | 11.0 | ns |
| Body weight (g) | 2294 | 1104 | ••• |
| Weight gain (g over 5 days) | 150 | 66 | ••• |
| Food intake (g day$^{-1}$) | 172 | 97 | ••• |
| Time spent feeding (min day$^{-1}$) | 89 | 168 | • |
| Rate of eating (g min$^{-1}$) | 2.4 | 0.8 | • |
| Number of meals per day | 49 | 41 | •• |
| Meal length (min) | 2.5 | 6.0 | •• |
| Intermeal interval (min) | 15.3 | 14.7 | ns |
| Meal weight (g) | 3.5 | 2.4 | •• |

ns, Not significant.
$^*P < 0.05$; $^{**}P < 0.01$; $^{***}P < 0.001$.

device that animals adjust to exploit the available resources in their current habitat efficiently'. As mentioned above, Savory (1989) has suggested that feeding behaviour should be studied in conditions where birds have to do a modest amount of work to get food as this provides more clearly defined meals than when food is easily available all the time.

Although broiler chickens eat almost twice as much as layers of the same age, they spend only half as much time eating and take more meals of shorter duration (Masic *et al.*, 1974). Table 2.1 gives the main features of feeding behaviour for chickens of the two strains.

*Pigs*

De Haer and Merks (1992) used an objectively derived critical intermeal interval of 5 min. Table 2.2 gives the characteristics of feeding for group-housed animals, whose behaviour was monitored by an automatic feeding system, and for individually penned littermates. In groups, 69% of meals accounted for 87% of intake and 83% of eating time. With individual housing, 39% of meals contributed 90% of the food eaten and 79% of the feeding time. In other words, there were a lot of small, short meals when pigs were kept individually, compared to when they were in groups. The repeatabilities of day-to-day recordings of intake traits were high within 2-week periods compared to within months or the whole fattening period, indicating a steady change in feeding behaviour as pigs grow. The diurnal pattern of eating is shown in Fig. 2.6 for pigs in the two housing situations.

**Table 2.2.** Feeding behaviour of group-housed and individually penned growing pigs (de Haer and Merks, 1992).

|  | Group | | Individual | |
| --- | --- | --- | --- | --- |
|  | Mean | s.d. | Mean | s.d |
| Length of meal (min) | 6.9 | 1.8 | 4.2 | 1.6 |
| Weight of meal (g) | 225 | 59 | 110 | 38 |
| Rate of eating (g min$^{-1}$) | 32 | 5.0 | 27 | 5.0 |
| Meal number (day$^{-1}$) | 9.2 | 2.4 | 21.0 | 4.9 |
| Total food intake (g day$^{-1}$) | 2043 | 291 | 2203 | 200 |
| Total eating time (min day$^{-1}$) | 63 | 13 | 84 | 15 |

s.d., Standard deviation.

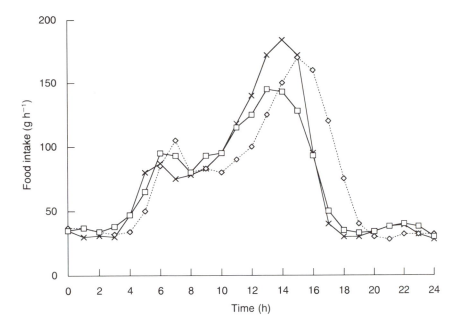

**Fig. 2.6.** Diurnal patterns of feed intake in group-housed growing pigs (de Haer and Merks, 1992). The three lines represent different batches of animals.

## Cattle

By using a critical intermeal interval of 7 min it was found that lactating Friesian–Holstein cows ate an average of 15 meals per day, irrespective of whether the supplementary compound food was high in starch or high in digestible fibre (Jackson *et al.*, 1991). The daily intakes of silage for the two supplement types were 10.8 and 13.0 kg dry matter (DM), respectively, eaten in 209 and 229 min. Thus the higher silage intake was achieved on the digestible fibre supplement by eating larger, longer meals. Intake reached a peak in mid-lactation whereas the number of meals per day reached a nadir around week 15 of lactation (Fig. 2.7). Figure 2.4 shows an example of a 24 h meal pattern of one cow. In this case nine meals of silage were taken and three allocations each of 2 kg concentrates were dispensed. At 230 min she tries to get concentrates but is not allowed and diverts her attention to eating silage. Some of the silage meals are protracted and fragmented

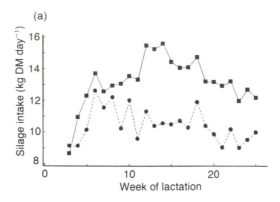

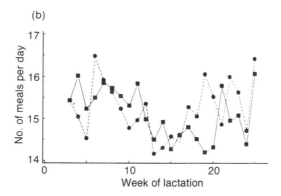

**Fig. 2.7.** (a) Intakes and (b) number of meals by cows fed supplements with high digestible fibre (■) or high starch (●) during the first 25 weeks of lactation (Jackson *et al.*, 1991).

(e.g. that at 650–750 min) whereas others are continuous (e.g. that starting at 840 min).

Steers fed a 70% concentrate:30% hay diet took about 30 feeding bouts per day (Morita and Nishino, 1991).

*Sheep and goats*

Dulphy *et al.* (1980) report a mean total eating time of 305 min day$^{-1}$ for wether sheep fed fresh-cut green forages with a mean rate of eating of 4.3 g DM min$^{-1}$. These animals took 7.5 meals day$^{-1}$ and spent an average of 537 min day$^{-1}$ ruminating.

**Table 2.3.** Parameters of eating by pygmy goats (Langhans *et al.*, 1988).

| | 12 h light | | 12 h dark | | Total | |
|---|---|---|---|---|---|---|
| | Mean | s.e. | Mean | s.e | Mean | s.e. |
| Number of meals (per 12 h) | 8 | 0.9 | 4 | 0.3 | 12 | 0.7 |
| Meal weight (g) | 43 | 4 | 62 | 5 | 49 | 4 |
| Meal length (min) | 22 | 3 | 28 | 7 | 24 | 4 |
| Intermeal interval (min) | 63 | 6 | 170 | 13 | 87 | 6 |
| Total intake (g) | 384 | 14 | 226 | 15 | 610 | 21 |

s.e., Standard error.

The feeding behaviour of pygmy goats has been monitored by Langhans *et al.* (1988) who noted that about twice as many meals were taken in the 12 h day than at night (Table 2.3). Meal weight was smaller in the day than at night so that food intake was not quite double in the day, compared to the night.

## Abnormal Feeding-related Behaviour

In intensive husbandry it is not uncommon to observe abnormal feeding-related behaviours. Although these have been ascribed to boredom it is also possible that such behaviours as tail-biting and feather-pecking are expressions of a desire to obtain nutrient(s) not provided in sufficient quantities by the diet.

A stereotypy is 'a repeated, relatively invariate sequence of movements which has no obvious purpose' (see Fraser and Broom, 1990, Chapter 32), such as repeated chewing of metal bars by individ-ually penned sows. They are mostly performed during the post-feeding period and are initiated by giving a small amount of feed. This, and the fact that they are not normally elicited by non-food-related stimuli, suggests that they are due to underfeeding and exacerbated by the lack of alternative possibilities for exploration and activity.

Excessive water consumption is sometimes seen in poultry, pigs, sheep and horses, the latter taking up to $140\,l\,day^{-1}$. When this occurs it is usually in confined animals and can be overcome by provision of more space and exercise. Often the apparently high consumption of water is due to excessive waste as bored animals stand with their noses on nipple drinkers.

*Poultry*

Feather-pecking can occur in all types of poultry, especially if insufficient trough space is provided (Fraser and Broom, 1990, Chapter 34).
This can be alleviated by giving birds something to search for, e.g. by
giving some whole grains in the food or on the floor. Feather-pecking
sometimes leads to body-pecking and wounding.

Egg-eating by hens may be an indication of mineral deficiency in
the diet as it is reduced by providing grit, although this again may be
a question of lack of variety of activities rather than a nutrient
deficiency. Birds eat shavings on which they are bedded if they have
not enough trough space; this can result in gizzard compaction and
eventual death if not forestalled by increasing the availability of food.

Pecking at metal or wood in a stereotypic manner is sometimes
observed in birds, again when the environment is monotonous. Kostal
*et al.* (1992) found that the amount of time spent stereotypically pecking
was negatively related to plasma corticosterone levels and they
suggested that such activity relieves stress.

*Pigs*

It is natural for newly weaned animals to explore their environment
and they often lick and chew objects, including other animals (Fraser
and Broom, 1990, Chapter 33). However, this sometimes develops into
biting each other's tails if pigs are heavily stocked in a boring
environment. The use of straw bedding and/or the provision of 'toys'
is helpful as it gives the pigs more interest and activity. Belly-nosing in
early weaning piglets is a response to the lack of the mother. Pigs also
show increased tail-biting when the diet is salt- or protein-deficient.
this is probably a general increase in oral activity rather than a specific
alleviation of the nutrient deficiency as the little blood obtained would
not significantly improve their salt or protein status (Fraser and Broom,
1990).

Bar-chewing or sham-chewing in sows, common in individual
pens or stalls, is usually reduced if straw or sawdust is provided
(Lawrence *et al.*, 1993). Sows often eat dead piglets but occasionally a
sow may attack, kill, and eat a piglet. Usually only first litters are
affected and in the first few hours after parturition.

*Cattle*

Calves spend about an hour per day sucking naturally from their
mothers but can drink milk replacer much more quickly than this,
leading to boredom and sucking of other calves, particularly the navel.

The use of dispensers which deliver the milk slowly to simulate natural suckling is helpful as is the provision of straw bedding.

Many calves in crates lick their own hair, a symptom of boredom and possibly of nutrient deficiency. This often creates hair-balls in the stomach which can occasionally become so large that they block the digestive tract.

*Sheep and goats*

Sheep will pull and eat the wool of others if too tightly penned but this can usually be prevented by providing roughage for them to chew. Agile, young goat does can also suck their own teats.

Marsden and Wood-Gush (1986) fed individually penned lambs aged 8 weeks either high (174 g kg $DM^{-1}$) or low (110 g) protein feeds *ad libitum* or restricted to 1 kg $day^{-1}$. More time was spent in abnormal activities (such as biting empty feed bins, wood or wool, 'star-gazing') by those on the restricted level of food but when hay was offered in addition there was much less abnormal behaviour. Blackface lambs chewed wool more when on low protein than when on high protein food whereas there was no difference in Suffolk crosses. The former spent less time eating than the latter when on *ad libitum* feeding and more time in abnormal food searching. These animals fed *ad libitum* grew at a very high rate, thus showing that high performance is not necessarily an indication of good welfare.

# Rate of Eating

When it is possible to measure intermediate weights of the food during the course of a meal it can be seen that rate of eating sometimes declines towards the end of a meal. This has been studied systematically in rats by Davis and Smith (1988) who showed that rate of eating declines steadily during a meal and that faster initial rates are associated with more palatable foods.

*Poultry*

Growing broilers eat faster than layers of the same age (Masic *et al.*, 1974, Table 2.1): 15-week-old layer cockerels ate a standard grower food at an average speed of 0.3 g $min^{-1}$ (Rusby *et al.*, 1987) whereas layer pullets ate at about 0.4 g $min^{-1}$ (Savory and Hodgkiss, 1984).

Rates of eating were significantly faster for pellets than for the same food in powdered form and declined during the 30 min after giving food after a 0–4 h fast (Savory, 1988). The weight eaten in the

first 5–10 min was proportional to the length of the previous deprivation period (see below).

*Pigs*

Auffray and Marcilloux (1983) observed a deceleration in rate of eating
as the meal progressed. 'Unpalatable' foods are eaten more slowly than
'normal' ones and rate of eating often increases over a period of several
weeks as the animals learn that the food is completely safe.

It had been assumed that rate of eating would be influenced by the
bitter-tasting glucosinolates present in rapeseed meals but Lambert *et
al.* (1992b) showed that the food eaten most slowly was that lowest in
glucosinolate.

*Cattle*

Faverdin (1985) (quoted by Dulphy and Faverdin, 1987) observed that
the rate of eating of a complete food by a lactating cow increased
linearly from 50 g min$^{-1}$ in the first few days of lactation to 90 g min$^{-1}$
in week 9 of lactation. The rate declined as a large meal proceeded, from
120 to about 50 g min$^{-1}$ due to longer pauses in actual chewing as the
meal progressed.

Suzuki *et al.* (1969) found that the mean rate of eating of DM by
lactating cows was greater for silage, at around 100 g DM min$^{-1}$,
compared with hay (40 g min$^{-1}$). The figure for silage is higher than that
observed by other workers and this is probably accounted for by the
fact that Suzuki's cows were not fed *ad libitum* and were therefore
eating after a period without food. Rate of eating declined as the meal
progressed but this was not simply due to jaw fatigue as unpublished
work quoted by Suzuki *et al.* (1969) was reported to show that giving
fresh silage half-way through a meal resulted in a resumption of eating
at the maximum rate.

The mean rates at which lactating mature cows ate grass silage (50
or 57 g DM min$^{-1}$; Jackson *et al.*, 1991), were very similar to that for
lactating heifers eating a complete silage/concentrate mixed food with
an average rate of approximately 50 g DM min$^{-1}$ (B. McGuirk and J.M.
Forbes, unpublished observations).

Presumably in systems where food is limited, e.g. dairy cows fed
concentrates in a group, the fastest eaters will consume more and
produce more milk, thus rendering themselves more likely to be
selected as the mothers of future cows, i.e. selection for fast rate of
eating. However, the rate of eating by cows low in the dominance order
was found by Kenwright and Forbes (1993) to be significantly faster
during the 40 min peak periods after each milking (300 g fresh matter

min$^{-1}$) than at a quiet period (10.00–12.00 h) (200 g min$^{-1}$) and the time spent eating significantly less (14.6 vs. 18.7 min). The most dominant animals did not eat significantly faster during these peak times than at other times of day (270 vs. 250 g min$^{-1}$) but spent a little more time eating than at other times of day (19.9 vs. 17.6 min). Thus, the dominant cows did not feel under pressure to eat quickly at busy times as they were confident of being able to continue eating when they were hungry.

Rate of eating of concentrates is particularly important when cows are fed at milking time. Any cow not finished eating when her group have finished milking will hold up the whole group, or miss part of her ration which will then be eaten by the next cow to come into that position in the milking parlour. Inclusion of rapeseed meal in a dairy compound food slows rate of eating but only to a marked extent during the first two or three feeds after the rapeseed is introduced (Frederick *et al.*, 1988). A mixture of flavours incorporated in the food successfully prevents this initial slow rate of eating.

Wet food is eaten faster than the same food given in the dry form and Clough (1972) found that cows which ate loose meal at 323 g min$^{-1}$ ate pellets at 455 g min$^{-1}$ and slurry at 1670 g min$^{-1}$; even though the slurry contained water, the rate of DM intake was considerably higher with the food in this form.

## Sheep

Pregnant ewes fed throughout on a complete, pelleted food ate at an average rate of 15 g min$^{-1}$ and this increased to around 20 g min$^{-1}$ during lactation and to over 30 g min$^{-1}$ after weaning (Forbes *et al.*, 1989).

Rates of eating during the first 30 min of the large meal taken after offering fresh hay, chopped dried grass or pelleted dried grass were 7.3, 9.4 and 10.8, respectively (Forbes *et al.*, 1972). During the second and third 30-min periods there were progressive reductions in rate of eating. In a further experiment the same authors penned ewes either singly or in groups of six and fed them on hay either *ad libitum* or at two-thirds of *ad libitum*. Rate of eating in the 30 min after giving fresh hay was significantly higher for the lower level of feeding (9.7 g min$^{-1}$) than for *ad libitum* (8.4 g min$^{-1}$), but only slightly higher for group-fed ewes (9.3 g min$^{-1}$) than those penned individually (8.8 g min$^{-1}$). The fact that restricted-fed sheep ate more quickly than those fed *ad libitum* shows that the latter were not eating at their maximum rate and therefore that neither jaw fatigue nor lack of saliva was likely to have limited *ad libitum* intake.

# Circadian Rhythms

Rats eat more frequent and larger meals at night than during the day as they are nocturnal animals, whereas farm mammals are more active during the day when they eat a greater proportion of their meals than at night.

## Poultry

Unless the nights are very long poultry do not eat during the hours of darkness so there is a very marked diurnal rhythm of feeding. Savory (1979) observed a peak of feeding activity and intake during the hour before dusk, presumably to fill the crop as a reservoir of food to last the bird through the night. It is not necessary for the light to dim slowly for this feeding to occur as the peak of feeding still occurs when the lights are extinguished abruptly. In order to see the extent to which birds learn to anticipate a fast, Petherick and Waddington (1991) housed pullets individually in a circadian-free environment and on days 17–47 half were shown a coloured card during the final hour of food availability, prior to food deprivation of 8 or 12 h. There was no indication of increased intake during this period and so no suggestion that they could learn to use the colour cue to anticipate a fast. Do they learn when dusk is approaching by the number of hours since dawn?

## Pigs

There are two peaks of feeding, one in the morning and one in the early afternoon (de Haer and Merks, 1992) but Fig. 2.6 shows that the evening one is by far the greater. Note that some feeding still takes place at night and that there is little effect of single vs. group penning.

## Cattle

A high level of feeding activity is usually observed after fresh food is offered. A smaller peak often occurs before sunset and another just after midnight. Data from individual young bulls fed from automatically recording feeders showed that the sunset peak moved according to the time of year and that the night-time quiet period was longer in the winter (Stricklin, 1988). In another trial, cattle were either trough-fed or fed from a single automatic feeder. Whereas those fed from the trough showed a normal diurnal pattern of feeding, those on the single-space feeder ate at any time of day or night, presumably due to competition. Trough-fed cattle spent about 120 min day$^{-1}$ feeding compared to 80 min for those on the single feeder.

Under conditions where little competition for feeder space exists, dairy cows eat few meals from around 01.00–06.00 h. When there are more animals than feeder spaces there is strong competition at busy times, particularly after milking and when fresh food has been delivered. Kenwright and Forbes (1993) observed a clear triphasic pattern of eating in cows milked three times per day, peaks of feeding activity occurring during the periods after return from milking including large meals which shows that some cows were monopolizing feeders thereby preventing others from eating at this time. The 01.00–06.00 h period was relatively quiet with 13% of the total number of meals taken in 15% of the total time spent eating. The more dominant animals ate less at night (01.00–06.00 h) than those at the bottom of the order. Therefore heifers low in the social dominance order were not able to satisfy fully their desire to eat when the level of competition for feeding space was high. The high incidence of aggressive interactions during the period immediately after return from milking has implications for the health and nutrition of the animals.

The fact that lower yielders were lower in the dominance order (calculated according to Rutter *et al.*, 1987) than high yielders but ate more at night suggests that high demand for nutrients was not the prime cause of nocturnal eating, although it is possible that low dominance caused low intake which resulted in lower milk yield. It is more likely that those lower in the dominance order were prevented from meeting their needs during the day and were thus forced to satisfy their requirements by eating in the middle of the night. When they did manage to eat at the most popular times of day it was in short meals, eaten at a rapid speed and presumably terminated by the arrival of a more dominant animal.

What are the implications of these findings for the management of dairy herds? Jackson *et al.* (1991) suggested that up to a ratio of 3.5 cows per feeder there was no effect on daily intake of silage whereas P. Elizade and S.C. Mayne (personal communication) have shown that, although feeding behaviour is affected with five or more cows per feeder (increased rate of eating and shorter total feeding times), it is not until there is a ratio of seven cows for each feeder that daily intake of silage becomes depressed.

*Sheep*

Sheep show similar light-entrained circadian rhythms of feeding to cattle (Fig. 15.4). Another factor affecting feeding rhythms is environmental temperature; sheep do not eat in the hottest part of the day when the heat load is so great that they must seek shelter (Johnson, 1987).

# Hunger and Satiety Ratios

If there is a high degree of correlation between the size of meals and the length of the preceding intermeal intervals this implies that there is a mechanism which determines when feeding should stop, i.e. that satiety mechanisms predominate. Conversely, a significant correlation between meal size and postmeal interval implies that there is a mechanism for determining when feeding should start, i.e. a hunger mechanism. Le Magnen and Devos (1980) found a good correlation between the weight of food eaten by rats in a meal and the interval to the next meal during the night, but no correlation with premeal interval, and concluded that the size of a meal is not determined by the metabolic deficit incurred prior to the meal. It was deduced that it is the size of a meal which determines the length of the subsequent interval and therefore that the satiety ratio is more important than the hunger ratio.

The hunger ratio has usually been found to be more important than the satiety ratio in chickens, as in rats. Kaufman and Collier (1983) and Savory (1989) suggest that using a fixed schedule operant situation gives more 'normal' feeding patterns with more reliable hunger ratios.

In cattle, however, Metz (1975) found a positive correlation between meal size and the length of the premeal interval as did Baile (1975) with sheep offered a 0.6 concentrate:0.4 forage mixture, i.e. the hunger ratio was thought to be more useful than the satiety ratio. Chase *et al.* (1976) analysed 968 meals of a complete feed (a single food which contains all the required nutrients in the correct ratio) taken by cattle at all times of day and found no significant correlation between the weight of a meal and either the pre- or postprandial interval.

# Food Restriction and Fasting

Periods without food leave the animal in a different state than when fully fed. It is important to measure fully this state in order to predict how the animal will respond when fully fed again (Kyriazakis and Emmans, 1992). Care needs to be given to the choice and description of the treatment(s) during the rehabilitation period.

*Poultry*

Pecks at food become faster, stronger and less accurate after increasing periods of deprivation (Wood-Gush and Gower, 1968) but when food is unavailable for 1 day in 5 there is complete compensation of intake and growth (Sherwood *et al.*, 1964). Petherick *et al.* (1992) trained hens to run down a 14.4 m alley for food after being deprived for 0, 6, 12 or 18 h. The speed of running was significantly increased by deprivation, but there was no difference between deprivation periods (0.29, 0.62, 0.65, 0.57 m s$^{-1}$ respectively).

Food restriction is sometimes used to delay puberty in pullets. When pullets were subsequently restricted to that weight of food eaten voluntarily at 6 weeks of age (45 g day$^{-1}$) (Savory and Fisher, 1992) the birds ate and pecked at empty feeders for the same amount of time per day as *ad libitum* controls spent eating, i.e. there was no increase in attempts to get food, as is seen in more severe types of underfeeding.

Broiler breeder stock are usually restricted to between one-half and one-quarter of *ad libitum* intake, depending on whether birds of the same weight or the same age are compared. Such animals have a high rate of working for food, even just after their ration has been consumed. Birds fed a commercial daily ration, or twice that amount, are highly motivated to eat at all times (Savory *et al.*, 1993).

When food was returned to cockerels of an egg-laying strain after food deprivation the rate of eating was higher after a 24 h fast than after a 2 h fast but there was no further effect of 48 h (Wood-Gush and Gower, 1968). It is likely that the size of the first meal after a long fast is limited by the capacity of crop which acts as a storage organ, distension of which inhibits feeding (Richardson, 1970b).

Rather than restrict intake by offering weighed amounts of food, it is often more convenient to give access to unlimited amounts of food for limited periods of time. Cockerels of a layer strain allowed food for one or two periods of 2 h each per day ate 65 and 80% of the amount eaten by control groups with 24 h day$^{-1}$ access (Barach *et al.*, 1992).

In a review of the welfare of poultry in modern production systems Mench (1992) discusses food deprivation and restriction which poses a welfare dilemma, as if fed *ad libitum*, broiler breeders experience reduced fertility and health problems.

## Pigs

There was a linear increase in the weight of food eaten by growing pigs during the first meal after deprivation of 1–6 h (M. Corbett, S. McNicholas and J.M. Forbes, unpublished observations).

Restriction of protein intake in pigs has been shown to cause increased rooting and general activity suggesting that specific nutritional needs increase foraging motivation (Lawrence *et al.*, 1993). Restriction of food intake gives rise to increases in 'working' for food in an operant conditioning situation but normal farm environments do not provide facilities for foraging. Therefore animals develop stereotypies such as chewing chains; ingestion of even a small amount of food stimulates such activities. Pregnant sows are usually restricted to about 60% of their *ad libitum* intake and such animals have a high rate of working for food, even just after their ration has been consumed (Lawrence *et al.*, 1988). In order to give sows a more natural way of getting food by working for it, Young *et al.* (1993) have developed a feeding ball which delivers food pellets at random intervals if it is rolled around. The lower the level of feeding the more sows push the ball around.

Quite severe food restriction of boars made them much more willing to press a button to obtain small rewards of food, compared with those fed almost *ad libitum* (Lawrence *et al.*, 1989). When the bulk of the restricted ration was increased by incorporating straw there was no reduction in operant responding showing that the mere presence of bulk in the digestive tract was not satiating.

Pregnant gilts and sows given restricted amounts of food with different levels of fibre showed a significant reduction in stereotypies with higher fibre foods (Robert *et al.*, 1993). These authors conclude that bulky food may be beneficial for welfare of pregnant sows.

*Cattle*

The intake of hay by cows increased by 20% as the increase in time of access to food was increased from 5 to 24 h day$^{-1}$, in contrast to an 80% increase in intake when the food was a concentrate mixture (Freer and Campling, 1963). Daily access for at least 6 h is necessary for maximum intake of silage by beef cattle (Wilson and Flynn, 1974). Dry cows ate 8.0 kg day$^{-1}$ when given access to silage for 5 h day$^{-1}$ whereas those with continuous access ate 10.1 kg (Campling, 1966a).

*Sheep*

When sheep were given access to hay cubes for 3, 6, 12 or 24 h day$^{-1}$ intakes were 1502, 1869, 2086, and 2413 g day$^{-1}$ (Hidari, 1981). With shorter fasts of 1 to 6 h, sheep fed on a pelleted 0.5 dried grass:0.5 barley compound food compensated for the fasting period in the first two or three meals after the food had been replaced and there was no effect on daily intake (J. Black, F. Carey-Wood and J.M. Forbes, unpublished observations).

## Conclusions

There are various ways of monitoring food intake but some of the indirect ones have a large amount of variability associated with them.

Automation allows the collection of large amounts of data without the presence of a human observer to disturb the animals. It is now possible to monitor the feeding behaviour and food intake of individual animals kept in a group which allows monitoring under realistic farm conditions. This has paved the way for the use of food intake and efficiency of utilization in selecting breeding stock.

The feeding behaviour of an animal in a barren experimental environment might be quite different from that of the same animal in more natural surroundings and it has been suggested that the use of operant systems which make the animal work to obtain food make the animal adopt a more natural feeding pattern. Unnatural feeding-related behaviour is seen in animals which are frustrated, either by lack of food or by being kept in a restricting environment.

There are strong circadian rhythms of feeding but these are not inflexible; for example, chicks will eat during the dark if that is the only time food is available, even though they normally eat nothing at night. Short periods without food can be compensated for when food becomes available but longer periods of fasting result in a significant reduction in daily intake.

# 3 FEEDBACK SIGNALS

- Oropharyngeal receptors
- Stomach receptors
- Intestinal receptors
- Liver receptors
- Conclusions

In searching for hunger/satiety signals we are looking for changes in the body that go in one direction during a meal, may continue in that direction for some time after the meal, but eventually return to the premeal level. There are numerous changes which fit these criteria, including physical and chemical factors in the gastrointestinal tract, and hormones and metabolites in the bloodstream. Because of the large amount of work done with ruminants to study the role of the reticulorumen in the control of feeding, this topic is dealt with separately (Chapter 4).

Most theories of the control of intake include the idea that ingestion of food causes changes in the body which are monitored by the brain and used to determine when feeding should cease. These changes, and the routes by which information concerning them is carried to the brain, are referred to as negative feedback pathways. It is unlikely that, under normal circumstances, only one factor is involved in the termination of feeding, or satiety. Rather, satiety occurs when the combined strength of signals from gastrointestinal and liver receptors reaches a threshold (see Chapter 7). Even this is a simplification, however, as it does not allow for long-term balancing of food intake with requirements; in order to achieve this match, feeding must terminate long before the animal knows how much of the various nutrients has been absorbed. In order to provide ways of predicting nutrient availability, learned associations between the organoleptic properties of a food and its eventual nutritive value are developed (see Chapter 12). Also, there are learned associations between the gastro-intestinal effects and eventual yield of nutrients and learned associations between the early metabolic effects of the nutrients absorbed from a meal on liver and brain, and eventual nutrient yield. It is not anticipated that the total of all these mechanisms could be accurate, however, so that feedbacks from the regulated stores of nutrients are required in addition to the above-mentioned immediate effects of a meal on feeding. Therefore, satiety is induced and feeding ceases at a point at which the total of all the signals, from both direct physical and chemical stimuli and from learned associations, reach a satiating level.

## Oropharyngeal Receptors

Receptors in the buccal cavity and throat are important in the animal's sensory perception of food; the sensory properties of a food are as likely to encourage further feeding as they are to cause feeding to stop. Zeigler (1975) has shown that deafferentation of the buccal region in the pigeon, by section of the trigeminal nerves, leads to loss of interest in food although drinking and grooming were unaffected; clearly in this species the taste and texture of food in the mouth is an important reinforcer of feeding.

It has been suggested that the jaw muscles become fatigued in species such as ruminants which have to spend a long time chewing each day, leading to slowing of the rate and eventually to the cessation of eating. Such fatigue is not of importance in normal satiety, however, because rats (Gibbs *et al.*, 1973a) and cows (Campling and Balch, 1961) continued to eat for much longer than usual when ingested food was removed via a gastric fistula. It is not appropriate, therefore, to consider the mouth as a generator of negative feedback signals except in helping the animal to identify the food with learned associations.

## Stomach Receptors

The first internal changes to be correlated with feelings of hunger were the so-called hunger contractions of the stomach. However, vagotomy, which abolishes these contractions, does not seriously interfere with the regulation of food intake. In the chicken, hunger contractions occur in the crop (Patterson, 1927) and in the proventriculus and gizzard

(Ashcraft, 1930) whereas with ruminants there is a decrease in the frequency of contractions during periods without food (Church, 1975).

Distension of a balloon in the stomach depresses intake, but does not completely abolish feeding in dogs (Share *et al.*, 1952). Intragastric administration of the amount of food normally taken in a meal also depresses, but does not totally inhibit, feeding (Janowitz and Hollander, 1955) showing that stomach distension is not the only controller of intake. If ingested food is not allowed to accumulate in the stomach, dogs (Janowitz and Grossman, 1949) and rats (Antin *et al.*, 1975) continue eating for longer than normal. Clearly the presence of food in the stomach and/or its passage through and absorption from the intestines are important factors in inducing satiety.

If distension of some part of the digestive tract were the main controlling factor, then dilution of food with inert material would not be compensated for by any increase in intake. However, in simple stomached animals dilution stimulates intake (rats, Adolf, 1947; pigs, Owen and Ridgman, 1968; chickens, Hill and Dansky, 1954) although with excessive dilution (above about $300 \, g \, kg^{-1}$) the same digestible energy intake cannot be maintained (Chapter 10).

Non-nutrients, or 'dietary bulk' reduce the concentration of nutrients in the food so that more food is eaten before nutrient-induced satiety occurs. However, the volume accumulating in the stomach, and later passed to the intestines, may be limited by the capacity of these viscera and a physical, distension-induced satiety may result. This is particularly true in ruminant animals with foods high in fibrous constituents which have to stay in the rumen for many hours. Chapters 4 and 10 discuss this aspect in more detail. Gastrointestinal involvement in intake control has recently been reviewed by Rayner (1992).

*Poultry*

Stimulation of the crop by filling it with water, saline or a balloon, or cooling the crop, all cause electroencephalograph arousal (Gentle and Richardson, 1972) and depress food intake (Richardson, 1970b). Distension of the crop by introducing 10 ml of a $180 \, g \, l^{-1}$ solution of glucose via a stomach tube had no effect in birds fasted for 22 h, but significantly depressed intake in unfasted birds; this was thought to be due to osmotic effects (Richardson, 1970b). Such treatment involves considerable disturbance and there would have been less stress if the crop were loaded via a surgically implanted cannula. Introduction of 12 or 10 ml of a paste of food into the crop via a cannula depressed food intake (Shurlock and Forbes, 1981a). To determine whether bulk or nutrients were involved in this response, glucose solutions were given into the crop. Amounts greater than 1.5 g in 10 ml of water significantly

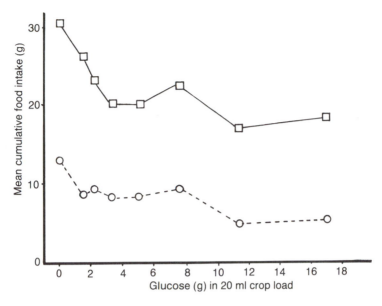

**Fig. 3.1.** Food intake during 1 h (○) and 3 h (□), after loading the crop of chickens with various amounts of glucose dissolved in 20 ml of water (Shurlock and Forbes, 1981a).

depressed food intake during the hour after injection, whereas at least 3.8 g was necessary to depress intake over a 3-h period (Fig. 3.1). Note that the effect of additional amounts of glucose is greatest with loads of up to 4 g and that with greater weights there was little additional effect on food intake, suggesting that the receptor(s) involved are maximally stimulated by 4 g. Even so, intake was only depressed by half of control during the hour after injection and by one-third during the 3 h after.

Although the results of this experiment might indicate the presence of receptors sensitive to glucose in the crop, or lower down the digestive tract or postabsorptively, they do not rule out the possibility of distension receptors because more concentrated solutions take up more water and therefore occupy more space; osmoreceptors might also be present. Shurlock and Forbes (1981a) therefore compared the effects on feeding of glucose and the non-absorbable substances, sorbitol and potassium chloride, all at an osmolality of 3 osmol l$^{-1}$. During the 3 h after injection into the crop the food intakes were depressed to an equal extent by all three solutes. It was concluded that glucose introduced into the crop was probably not, therefore, influencing intake by stimulating postabsorptive receptors, but by an osmotic effect.

Mechanoreceptors are to be found in the muscular stomach of the chicken and both the crop and the gizzard are well innervated by branches of the vagus nerve (Hill, 1979). Crop distension causes increased frequency of impulses in the vagus nerve (Hodgkiss, 1981) which clearly demonstrates a neural pathway to the central nervous system. The crop is, however, a diverticulum and food often bypasses it; thus it cannot be the main controller of meal size. Following surgical removal of the crop, daily intake is normal once the immediate effects of surgery and the adaptation period are over (Smith and Pilz, 1970; Savory, 1985). Cropectomy is followed by decreased meal size and increased feeding frequency, although eventual oesophageal dilation often leads to a gradual return to normal meal frequency.

Distension of the stomachs by constriction of the duodenum (Richardson, 1972) depressed voluntary intake to a marked extent in birds with free access to food.

## Pigs

Indirect evidence of a physical limit to intake in the pig has been obtained from observations of the effects of dietary dilution. Wangsness and Soroka (1978) found that baby pigs attempted to compensate for dilution by increasing their intake of a liquid diet when its energy content was reduced, but could not maintain energy intake and weight gain at the greatest dilution. They postulated that complete compensation was prevented by gastric distension. Although there appear to be no reports in the literature of balloon inflation in the stomach of pigs, loading young pigs with hypertonic saline or water, equal in volume to the volume of milk taken voluntarily after a 3 h fast (40 ml), depressed intake (Houpt *et al.*, 1977). Stomach loading with milk or solutions of sugars also depresses intake but this can be ascribed to chemical as well as to osmotic and mechanical effects. As pigs grow older they can compensate more for diet dilution (Chapter 10). Pekas (1983) loaded the stomachs of young pigs daily through a cannula which led to a reduction in voluntary intake which almost exactly compensated for the weight of food introduced. When loading was carried out on four days per week compensation was incomplete on these days so that total intake increased. However, a reduction of voluntary intake on the other three days of each week led to weekly intakes, growth rates and carcass compositions which were indistinguishable from controls.

The rate at which the stomach discharges its contents into the duodenum has an important influence on the signals generated by that part of the intestine and is partly controlled by the quantity and quality of duodenal contents. In the pig Gregory and Rayner (1987) infused fats and products of lipolysis into the stomach, duodenum or ileum; as the amount of fat infused into the stomach was compensated almost exactly by reduced food intake they concluded that the rate of stomach emptying plays a major part in determining meal size. Glucose infusions into the stomach similarly depressed intake (Gregory *et al.*, 1987) but this effect was ascribed to intestinal osmotic or caloric effects of the glucose which delayed stomach emptying and prolonged stomach distension.

*Ruminants*

As mentioned in Chapter 1, a considerable body of evidence had been built up by about 1960 to support the concept that the food intake of ruminants was restricted primarily by rumen capacity; this has been reviewed by Balch and Campling (1962). Evidence for the physical limitation of intake comes from observations of a positive relationship between voluntary intake and digestibility (Crampton *et al.*, 1960; Balch and Campling, 1962) or digestible energy concentration (Blaxter *et al.*, 1961).

A detailed coverage of rumen receptors is to be found in Chapter 4 while dietary effects on intake which are mediated by the rumen are covered in Chapter 10.

*Horses*

Ralston and Baile (1982) studied gastrointestinal stimuli in the control of food intake in ponies by giving 2 l of water with 300 g glucose, cellulose or kaolin into the stomach. Glucose delayed feeding for 113 min during which period the ponies exhibited normal satiety behaviours. When 100 or 200 g glucose was given, the effects on feeding were dose-related. There was no immediate effect of bulk as the cellulose load given into the stomach did not reduce intake until 3–18 h post-treatment, suggesting that it might be distending the lower intestine.

# Intestinal Receptors

Chyme is likely to reach the jejunum before the end of the meal and the distension which results may play a part in the initiation and maintenance of satiety. Slow infusion of a liquid diet into the jejunum of rats caused a reduction in food intake which was not due to discomfort as no aversion to a flavour paired with this infusion was apparent (Canbeyli and Koopmans, 1984). Jejunal infusion was more effective than duodenal infusion which was, in turn, more effective than infusion of the same amount of liquid food into the stomach. As it is likely that the yield of absorbed nutrients was at least as high following gastric or duodenal infusion it seems reasonable to interpret these results in terms of physical distension of the small intestine. Distension of a jejunal loop in the pig prevents feeding (Houpt, 1985).

The effects of digesta reaching the duodenum and jejunum could be mediated by stretch receptors, osmoreceptors or chemoreceptors. Although there is adequate neurophysiological evidence for receptors sensitive to several chemical types, that for osmoreceptors is weak (Mei, 1985 and Chapter 4) despite much circumstantial evidence that they are important in the control of food intake.

*Poultry*

Hodgkiss (1984) has shown that the intestinal nerve can transmit impulses centrally and may thus be in a position to relay information on intestinal distension. It has proved to be very difficult to study this nerve as it makes multiple connections with the sympathetic ganglia.

Duodenal infusion of glucose solutions inhibits feeding (Shurlock and Forbes, 1981a) but potassium chloride and sorbitol solutions, which are not absorbed, have a more prolonged effect (see below) suggesting that it is the physical presence rather than the chemical nature that is important.

Distension of the cloaca or rectum also results in reduced food intake (Sturkie and Joiner, 1959) so that it seems safe to conclude that stimulation of stretch receptors at any point along the digestive tract will result in hypophagia, and that this distension during and after meals is a factor in the control of meal size and frequency. Some of the solutions injected into the crop in the experiments of Shurlock and Forbes (1981a) probably found their way further along the digestive tract and might have effected food intake by means of gastric or intestinal stimulation. This was investigated by slowly injecting 10 ml of 3 osm solutions of glucose, sorbitol or potassium chloride into the duodenum of cockerels through permanently implanted cannulae. Compared with control (no injection), neither water nor glucose had any effect on intake, whereas sorbitol and potasium chloride caused highly significant decreases in intake. Intraduodenal glucose infusions were also shown not to affect food intake in the work of Lacy *et al.* (1986b). Glucose is absorbed quickly from the small intestine and would not be present for long enough to result in prolonged stimulation of gut distension- or osmoreceptors whereas the non-absorbed solutes would continue to stimulate these receptors, resulting in depressed voluntary intake. In birds which were fasted overnight before these same treatments were given, glucose injection into the duodenum did significantly depress feeding, perhaps because the liver content of glycogen was depleted so that it took up glucose which stimulated liver receptors (see below).

Vagotomy at the level of the proventriculus prevented the effects of glucose solutions infused at up to 90 mg min$^{-1}$ into the duodenum of chickens (Shaobi and Forbes, 1987) but as the nerve section included fibres to and from the liver and pancreas as well as the duodenum it is not completely clear whether the glucose was acting primarily on the duodenum or at another site. It seems likely that osmoreception is important in birds although it is possible that the effects of hypertonic solutions are due to physical distension of the duodenum by the increase in volume as water is drawn from the blood. It is also worth nothing that hypertonic solutions stimulate gut motility which is likely to stimulate mechanoreceptors in the gut wall.

*Pigs*

Food intake by hungry growing pigs was reduced by injection of 250 ml of a 150 g l$^{-1}$ solution of glucose into the duodenum. When the treatment was given 3 min after food had been offered following an overnight fast, intake was 445 g compared with 782 g for control whereas 250 ml of a 15% solution of neutral fat or a 10% solution of amino acids had no effect (Stephens, 1980). This suggests that there are specific glucose receptors in the duodenum rather than osmo- or distension receptors. The effect of 250 ml of a 150 g l$^{-1}$ glucose solution into the duodenum was prevented by prior bilateral thoracic vagotomy (Stephens, 1985), confirming that there is a neural link with the central nervous system (CNS) rather than a humoral one in this context. 2-Deoxy-D-glucose (2DG, a glucose antimetabolite) did not affect feeding when given just after the start of the meal but it did block the effect of glucose, suggesting that some of the hypophagic effect of glucose solutions infused into the duodenum is not osmotic unless, of course, the glucose has to be absorbed before gaining access to the osmoreceptors.

Loading the duodenum of young pigs fasted for the previous 6 h with hypertonic saline or glucose solutions depressed the size of the next meal (Fig. 3.2), an effect that was blocked by vagotomy (Houpt, 1983a). The fact that glucose and saline had almost identical effects when given at the same osmotic concentrations strongly suggests that the glucose solutions are acting on osmoreceptors rather than gluco-receptors.

Intraportal infusions of these solutions were ineffective (Houpt *et al.*, 1979) and it was suggested that the effects of duodenal loading were mediated by stretch and/or osmoreceptors in the duodenum rather

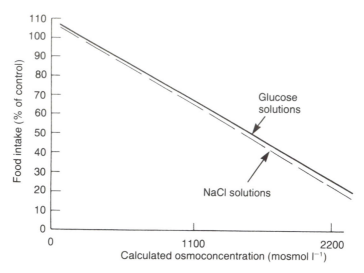

**Fig. 3.2.** Effect of loading the duodenum of growing pigs with glucose or saline solutions on the size of the subsequent meal (Houpt, 1983a).

than by chemoreceptors in the liver. This conclusion was supported by the fact that duodenal infusions of solutions of non-absorbable sugars such as mannitol had a more prolonged action than glucose. A 400 g $l^{-1}$ solution of glucose infused into the duodenum had a small but significant depressing effect on intake; a fat emulsion also depressed intake but this was blocked by local anaesthetic (Rayner and Gregory, 1985). Local anaesthetics also blocked the effect of glucose given into the duodenum (Houpt *et al.*, 1979) and also largely prevented the depression of intake caused by glucose infusion into the stomach (Gregory *et al.*, 1987) which suggests that some of the effects of stomach loading are due to flow of the infusate into the duodenum. Houpt (1983a) showed that a large increase in the osmolality of duodenal contents occurs during a normal large meal so that these receptors could be of physiological importance in the termination of meals. Osmotic effects might be mediated by distension receptors stimulated by the increased intestinal distension due to water drawn into the lumen of the gut by its hypertonic contents as distention of a jejunal loop prevented feeding in pigs (Houpt, 1985).

Xylose solutions, which are not absorbed, were less effective than glucose or sodium chloride when given into the duodenum (Houpt *et al.*, 1983) which suggested that the osmoreceptors were not on the surface of cells exposed directly to the infusate. Most of these effects could be blocked by a local anaesthetic given in the infusion so the receptors were not thought to be deeper than the mucosal layer.

Houpt *et al.* (1983) suggested that good control over food intake in the pig could be exerted by a combination of three factors working largely in the duodenum: (i) osmotic sensitivity, which is precise but not directly related to nutritive value (ii) cholecystokinin (CCK) responses to protein and fat in duodenal digesta; (iii) glucoreceptors in the intestine. On the basis of their experiments, Houpt *et al.* (1979) have partitioned the satiating effect of glucose infused into the duodenum of young pigs, suggesting that 20% of the effect is due to fluid movements from blood to gut, 55% is osmotic within the gut, and the remaining 25% is hormonal, perhaps involving CCK.

Despite this emphasis on osmolality as a major factor in intake control in pigs (Houpt *et al.*, 1983), Rayner and Gregory (1989) found that with normal feeding, osmolality of duodenal fluid never exceeded 300 mosmol kg$^{-1}$. Therefore, they gave glucose at low rates (30–60% of the normal rate of production) to avoid hypertonicity. A 40%, glucose solution reduced food intake at a meal when infused at 4 ml min$^{-1}$ or more and a very similar result was found with an equivalent amount of hypertonic saline, confirming the importance of osmolality. The response to stomach infusion was partly blocked by duodenal infusion of local anaesthetic suggesting a duodenal neural response.

Protein infused into the stomach or protein hydrolysate into stomach, duodenum, jejunum or ileum all decreased intake approximately in proportion to the amount of energy infused. Glucose infusion into the duodenum slowed gastric emptying so that the total flow of energy through the duodenum was unchanged but the mechanisms for this apparent control of energy flow are not understood. Infusion of fat into the stomach or duodenum, or fat, bile salts and lipase into the upper jejunum depressed intake in pigs (Rayner and Gregory, 1989). Fat, bile and lipase into the ileum had no effect on that meal but did tend to reduce the size of the next meal. Older pigs, over 60 kg body weight, still respond to glucose and fatty acid infusions, so their 'overeating' is not due to lack of sensitivity to nutrients in the gastrointestinal tract.

The role of gut hormones such as CCK is covered in Chapter 5.

## Liver Receptors

The liver is well placed to monitor the uptake of nutrients from the digestive tract and, given its role in smoothing out this erratic supply to maintain more stable plasma levels, it must be able to detect concentrations or rates of uptake of metabolites such as glucose and amino acids. There are important nervous links between the liver and the CNS (Anil and Forbes, 1987) and it is perhaps surprising that little serious attention was paid to the role of the liver as a source of signals for controlling food intake until the early 1970s, following Russek's (1963) original suggestions. He observed that infusion of glucose into the hepatic portal vein of the dog depressed food intake whereas the same infusion into the jugular vein had no effect, nor did the infusion of saline into the portal vein. The potent effect of portal glucose infusion is reduced by liver denervation (Novin, 1976) showing that there is an involvement of the nervous system. Schmitt (1973) showed that electrical activity was induced in some neurons in the lateral hypothalamus in rats by portal infusion of glucose. The activity was modified by either vagotomy or splanchnectomy. Further evidence for glucose-sensitive liver receptors was provided by Niijima (1969) working with isolated liver from guinea pig. He showed that the frequency of impulses in the vagal branch from the liver was inversely proportional to the glucose concentration in the perfusate. Recent studies have failed to find nerve endings in liver parenchyma but Berthoud *et al.* (1992) have demonstrated many nerve endings in the wall of the portal vein and superfusion of the exposed inner wall of the hepatic portal vein with glucose solution decreases firing of vagal fibres whereas mannose had no effect (A. Niijima, personal communication).

Glucose uptake by the liver can be blocked by 2DG and Novin *et al.* (1974) found that the food intake of rabbits was stimulated by infusion of 2DG into the hepatic portal vein whereas infusion into the jugular vein had much less effect; vagotomy reduced the effect of portally introduced 2DG. There is now considerable evidence that the supply of oxidizable substrates to the liver is monitored in simple-stomached animals with transmission of information to the central nervous system via the nerves of the hepatic plexus (Anil and Forbes, 1987) and that this plays a part in the control of feeding (Forbes, 1988b).

The liver is an important site of fat metabolism in mammals where in the rat the intake-depressing effects of fatty acids are blocked by substances which block fatty acid oxidation. Inhibition of fatty acid oxidation with mercaptoacetate increased intake of a food containing 18% fat but had no effect when the diet contained only 3% fat (Scharrer and Langhans, 1986). Presumably rats on the former food were accustomed to obtaining a significant proportion of their energy from fat so that when this source was denied them they ate more food, whereas in the low fat diet fatty acids provided such a small proportion of their energy that there was no need to eat significantly more when fatty acid oxidation was inhibited. Vagal section prevented the effect of mercaptoacetate on the medium-fat diet (Langhans and Scharrer, 1986), further strengthening the belief that fatty acids can play a significant role in satiation via the liver.

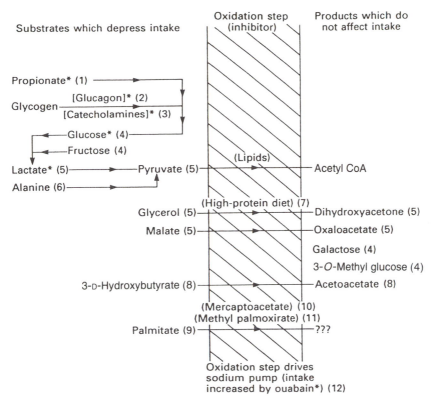

**Fig. 3.3.** Outline of some metabolic pathways in the liver and the manipulations which have been found to influence food intake. (1) Anil and Forbes, 1980a; (2) Weatherford and Ritter, 1986; (3) Russek, 1981; (4) Booth, 1972b; (5) Langhans *et al.*, 1985a; (6) W. Langhans, unpublished results; (7) Langhans *et al.*, 1984b; (8) Langhans *et al.*, 1985b; (9) Vandermeerschen-Doize and Paquay, 1984; (10) Scharrer and Langhans, 1986; (11) Friedman *et al.*, 1986; (12) Langhans and Scharrer, 1987; *, effects which have been blocked by vagotomy (Forbes, 1988b).

Langhans *et al.* (1985a) have shown that the hypophagic effect of metabolites is linked to a particular step in their metabolism, principally in the liver. The results of the relevant experiments are shown in Fig. 3.3. Whereas glycerol and malate depressed intake, their oxidation products dihydroxyacetone and oxaloacetate did not, indicating that the oxidation process itself is important. Lactate and its product of metabolism, pyruvate, depressed intake to an equal extent and as lactate is metabolized to pyruvate and as pyruvate itself is oxidized to acetyl coenzyme A (CoA) the importance of the oxidation step is supported. When a high-fat diet was offered lactate and pyruvate no longer showed the intake-depressing effect but fat is known to depress pyruvate oxidation; it is likely that such a depression occurred in this experiment because blood levels of these metabolites remained elevated for longer after injection in rats fed the high-fat diet compared to those on a high-carbohydrate diet.

For a detailed discussion of the way in which liver metabolism might be involved in the control of food intake, see Forbes (1988b).

Several studies have failed to confirm an important role for the liver in sensing nutrients and transmitting the information via the nervous system. Total denervation of the liver of rats did not change any parameters of spontaneous feeding between 3 and 9 days after surgery, nor daily intake and body weight gains during the next six months (Bellinger *et al.*, 1984). However, abdominal vagotomy increased meal size and reduced meal numbers in rabbits (Geiselman *et al.*, 1980) and section of the hepatic branch of the vagus of rats reduced the nocturnal bias of feeding while not affecting total daily intake (Friedman and Sawchenko, 1984). Thus, despite several failures to demonstrate a role for the liver in the control of feeding (Tordoff and Friedman, 1986), work is continuing to resolve the many unanswered questions. M.G. Tordoff and M.I. Friedman (personal communication) have noted that those experiments, in which there has been no effect on feeding of increasing nutrient flow to the liver, have exposed animals to different, contrasting, treatments at short intervals, thus confusing them by not allowing adequate time for them to learn the effects of different infusions (Chapter 12). Despite the evidence presented here, there is still considerable controversy as to whether the liver is important in the control of intake under physiological conditions.

*Poultry*

Several experiments investigated the glucostatic theory of intake control in birds (Chapter 5) without finding any significant depression due to glucose injections or infusions. In the first recorded infusions of glucose solutions into the coccygeo-mesenteric vein (leading into the liver) of chickens Shurlock and Forbes (1981b) infused a solution of 60 g glucose $l^{-1}$ at a rate of 1.2 ml $min^{-1}$ into cockerels over a period of 3 h. Even though this high rate of infusion had no effect on food intake when given into the jugular vein (32 vs. 28 g 3 $h^{-1}$), it almost completely suppressed feeding when given into the liver (34 vs. 2 g 3 $h^{-1}$). Further, when a range of solutions from 1 to 60 g $l^{-1}$ was given, there was a highly significant negative correlation between the concentration of glucose in the solution and the weight of food eaten during the infusion (Fig. 3.4). The slope of the relationship is steep at lower concentrations, which is the physiological range, suggesting that liver sensitivity to

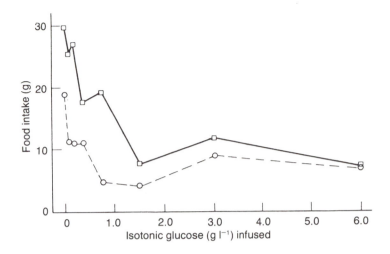

**Fig. 3.4.** Effect of glucose infusion into the liver of cockerels on food intake over 1 h (○) and 3 h (□) periods (Shurlock and Forbes, 1981b).

glucose has the potential to exert a powerful control over feeding in the normal chicken.

The effects of overnight fasting on the response of cockerels to portal infusion of glucose were investigated by Shurlock and Forbes (1981b). Intake was depressed only by the highest dose of glucose when access to food was allowed during the infusion. When food was withheld until the end of the infusion there was a large dose-dependent inhibition of voluntary intake. This result, together with observations made during the post-infusion period in previous experiments, showed that the effect of glucose lasted beyond the infusion period and was more likely to be a result of changes in liver glycogen or glucose content rather than simply an effect of the concentration of glucose in the blood perfusing the liver.

An amino acid mixture infused into the portal vein also depressed intake whereas jugular introduction at the same rate had a much smaller effect (Shurlock and Forbes, 1984); effects of glucose and amino acids were additive (Rusby *et al.*, 1987; Fig. 3.5) and possibly affected the same system in the liver. Lysine infused at 50–150 mg 3 h$^{-1}$ caused a reduction in intake during the 3 h treatment whereas ammonia at an equivalent rate did not and leucine had a delayed effect (Rusby and Forbes, 1987). Vagotomy at the level of the proventriculus blocked these effects of portal infusion of glucose and lysine (Rusby *et al.*, 1987; Fig. 3.5.). Lacy *et al.* (1986a) could find no effect of amino acids infused into the liver at about 75% of the rate at which amino acids would normally

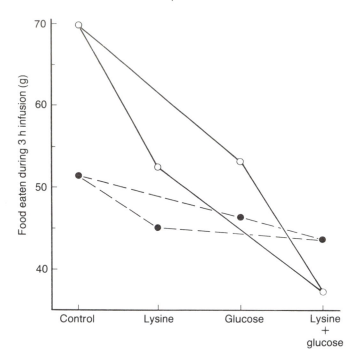

**Fig. 3.5.** Food intake during 3 h infusions of glucose and/or lysine solutions into the liver of intact (○) or vagotomized (●) chickens (Rusby *et al.*, 1987).

be absorbed during 30 min in either cockerels of an egg-laying strain or broilers.

Adrenaline injected into the hepatic portal vein at low doses of up to 0.1 mg kg$^{-1}$ depresses intake, an effect which is blocked by section of the hepatic branch of the vagus nerve (Howes and Forbes, 1987a). As adrenaline causes glycogenolysis, these results suggest that it is glucose concentration in or around hepatocytes which is important rather than the direction of flow of glucose through the hepatocyte membrane. In order to study the mode of action of adrenaline, an α-adrenergic blocker, phenylephrine, was given into the liver at a wide range of doses, but without effect; a β-blocker, salbutamol, depressed intake but the range of doses used (500–2000 μg) was probably too high to achieve its effect just by a physiological blocking of endogenous adrenaline. The intake-depressing effect of injecting glucagon into the liver of chickens is also blocked by vagal section (Howes and Forbes, 1987b), but whether the dose used was physiological is open to question.

In birds, most fat synthesis occurs in the liver and plasma levels of triglycerides are much higher than in mammals. Lacy *et al.* (1986a) found that cockerels of an egg-laying strain were sensitive to fat infused into the hepatic portal vein, but not into the jugular vein, whereas in broilers there was no effect, irrespective of site of infusion. Has selection of meat-type chickens bred out some of the liver's sensitivity to metabolites?

If the liver is important in the control of food intake it would be expected that liver denervation would disrupt feeding behaviour. Local denervation has not been undertaken in the chicken but section of both vagus nerves as they cross the proventriculus (the equivalent of subdiaphragmatic vagotomy in mammals) has been carried out which affects many visceral organs, not just the liver. It is perhaps surprising, therefore, that Savory and Hodgkiss (1984) found no differences in feeding behaviour between vagotomized and sham-vagotomized chickens although Rusby *et al.* (1987) observed significantly fewer meals, each of a larger size, but there was no effect on total daily intake. If, as suggested in Chapter 7, many feedback factors are integrated by the CNS, the loss of some of these would not necessarily result in a change in daily intake but would be likely to result in larger meals.

## Pig

Stephens and Baldwin (1974) found no effect of intrajugular or intraportal injections of glucose or amino acids on food intake of pigs. In further work infusion of a solution of 150 g glucose $l^{-1}$, or of 250 ml of a solution of 100 g amino acids $l^{-1}$ into the jugular vein or hepatic portal vein during feeding had no effect on the voluntary intake of pigs trained to eat in one session per day under operant conditions (Stephens, 1980). These results are in contrast to those with other mammals and birds but there is no *a priori* reason why the pig should be different from other mammals as its liver metabolism is similar to that of the rat. It seems likely that the feeding regime used in experiments with pigs, with only one or two periods of access to food per day, makes then reliant on different stimuli to terminate feeding compared with animals with continuous access to food. Perhaps the large amount they must eat in the short period of access emphasizes the physical aspects of gut-fill as a limit to meal size.

## Cattle

Ruminant animals absorb most of their energy from the digestive tract in the form of volatile fatty acids (VFAs), of which propionate is gluconeogenic and has been shown to depress intake in sheep (see below). The only direct study involving infusions into the hepatic portal vein of cattle was that of Elliot *et al.* (1985) who noted reduced intake during 10 out of 30 infusions of between 20 and 50 mmol min$^{-1}$ of sodium propionate into the portal vein of growing cattle; they ascribed the variability of their results to their method of feeding which was restricted to 0.025% of body weight per day, given in 24-hourly meals.

*Sheep*

Baile (1971) found the propionate depressed intake to a greater extent when infused into the ruminal vein than into other vessels and proposed the existence of propionate receptors at that site. However, Anil and Forbes (1980a) showed that a 3-h infusion of 1.2 mmol min$^{-1}$ of sodium propionate into the hepatic portal vein almost completely prevented feeding in sheep whereas the same rate of infusion into the jugular vein had little effect. It seems highly likely, therefore, that the ruminant liver is sensitive to its rate of utilization of propionate.

The route(s) taken by information from the liver to the CNS have been studied by sectioning the hepatic plexus of nerves, by sectioning or anaesthetizing the splanchnic nerves, and by sectioning the hepatic branch of the vagus nerve (Anil and Forbes, 1980a, 1988). Almost complete section of the hepatic plexus, bilateral splanchnotomy or temporary blockade of nervous transmission in the splanchnic nerves all prevented the intake-depressing effect of 3 h infusions of sodium propionate into the hepatic portal vein at 1.2 mmol min$^{-1}$ (Fig. 3.6). The paradoxical situation whereby either one of the two likely routes for transmission of afferent information from liver to CNS results in blockage of the effects of propionate given into the liver has not been resolved but may be due to some efferent involvement with the control of blood flow or enzyme activity (e.g. Anil *et al.*, 1987) which is prevented by nerve section.

These clear-cut effects on feeding of propionate infusion into the portal vein of sheep have not always been seen by other workers. de Jong *et al.* (1981) infused a mixture of the sodium salts of VFAs into the hepatic portal vein of goats at a rate similar to that used for sheep by Anil and Forbes (1980a) but found no change in food intake despite a doubling of plasma levels of VFAs. The protocols used by the two groups were very similar and it seems unlikely that there is a fundamental difference between such closely related species. The effect observed in the sheep is not likely to be simply osmotic because sodium acetate infused into the portal vein at 4 mmol min$^{-1}$ (i.e. more than three times the osmotic load of the sodium propionate infusion) had no effect on feeding (Anil and Forbes, 1980a). Peters *et al.* (1983) failed to influence feeding in sheep by intraportal infusion of propio-

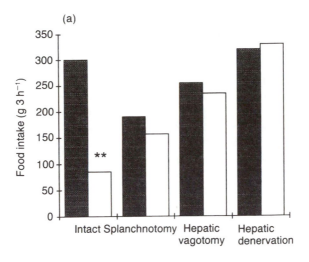

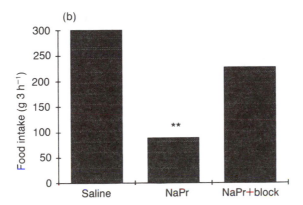

**Fig. 3.6.** The prevention of the intake-depressing effect of saline (■) and sodium propionate solution (□) infused into the hepatic portal vein of sheep by (a) bilateral splanchnotomy, splanchnic blockade with anaesthetic, section of the vagal innervation of the liver, or total liver denervation or (b) splanchnic blockade with anaesthetic (Anil and Forbes, 1988). **, Highly significant effect of propionate infusion.

nate at 1.0 mmol min⁻¹, which was thought to be within the physiological range. However, their animals were not fed *ad libitum*.

Denervation of the liver does not affect daily food intake in several species, including sheep, and this has been picked on as evidence that the liver does not play a role in the control of food intake. However, the meals are larger and less frequent than those of normal animals (Anil and Forbes, 1980) as would be expected if some, but not all, of the negative feedback information from the visceral organs had been cut off.

A nervous pathway from liver to the nucleus of the solitary tract in the medulla oblongata via the vagus nerve has been identified (M.H. Anil, P. Chaterjee and J.M. Forbes, unpublished observations) and it would appear that the sheep is similar to the rat in that both vagal and splanchnic afferent pathways are involved in the transmission of information from liver to brain (Anil and Forbes, 1988).

Attempts to study vagal discharges from chemoreceptors in the liver of the sheep have not revealed any consistent responses to propionate injected into the hepatic portal vein (M.H. Anil and J.M. Forbes, unpublished observations). Nor have we been able to find receptors in liver tissue of sheep or chickens by electron microscopy (P. Chaterjee, M.H. Anil and J.M. Forbes, unpublished results). This is in line with the failure clearly to demonstrate receptor nerve endings in the parenchyma of the liver of several other species, including the rat (see above). Structures with the appearance of chemoreceptors have, however, been located in the hepatic portal vein of the rat so further studies are required in farm animals.

Ingestion by sheep of the plant *Lantana camera* leads to rumen stasis and anorexia which McSweeney and Pass (1983) showed to be due to liver damage rather than to direct effects of the toxin on receptors in the reticulorumen. Liver denervation of intoxicated animals reduced the severity of the reduction in rumen muscular activity and it was concluded that the effects of lantana poisoning on the rumen were indirect and that the rumen stasis was reflex in nature, the primary lesion being in the liver.

## Conclusions

There are stretch receptors in most or all parts of the gut which relay information on fill to the brain via the nervous system to inhibit feeding. Hypertonic solutions infused into the gut inhibit feeding but it is not certain whether there are osmoreceptors or whether water drawn in by the hypertonic solution stimulates the stretch receptors. There is evidence for chemoreceptors in the duodenum but the relative importance of distension, stretch or chemical effects probably varies depending on the type of food.

The liver is sensitive to oxidizable nutrients including glucose (propionate in the ruminant), especially when glycogen has been depleted by a period of fasting. The effects of infusion of glucose or propionate into the liver can be blocked by local section of the vagus and/or splanchnic nerves showing that the information to the brain is transmitted via the autonomic nervous system. A major role of the liver is to prevent the uneven flow of nutrients from the digestive tract causing undue fluctuations in the energy supply to the rest of the body, especially the CNS, so it is well placed to play a major role in the control of feeding.

# 4 RUMINANT GASTROINTESTINAL TRACT

- Physical aspects
- Chemoreceptors
- The omasum
- The abomasum
- Intestinal receptors
- Interactions between different families of receptor
- Conclusions


Ruminant animals have evolved a complex set of stomachs in which digesta are stored for many hours for microbial fermentation (Appendix 1). This long period of storage makes the physical capacity of the stomachs a potential limiting factor to intake and gives considerable importance to the rates of digestion, breakdown and onward passage of particles of food. In addition, there are several unusual products of digestion, particularly the volatile fatty acids (VFAs), which the host animal must metabolize and which are therefore potentially important controllers of voluntary intake.

Altering the digestibility and rate of passage of a forage food causes parallel changes in intake (Van Soest, 1982). For example, supplementation of low protein forages with urea increases the rates of digestion and passage and allows a greater intake. Grinding a forage food also increases its rate of flow out of the rumen and allows increased voluntary intake (Balch and Campling, 1962; Minson, 1963). Although the digestibility of the food is reduced by grinding, since the food is in the rumen for a shorter time, the total weight of nutrients absorbed daily is increased. Such treatment of poor forages, accompanied by pelleting, is sometimes practised commercially.

Relationships between the digestible energy concentration of food and level of intake by ruminants are discussed in Chapter 10. In the present chapter no attempt is made to separate results from experiments with cattle from those with sheep and goats.

## Physical Aspects

### Correlations between rumen capacity and intake

Not only is intake affected by the rates of digestion and passage but also by the capacity of the digestive tract, principally the rumen. For example, Purser and Moir (1966) with sheep found:

$$FI = 540 + 36RC \tag{4.1}$$

Where FI is forage intake (g day$^{-1}$) and RC is rumen capacity (l water)

Positive correlations have been found between level of intake and the weight of the empty reticulorumen in lambs (e.g. Wardrop, 1960) but cause and effect are difficult to establish because there is a positive relationship between rumen weight and level of intake in animals offered less than *ad libitum* levels of feed. There are positive correlations between the weight of voluntary intake of forage just before slaughter and the weight of rumen contents at slaughter in older cattle (Makela, 1956; Tayler, 1959) but again the causality cannot be established with certainty.

Increases in the volume of other abdominal organs, such as abdominal fat or the pregnant uterus, can apparently cause compression of the rumen and a reduction in food intake. Tayler (1959) found a negative correlation between the weight of abdominal fat and the intake of herbage in cattle. In late pregnancy, although there is an increase in the girth of the abdomen, this is not always great enough to accommodate the growth of the uterus. Although the rate of passage of particles of forage food through the digestive tract is increased during pregnancy (Forbes, 1970), under some circumstances this is not enough to prevent a limitation of voluntary intake (Chapter 9).

For animals of any given size the fatter they are the heavier they are, so intake is often inversely correlated with body weight. On the other hand, there is a positive relationship between intake and body weight in growing animals, and between mature animals of different skeletal sizes but of equal fatness.

Ulyatt *et al.* (1967) observed that the volume of liquid in the rumen, measured by a marker-dilution technique and at slaughter, was relatively constant despite widely different voluntary intakes of dried grass, medium quality hay or poor hay and suggested that this was because of a capacity limit to rumen fill.

## Addition of material to the rumen

In the early 1960s Campling and Balch conducted a series of experiments involving a more critical approach. One of their methods was to insert balloons via a fistula into the rumen of non-pregnant, non-lactating mature cows; the balloons were then filled with water and the effect on intake during a 4-h period of access to food was noted. When 50–100 l of water-filled balloons were introduced for 10–14 days there was a 0.54 kg day$^{-1}$ decrease in dry matter intake for each 10 l of water (Balch and Campling, 1961). If the water was added directly into the rumen of cattle there was no effect on intake even when large quantities were involved (45 l). With sheep, addition of 8 l of water into the rumen had no effect on forage intake whereas inclusion of only 2 l in a balloon depressed intake by 27% (Davies, 1962). Adding water to hay before eating did not affect intake (Hillman et al., 1958). There is often a negative relationship between the water content of grass or silage and voluntary intake; water in stems and leaves acts more like water in balloons than free water.

There is extensive circumstantial evidence for physical limitation of food intake in the ruminant but it is likely that physical aspects were unduly emphasized as a result of the approach adopted in the work of Balch and Campling, because the 20 h fast that preceded each feeding period would leave the animals in considerable nutrient deficit causing them to need to eat a larger amount than would otherwise be eaten during such a small part of the day. Also, the use of rumen dry matter (DM) as a measure of fill is inappropriate as volume is related more closely to total weight, that is the wet weight of the rumen contents.

More recent studies using balloons in the rumen of lactating cows fed grass silage (Anil et al., 1993) showed that there was a 70 g DM decrease in intake for every additional litre of water put in the balloon over a 3-h period, and that this response was approximately linear over the range 0–25 l. This is similar to the 54 g DM$^{-1}$ decrease noted by Campling and Balch (1961) with non-lactating cows fed on hay. This approach has been extended to include gradual increases in the volume of balloons in the rumen of cattle by Mowatt (1963) who found little evidence of a compensatory increase in rumen capacity. In longer-term studies Bines et al. (1973) placed bags with 33 l of water in the rumen of a cow for 17 weeks; intake was depressed for the duration and rose again as soon as the bags were removed, giving no evidence for adaptation or hypertrophy of the rumen. Some recovery of food intake towards pretreatment levels was seen in sheep with balloons in the

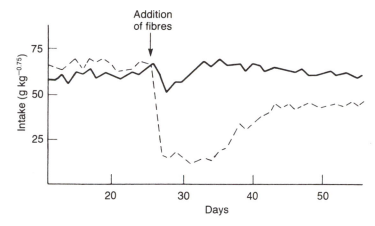

**Fig. 4.1.** Intake of hay by sheep with or without the addition of 150 g of polypropylene fibres to the rumen on day 26 (Welch, 1967).

rumen when fed on a pelleted diet, but not on straw (Egan, 1972). It seems likely that a consistent increase in rumen capacity occurs only when nutrient requirements are increased, as during lactation.

As an alternative experimental technique for demonstrating effects of rumen fill on intake Welch (1967, Fig. 4.1) introduced into the rumen via a fistula 150 g of polypropylene fibres, each 30 cm in length, which were too long to leave the rumen. Intake of hay was depressed to 33% of control values and remained low. With shorter fibres (3.5 or 7 cm) regurgitation was possible so that the fibres were broken down and fragments were found in faeces; intake was initially depressed but recovered during the few weeks after administering the fibres.

## Rumen mechanoreceptors

In order for rumen capacity to impose a limit on feeding it is necessary for there to be mechanoreceptors in the wall of the rumen with afferent fibres to the central nervous system (CNS). The ruminant fore-stomachs are innervated by branches of the vagus and splanchnic nerves (see Leek, 1986, for detailed review). Leek and Harding (1975) have described rapidly adapting mechanoreceptors in the epithelial lining of the reticulorumen, concentrated in the anterior dorsal rumen and the reticulum. There are slowly adapting tension receptors in the muscular layers throughout the gastrointestinal tract (Cottrell and Iggo, 1984b). One important role of mechanoreceptors is in the control of gastrointestinal motility (Crichlow, 1988). However, since the epithelial receptors found in the reticulorumen and duodenum also respond to chemical stimuli (see below), it is likely that chemical effects are also involved in the control of motility.

Central projection of these receptors is to the gastric centres of the medulla oblongata which have afferent fibres projecting to the nucleus of the solitary tract of the hind brain in the rat (Ritter and Edwards, 1986), but there is no evidence of this in the sheep (Harding and Leek, 1973).

*Reticuloruminal motility*

There are spontaneous biphasic cyclic contractions of the rumen which mix the digesta, the contractions being weaker when ground and pelleted diets are fed than with long forages (sheep, Reid, 1963; cattle, Colvin *et al.*, 1978). Reduction in the strength or frequency of rumen contractions does not necessarily mean a decrease in tension, however. Pentagastrin infused into the coeliac artery caused an increase in reticular tension receptor activity without an increase in pressure as measured by a balloon in the lumen. Intraruminal pressure is, therefore, not a reliable indicator of tension.

If the reticulorumen were an inert elastic sphere then it would be a simple matter to calculate the degree of stretch for any given load of digesta. However, the muscular activity of the rumen wall complicates the situation, especially as eating (or even teasing with food) stimulates more frequent contractions. If stimulation of the in-series stretch receptors by distension of the rumen depresses voluntary food intake then this increased muscular activity during feeding will act to inhibit feeding. However, increased motility, as during feeding, increases the rate of outflow of digesta leading to decreased distension and, potentially, to increased food intake.

Rumination increases the breakdown of particles of food and thus increases the rate of emptying of the reticulorumen. When rumination was prevented with a face mask to impair jaw movements (10 h on and 2 h off, successively for 4 days), food intake in steers was significantly reduced (Welch, 1982). Rumination is also accompanied by increased ruminal muscular activity and therefore helps to maintain voluntary intake by reducing the bulk of digesta in the reticulorumen.

To test whether drug-induced changes in rumen motility affect intake, clonidine, xylazine or $PGF_{2\alpha}$ were given to dwarf goats by Van Miert and Van Duin (1991). Although they caused bradycardia and inhibited rumen contractions they did not affect food intake. Oxytocin, vasopressin, octapressin or $PGE_1$ did not affect feeding behaviour whereas in previous studies they were found to affect rumen motility. The PG analogues etiproston, luprostiol or tiaprost induced hypophagia but stimulated intestinal propulsion. Therefore, there is no connection in these studies between gut motility and feeding.

*Tactile responses*

Muscular activity of the reticulorumen causes particles of digesta to rub against the papillae stimulating the epithelial receptors but the role of these receptors in the control of feeding is unclear. Baumont *et al.* (1990a) placed blocks of expanded polystyrene in the rumen which floated on top of rumen fluid so that they would stimulate tactile responses as well as increase the bulk of rumen contents. Hay intake was significantly reduced by 2 l of cubes but there was no effect on the frequency of reticulorumen contractions during eating. However, the frequency of contractions during rumination was increased and more periods of rumination occurred. The polystyrene blocks became rounded during their stay in the rumen showing that they must have been rubbing on the rumen papillae but their bulk meant that they were also likely to have been stimulating the distension receptors.

In order to stimulate tactile receptors without a distension effect, Baumont *et al.* (1990a) fed sheep by infusion with a liquid diet and stimulated the rumen wall with a stiff brush. This induced pseudorumination and extrareticular contractions, as did a small amount of hay or 1 l of polystyrene cubes. On the other hand, insufflating the rumen with air for 5 min or adding 2 l of buffer, which would cause distension but not stimulate tactile receptors, had no effect on contractions and did not induce pseudorumination. These results suggest that the use of a balloon in the rumen might not mimic all of the effects of forage, especially if, as is often the case, the balloon gets dragged down into the rumen away from the sensitive anterior dorsal areas.

## Chemoreceptors

Acids affect the epithelial receptors according to their titratable acidity and molecular size (but not pH) to cause rumen stasis. Butyric acid has a more potent effect than would be predicted from the effects of a mixture of VFAs. Leek (1986) questioned whether epithelial receptors have a physiological role as chemoreceptors in view of the high concentration of chemicals required to activate them and their long response times. However, the inhibition of reticuloruminal motility caused by intraruminal infusion of VFAs or arising pathologically during the ruminal acidosis syndrome is undoubtedly attributable to reticuloruminal epithelial receptor excitation. Crichlow and Leek (1981) and Crichlow (1988) have reported that ruminal fluid samples taken from sheep, immediately after the contractions of the reticulorumen had been inhibited by intraruminal infusion of VFAs, were able to elicit responses in the ruminal epithelial receptors of another anaesthetized sheep. Decreasing the pH enhanced the potency of this fluid, whereas raising it decreased activity, showing that it was undissociated acid affecting the receptors. VFAs are transported through the ruminal epithelium mainly as unionized molecules and the pH partition hypothesis of membrane permeability predicts faster transport for unionized substances which suggests that weak organic acids have to diffuse through cell membranes in order to affect epithelial receptors.

## Volatile fatty acids

It has been reported many times that VFAs, particularly acetate, can depress food intake when infused into the rumen (Baile and Forbes, 1974; de Jong, 1986). As the effect was either greatly reduced or absent when the VFAs were infused into the jugular vein it was assumed that they were sensed by receptors in the ruminal wall. This idea was strengthened when it was demonstrated that a local anaesthetic, when infused into the reticulorumen along with acetate, prevented most of the intake-depressing effect of the latter (Martin and Baile, 1972). However, the effect of the anaesthetic need not have been on 'acetate receptors' but on 'osmoreceptors' (see Osmolality below).

A mixture of VFAs in physiological proportions (0.55 acetate, 0.30 propionate, 0.15 butyrate), infused intraruminally during spontaneous meals, had a dose-related effect on intake by sheep or goats (Baile and Mayer, 1969) and similarly in cattle (Simkins *et al.*, 1965). Faverdin (1990) observed that 3 or 6 mol of mixed VFAs infused into rumen during 3 h of feeding depressed DM intake by 1.5 kg in lactating cows and by 0.8 kg in dry cows. These differences occurred in the second and third hours and the deficit was not recovered during the rest of the day.

Baile and colleagues (e.g. Baile and Mayer, 1969) infused VFA mixtures into the rumen or other sites during spontaneous meals by means of pumps triggered by their sheep breaking light beams as they ate. They observed significant relationships between the amount of VFAs infused, in the range 2.5–20 mmol min$^{-1}$, and the depression in food intake:

$$DEPR = 0.38VFA + 8.74 \qquad (4.2)$$

where DEPR is the percentage reduction in intake, compared to pretreatment control periods and VFA is the mean amount of a mixture of the three salts infused (mmol per meal).

Separate infusion of the three acids showed that the effect of the mixture was due mainly to acetate and propionate.

*Acetate*

The effects of intraruminal acetate have been shown many times (Baile and Forbes, 1974); for example with sheep (Baile and Mayer, 1969):

$$DEPR = 0.39Ac - 5.18 \tag{4.3}$$

Where DEPR is the depression in intake (%) and Ac is the amount of acetate infused (mmol per meal), and for dairy cows (Anil *et al.*, 1993):

$$HAY = 2.85 - 0.085Ac \tag{4.4}$$
$$SILAGE = 2.25 - 0.07Ac \tag{4.5}$$

where HAY and SILAGE are the weights of food eaten during the infusion (kg DM $3h^{-1}$) and Ac is the amount of acetate infused (mol $3h^{-1}$).

Intravenous injection of acetate has less effect than intraruminal administration in cattle and no effect on the intake of sheep, suggesting that receptors to acetate are in the rumen wall. Baile and McLaughlin (1970) made selective infusions into different areas of the rumen and found that the biggest effect on intake was in the dorsal part; infusion of acetate into isolated 'Pavlov' pouches made of 5% of the rumen was sufficient to depress intake significantly (Martin and Baile, 1972). Direct comparison of intraruminal versus jugular infusion in goats (Baile and Mayer, 1968a), and of intraruminal versus ruminal vein infusion in sheep (Baile, 1971) confirmed that the main effect of acetate is on the rumen wall.

Evidence for neural receptors sensitive to acetate comes from the observation that local anaesthetic infused into the rumen of sheep along with acetate prevented most of the intake-depressing effect of the latter (Martin and Baile, 1972). Infusion of local anaesthetic around the ruminal vein had a similar effect in goats and Martin and Baile (1970) concluded that signals transmitted in response to increased rumen acetate concentrations were neurally transmitted to the CNS. It is now accepted that the major effect of acetate on intake in ruminants is via receptors in the rumen wall. However, de Jong *et al.* (1981) have shown that the type of infusion used by Baile and others induces large, probably unphysiological, changes in rumen fluid and blood composition and de Jong could not reproduce the results of Baile's group with infusions made so that these unphysiological changes were avoided.

Continuous infusion of sodium acetate for 3 h into the rumen of lactating cows had small and non-significant effects when the doses were less than the rate at which it is calculated that acetate is normally produced even though this led to greatly elevated concentrations of acetate in ruminal fluid (Anil *et al.*, 1993). The depression in intake only became obvious and significant at rates of infusion considerably above the normal production rate which elevated the concentration of rumen acetate to at least twice the normal. However, the significant, linear relationship between the dose of acetate administered and the depression in food intake suggests that the effect of physiological amounts is real.

Prolonged infusion of VFAs into the rumen of cattle for several weeks at rates up to 20 MJ day$^{-1}$ did not affect voluntary intake (Rook *et al.*, 1965) suggesting that the receptors for short-chain fatty acids or the control centres to which they are linked adapted to the changed conditions. This, together with the fact that changes in short-chain fatty acid production are small during and after the relatively small meals which are taken with *ad libitum* access to food (cattle, Chase *et al.*, 1977; sheep, Adams and Forbes, 1982), has been used as evidence that short-chain fatty acids are not important in the physiological control of intake in ruminants.

Infusion of acetate into the rumen avoids oral effects during ingestion. However, when rumination occurs there will be a higher concentration of acetate than normal in the regurgitated bolus. Buchanan-Smith (1990) and Gherardi and Black (1991) have recently shown that acetate added to food reduced the rate of eating of that food and, by implication, its acceptability. The former author avoided the complication of ruminal effects of acetate by working with oesophageally fistulated animals which, during the test periods, had the fistulas open so that none of the treated food entered the rumen. The latter used a sophisticated method whereby the effects of additions of a range of levels of acetate on rate of eating were compared with several foods. Surveys have shown a negative relationship between the acetate content of silages and their daily intake by ruminants (Tayler and Wilkins, 1976) but, at the present time, we have no way of knowing the relative significance of oral and ruminal effects of acetate. In general, however, oral effects are of little significance when only one food is on offer; palatability effects come into play in determining the food to be eaten when a choice is available (Chapter 13).

A further complication in ascertaining the effects of acetate on food intake arises from the fact that acetate has been shown to inhibit ruminal motility (Crichlow, 1988), which would be likely to reduce the intake of forage foods by reducing rate of passage and increasing the occupancy of the rumen (see above). However, infusions of acetate which significantly depressed silage intake in cows did not affect the frequency or amplitude of rumen contractions (S.B.J. Dunne, M.H. Anil and J.M. Forbes, unpublished results).

*Propionate*

Propionate was approximately as effective as acetate in depressing intake when infused into the rumen of sheep (Baile and Mayer, 1969):

$$DEPR = 0.36Pr - 0.27 \qquad (4.6)$$

where DEPR is the depression in intake (%) and Pr is the amount of propionate infused (mmol per meal). However, propionate was rather more effective than acetate when infused into the rumen of lactating cows (Anil *et al.*, 1993):

$$HAY = 2.61 - 0.13Pr \qquad (4.7)$$
$$SILAGE = 2.09 - 0.14Pr \qquad (4.8)$$

where HAY and SILAGE are the weights of food eaten during the infusion (kg DM $3\,h^{-1}$) and Pr is the amount of propionate infused (mol $3\,h^{-1}$).

Sodium propionate is particularly effective in depressing intake when incorporated into feeds for sheep (Hovell and Greenhalgh, 1978). Seeking its site of action Baile and McLaughlin (1970) infused propionate into the dorsal rumen, ventral rumen, abomasum or duodenum of goats; intake was depressed to the same extent by each infusion, which shows that, in contrast to those for acetate, the receptors are not specifically in the rumen. Comparison of infusion into the lumen of the rumen, ruminal vein, mesenteric vein, portal vein and carotid artery showed the biggest effect on voluntary intake with ruminal vein infusion and Baile (1971) concluded that receptors sensitive to propionate were in the wall of this vessel. In the light of later work this seems unlikely, as sensitivity to propionate has been demonstrated in the liver (Chapter 3).

*Butyrate*

When injected intravenously or intraruminally, butyrate has smaller and more variable effects on feeding than acetate or propionate (Baile and Mayer, 1979):

$$DEPR = 0.17Bu + 11.4 \qquad (4.9)$$

where DEPR is the depression in intake (%) and Bu is the amount of butyrate infused (mmol per meal).

Although intravenous infusion of butyrate sometimes reduces feeding this is probably of little physiological significance as butyrate is produced by fermentation at a much slower rate than acetate; it is converted into 3-hydroxy butyrate in the rumen wall so that plasma levels are very low.

For these reasons there have been few studies of the effects of butyrate on voluntary intake. However, butyrate appears to be more slowly absorbed from the rumen than acetate or propionate and is more effective in causing rumen stasis. Butyrate improves the acceptability of foods to which it is added (Buchanan-Smith, 1990; Gherardi *et al.*, 1991). It is not possible to say whether the positive effect of butyrate on palatability might override its negative effect on rumen chemoreceptors nor, indeed, whether its attractiveness to sheep is due to its metabolic effects.

### Difficulties of interpretation of work with sodium salts of VFAs

Most studies of the effects of VFAs on feeding have used infusions of their sodium salts. In addition to elevating the concentrations of the VFA(s) in question, they also elevate sodium levels and osmolality in rumen fluid. The use of the acids themselves has been restricted by the discomfort apparently induced in the experimental animals. Thus, there has been considerable confounding of the specific effects of VFAs and the more general osmotic effects of intraruminal infusions. Grovum (1987) has been particularly active in highlighting doubts about the specificity of VFA effects on feeding and the effects of rumen osmolality are reviewed below.

Duranton and Bueno (1985) have cast further doubt on the relevance of VFA concentrations in the rumen on the control of meal size. They fasted sheep overnight, then gave a meal of concentrates 30, 60 or 120 min before hay was offered *ad libitum*; there was no effect on the intake of hay in the 1 or 3 h following despite different levels of rumen VFA concentrations when hay was offered. However, the daily intake of hay was significantly reduced.

VFA mixtures were infused continuously into the rumen of sheep at 0, 0.47, 0.68, 0.94 or 1.14 mmol min$^{-1}$ for 5 days, 0.47 mmol being the equivalent of the products of fermentation of 50 g of digestible organic matter in 24 h (Lopez and Hovell, 1993). There was no effect on rumen VFA concentrations or on voluntary intake of ground pelleted barley straw with a digestibility of 340 g kg$^{-1}$, which the authors suggested as being primarily due to the low digestibility of the food. The fact that the VFA mixtures used were in the normal proportions of acetate:propionate:butyrate, i.e. balanced, might be the reason they were absorbed quickly (there was no significant effect of treatment on rumen VFA concentrations) and did not affect intake (Chapters 7 and 18).

Another concern is the rate at which VFAs are infused. In much of the work of Baile and his colleagues infusion into the rumen was carried out at a high and unphysiological rate for the duration of each spontaneous meal and this would cause a very rapid elevation in VFA and sodium concentrations. It is more appropriate to use continuous infusion for several hours at lower rates in order to achieve increases similar to those occurring naturally.

Experimental addition of material into the rumen via a fistula is a widely used technique which appears to avoid sensory evaluation by the animal. However, we rarely consider the effects of such materials on the taste, smell and physical form of the boluses of digesta regurgitated during rumination. In assessing the effects of the characteristics of the food on intake we must be careful to differentiate between their influence on the taste of the food and its post-ingestional effects.

Despite these difficulties, the facts that (i) VFA concentrations, osmolality and distension increase during feeding, (ii) food intake is depressed by experimentally increasing VFA concentrations, osmolality or distension in the rumen and (iii) there are receptors which are sensitive to these changes, encourage the belief that there is a physiological role for gastrointestinal receptors in the control of food intake in ruminants.

### Lactate

Lactic acid is present in silage (grass conserved by the acids produced by fermentation) at concentrations of up to 8% of the organic matter as well as being a product of rumen fermentation. The evidence for lactate affecting voluntary intake is somewhat controversial as 0.16 mol of sodium lactate infused intraruminally to goats over 5 h did not affect intake (de Jong, 1981a) whereas intraruminal infusions of 35 mmol during each of about 10 meals per day reduced food intake in goats by almost half but had a smaller effect in sheep (Baile, 1971). Compared with VFAs, infusion of lactate had a prolonged after-effect on intake.

When a high physiological concentration of lactic acid was infused into the duodenum of sheep the intake of concentrates was reduced (Bueno, 1975), probably related to the reduction in stomach motility or to the involvement in propionate metabolic pathways.

### Nitrogenous compounds

The intake of silage is often lower than that of hay made from the same grass (Chapter 16). Numerous possible reasons for this have been put forward and several of these are likely to act together to reduce intake. Clancy *et al.* (1977) infused lucerne silage juice into the rumen of sheep and found decreases in hay intake but the effect could not be attributed to any particular component of the extracts as VFAs, lactate, several nitrogenous compounds and osmolality of the ruminal fluid were all greatly elevated.

Intake of silage is inversely related to the content of ammonia-N (expressed as a proportion of total N) (Wilkins *et al.*, 1971; Lewis, 1981) but infusion of ammonium salts into the rumen has to be at rates that are toxic in order to depress intake significantly. Urea enters the rumen in the saliva in large quantities and much of this is metabolized to ammonia; urea infusion into the rumen of goats during spontaneous meals depressed intake but was less effective, mole for mole, than ammonium salts (Conrad *et al.*, 1977).

Small amounts of numerous other nitrogenous compounds are produced by fermentation, both in silage and in the rumen. Neumark *et al.* (1964) found that, of the products of silage fermentation they examined, formaldehyde was the only one that markedly reduced food intake in sheep and a goat, although histamine enhanced this effect. This was supported by further work in which 1 g of histamine per day infused into the rumen did not affect silage intake unless formic acid was also added (Neumark, 1967) and then only when the solutions were given by stomach tube and deposited in the anterior rumen. Direct infusion of histamine into the abomasum caused a reduction in intake, but the increase in respiration rate indicated that it had a systemic effect and Neumark (1967) concluded that it would require a very rapid passage of dietary formate or histamine into the abomasum to obtain the observed low intake of silages.

Buchanan-Smith and Phillip (1986) infused into the rumen of sheep extracts of three different silages as well as high rates of infusion of various amines or organic acids. All these treatments depressed intake and the authors concluded that, although soluble constituents of silage can inhibit intake, no single constituent is primarily responsible for the control of silage intake.

Although under some circumstances ammonia or amines depress intake there is as yet insufficient information about their site(s) of action or the receptors which might be involved, although many of these compounds are of types that are known to be biologically active.

## pH and acidity

It has been suggested that the fall in rumen pH towards the end of large meals is involved in the cessation of feeding. Leek and Harding (1975) have demonstrated the existence of chemoreceptors in the anterior rumen and reticulum, the activity of which is changed according to the pH of rumen fluid, irrespective of the type of acid applied (Crichlow and Leek, 1981). However, Baile and Mayer (1969) found a similar depression of intake by sheep whether the pH was lowered by acetic acid or with infusion of sodium acetate which did not affect rumen pH. This specificity agrees with the work of Ash (1959) who reported that VFAs, but not lactic, citric or hydrochloric acids given into the reticulum at concentrations of 100–200 mM inhibited rumen contractions. However, from a comparison of effects of acetic acid with potassium acetate given intraruminally Hutchinson and Wilkins (1971) concluded that pH is important because the acid depressed intake but there was no effect of the salt. When rumen pH falls below about 5.0 rumen stasis occurs and the hypophagia that follows is more likely to be due to rumen stasis than to low pH *per se.*

Bhattacharya and Warner (1967) infused various acids including phosphoric, lactic, and citric acids, into the rumen of steers, maintaining the rumen pH at about 6.0. They observed significant reductions in food intake but this effect might be an indirect one because acidity, even when pH is maintained within the normal range for the rumen, is known to have strong inhibitory effects on reticuloruminal motility.

It is therefore likely that the titratable acidity of silage is more important than pH (McDonald, 1981) and attempts to stimulate the intake of concentrates by incorporating buffers in the food have not always been successful. The inclusion of sodium bicarbonate (25 kg tonne$^{-1}$) in concentrates for dairy cows increased hay intake and the fat content of milk, with no effect on total milk yield (Edwards and Poole, 1983). Inclusion at 20 kg tonne$^{-1}$ of a complete food in another experiment increased intake (13.9 to 14.9 kg day$^{-1}$) and reduced weight loss but no effect on milk yield or composition was observed (Edwards and Poole, 1983). Bhattacharya and Warner (1968b) included calcium hydroxide at 25 g kg$^{-1}$ in a complete food containing 30% hay and 70% concentrates. Intake by sheep increased significantly from 920 to 1120 g day$^{-1}$ whereas in cattle the increase was from 14.1 to 16.3 kg day$^{-1}$. Sodium carbonate (25 g kg$^{-1}$) and sodium bicarbonate (50 g kg$^{-1}$) were as effective as calcium carbonate in cattle but less so in sheep. Other experiments have not always shown an effect, however, and these additives are not widely used in practice.

There has been much recent activity to develop methods of improving the nutritional value of straw, mainly by treatment with alkalis. The resulting improvement allows increased intake by ruminants, as detailed by Nicholson (1984).

## Osmolality

Many of the effects which have been attributed to chemoreceptors could be due to osmotic effects rather than specific chemical effects on the gut wall. There are significant changes in the osmolality of rumen contents depending on the intakes of DM and water. In general, osmolality increases during and after a meal. Osmolality of the ruminal contents has been reported to increase from a pre-feeding level of 250–300 mosmol $kg^{-1}$ to as much as 500 mosmol $kg^{-1}$ in a few hours after a large meal (Warner and Stacy, 1968) and thus it must be considered as a candidate for involvement in the control of food intake.

Several authors have studied, directly or indirectly, the effect of changes in rumen osmolality on food intake by ruminants. Although the methodology used has differed quite widely, all the following studies have reported decreases in food intake after different infusions into the rumen of sheep.

Bergen (1972) raised ruminal osmolality to 400 mosmol $kg^{-1}$ by injecting sodium chloride or sodium acetate solutions into the rumen just prior to feeding and observed a reduction of food intake. It is not possible to compare directly the effects of the two salts as sodium chloride was given in larger amounts than sodium acetate, produced a larger rise in rumen fluid osmolality and a greater depression in the intake of a complete food. A local anaesthetic given with either the chloride or the acetate blocked the inhibition of feeding whereas the anaesthetic given alone had no effect. Bergen concluded that osmolality does not play a significant role in the control of food intake unless it is increased above the physiological range. However, in a critical review of the control of food intake, Grovum (1987) suggested that osmolality can account for many of the effects of intraruminal or intravenous infusions of VFA salts on food intake.

Phillip *et al.* (1981b) infused into the rumen of sheep extracts from fresh and ensiled maize adjusted with NaCl to osmolalities within the range 200–1600 mosmol $kg^{-1}$. They found a reduction in food intake during the first 30 min directly proportional to the osmolality of the infused solution; similar effects were observed when the infused solutions contained only NaCl to achieve the same osmolalities. Drinking water was not withheld during the experimental period and there were no effects of treatment on the frequency of rumen contractions.

Infusion of hypertonic solutions of polyethylene glycol (PEG, an unabsorbed, osmotically active molecule), potassium chloride or sodium chloride into the rumen of sheep during meals depressed intake but the correlations between intake and sodium or potassium concentrations were closer than that with osmolality (Kato *et al.*, 1979). This suggests that osmolality *per se* was not the primary cause of the reduction in food intake. However, by increasing the osmolality of rumen contents with either sodium chloride or PEG, Carter and Grovum (1990) found a decrease in food intake directly related to the osmolality of rumen contents (Fig. 4.2). After loading the rumen with

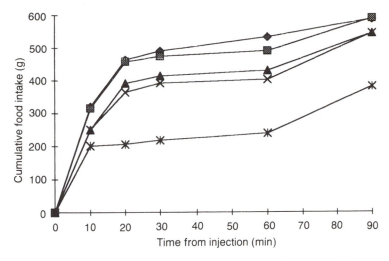

**Fig. 4.2.** Decreasing food and water intakes of sheep injected with 2.37 (♦), 6.25 (■), 12.5 (▲), 25 (X) or 50 g (✳) sodium chloride into the rumen (Carter and Grovum, 1990). From 0−60 min they were deprived of water whereas from 60 to 90 min water was available.

sodium chloride or PEG, there was a linear reduction in food intake during first 10 min of 3.49 g food $g^{-1}$ NaCl. The local anaesthetic lidocaine injected intraruminally just before the sodium chloride did not reduce the response. When given into the abomasum, sodium chloride had no effect in the first 10 min and there was no consistent relationship between osmolality of plasma collected from the jugular vein and the reduction in intake following either loading or drinking. Thus, it was concluded that osmolality is sensed in the rumen rather than in the abomasum or vascular system.

The importance of osmolality in the rumen has been further stressed by Grovum and Bignell (1989) who studied the effects of loading the rumen with solutions containing 0.4 or 0.8 osmol of sodium chloride, sodium acetate, sodium propionate or PEG. The result depression in food intake during the next half-hour was directly related to the osmotic load, with no difference between isosmotic amounts of the four substances, leading the authors to conclude that the effects of salts of VFAs have no effect on intake other than through their osmotic properties. One difficulty in interpreting these results is that raised rumen tonicity normally stimulates voluntary drinking (Fig. 4.2), thereby attenuating the effects of the infusion, but can only do so if animals have access to water. As Carter and Grovum (1990) and Grovum and Bignell (1989) withheld water during their experimental periods, it is understandable that Grovum should place such emphasis on the importance of osmolality of rumen fluid as a controller of food intake. Grovum and Bignell (1989) noted a resumption of feeding at the end of their experimental period, when access to water was given, similar to the observations by Barrio *et al.* (1991).

In the experiments of Baile and Mayer (1969) infusions of sodium salts of VFAs into the rumen reduced voluntary food intake but stimulated water intake; there was no effect on drinking when the acids were infused. Because VFAs are naturally produced in the rumen without such large increases in tonicity as have been induced by most experimental manipulations, it is essential that future research addresses this problem under conditions of natural feeding.

In most experimental work with VFAs the sodium salts have been used because the acids cause irritation of the rumen mucosa. When acetic acid was infused into the rumen of sheep at 60 g in 3.5 l of water over 4 h there was no change in the intake of a pelleted diet, rumen osmolality or pH (Phillip *et al.*, 1981a). In relation to the amount of acetate produced by fermentation in the rumen this is not a high rate of infusion and does not prove that acetic acid is less effective than sodium acetate in inhibiting feeding. In comparisons between equimolar sodium acetate and sodium chloride infusions into the rumen of cows and sheep, Forbes *et al.* (1992) and Azahan and Forbes (1992), respectively, have shown a somewhat greater inhibitory effect of the former.

A possible mechanism for osmotic effects on feeding has been found by Meyer *et al.* (1989) who have shown that intraperitoneal injection of arginine vasopressin reduces feeding in goats by reducing the weight eaten during the first meal after injection and prolonging the first intermeal interval. There do not appear to have been measurements of vasopressin concentrations in relation to feeding in ruminants but it is reasonable to assume that there is a rise in view of the marked changes in renin and angiotensin (Blair-West and Brook, 1969).

Raising the osmolality of rumen contents results in increases in the osmolality of digesta further down the gastrointestinal tract and of blood, either of which might mediate the effects on intake. Osmoreception in the rumen seems to be of primary importance, however, as Carter and Grovum (1990) showed that infusions into the abomasum had little effect on intake, even though they resulted in larger increases in blood osmolality than did rumen infusions.

Despite these demonstrations of osmotic effects on feeding there is no consistent experimental evidence of osmoreceptors located in the ruminal wall and/or duodenum (B.F. Leek, personal communication). One explanation for this, proposed by Forbes and Barrio (1992), is that osmotic changes in the rumen induce changes in the concentration of sodium and potassium in the extracellular fluid of the rumen mucosa.

An increase in extracellular sodium, as would occur during and for some time after an infusion of sodium salts into the rumen, should increase the likelihood of transmission of an action potential in view of the fact that removal of sodium from the extracellular fluid abolishes transmission (Hodgkin and Katz, 1949). Thus, osmolality would only affect the frequency of afferent impulses in the vagus nerve if the receptors were themselves being stimulated. Under the conditions of Leek's experiments, in which solutions were gently sprayed onto the exposed rumen mucosa of anaesthetized sheep, there would be little nervous activity and therefore little chance to show a modifying effect of osmolality. In the conscious sheep, on the other hand, in which epithelial receptors are being continually stimulated, both physically and chemically, there is plenty of opportunity for osmotic changes to attenuate or amplify the action potentials passing along the axons, hence the observed osmotic effects on feeding.

An indirect effect of osmotic changes in the rumen on intake might be by inhibition of ruminal microfauna, but this is not likely to be important in short-term responses to treatments. Nevertheless, a normal rumen osmotic pressure near 260 mosmol $kg^{-1}$ is favourable for ciliate protozoan activity (Church, 1975), and, as noted by Bergen (1972), cellulose degradation is inhibited *in vitro* at osmolalities above 400 mosmol $kg^{-1}$.

Almost all experiments involving infusion of salts into the reticulorumen have been performed using sodium salts, other cations being rarely used (Kato *et al.*, 1979). However, Warner and Stacy (1965) stated that the post-feeding rise in rumen osmotic pressure, when sheep were fed on equal amounts of lucerne chaff and wheaten chaff, was largely due to increases in the concentration of potassium and, to a lesser extent, ammonium. J.P. Barrio, S.T. Bapat and J.M. Forbes (unpublished results) have observed a closer relationship between osmolality of rumen fluid and potassium concentration than between osmolality and sodium concentration in sheep with free access to a pelleted, complete diet and drinking water.

Ternouth and Beattie (1971) infused sodium chloride, potassium chloride or sodium salts of acetate, propionate and butyrate into rumen-fistulated sheep accustomed to eating their daily ration in 2 h; the reduction in food intake was related to osmolality of the added fluid but not with the energetic content, and the reduction was more significant when potassium chloride was infused than with sodium chloride; this is probably related to the slower absorption of potassium compared with sodium. When water was infused into the reticulorumen, thus decreasing its osmolality, food intake increased, further suggesting a role for ruminal osmoreceptors in the control of feeding. Given a salty food to eat, sheep ate more after loading the rumen with water (Ternouth and Beattie, 1971). Mbanya (1988) also found a tendency for cows to eat more silage during three hours of infusion of water than when no infusion was given, as did Azahan (1988) with sheep. It seems likely, therefore, that osmotic effects in the rumen wall play a major role in controlling intake, even though osmoreceptors have not been clearly demonstrated.

Ruminal osmolality can indirectly affect voluntary food intake by altering salivary secretion. Large amounts of saliva are secreted and swallowed by the ruminant in order to keep constant the ruminal pH which tends to be lowered by the continuous production of VFAs. When strongly hypertonic solutions of sodium or potassium salts were infused into the reticulorumen of sheep, or sodium salts or urea were infused into the bloodstream, saliva production was found to decrease (Warner and Stacy, 1977). Marked decreases in plasma volume have been shown during feeding (Blair-West and Brook, 1969; Christopherson and Webster, 1972). The state of hydration of the body probably plays a part in the control of feeding as giving a diuretic before feeding reduced food intake whereas a preload of isotonic saline given intraperitoneally in sheep increased intake (Ternouth and Beattie, 1972). It is concluded that the relative importance of osmolality as a satiety factor in ruminants is still uncertain.

*Temperature receptors*

Increasing the temperature of rumen contents from 38.0 to 41.3°C by means of heating coils in the rumen depressed intake of cattle by 15% (Gengler *et al.*, 1970). Bhattacharya and Warner (1968b), by adding cold water to the rumen of cattle for 6 h, reduced intraruminal temperature by about 10°C and tympanic temperature by 0.2°C and caused an increase in the intake of a pelletted diet of 24%. Addition of warm water to raise rumen temperature by 2°C then depressed intake by 9%. Rawson and Quick (1971) demonstrated temperature receptors in the abdomen of sheep with the afferent fibres in the splanchnic nerves. This may be the way in which ruminal heating or cooling affects intake.

# The Omasum

The reticulo-omasal orifice is very sensitive to mechanical stimuli and its distension evokes rumination and parotid salivary secretion (Ash and Kay, 1957) via the vagus nerves. As the only exit for particles of food not digested in the rumen is via this orifice, and in view of its small size, it might be thought that control of rumen emptying, and thus of voluntary intake, could reside at this site. Laplace (1970) observed a correlation between feeding and omasal activity and proposed a role for the omasum in the control of food intake and rumination.

## The Abomasum

Mechano- and chemoreceptors are to be found in the stomach of non-ruminants and the abomasum, as the equivalent organ in the ruminant, also possesses such sensitivity. Harding and Leek (1972) described mechanoreceptors in the epithelium of the abomasum, which give a rapidly adapting response to stimulation but continuous discharge if sufficient stimulus is provided. These abomasal receptors also respond to chemicals. The effects of acids on abomasal mucosal receptors are very similar to those in the rumen (Leek, 1977), being positively related to their titratable acidities rather than to pH and inversely related to molecular mass. Thus acetic acid had the same effect whether buffered or unbuffered. Alkalis also stimulate these receptors as do hyper- and hypotonic solutions and water. The effect of tonicity is very variable, however, application of the same stimulant to the same unit generating different latent periods on successive occasions.

Bolton *et al.* (1976) showed that intra-abomasal infusion of VFAs reduced abomasal activity and emptying, butyric acid being the most potent. This suggests that total VFA content and the relative proportions of VFAs may be important factors in the induction of the abomasal hypomotility preceding abomasal displacement in dairy cattle. Whether the composition of abomasal fluid and the degree of activation of the receptors has any influence on rumen emptying and food intake is not clear. Infusion of fat into the abomasum of sheep reduces food intake (Titchen *et al.*, 1966), presumably by inhibiting rumen outflow.

Abomasal motility is increased during rumination (Laplace, 1970) which might account for the increased rate of outflow from the rumen during the night (Thiago *et al.*, 1992), which is when most rumination takes place.

## Intestinal Receptors

There are tension receptors with vagal afferent fibres in the duodenum of the sheep which also respond to chemicals (Cottrell and Iggo, 1984a). In view of the evidence of important roles for intestinal mechano- and chemoreceptors in the control of food intake in other classes of animal

(Chapter 3) it is likely that such receptors are also important in the ruminant. There are two different types of duodenal chemoreceptor, one excited by potassium chloride solutions, the response increasing with the concentration of the salt (12.5–450 mM), whereas the other is insensitive to potassium chloride but excited by acetic, butyric or propionic acids (10–150 mM) (Cottrell and Iggo, 1984a). The responses elicited were directly related to molecular weight but not to pH or osmolality; both were excited by sodium hydroxide solutions but not usually by sodium bicarbonate. Considerable quantities of potassium ions and VFAs leave the rumen and might, therefore, be expected to stimulate the duodenal chemoreceptors and act in the negative feedback control of feeding.

Dynes (1993) studied the effect of duodenal osmolality on feeding in sheep by injecting 5 ml kg$^{-1}$ of 6.5% NaCl or mannitol into the duodenum 5 min before feeding without drinking water. There was almost complete inhibition of feeding in the first 15 min, an effect which was not alleviated by local anaesthetic. When water was made available 30 min after feeding started, the sheep immediately drank a large volume and between 1.5 and 3 h food intake was significantly higher than when water was not available. The amounts of salt, mannitol and anaesthetics were similar to those used by Houpt et al. (1983) who did observe reversal of intake depression by anaesthetic in pigs. It seems unlikely that there would be basic differences between the intestinal physiology of pigs and sheep but no explanation has been proposed for these different experimental results.

In adult ruminants offered dry feeds osmolality can be up to 585 mosmol kg$^{-1}$ in the duodenum but not so high further down the intestines (Maloiy and Clemens, 1980). The osmotic effect of digesta in the duodenum could be an important contributor to satiety under many circumstances, but little relevant research has been carried out with ruminants.

Although there have been suggestions on several occasions that flow through the intestines limits voluntary intake by ruminants (e.g. Demarquilly et al., 1965, quoted by Van Soest, 1982) this is not a generally important factor. Egan (1972) added sawdust equivalent to a quarter of the daily food intake into the rumen of sheep. This increased faecal output but had no effect on food intake. Grovum and Phillips (1978) infused methylcellulose into the abomasum at rates which doubled the volume of faecal production, but without effect on voluntary food intake. They concluded that intestinal capacity is not a limiting factor in feeding.

# Interactions between Different Families of Receptor

There are several instances of stimulation of receptors in one part of the digestive tract having consequences elsewhere which might influence voluntary intake indirectly. Chemical or acid factors in the rumen affect motility and therefore the stimulation of mechanoreceptors by local contractions so that, for example, loss of reticuloruminal motility occurs when epithelial receptors in the rumen become stimulated by high levels of VFAs (Leek, 1983). Lactic acid may facilitate the inhibitory effects of VFAs, as Crichlow (1988) reported activation of reticuloruminal epithelial receptors by low levels of undissociated VFAs after exposure of the luminal surface to DL-lactic acid. Thus the intake-depressing effects of lactic acid on food intake (Baile and Mayer, 1969) may be indirectly related to the inhibition of reticuloruminal motility.

There is presumably a concentration gradient in digesta for such things as VFAs, with the highest levels in the centre of the rumen and lower levels at the rumen wall, from where they are absorbed. Such a gradient is difficult to confirm experimentally in view of the contractions which move the tips of sampling tubes, and may be quite small in magnitude. However, the increase in frequency of rumen contractions during feeding, speeding up the mixing of rumen contents, may significantly increase the level of intake-depressing activity at the rumen wall.

Leek (1977) points out that one stimulus excites several types of receptor and one type of receptor is excited by several types of stimulus. Thus, no single stimulus/receptor combination is likely to explain the effects of the physical and chemical properties of digesta in the gastrointestinal tract on motility and food intake. The experimenter measures fullness of a part of the tract as the volume of its contents whereas to the CNS this may be:

> a composite quality depending not on the absolute volume of the contents but on the rate of change of volume, the tonic state of the visceral muscle, the texture and chemistry of the contents and the extent to which the contents displace the viscus on its mesenteric attachment. such possibilities illustrate the difficulty of defining and quantifying a visceral stimulus.
>
> (Leek, 1977)

If these are the difficulties involved in understanding receptor involvement in signalling to the CNS, how much more difficult will it be to understand the control of voluntary food intake, in which many more factors must be taken into account?

# Conclusions

The capacity of the rumen to hold digesta clearly sets a limit to how much the ruminant can eat but rarely is this the only factor controlling food intake. Those receptors in the ruminal mucosa which are sensitive to chemical influences cannot be envisaged as ceasing to inform the CNS about pH, VFA concentration and osmolality when the mechanoreceptors are being strongly stimulated. In fact chemo- and mechanoreception are properties of the same neurones and it seems likely that chemical and stretch information are dealt with in an additive manner.

The osmolality of rumen contents has an important influence on feeding when it is raised above the normal range and this changes the interpretation of results from experiments in which the sodium salts of the VFAs were infused. The situation is clouded by the difficulty of demonstrating receptors sensitive to osmolality and new experimental approaches will have to be developed to resolve this difficult area.

We can rarely be sure of the exact mechanism(s) being brought into play when intake is affected by a change of diet or an experimental treatment. It is difficult to design experiments to isolate one factor at a time but such experiments are necessary if progress is to be made in understanding more fully the control of food intake. It might be technically possible, for example, to manipulate the composition of rumen fluid while maintaining normal conditions in the rest of the tract by preventing the flow of digesta from the rumen and infusing artificial digesta of normal composition into the abomasum. However, a multiplicity of cannulae and tubes, even if ethically acceptable, will undoubtedly increase the risk of inappetence in the experimental animals.

# 5 | METABOLITES AND HORMONES

- Glucose
- Fats and related metabolites
- Amino acids
- Metabolic hormones
- Gut peptides
- Other gut hormones
- Other hormones
- Hormones involved in reproduction and growth
- Conclusions

Digesta in the stomach(s) and intestines stimulate mechano- and chemoreceptors (Chapters 3 and 4) but it is unlikely that the total of the information from these receptors is sufficient for the central nervous system (CNS) to gain a complete picture of the quantities of nutrients ingested in order to balance intake with output. As we have seen in Chapter 3, the liver is the first point at which most of the absorbed nutrients can be monitored by a single organ but, even then, lipids are absorbed via the lymphatic system and bypass the liver. The general circulation transports nutrients between organs and also is the medium whereby hormones, secreted from endocrine organs, pass to their target organs. Many of the hormones have metabolic functions and have been implicated in the control of food intake (e.g. insulin) whereas others have primary roles in other bodily functions but influence intake secondarily (e.g. oestrogens).

Early theories of food intake control gave a prominent place to the monitoring of blood metabolite levels such as glucose, suggesting that they were sensed by the CNS. However, many of the functions of the body have evolved to protect the CNS from fluctuations in its supply of nutrients. A parallel can be made with the regulation of body temperature, where it is now believed that the temperature sensors in the periphery are more important than central receptors so that the CNS is made aware of potential changes in deep body temperature and can set in motion actions to balance environmental changes before brain temperature itself has changed. So with nutrient supply we can envisage a more important role for peripheral receptors with those in the CNS only being stimulated under severe conditions of nutrient shortage or excess. This will be explored further in Chapter 6 and it is sufficient here to say that blood concentrations of metabolites or hormones are unlikely to be the only factors taken into account by the CNS circuits controlling voluntary intake.

This is not to say that blood-borne nutrients and hormones cannot exert marked influences on feeding as changes in concentrations induce changes in the metabolism of tissues and organs. Evidence of an important role for a factor(s) carried in blood was obtained by Hervey (1959) working with parabiotic rats (pairs of animals joined by skin and therefore exchanging blood). When one of a pair was subjected to lesioning of the ventromedial hypothalamus it gained weight rapidly while its unlesioned partner lost weight and would have eventually died. It was postulated that a blood-borne satiety factor produced in excess by the obese animal could not be sensed by its brain because of the lesions in critical circuits but was sensed by the circuits of the intact partner which was thus inhibited from feeding. Such an hypothesis depends on the signalling chemical having a much longer half-life in the bloodstream than nutrients, otherwise the latter could have been carried in adequate amounts from fat to lean partner, preventing the inanition of the latter.

No attempts have been made to make parabiotic preparations with farm animals. There have, however, been a few experiments in which exchange of blood has been achieved between sheep. Satiated sheep began to eat soon after the start of blood exchange with hungry donors; the intake of hungry sheep was reduced when blood was exchanged with satiated donors (Seoane *et al.*, 1972).

Exchange of blood was also carried out in chickens by Savory and Smith (1987) but with equivocal results as far as food intake is concerned.

The levels of many metabolites and hormones in the blood have been suggested as informing the brain of the animal's metabolic state and being involved in the control of feeding (Forbes, 1988b). Of these, insulin and glucagon are the most likely candidates despite the attention that has been directed at other hormones, particularly cholecystokinin (CCK).

# Glucose

Mayer (1953) suggested that voluntary intake is controlled by blood glucose levels. He pointed to the fact that blood glucose concentration rises after a meal, then falls before the next meal and that injection of gold thioglucose into mice caused hyperphagia and obesity. At autopsy gold was found in the ventromedial hypothalamus which was damaged by its toxic effects: this was used as evidence that glucose was taken up by this part of the brain. It was later shown that the uptake of gold thioglucose into the ventromedial hypothalamus is dependent on the presence of insulin. These findings supported the theory that the hypothalamus monitored blood glucose concentration in order to control intake.

A small fall in blood glucose concentration normally occurs just before a meal, reaching a nadir around 5 min before the start of the spontaneous meal. Preventing this in rats by infusion of a small amount of glucose intravenously maintained satiety so that animals which would have otherwise started to eat 12 min later actually waited 318 min before starting to eat (Campfield and Smith, 1986). Withholding of food during the preprandial trough of blood glucose prevented feeding until the next spontaneous decline in blood glucose about 1 h later so that it appears as if it might be the actual fall in glucose which triggers feeding.

These observations suggest that the glucose fall is causally involved in the initiation of a meal in the laboratory rat but Strubbe *et al* (1977) found no effect of glucose infused between spontaneous meals on meal size or duration. However, when insulin accompanies the glucose infusion suppression of feeding results and insulin levels have been found to be at their lowest just before meals in rats. It seems, therefore, that glucose needs to be taken up by insulin-sensitive tissue in order to be effective in depressing intake but that only a small amount of energy-yielding nutrient causes a very great prolongation of the intermeal interval demonstrating a very sensitive means of monitoring energy status of the body.

Glucose introduced into the stomach has a much greater effect on the size of a subsequent meal than the same amount of the unabsorbable analogue of glucose, 3-O-methylglucose (Booth, 1972a), showing that the metabolic effect of glucose is more important than the osmotic effect. Fructose, which is used by the liver, was as effective as glucose in suppressing feeding (Booth, 1972b); galactose was ineffective as it is utilized very inefficiently by the liver. These results demonstrate a postabsorptive effect of glucose on feeding in which the liver and the CNS have been particularly implicated as sensors.

Glucose is not the only factor which controls intake: for example rats eat more at night than during the day but their blood glucose levels are higher at night. As a result of this and many other considerations the glucostatic theory was modified to say that the rate of glucose utilization was the controlling factor rather than its concentration in the blood.

More recent evidence shows that the brain is not the only part of the body sensitive to glucose and may not even be the major one. As detailed in Chapter 3, work with laboratory animals shows that the liver is sensitive to glucose (Russek, 1976).

However, it is clear that certain regions of the brain are also sensitive to glucose shortage and that both play their part in the control of intake in a manner analogous to the integration of peripheral and central temperature receptors in the control of body temperature. It is not fully understood whether the brain's sensitivity to lack of glucose is called into play under normal circumstances, or whether the peripheral mechanisms which normally protect the brain from fluctuations in glucose supply mean that the central mechanism for detecting glucose is only called upon in emergencies.

There are glucose-sensitive neurons in the lateral hypothalamus which decrease their firing rate in the presence, locally, of glucose. Most of these decreased their rate of firing when glucose was infused into the hepatic portal vein (Shimizu et al., 1983) and therefore appear to be linked to the 'metabolic sensors' of the liver.

Glucoprivation causes activation of the sympathetic nervous system leading to release of catecholamines, glucocorticoids, growth hormone and glucagon, as well as inhibition of insulin secretion, all of which mobilize glucose and protect the brain (Ritter, 1986). Experimentally, insulin injection to increase glucose uptake by peripheral tissues, 2-deoxy-D-glucose (2DG) to block glucose entry into cells, activate a cerebral response which results in feeding; for example, a dose of 2DG too small to have any effect when given into the general circulation causes a marked feeding response in rats when given into the cerebroventricles (Miselis and Epstein, 1975). Ventromedial hypothalamus (VMH) lesions (King et al., 1979) block the ability of intraventricular 2DG to stimulate feeding, but lesions in other sites in the brain also have this effect, suggesting that the VMH is not the only glucose-sensitive site. Also, direct injection of 2DG into the VMH does not stimulate feeding (Miselis and Epstein, 1975). Glucose-sensitive neurons have been identified in the brain (Oomura, 1976) but little is known about their characteristics other than that they are probably activated by lack of glucose within the cell rather than on its surface. It might be more appropriate to talk of energoprivation rather than glucoprivation because D-3-hydroxybutyrate, which is used by brian cells when glucose is unavailable, prevents the feeding induced by 2DG (Bellin and Ritter, 1981).

*Poultry*

Infusion of glucose into peripheral veins has no effect on intake, even when plasma levels of glucose are increased to over $500 \, mg \, l^{-1}$ (Richardson, 1970a); it tends if anything to stimulate intake in the chicken (Smith and Bright-Taylor, 1974) except when infused into the hepatic portal vein, when it has a potent suppressing effect (Shurlock and Forbes, 1981b; Chapter 3). Intracerebroventricular infusion of 120 mg glucose over a period of 1 h depressed voluntary intake (Matei-Vladescu *et al.*, 1977) but this might well have been a non-specific osmotic or stress effect as no suitable control was used. Mannoheptulose, a seven-carbon sugar which induces a diabetes-like state in mammals, depressed intake from 8.5 to 6.0 g during the 3 h following injection intraperitoneally or intracardially in chickens (Smith and Baranowski-Kish, 1976).

The quantities of glucose required to depress intake when infused into the portal vein are within the physiological range (Shurlock and Forbes, 1981b) and the effects are blocked by bilateral vagotomy at the level of the proventriculus (Rusby *et al.*, 1987). This shows that the flow of glucose from the digestive tract is monitored by the liver which relays its information to the CNS via peripheral nerves. The liver is the first organ to be presented with an overall picture of what is being absorbed; also, with its role as a buffer in the maintenance of blood glucose concentration, the liver takes up glucose from the portal blood when it is in excess of the requirements of the rest of the body and releases it when necessary. Thus, it can transmit a signal which contributes to satiety when glucose (and other metabolites such as amino acids) are becoming available in excessive quantities, this signal being reduced or reversed in times of need.

Although blood glucose levels fluctuate in relation to fasts of several hours (e.g. Lepkovsky *et al.*, 1967) it has proved to be difficult to affect feeding in chickens by manipulation of blood glucose concentrations with insulin. Injection of mammalian insulin, for example, caused a decrease in blood glucose in birds, but intake was depressed (chickens, Smith and Bright-Taylor, 1974; ducks, Evans, 1972; geese, Nir and Levy, 1973) rather than elevated as in mammals. This is still true when repeated injections are given to chickens over 6 days (Lepkovsky *et al.*, 1967); perhaps avian insulin would give different results.

In the chicken, gold thioglucose given systemically did not cause hyperphagia (Gentle, 1976), nor when implanted directly in the hypothalamus (Walker *et al.*, 1981). Only 5 out of 18 hens became hyperphagic when gold thioglucose was implanted in the median eminence (Sonoda *et al.*, 1974) and the significance of this finding is not clear.

2DG, which prevents the uptake and utilization of glucose in mammals and stimulates voluntary intake because of glucoprivation, actually depresses feeding in the chicken (Smith *et al.*, 1975; Rusby and Forbes, 1985); unfortunately it is not yet known whether 2DG has the same metabolic effects in birds as in mammals.

Incorporation of 100 g of glucose per litre in the drinking water for growing chickens does not depress food intake, nor does it increase live weight gain. There is, however, an increase in carcass fatness (Azahan and Forbes, 1989). Thus, apart from osmotic effects, only hepatic infusion of glucose suggests that it is specifically involved in the control of intake in chickens.

*Pigs*

Glucose infused into the jugular vein or hepatic portal vein had no effect on the food intake by young pigs (Houpt *et al.*, 1979) but the conditions of the experiment (10 min access to food after an overnight fast) would not necessarily allow an effect to be shown. In the young pig 1 unit insulin $kg^{-1}$ causes increased intake during the 6 h after injection (Houpt and Houpt, 1977).

Infusion of glucose solution into the duodenum of fasted pigs depresses intake (Chapter 3) but the effect is not specific to glucose as similar depression of intake was induced by infusion of hypertonic saline. Thoracic vagotomy, or concurrent infusion with local anaesthetic, largely blocked the effect of duodenal infusion of glucose. Thus, there is a mechanism for sensing of duodenal osmotic pressure with nervous transmission to the CNS but once absorbed glucose seems to have no effect under the conditions of the work done so far, in which food was only available for short periods each day.

*Cattle*

Plasma glucose concentrations in ruminants are much lower than those in simple-stomached animals and the fluctuations are smaller. However, because of the major role of glucose as a fuel in the non-ruminant and the prevalence of the glucostatic theory of control of intake, there were several investigations in the 1960s of effects on feeding of manipulation of blood glucose levels in ruminants. Glucose had no effect whether given intraruminally or intravenously in cows (Dowden and Jacobsen, 1960) or intracerebroventricularly in calves (Peterson *et al.*, 1972).

*Sheep and goats*

Intravenous infusion of glucose to raise the plasma glucose concentration above that normal in non-ruminants depressed intake in sheep (Boda and Riley, 1961; Stone, 1975) but lower rates of infusion had no effect (Manning *et al.*, 1959; Holder, 1963). Insulin infusion, at a rate sufficiently high to depress the concentrations of glucose and acetate in plasma, had no effect on feeding in goats (Baile and Mayer, 1968c).

Intracerebroventricular injection of glucose did not affect intake (goats, Baile and Mahoney, 1967; sheep, Seoane and Baile, 1972a). Thus there is no good evidence for involvement of glucose in negative feedback pathways in the control of food intake in ruminants.

Although a very large dose (19,806 mU) of insulin given into the jugular vein depressed intake, lower amounts had no effect (Muller and Colenbrader, 1970; Deetz and Wangsness, 1980). However, a relatively slow rate of infusion (6 mU min$^{-1}$ for 15 min) into the hepatic portal vein depressed intake (Deetz *et al.*, 1980). Moreover, infusion of glucose to prevent insulin-induced hypoglycaemia blocked the intake-stimulating effect of that hormone (Houpt, 1974). Gold thioglucose did not affect intake in ruminants, even when given with insulin to ensure sufficient uptake of the drug to cause severe damage to liver and kidneys (Baile *et al.*, 1970). Injection of 2DG into the cerebroventricles together with insulin did depress intake (Babapour and Bost, 1973), a paradoxical result as 2DG inhibits glucose uptake and would be expected to stimulate intake by causing glucoprivation in hypothalamic cells. However, Houpt (1974) showed that 2DG given intravenously induced hyperphagia in sheep, even when hyperglycaemia was prevented by adrenalectomy.

From this evidence it can be concluded that glucose is not likely to be specifically involved in the control of feeding in sheep, although energy status is of significance.

VFAs do affect intake, however, and the whole subject of receptors and the role of the reticulorumen in the control of feeding has been covered in Chapter 4.

## Fats and Related Metabolites

Fat is stored in the body in large quantities, with continuous turnover which involves the release of fatty acids, glycerol and ketones such as D-3-hydroxybutyrate. There is particular interest in ways in which adipose tissue might affect feeding in view of the practical significance of preventing or reversing over-fatness, both in humans and in farm animals (Chapter 8).

Addition of fat improves the palatability of food for rats and it is not easy to separate the hedonic from the metabolic effects of fat on intake. In a commendable attempt to divide the two Jen et al. (1985) trained monkeys to suck liquid diets from a tube which activated an intragastric infusion. Thus, the ratio of fat to carbohydrate entering the stomach could be varied independently of that in the diet being taken by mouth. Gastric infusion depressed oral intake but varying the carbohydrate content of the whole food entering the stomach between 280 and 770 g kg$^{-1}$ and the fat between 160 and 650 g kg$^{-1}$ had no further effect. This suggests that the hedonic properties of high-fat diets are more important than the metabolic effects in stimulating intake.

Dietary fat is absorbed into the lymphatic system rather than into the venous drainage of the intestines in mammals and thus bypasses the liver. However, the liver is an important site of fat metabolism in mammals and especially in birds. Intravenous infusion of fat emulsion depresses intake, an effect that is not accompanied by changes in plasma glucose or insulin concentrations. As animals fatten there is a gradual increase in plasma insulin concentration and Woods et al. (1986) have reviewed the impressive evidence that this is reflected in increased concentrations of insulin in the cerebrospinal fluid which inhibit intake thus acting as a homeostatic mechanism for body fat.

## Poultry

The site(s) of action of fats on intake has not been adequately studied in chickens. If the situation is similar to that in mammals then one of the effects of fat in the diet is to slow the rate of emptying of the stomach and this has been confirmed in hens (Mateos et al., 1982) but not in young broilers (Golian and Polin, 1984). If a reduction in rate of passage does occur it might in turn depress food intake by a stomach distension mechanism. In view of the discussion above, there is clearly a lot of scope for studies on the involvement of lipids in the mechanisms which control intake in the chicken.

The chicken seems to be particularly sensitive to the effects of infused fat on feeding which may be related to the fact that most lipid synthesis occurs in the liver and the lipid is then transported in the bloodstream. Lacy et al. (1986a) found that as little as 100 mg of lipid given in suspension into the hepatic portal vein of cockerels of an egg-laying strain over a 30-min period depressed subsequent intake to half of control levels whereas a similar infusion into the jugular vein was without effect. However, a much larger amount was without effect in broiler chickens of the same weight (but younger age) and these birds were also insensitive to glucose infused into the hepatic portal vein (Lacy et al., 1986a). Broilers have been selected for high food intake but whether this has involved reduced sensitivity to metabolites is not yet understood (Forbes, 1988b).

*Sheep*

Abomasal infusion of peanut oil reduced intake in sheep but only at high rates (100–150 ml h$^{-1}$) which are probably unphysiological (Titchen *et al.*, 1966).

## Free fatty acids

Palmitate increases liver cell membrane potential and this could be a way in which fat metabolism influences feeding. Injection of mercaptoacetate (inhibits fatty acid oxidation) intraperitoneally in rats had no effect on the intake of a low-fat (30 g kg$^{-1}$) diet but greatly increased the intake of a medium-fat (180 g kg$^{-1}$) food (Scharrer and Langhans, 1990). This effect was more potent during the day than at night perhaps because the rate of fatty acid oxidation is normally higher during the day. It may be that another inhibitor of fatty acid oxidation, pent-4-enoate, did not affect intake because the diet used in that experiment was quite low in fat. Section of the hepatic branch of the vagus almost completely prevented the increase in intake of the medium-fat diet whereas atropinization did not block the effect, which again suggests that it is the afferent (rather than efferent) fibres of the vagus which are important in the feeding response to modification of fatty acid metabolism. Diabetic rats can oxidize dietary fat but not glucose; whereas normal rats showed no preference for a flavour which had been paired with glucose, compared with a flavour paired with oil, diabetic rats preferred the flavour which had been paired with oil (Tordoff *et al.*, 1987), which they associated with an oxidizable (and therefore satiating?) substrate.

*Sheep*

Although a positive correlation between plasma levels of total fatty acids and the amount of food eaten voluntarily has been found in sheep (Thye *et al.*, 1970) there is no proof that the fatty acids were directly stimulating food intake. Work with sheep by Vandermeerschen-Doize and Paquay (1984), in which long-chain fatty acids were infused intravenously, does not clarify the situation because, although intake was depressed by physiological amounts of stearate, the albumin to which the fatty acids were coupled was of bovine origin and might have caused an allergic response. However, oleic acid esters (5 g day$^{-1}$) infused into the jugular vein depressed the intake of sheep compared with albumin alone (Paquay and Vernaillen, 1984), supporting the idea that the effect is physiological.

## Volatile fatty acids

Although plasma levels of the VFAs increase in ruminants after large meals the changes in peripheral blood during and between small spontaneous meals are not clear-cut. The available evidence indicates that acetate affects receptors in the rumen wall (Chapter 4) and propionate affects the liver (Chapter 3); transport in the general circulation is not considered to be very important as a negative feedback signal.

## Glycerol

The release of glycerol from adipose tissue is proportional to the mass of fat and the size of adipocytes. As exogenous glycerol depresses food intake (Wirtshafter and Davis, 1977a) it is possible that a lipostatic influence on feeding could be exerted by glycerol concentration in plasma or uptake by a responsive tissue. However, the dose of glycerol required to depress intake is supraphysiological but further study of the phenomenon might lead to better understanding of physiological control. Langhans et al (1984) used a dose of glycerol (6.3 mmol kg$^{-1}$) that was high enough to depress intake in rats and found plasma glucose and liver glycogen concentrations to be unaffected. This suggested that it might be the oxidation of glycerol rather than the glucose produced subsequently which was important. This idea was supported by the observations that glycerol had no effect on intake when a high protein diet was offered; such diets are known to depress the activity of glucose-3-phosphate dehydrogenase in the liver which would reduce the rate of glycerol oxidation in that organ. While observing that plasma levels of free fatty acids, glucose, insulin and catecholamines rose during meals in the rat, Steffens et al. (1986) noted that glycerol concentration did not change and concluded that lipolysis did not increase at this time. This does not rule out a long-term effect of glycerol, added to the meal-related short-term changes in metabolism which primarily control meal size.

## Sheep

Glycerol was infused into the portal vein of three castrated male sheep in medium body condition at the rate of 0.3 mmol min$^{-1}$ for 3 h and no effect on food intake was observed. There was no increase in peripheral concentrations during treatment, indicating that the infused glycerol was rapidly removed from the circulation. In the same experiment

1.2 mmol min$^{-1}$ of propionate completely suppressed feeding (P.M. Driver and J.M. Forbes, unpublished results).

### Ketones

D-3-Hydroxybutyrate (10 mmol kg$^{-1}$ subcutaneously) depressed food intake in rats whereas its metabolic product, acetoacetate, did not (Scharrer and Langhans, 1990) even though it appeared to be utilized more rapidly than D-3-hydroxybutyrate. This is consistent with the hypothesis that it is the process of oxidation of hydroxybutyrate to acetoacetate (which occurs primarily in the liver) which generates a satiating signal, analogous with the effects of oxidation of other substrates reviewed in Chapter 3.

## Amino Acids

Amino acids stimulate gut receptors (Mei, 1985), but whether these are osmoreceptors or whether there are specific aminoreceptors is not clear. Once absorbed, amino acids reach the liver and some metabolism takes place, including deamination and oxidation of those present in excess. An imbalance in the proportions of amino acids relative to the requirements invariably leads to reduction in food intake (Chapter 11).

The liver of the chicken is sensitive to lysine, as infusion into the portal vein causes a much greater depression of intake than infusion at the same rate into the jugular vein (Rusby and Forbes, 1987); the liver effect is blocked by vagotomy in the same way as the effect of portally infused glucose (Rusby *et al.*, 1987).

The evidence for a direct effect of amino acids on the brain is stronger than for glucose. Tobin and Boorman (1979) fed chickens on a histidine-deficient diet and found that infusion of histidine into the carotid artery, which goes directly to the brain, reversed the effect of the amino acid imbalance whereas infusion into the jugular vein had no effect. Thus, histidine appears to act directly on the brain to alleviate the intake-depressing effects of deficiency rather than more generally in the whole body.

## Metabolic Hormones

### Insulin

At meal onset there is an initial spurt of insulin secretion which, in the sheep, can be induced by the sight of the food (Bassett, 1975) and this is also true of cattle (Vasilatos and Wangsness, 1980; Faverdin, 1986a). One effect of the insulin is to cause a short-lived decline in plasma glucose concentrations at the start of the meal.

The initial surge of insulin at the start of the meal continues as a prolonged, nutrient-related secretion which serves to maintain a fairly stable concentration of glucose in the blood. Insulin injection results in the termination of sham feeding in rats and this satiety seems to be a pleasant sensation because when the insulin was paired with a flavour the rats subsequently preferred that flavour (Oetting and Vander-weele, 1985). Thus, the surge of pancreatic insulin during feeding is an important part of the satiating signal. The hyperglycaemia caused by glucose infusion can be suppressed with appropriate doses of insulin but intake is still depressed (Woods *et al.*, 1984), further confirming that it is insulin that is required to induce glucose uptake in order to affect intake. Insulin is particularly effective in suppressing intake when infused into the third ventricle of the brain and it has been proposed that this is an important physiological action of insulin (Chapter 6).

In contrast to these observations, chronic treatment with insulin increases the rate of fat deposition and stimulates food intake. It seems as if insulin depresses intake in the presence of high rate of supply of nutrients but stimulates intake when the availability of nutrients is insufficient to match the increased demand created by insulin treatment; there was only a 40% reduction in intake when glucose alone was infused intravenously at 170% of the normal rate of utilization, but a 70% reduction when insulin was also administered (Even and Nicolaidis, 1986); insulin alone stimulated intake.

In farm animals also, the effects of insulin administration have sometimes been to depress food intake and sometimes to stimulate it. In the chicken, mammalian insulin depresses intake, but avian insulin is structurally different from that of mammals and future work will need to use chicken insulin. Insulin (0.7 µg kg$^{-1}$) given intravenously at the beginning of a meal depressed food intake during the following 30 min by 14% when given to cows deprived of food for 11 h but not in those fed 4 h before (Faverdin, 1986a). Thus the role of insulin in short-term control of intake depends on nutritional status in ruminants as well.

Exogenous insulin has been shown to stimulate voluntary intake of pigs under some circumstances (Houpt and Houpt, 1977). Similarly, some experiments with sheep have shown increased intake (e.g. Houpt, 1974) whereas others have not (e.g. Baile and Martin, 1971).

Evidence that insulin does play an important physiological role in maintaining food intake in ruminants comes from the observation that alloxan-induced diabetes causes inappetence and death in sheep (Reid *et al.*, 1963). This is due to the lack of insulin rather than to the general

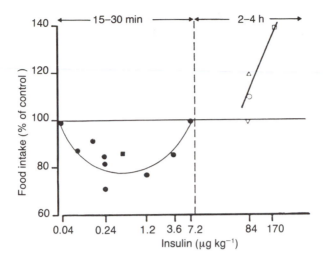

**Fig. 5.1.** Effects of insulin on food intake by cattle and sheep (Dulphy and Faverdin, 1987).

toxic effects of alloxan, because replacement therapy with insulin maintains intake at normal levels.

A collation of data from the literature on effects of intravenous insulin (Dulphy and Faverdin, 1987) shows that in the short term (15–30 min after injection) doses up to about 0.5 µg kg$^{-1}$ depress feeding but above this have less effect; higher doses (84–170 µg kg$^{-1}$) stimulate intake from 2–4 h (Fig. 5.1).

### Glucagon

Glucagon has also been found to increase in blood during feeding and the rapidity of this increased secretion by the pancreas suggests that it is induced by the autonomic nervous system and/or gut hormones rather than by changes in blood glucose concentration. Suggestions that glucagon might be involved in satiety came initially from effects of exogenous glucagon on feeding but it has been concluded that these effects were pharmacological. Small quantities of glucagon injected into the cerebral ventricles depressed intake and it has been proposed that glucagon entering the brain could participate in normal satiety. Are the doses of glucagon which have been used experimentally within the range of rates of secretion seen during spontaneous meals? Langhans *et al.* (1984) monitored the levels of pancreatic glucagon in the hepatic portal and hepatic veins and found that during the large meal following a 12 h fast the concentration in the hepatic portal vein doubled whereas that in the hepatic vein was little changed. Thus, most of the glucagon produced under physiological conditions is taken up by the liver and is presumably partly responsible for the rapid fall in liver glycogen content that occurs during a meal, although the catecholamines and gut hormones which are released during feeding will also play their part. Thus the liver should be the focus of attention for effects of this hormone on feeding. Injections into the portal vein are more effective in depressing feeding than into the general circulation and hepatic vagotomy blocked the effect of glucagon given portally. Atropine does not block the effect of glucagon on feeding showing that it is afferent rather than efferent fibres in the vagus which are important.

*Poultry*

Howes and Forbes (1987b) injected glucagon into the portal vein of cockerels at doses of 5 or 50 µg and found a dose-related depression in food intake during the subsequent 90 min. This effect was prevented by vagotomy (Fig. 5.2) although interpretation of the results was somewhat clouded by the fact that control levels of feeding at the time of day the experiments were carried out were lower in vagotomized birds than intact birds. The reason for this is probably that vagotomized chickens eat fewer meals and the infusion period happened to include fewer meals after vagotomy.

The accumulated evidence is thus for a meal-induced rise in pancreatic glucagon secretion to cause glycogenolysis in the liver and activation of a vagal pathway to the brain.

### Growth hormone

Vasilatos and Wangsness (1980) collected blood samples from the jugular vein of lactating cows at frequent intervals and showed that the concentration of growth hormone (GH) tended to fall during spontaneous meals. In the sheep spontaneous meals of a highly digestible food were preceded by peaks of GH in plasma, as shown in Fig. 5.3 (Driver and Forbes, 1981). GH secretion is a sensitive index of nutritional status and this suggests that the premeal peak is an indication of the need to replenish body stores, rather than a direct cause of eating. Injection of growth hormone to mimic spontaneous peaks has no effect on feeding behaviour (P.M. Driver and J.M. Forbes, unpublished results) so that the release of growth hormone from the anterior pituitary (under the control of the hypothalamus) and the onset of feeding seem to be independent consequences of a relative shortfall in nutrient supply from the digestive tract. Tindal *et al.* (1978) failed to find similar synchrony of GH secretion and spontaneous meals in goats.

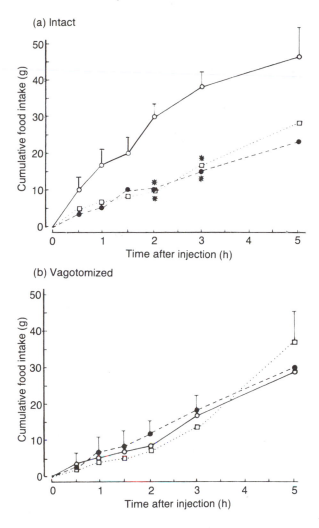

**Fig. 5.2.** Effect of vagotomy on the feeding response of chickens to 0 (○), 5 (●) or 50 (□) μg glucagon injected into the liver (Howes and Forbes, 1987a). ∗, significantly different from zero dose (P<0.05).

## Adrenaline

Eating stimulates the sympathetic and parasympathetic branches of the autonomic nervous system causing the release of adrenaline from both the adrenal medulla and the sympathetic nerve endings in the liver (Steffens *et al.*, 1986) which, in addition to causing the insulin spurt referred to earlier, might contribute to satiety via actions on the liver. α- and β-receptor blockers prevented the intake-depressing effects of

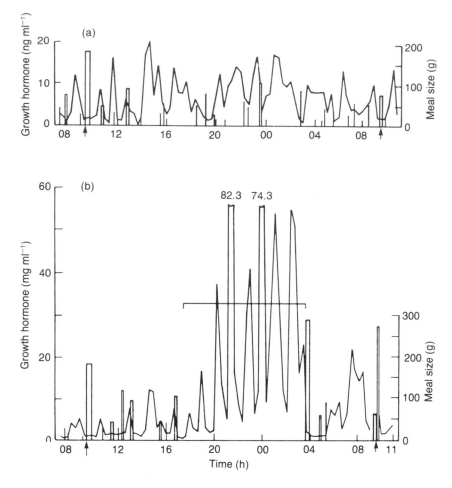

**Fig. 5.3.** Plasma growth hormone concentrations and meal sizes during 27 h periods in a sheep: (a) with free access to food throughout; (b) food removed from 1730 to 1330h (Driver and Forbes, 1981).

exogenous adrenaline (Langhans *et al.*, 1985c) but there were no effects on spontaneous feeding. The intake-depressing effects of adrenaline infused into the hepatic portal vein of the rat are blocked by abdominal vagotomy, but not by hepatic vagotomy (Tordoff and Novin, 1982) showing that it is not principally the liver which is mediating the intake-depressing effects of adrenaline. Adrenaline led to abnormal behaviour, including the termination of feeding, whereas injections of glucagon caused apparently normal satiety (Hinton *et al.*, 1987).

It can be concluded that the status of peripheral catecholamines as regulators of feeding behaviour in response to metabolic signals is uncertain.

*Poultry*

Intramuscular injection of adrenaline at doses of 0.2–1.0 mg per bird caused hypophagia for several hours (Sykes, 1983). This inhibition of feeding was not overcome by prior starvation for 24 h but pretreatment with 1.5 mg phentolamine or 0.4 mg propranolol (α-adrenergic antagonists) completely blocked this effect.

Injection of up to 2500 μg adrenaline into the hepatic portal vein of cockerels depressed intake in a dose-related manner, but the effect of the highest dose was not attenuated by vagotomy at the level of the proventriculus (Howes and Forbes, 1987a). Phenylephrine, a pure α-blocker, given intraportally at doses of up to 3000 μg had no effect on food intake whereas the β-blocker, salbutamol, gave a dose-related depression, whether or not the vagus nerves were intact. The biological significance of these results is in doubt, however, as the doses used are likely to be well above the physiological range.

*Sheep*

When adult sheep were infused with noradrenaline intravenously for 40 h at a rate sufficient to cause a large elevation in plasma free fatty acids, a reduction in the intake of straw and a halving of plasma GH concentration were observed suggesting either that noradrenaline is satiating or, more likely, that the increased availability of free fatty acids reduced the need for nutrients and thus the secretion of GH.

# Gut Peptides

The secretion of several gut hormones is increased during feeding and subsequently as digesta passes through the stomach and duodenum. Of these, CCK is perhaps the most studied as a satiety signal, but others, such as bombesin and gastrin are also likely to be involved (Rayner, 1992; Read, 1992).

CCK is produced principally in the duodenum. If its secretion in response to the presence of food is important in the control of intake then nutrients infused into the duodenum should be more satiating than when infused lower in the small intestine. Glick (1979) found no difference in the satiating effects of glucose solutions, saline or liquid food infused into these two sites and concluded that CCK is not necessary for normal responses to the presence of chyme in the intestines. However, strong evidence that endogenous CCK is important in the limitation of feeding has been provided by autoimmunization of rats to CCK which increases food intake and weight gain (McLaughlin *et al.*, 1985) and by the conditioning of a flavour preference to CCK with very low dose (Perez and Scalfani, 1991); higher doses condition an aversion.

The receptors for CCK which are involved in the feeding response were initially assumed to be in the brain, but Smith *et al.* (1981) have shown that there are also receptors in the stomach as gastric vagotomy prevents the effects of exogenous CCK on intake.

After feeding rats typically display a sequence of behaviour starting with exploring and grooming and continuing with resting or sleeping. This sequence is seen following CCK-induced termination of feeding (Antin *et al.*, 1975) and after the ingestion of glucose solutions (Kushner and Mook, 1984).

The major effect of peripheral injection is probably on the digestive tract, stimulated to contract and thereby activate mechanoreceptors whose information is relayed to the CNS via the vagus nerves. The effect of injection into the brain is direct and the effect on feeding is probably independent of that on the gastrointestinal tract (Chapter 6).

## Poultry

Intravenous injection of CCK in chickens reduced food intake (Savory and Gentle, 1980), depressed gizzard motility and stimulated muscular activity in the duodenum (Savory *et al.*, 1981). In later experiments it was found that intravenous infusion of CCK had less effect in birds offered diluted food and it was suggested that CCK may induce gastrointestinal responses which lead to abdominal discomfort; these are reduced when the motivation to feed is higher (Savory and Gentle, 1984). Savory (1987) used conditioning tests to demonstrate that bombesin or CCK-8 at $1–10\ \mu g\ kg^{-1}$ was mildly aversive, increased heart rate and induced abnormal gastrointestinal motility. CCK was less effective when arousal was reduced with reserpine, when the birds were very hungry or when their attention was distracted, all these points being used to support the contention that CCK acts by inducing abdominal discomfort rather than normal satiety.

Covasa and Forbes (1994a) confirmed the effects of CCK in broiler chickens by intraperitoneal injection and demonstrated a learned aversion to the colour of food offered for 2 h after injections of CCK $(14\ \mu g\ kg^{-1})$ compared to saline. Vagotomy at the level of the proventriculus (equivalent to subdiaphragmatic vagotomy in the mammal) prevented the effect of CCK on feeding and the learned aversion to

CCK-paired coloured food. A very low dose of CCK ($2\,\mu g\;kg^{-1}$) had no significant effect on feeding and did not elicit a preference for the colour paired with the injection, in contrast to the results with rats referred to above (Perez and Sclafani, 1991).

The CCK-blocker MK-329, at doses of $9\,\mu g\;kg^{-1}$ or above, significantly increased food intake in the next 2 h whereas when given intravenously somewhat lower doses were effective (Covasa and Forbes, 1994b). Doses of 8.0, 16.0 and 32.0 mg $kg^{-1}$ of MK-329 did not affect food intake and failed to condition a preference or aversion for the colour of food given for 2 h after the injection. CCK ($14\;mg\;kg^{-1}$) caused a reduction in feeding but this effect was not blocked by pretreatment with intraperitoneal injection of MK-329 (32, 90, 180 and 360 mg $kg^{-1}$) thus questioning the role of endogenous CCK in satiety, in chickens. A logical next step is to see whether MK-329 still stimulates intake when given intraperitoneally in vagotomized birds.

## Pigs

CCK is thought either to constrict the pylorus, reducing stomach emptying, or to increase the sensitivity of vagal afferent receptors. CCK given into the jugular vein of pigs at a rate sufficient to depress food intake by 25% did not affect gastric emptying, suggesting that an effect on stomach motility is not necessary for CCK to exert at least some of its effect on feeding. This is confirmed by the observation that MK-329 reverses the depression of intake caused by fat infusion but does not reverse the effect on gastric emptying (Rayner *et al.*, 1991). MK-329 increases intake in operant-fed pigs (Ebenezer *et al.*, 1990) and also in pigs given a single meal after an overnight fast (Rayner *et al.*, 1991). Another CCK antagonist (L-364,718) blocked the inhibition of food intake induced by jugular or abdominal aorta infusion of CCK or duodenal infusion of emulsified fat or monoglyceride whereas the responses to duodenal glucose, glycerol or oleic acid were not blocked.

Feeding in the pig is depressed by infusion of CCK into the general circulation but not into the hepatic portal vein or gastric artery. Probably, CCK is most active in the upper intestine as it was most effective when given into the mesenteric circulation going to this part of the intestine (Houpt, 1983b). It was concluded that the site of action was in the intestines but it is not yet known whether this is dependent on vagal innervation (Houpt, 1983b). The fact that duodenal infusion of phenylalanine or tryptophan in pigs increased plasma concentrations of CCK, but did not affect feeding (Rayner and Gregory, 1985) casts further doubt on the role of CCK as a true hormone of satiety.

However, pigs immunized against CCK increased their intake by 8.2% and their growth by 10.6% (Pekas and Trout, 1993), strong support for a physiological role for CCK in the control of food intake.

Baldwin *et al.* (1983a) have suggested that exogenous CCK causes a general malaise in the pig. They trained pigs by operant conditioning to respond for food, water, sucrose solution or heat. Doses of 20 or 40 units of CCK octapeptide given intravenously transiently reduced responding for food, water or sucrose but had no effect on responses for heat. These results show that CCK affects several types of behaviour and is thus unlikely to be a specific food satiety factor. However, the CCK receptor antagonist MK-329 caused a dose-related increase in food intake during two hours after intravenous injection and MK-329 also abolished the intake depression caused by CCK (Ebenezer *et al.*, 1990).

It is likely that the doses of exogenous CCK mostly used have been above physiological levels and have caused malaise but the recent work with low doses of exogenous CCK, with antagonistic drugs and with immunization against CCK provides very strong evidence for a role for CCK in normal satiety.

In ruminants and chickens there are delays between eating and the arrival of food at the CCK-producing sites. Thus, CCK might be less important in these types of animal than in those such as the pig in which the simple stomach releases digesta into the duodenum as soon as a meal starts.

*Ruminants*

Grovum (1981) infused CCK into several blood vessels in sheep and found that there was no greater effect on food intake when infusion was into the carotid artery or portal vein than when it was into the jugular vein. He concluded that neither the brain nor the liver was involved in the reduction of food intake in response to CCK. The main effect is probably on the digestive tract. However, the flow of digesta through the duodenum is relatively constant in free-feeding ruminants and Furuse *et al.* (1991) found no significant fluctuations in plasma levels of CCK in cows either with concentrate or roughage feeding. Without such meal-related fluctuations it is difficult to see how CCK can be involved in the control of feeding.

## Other Gut Hormones

Pentagastrin depressed food intake of sheep whether given into the jugular vein (Grovum *et al.*, 1974) or portal vein (Anil and Forbes, 1980b) whereas secretin had no effect by either route.

Two other gut peptides, somatostatin and bombesin, also depress food intake and the former has many properties which make it a possible satiety hormone (McCoy and Avery, 1990). The effect of somatostatin is blocked by gastric vagotomy but that of bombesin is not (Baile *et al.*, 1983).

## Other Hormones

### Vasopressin

Vasopressin (0.75–3 µg kg$^{-1}$) given by intraperitoneal injection reduced food intake by goats in a dose-dependent manner (Meyer *et al.*, 1989). This effect was reversed by a $V_1$-receptor antagonist or an α-adrenergic antagonist. The vasopressin concentrations achieved in plasma as a result of the injections were similar to those seen during stress and it was suggested that this hormone might be involved in stress-induced anorexia.

### Endorphins

It has been suggested that endorphins are involved in the control of food intake (Margules, 1979) but it is unlikely that circulating β-endorphin is a controller of food intake (Wallace *et al.*, 1981). There is not yet enough information on the rates of secretion of these hormones, and whether they change with feeding state, to allow judgement on their roles in feeding control.

### Satietin

Satietin is a glycoprotein, found in the serum of many species, including avian and ungulate (Bellinger and Mendel, 1988), which has been proposed as a negative feedback signal from gut to brain. Repeated injections into the cerebroventricles depressed body weight but tolerance eventually developed, casting doubts as to whether satietin has a physiological role in the control of feeding.

## Hormones Involved in Reproduction and Growth

These are discussed in Chapters 8 and 9.

# Conclusions

This chapter cannot claim to do justice to the complex subject of the roles of metabolites and hormones in the control of voluntary food intake. Although the glucostatic theory in the form originally proposed by Mayer (1953) is no longer tenable, it is clear that animals can monitor the availability of energy-yielding materials and use this information to control their food intake. Because glucose is the major energy-yielding substrate in most non-ruminants its infusion causes a reduction in food intake, especially when given into the liver (Chapter 3).

Fats and proteins can also yield energy and therefore affect the energostatic control of intake in situations where they are oxidized. This utilization is influenced by metabolic hormones and the effect of metabolites is modified according to the insulin and glucagon status of the animal.

Most hormones, when given in large amounts, affect food intake but it is often difficult to decide whether they are acting directly on the CNS or peripherally and whether they are important under normal, physiological conditions. This is true for the gut peptides such as CCK, which act at both sites and whose natural sites and rates of secretion are difficult to mimic experimentally.

# 6 | CENTRAL NERVOUS CONTROL

- Lesioning studies
- Electrical stimulation
- Chemical stimulation
- Thermostatic control
- CNS sensitivity to metabolites and hormones
- Possibilities of pharmacological manipulation of food intake
- Conclusions

The central nervous system (CNS) is clearly the integrator of most of the actions of the animal and as such plays a vital role in the control of voluntary food intake as well as growth, fattening and reproduction. It is axiomatic that information from receptors in other parts of the body, including the special senses, is relayed to the brain which integrates this with what it has previously learned about the consequences of feeding and makes decisions whether or not to seek and eat food.

The centres in the brain which are involved in feeding control were originally thought to be in the hypothalamus, a region with a volume of about 0.5 cm$^3$ in the sheep, lying just above the pituitary gland and optic chiasma at the base of the brain (Fig. 6.1). These centres have been associated with the glucostatic, thermostatic and lipostatic theories of control of feeding (Chapter 1). The ventromedial hypothalamus (VMH) is important in the control of anterior pituitary function as well as food intake, while the lateral hypothalamic area (LHA), being a part of the medial forebrain bundle, receives information both from the visceral receptors and from higher centres of the brain.

Early studies used lesioning techniques to destroy small parts of the brain followed by observation of changes in behaviour following recovery from the anaesthetic. Subsequently the effects of electrical

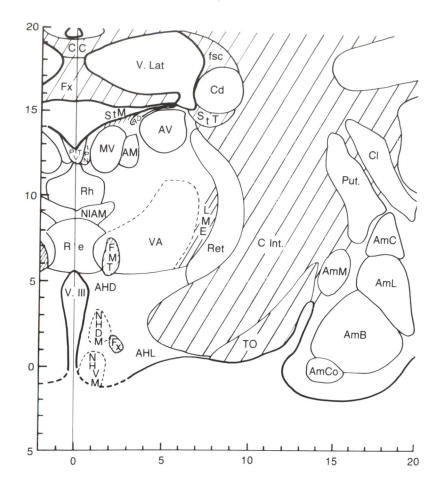

**Fig. 6.1.** Cross-section through the lower forebrain of the sheep (scale in mm). AHD, dorsal hypothalamic area – paraventicular nucleus lies between this and the third ventricle; AHL, lateral hypothalamic area; Fx, fornix; NHDM, dorsomedial hypothalamic nucleus; NHVM, ventromedial hypothalamic nucleus; TO, optic tract; V. Lat., lateral ventricle; V. III, third ventricle. (From Richard, 1967, reproduced with permission.)

stimulation were studied and more recently effort has been concentrated on the neurochemistry of intake control using techniques such as injection of drugs which mimic or block the effects of the naturally occurring brain chemicals. It is now accepted that feeding is organized by circuits and networks of neurons rather than by discrete 'centres' but the full picture is far from being complete.

The involvement of the brain in the control of food intake with particular respect to poultry is reviewed by Denbow (1985, 1989), whereas Forbes and Blundell (1989) have covered the subject for pigs and Baile and McLaughlin (1987) for ruminants.

## Lesioning Studies

The first evidence of a particular locus for feeding within the brain was based on hypothalamic tumours found in obese humans in the late 19th century. Then, in the early 1940s, it was found that abnormalities of feeding and/or body weight occurred when discrete electrolytic lesions were made in the medial and lateral hypothalamus of the cat. Further studies in the 1940s and 1950s confirmed that lesions of the VMH led to obesity and hyperphagia in the rat, and this area became known as the 'satiety centre'.

Lesions of the LHA, on the other hand, caused aphagia and death although rats kept alive by force-feeding did resume spontaneous feeding and survived, albeit at a lower body weight than normal; this area became known as the 'hunger centre'.

### Poultry

The VMH appears to be important in birds and lesions in this area have been reported to induce overeating and obesity (Wright, 1976). VMH lesions caused obesity in ducks (Hawkes and George, 1975) and geese (Felix *et al.*, 1980). The latter has been suggested as an alternative to force-feeding in order to get fatty livers for preparation of pâté de foie gras (Fig. 6.2).

However, the increased fatness of VMH-lesioned chickens in the study by Lepkovsky and Yasuda (1966) was not accompanied by hyperphagia (Sykes, 1983). Even the comprehensive work of Snapir *et al.* (1973a) does not include convincing evidence as to the exact site of obesity-inducing lesions neither does more recent work by the same group (Robinzon *et al.*, 1982).

Lesions of the hypothalamus in adult cockerels of an egg-laying strain caused a variable increase in fat deposition which was related to increased food intake (Lepkovsky and Yasuda, 1966). Not only do such lesions stimulate intake, they also increase fat synthesis (probably by depressing the secretion of growth hormone) and concentrations of fat in the liver so that these results do not help to unravel the causality of the relationship between fatness and intake. Snapir and Robinzon (1989) showed that lesions of the basomedial hypothalamus in chickens induce many changes, including hyperphagia, but that an increase of lipoprotein lipase activity preceded the increase in intake, suggesting

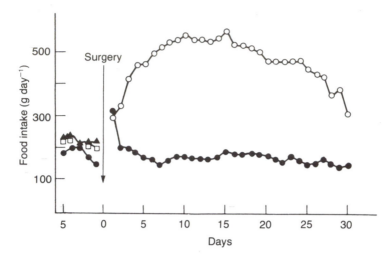

**Fig. 6.2.** Effect of electrolytic lesions in the ventromedial hypothalamus of geese. ●, controls; ○, lesioned. (From Auffray and Blum, 1970, reproduced with permission.)

that the hyperphagia was a response to altered fat metabolism rather than a primary effect of the lesions.

In a detailed review of nerve tracts involved in food intake control in birds, Kuenzel (1989) describes mechanoreceptors in the bill/beak which are innervated by the trigeminal nerve. However, lesions of the quintofrontal tract (the destination of the trigeminal nerve) in chicks only affect feeding for a few days, in contrast to the pigeon, which cannot recognize food for several weeks. Lesions involving the optic system cause several feeding problems, whereas olfaction was not so important. However, Robinzon *et al.* (1977) showed that removal of the olfactory bulbs caused an increase in food intake, but without obesity as metabolic rate was increased. Further evidence that obesity and hyperphagia are not always linked came from observations (Robinzon *et al.*, 1978) that septal lesioned cockerels overate but did not become obese.

Lesions placed in the mid-lateral hypothalamic region (equivalent to the 'hunger centre' of mammals) induced hypophagia and loss of weight in only a small proportion of individuals (Smith, 1969). Careful work by Kuenzel (1982), involving bilateral lesions in the LHA of the chick, showed hypophagia for only a few days; more posterior lesions gave more persistent effects.

Gold thioglucose, which causes hypothalamic lesions and hyperphagia in mice, had no effect in chickens whether given systemically (Gentle, 1976) or implanted directly into the hypothalamus (Smith and Szper, 1976).

Removal of the pineal gland from the brain of day-old chicks stimulates subsequent voluntary intake and weight gains (Injidi and Forbes, 1983; Chapter 15). However, Darre *et al.* (1978) did not find any effect of pinealectomy on subsequent food consumption when the operation was carried out at nine days of age.

*Pigs*

VMH lesions in pigs caused hyperphagia (Auffray, 1969; Khalaf and Robinson, 1972b). The latter study also showed that LHA lesions induced aphagia with no signs of recovery when the animals were kept alive by force-feeding. Lesions in the VMH of young pigs (5–6 weeks old) did not immediately induce hyperphagia although other metabolic effects were seen (Baldwin, 1985). This is similar to young rats where hyperphagia and fatness only occur after the infantile stage has been passed, both in VMH lesioned and genetically obese animals.

*Sheep and goats*

Holmes and Fraser (1965) and Tarttellin (1969) made small VMH lesions in sheep and saw no change in food intake. However, they may not have destroyed a large enough portion of the critical area because Baile *et al.* (1969), making larger lesions which destroyed the whole ventromedial part of the hypothalamus of goats, did observe overeating and excessive fatness.

Baile *et al.* (1968) and Tarttellin (1969) also made electrolytic lesions in the LHA of goats and sheep, respectively, which showed hypophagia, but not aphagia or death.

# Electrical Stimulation

Lesioning is obviously a clumsy technique and more sophisticated methods of studying brain function have been used since the original lesioning studies. Information is transmitted along nerve fibres electrically and between nerves by chemical transmitters and both electrical and chemical stimulation have been used experimentally.

*Poultry*

Although several species of bird have been tested for feeding responses to electrical stimulation, very few such responses have been obtained, even when the site of stimulation was the lateral hypothalamus (chicken, Tweeton *et al.*, 1973).

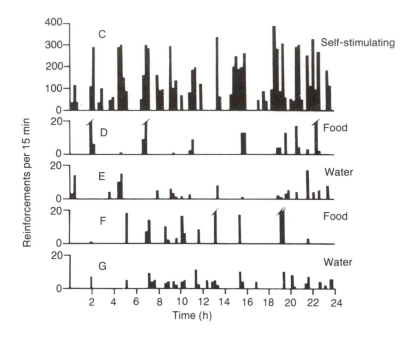

**Fig. 6.3.** Records of self-stimulation in the lateral hypothalmus, and responding for food and water in a pig. C, D, E, a 24 h period when the pig could self-stimulate, and respond for food and water; F, G, a 24 h period when the pig could respond for food and water but not self-stimulate. (From Baldwin and Parrott, 1979, reproduced with permission.)

*Pigs*

The only electrical stimulation which appears to have been done in the pig has been self-stimulation in which animals, aged 10–16 weeks, were trained to press a panel to stimulate the hypothalamus in addition to panels to obtain food and water (Baldwin and Parrott, 1979). After a 22 h fast there was a high rate of self-stimulation, compared to the rate after eating to satiation, in two out of four pigs, both of which had the electrodes in the lateral hypothalamus. Of six other animals tested on five consecutive days, four decreased their food and water intake when self-stimulation was available (Fig. 6.3), suggesting that the intake of food and/or water is pleasurable; these four had electrodes in the lateral hypothalamus whereas the other two were in other regions of the brain. The pigs did not starve themselves in favour of self-stimulation, however, indicating that there are more inputs to feeding control than simply the pleasure of eating.

*Sheep and goats*

Stimulation of the lateral hypothalamus for 60 s caused satiated sheep and goats to start eating again and to continue eating voraciously as long as the stimulus was applied (Larsson, 1954). Similar results were obtained by Baile *et al.* (1967) whereas stimulation of the ventromedial nucleus of goats reduced feeding activity (Wyrwicka and Dobrzecka, 1960).

# Chemical Stimulation

Although transmission of signals along nerves is primarily electrical, interneuronal communication is mainly chemical. Neurotransmitters, such as noradrenaline and acetylcholine, are released by the terminals of one nerve and stimulate the receptors on one or several other neurons which respond by an increase or decrease of firing rate. There is more scope for both physiological and pharmacological mechanisms to work at the synapse than along the nerve fibre and in recent years chemical stimulation of the brain has been used as the major experimental technique. The development of pharmacological antagonists to neural transmitters has also provided useful tools for the investigation of brain function.

Methods of introducing drugs into the brain include injection via cannulae implanted in the lateral ventricle, micro-injection via fine cannulae implanted or advanced through guides into brain tissue and by electrophoretic introduction (Myers, 1971). Invariably drugs must be injected in amounts which are greater than the amount normally present in brain tissue in order to cause a significant response, and the question arises as to whether results can be considered to be 'physiological'. Despite such methodological problems, it seems likely that substances in the extracellular fluid of the brain are involved with the physiological control of feeding. Martin *et al.* (1973) transferred 1 ml of cerebrospinal fluid (CSF) from fasted sheep into the lateral ventricle of recipients and found a fivefold increase in food intake during the following 15 min; CSF from satiated sheep had no effect.

*Anaesthetics*

By preventing neural transmission through affected parts of the brain, local anaesthetics are expected to have similar effects on feeding to lesions in the same areas. In general, this has proved to be the case.

Pentobarbital (a local anaesthetic) injected into the third ventricle of chickens caused intake to increase from 14 to 32 g during the hour after injection even though the birds were almost asleep; there was no effect when the injections were made into the posterior lateral hypothalamus (Snapir *et al.*, 1973b). Pentobarbital given into the basomedial hypothalamus resulted in increased feeding (Snapir and Robinzon, 1989).

A dose of 6.5 mg of sodium pentobarbital given into the LHA depressed intake in hungry pigs whereas in the VMH it stimulated intake in satiated animals (Khalaf and Robinson, 1972a). Infusion of pentobarbital into the cerebroventricles of pigs also caused an increase in the weight of food eaten during the following 30 min (Baldwin *et al.*, 1975).

Cerebroventricular injections of pentobarbital stimulated feeding in calves (Peterson *et al.*, 1972).

Similar observations were made with goats (Baile and Mayer, 1966) and sheep (Peterson *et al.*, 1972). More detailed studies with sheep, in which a range of barbiturates with different durations of action were compared, showed that long-acting ones were more effective than those with a short action in inducing feeding when injected into the third ventricle (Seoane and Baile, 1973). The effects of barbiturates were similar in a hot environment and at normal temperatures, and with high roughage and high concentrate rations (Beyea *et al.*, 1975). Micro-injection of barbiturates into the medial hypothalamus also stimulated feeding in sheep (Baile *et al.*, 1974a).

## Adrenergic agents

Substances such as anaesthetics are, of course, unnatural and a manipulation of the concentrations of substances found naturally in the brain have formed the basis of most recent work.

Since the original work with rats there has been ample confirmation of a major place for adrenergic transmitters in the control of intake and numerous experiments have demonstrated that noradrenaline given into the medial hypothalamus stimulates intake in several species, including farm animals. This effect can be prevented by prior injection of the appropriate blocker but blockers given alone do not stimulate feeding. Although work originally concentrated on the VMH and LHA, the detailed work of Leibowitz and colleagues (e.g. Leibowitz *et al.*, 1985) has identified the paraventricular nucleus (PVN) as the most sensitive site mediating the actions of adrenergic agonists on eating (Forbes and Blundell, 1989). It seems likely that the PVN and its $\alpha_2$-adrenergic receptors are important in the control of eating in response to deprivation and, possibly, to postingestional satiety signals.

Brain turnover of noradrenaline was increased by glucoprivation

(Bellin and Ritter, 1981b), a situation that could be reversed by providing substrates, either by ingestion or infusion, which could be used by the brain. This is evidence for a physiological role for noradrenaline in the control of feeding.

## Poultry

Denbow *et al.* (1982) reported that cerebroventricular injections of adrenaline or noradrenaline increased food intake in broiler-type chickens, whereas dopamine had no effect. However, the injection of adrenaline had no effect in birds of a layer strain. A differential response was also noted in response to cerebroventricular injections of 5-hydroxytryptamine (5-HT) which, in broilers, depressed food intake in fully fed birds but not in 24 h-fasted birds (Denbow *et al.*, 1983) whereas in layers 5-HT decreased food intake in both fully fed and 24 h-fasted birds.

Further studies by Denbow *et al.* (1986) with lines of broilers selected for fast and slow growth, showed that methoxamine (an α–adrenergic agonist) increased feeding in the fast- but not the slow-growing strain whereas 5-HT had no effect in fully fed birds but did depress intake in 24 h-fasted birds of both lines. Genetic selection for growth has been demonstrated to alter the meal pattern as well as alter the feeding response to intubations of amino acids and cerebroventricular injections of biogenic amines. Further studies are required to explore the mechanisms of these differences between breeds and strains.

Injection of 6-hydroxydopamine, which depletes noradrenaline, into the cerbroventricles (Auffray and Gallouin, 1971) or hypothalamus (Snapir *et al.*, 1976) not only increased food intake but also caused obesity and testicular atrophy in geese.

Fenfluramine is a well-known appetite suppressant in mammals and when incorporated in food it induced a dose-dependent reduction in food intake by broiler chickens (Hocking and Bernard, 1993).

## Pigs

In the pig noradrenaline injected into the hypothalamus stimulated feeding (Jackson and Robinson, 1971) whereas isoproterenol (a synthetic β-adrenergic agonist) caused temporary anorexia, which was blocked by propranolol (a synthetic β-adrenergic antagonist). The volume injected was large, however, so these results tell us little about the exact site of action.

*Cattle*

Lateral ventricular injection of noradrenaline in cattle depressed voluntary intake over a very narrow range of doses (50–200 nmol) whereas isoproterenol was effective over a broad range (500–2000 nmol) (Baile *et al.*, 1972).

*Sheep*

Baile and his colleagues have been particularly active in this field (see Baile, 1975). They found that intraventricular injection of noradrenaline at doses of 542 nmol induced hyperphagia for some 30 min after injection. The effect was blocked by prior injection of α-adrenergic blockers and it was later confirmed that intrahypothalamic injections had similar effects (Simpson *et al.*, 1975). At very low doses (4–16 nmol) the β-adrenergic agonist isoproterenol stimulated intake for about one hour and this was blocked by β- but not α-adrenergic antagonists. This suggests the existence of two classes of adrenergic receptors and adrenaline, which has both α- and β-adrenergic activity, stimulated intake at two dose ranges, presumably corresponding to optimum stimulation of the two types of receptor (Baile *et al.*, 1972). No increase

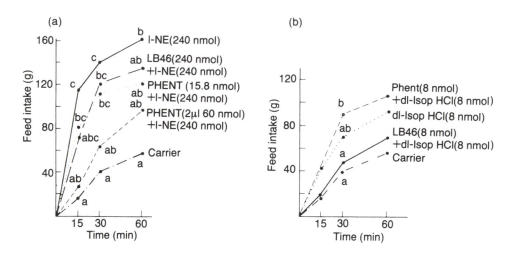

**Fig. 6.4.** Cumulative food intake of a pelleted food by sheep after intrahypothalamic injection of: noradrenaline (1-NE) alone or preceded by α- (phentolamine, PHENT) or β-adrenergic (LB46) blockers; and of isoproterenol (Isop) alone or preceded by α- or β-adrenergic blockers. At any time, means with the same superscript did not differ significantly. (From Baile *et al.*, 1974b, reproduced with permission.)

in voluntary intake was recorded in sheep injected with 593 or 1186 nmol of noradrenaline into the lateral ventricle (Driver *et al.*, 1979), perhaps because the overall level of feeding was much higher than in Baile's sheep.

A major drawback to ventricular injection is that the site of action cannot be determined because CSF secreted in the lateral ventricles transports the injected material through several parts of the brain. More precise injection can be achieved by implanting guides through the cranium which are directed towards certain loci in the brain. Using sheep prepared in this way it was shown that noradrenaline (240 nmol) and isoproterenol (8 nmol) had similar effects on feeding when given into hypothalamic tissue as they did when given intraventricularly (Baile *et al.*, 1974b). Again, effects of each were blocked by the appropriate blocking agent (Fig. 6.4) and the dose–response curve showed an optimum range with depression at high doses.

A brain locus sensitive to noradrenaline was not usually responsive to isoproterenol, and prostaglandins (PG) injected at loci which were sensitive to noradrenaline had different effects on feeding than at loci which were sensitive to isoproterenol (Baile and Martin, 1973; Baile *et al.*, 1974c). $PGE_1$ (14 or 28 nmol) depressed food intake when injected at loci that showed feeding in response to noradrenaline. A PG antagonist, polyphloretin phosphate, not only blocked the effects of subsequent PG injection but by itself significantly increased intake. Whether this means that $PGE_1$ normally inhibits feeding is not clear. At sites which responded to isoproterenol, $PGE_1$ significantly stimulated intake (Baile and Martin, 1973). This subject is complex and will not be properly understood until the full range of pharmacological and metabolic effects of these substances is known.

Duquette and Muir (1979) gave intramuscularly into lambs MK940, a drug which blocks noradrenaline re-uptake in the brain, and found a significant reduction in intake of a complete pelleted food due to a reduction in meal size.

## Serotonin (5-hydroxytryptamine, 5-HT)

In the mammalian CNS, 5-HT systems occupy a strategic anatomical location, projecting to, and passing through the hypothalamus. Experimental manipulations of 5-HT metabolism can, under certain conditions, produce marked changes in food intake, food preferences, and body weight, most obviously the suppression of food intake by experimental treatments that directly or indirectly activate 5-HT receptors. More controversial is the role of 5-HT in diet selection (Chapter 14).

5-HT binds to several distinct receptor types in peripheral tissues but although the significance of these receptor types in the CNS is uncertain, there is evidence linking them with effects on eating (Forbes and Blundell, 1989).

In chickens of an egg-laying strain 33–100 µg 5-HT injected intra-ventricularly depressed intake (Denbow *et al.*, 1983) whereas in broilers it had this effect only if the birds were satiated (Denbow *et al.*, 1982).

In sheep, 5-HT has smaller effects on feeding than noradrenaline and at fewer sites, the responsive ones being concentrated in the area of the anterior commissure (Baile *et al.*, 1979a).

## Dopamine

As is the case for noradrenaline, most information about brain dopamine and appetite arises from experiments on rats, from the results of which dopamine could be said to perform a 'permissive' rather than a central function in feeding (Blundell, 1988).

## Cholinergic agents

Acetylcholine is a neural transmitter which is found in significant amounts in the hypothalamus. In the rat, ventricular or hypothalamic injection of carbachol, a slowly metabolized cholinergic agonist, causes an increase in water intake but a consistent and large depression in food intake.

Carbachol injected into the hypothalamus at doses as low as 7 nmol stimulated feeding for 30–60 min (Forbes and Baile, 1974). When atropine, a cholinergic antagonist, was injected a few minutes before a 28 nmol dose of carbachol, the hyperphagia was prevented. Adrenergic antagonists did not attenuate the carbachol effect, showing that it was acting on cholinergic receptors in the hypothalamus rather than causing non-specific stimulation. However, atropine alone had no effect on intake which implies that endogenous acetylcholine is not involved in feeding control.

Baile and Martin (1974) showed that significantly increased feeding followed the injection of 50 nmol of carbachol into the lateral ventricle. However, in another experiment 56 or 109 nmol of carbachol given into the lateral ventricle of sheep almost totally prevented feeding for an hour, accompanied by significantly elevated plasma levels of growth hormone (Driver *et al.*, 1979); further research by Driver and Forbes (1982) confirmed that, under their conditions, 436 nmol carbachol caused inhibition of food intake and the discrepancy between the two sets of results cannot yet be elucidated.

It is unlikely that the carbachol-induced stimulation of growth hormone secretion directly caused the reduction in food intake because intrajugular growth hormone infusion to mimic peaks of this type had no effect on feeding behaviour in sheep (P.M. Driver and J.M. Forbes, unpublished results). It is equally unlikely that the low food intake following carbachol injection would give such a rapid response in growth hormone secretion; feeding and GH were probably affected independently by carbachol.

## Cyclic AMP

cAMP mediates the central actions of noradrenaline and dopamine and might thus be expected to influence food intake.

Within 60 s of giving cAMP at a dose of 50 nmol into the cerebroventricles of chickens there was head-shaking and preening lasting for 7–120 min (Mench *et al.*, 1986). With higher doses responses were more exaggerated and less coordinated, similar to the effects of electrical stimulation of the brain in chickens in that feeding was reduced but drinking increased.

## Gamma-aminobutyric acid (GABA)

Muscimol, the GABA-A receptor agonist, increased operant intake in pigs after injection into the lateral ventricles, an effect that was completely abolished by simultaneous administration of bicuculine, a GABA antagonist (Baldwin *et al.*, 1990). GABA itself at 800 and 1600 nmol increased intake and this was also abolished by bicuculine.

Seoane *et al.* (1988) also found that ventricular muscimol stimulated feeding in sheep and this was prevented by the GABA antagonist, γ-vinyl GABA; GABA itself, however, had little effect on feeding.

## Glutamine

Glutamine is important in brain development. If injected into the left cerebral hemisphere of chicks they do not subsequently select cereal grains from among pebbles (Rogers, 1986). The right eye is important in feeding, whereas the left eye is involved in responses to novelty. If the left eye is occluded, chicks can still differentiate between grain and pebbles, but not if the right eye is covered.

## Cholecystokinin (CCK)

CCK was first implicated in the control of feeding following experiments involving peripheral injections (Chapter 5). CCK is found in the brain and reduces food intake when injected intraventricularly. The possibility that CCK is a neurotransmitter involved in a physiological control is discussed by Baile *et al.* (1986).

*Poultry*

Savory and Gentle (1983) injected the cerebral ventricles of chickens with 0.1 and 0.4 µg CCK-8 kg$^{-1}$ (CCK-8 is the active moiety of CCK). This had no effect on gizzard or duodenal motility but caused drowsiness in some birds and reduced intakes by 20 and 31%, respectively, during the next 30 min. Dibutyryl cyclic GMP, a CCK receptor blocker, stimulated intake, supporting a physiological role for CCK. The mean concentrations of CCK-8 in different parts of the brain did not differ between fed birds and those fasted for 24 h (Savory and Gentle, 1983), however, but no measurements of turnover have been reported. Four-week-old broilers injected intracerebroventricularly with 100 and 150 ng of CCK-8 reduced intake for 60 and 105 min (Denbow and Myers, 1982). The fact that smaller amounts of CCK are required to depress intake by a given amount when injected into the brain, compared with peripheral injection, has been used to support the concept that brain CCK receptors are more important than gut CCK receptors, in the control of food intake.

*Pigs*

Parrott and Baldwin (1981) injected CCK octapeptide into the lateral ventricles of prepubertal pigs at doses between 149 and 1192 pmol following a 17 h fast. These doses were thought to be within the physiological range based on concentrations of CCK found in human CSF. They observed a dose-dependent reduction in food intake, cessation of feeding appearing to be similar to normal satiety, with no effect on drinking. Greater doses injected intravenously were without effect, strongly suggesting that the effect on feeding was on central mechanisms. However, Baldwin *et al.* (1983) subsequently suggested that exogenous CCK (given intravenously) causes a general malaise in the pig and thus depresses food intake non-specifically (Chapter 5).

*Sheep*

Infusions of CCK-8 into the lateral ventricles of sheep at 0.01 pmol min$^{-1}$ significantly depressed intake and rumen motility during a 3-h period and was much more effective than a single injection (Della-Fera and Baile, 1980). There was no effect on water intake or body temperature and increasing the time of fasting before the infusion reduced the magnitude of the effect. This experiment offers no proof of a physiological role for CCK in the central nervous control of feeding. However, lateral ventricular infusion of antibodies to CCK, which sequesters the natural CCK in the brain, significantly stimulated voluntary intake for two days (M.A. Della-Fera and C.A. Baile, personal communication); continuous ventricular infusion of dibutyryl cyclic GMP led to a large increase in food intake in the sheep (Della-Fera *et al.*, 1981). These two results both suggest that endogenous CCK in the brain is a natural satiety factor.

## Bombesin

This brain peptide is as effective as CCK in inhibiting feeding when given into the lateral ventricle of sheep (Della-Fera and Baile, 1980b) but in rats there is considerable evidence that it induces abnormal behaviour (Cooper, 1985). Vagotomy blocks the effects of CCK given intravenously, but not those of bombesin. Injected intracerebroventricularly at doses of 1.25–5 μg, bombesin also depressed food intake in the 17 h food-deprived young pig (Parrott and Baldwin, 1982) but the behaviour induced was not typical of normal satiety as the pigs appeared uncomfortable and occasionally vomited. In water-deprived pigs bombesin also inhibited drinking, showing that it, like CCK, was non-specific in its behavioural effects.

## Opioid peptides

It has recently been discovered that many peptides of the opiate family are synthesized in the brain; the existence of brain receptors for these peptides suggests that they have a physiological role. Among other effects the opiates have been found to stimulate feeding in rats and sheep after cerebroventricular injection (Baile *et al.*, 1981). Endogenous opioids might play a role in the regulation of food intake as the opioid antagonist naloxone decreases feeding in rats and in a variety of other species ranging from the slug to the wolf. It is likely that more than one opioid receptor and more than one brain site are involved in the opioid modulation of feeding (see review by Morley and Blundell, 1988).

Resistance to the inhibitory effects of naloxone on feeding occurs when animals are eating large amounts of food per kilogram of body mass and/or have high basal blood glucose concentrations. This strongly suggests that, although opioids play an important role in initiating food-seeking behaviours, they are not the only food-driven system. Much evidence has accumulated suggesting that stress-induced eating is driven by activation of the opioid system. Similarly, the hyperphagia associated with diabetes mellitus appears to have an opioid component.

*Poultry*

A stable analogue of met-enkephalin, D-ala$^2$-methionine enkephalina-
mide, stimulated food intake by pullets for 30 min after 2 and 8 μg kg$^{-1}$
given into the cerebroventricles, but had no effect when given intravenously at 15 and 60 μg kg$^{-1}$ (Savory *et al.*, 1989). Naloxone had no
effect after either cerebroventricular (50 and 200 μg kg$^{-1}$) or intravenous (1 and 4 mg kg$^{-1}$) injection. Nalmefene, a more potent and long-
lasting opioid antagonist than naloxone, inhibited feeding in a
dose-related manner at doses from 0.1 to 1.6 mg. It appears that central
release of endogenous opioids may reinforce feeding in birds.

*Pigs*

There was no effect on feeding of naloxone injected into the lateral
ventricles at doses of 0.4 or 0.8 mg, 10 min after access to food was given
following an overnight fast (Baldwin and Parrott, 1985). This was
attributed to the fact that the pigs were young and had been subjected
to a fast, and were therefore very highly motivated to feed.

More recently, however, Baldwin *et al.* (1990) found that 200 μg of
dynorphin (a natural endorphin) given into the lateral ventricles
resulted in a meal within a few minutes. Leumorphin and α-neo-
endorphin also elicted feeding but β-neo-endorphin did not. Administration after the start of a meal taken after 4 h of deprivation
increased the size of that meal. Naloxone (400 μg) significantly reduced
intake after 4 h of deprivation and abolished the effects of dynorphin.
It was concluded that dynorphin and related endogenous opioids are
involved in the regulation of food intake in pigs.

Feeding seems to induce an opioid-based analgesia as the latency
of tail-flick to a painful stimulus was longer after feeding than before,
and this was abolished by naloxone (Rushen *et al.*, 1990). However, sows
with marked behavioural stereotypies had shorter tail-flick latencies
after feeding.

*Sheep*

Opioid levels are elevated in the brain of sheep after a 4 h fast (Scallett
*et al.*, 1985), at which time the animal would be expected to be hungry,
and intracerebroventricular injection of several opioids stimulates
feeding. Baile *et al.* (1987), reviewing their work on involvement of
opioids in feeding control in sheep, concluded that more specific
agonists are needed before a full elucidation is possible.

Naloxone given intravenously prevents the feeding stimulated by
cerebroventricular injection of enkephalamide (Bueno *et al.*, 1983).

Many times more analogue were required to generate a similar effect on feeding when it was given intravenously compared to into the lateral ventricles, implying that the major site of action is the CNS.

## Calcitonin

Although it is well known that calcitonin is secreted by the thyroid gland and involved in bone accretion, it is also found in the brain and when given intraventricularly to rats in very small amounts (416 pg, Levine and Morley, 1981) it inhibits feeding. The fact that calcitonin levels in blood increase during feeding and that CCK stimulates calcitonin secretion suggests that the latter may be one of a whole complex of peptides which are involved in the control of feeding.

## Neuropeptide Y and peptide YY

The pancreatic polypeptide family consists of pancreatic polypeptide, neuropeptide Y (NPY), and peptide YY (PYY). Very low doses increase feeding when injected directly into the PVN, the magnitude of the increased food intake following NPY injections being much greater than that seen following central administration of opioid peptides or of noradrenaline (Williams *et al.*, 1991).

PYY has been shown to be a more potent stimulator of feeding than is NPY and when PYY is administered every 6 h for 48 h, it causes massive hyperphagia (80.5 g day$^{-1}$ compared to 31.1 g in the control group) and stomach distension, attesting to the fact that central factors can override the physiological satiety signals from the periphery.

## Poultry

NPY immunoreactivity has been found around the area of the PVN in chickens (Keunzel and McMurtry, 1988). Central (lateral ventricle) administration of NPY or PYY significantly stimulates feeding in chicks (Kuenzel *et al.*, 1987), possibly as a result of stimulation of insulin secretion.

## Pigs

In the only reported work with pigs, prepubertal animals were trained on an operant schedule with a fixed ratio of 5 to obtain reinforcements of 12 g of food (Parrott *et al.*, 1986). Between 25 and 100 µg of NPY injected into the lateral ventricles stimulated feeding in a dose-related manner, the highest dose causing a 12-fold increase in the number of reinforcements obtained in the 30 min after injection and reducing the

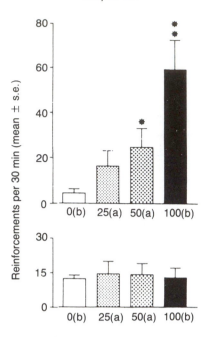

**Fig. 6.5.** Number of reinforcements obtained by pigs during 30 min after intracerebroventricular injection of 0, 25, 50 or 100 µg of NPY. *, $P < 0.05$; **, $P < 0.02$ compared with control. (From Parrott *et al.*, 1986, reproduced with permission.)

latency to feed from 17 min to 1.5 min. Both meal size and duration were increased and there were no aversive effects nor any influence on drinking (Fig. 6.5).

*Sheep*

A 10 µg bolus of NPY into the cerebral ventricles immediately stimulated feeding in sheep (Della-Fera *et al.*, 1990) whereas continuous infusion slowly increased feeding, but the cumulative effect was the same as the bolus injection.

A 3 nmol injection of NPY given intracerebroventricularly increased food intake by up to 150% over the next 30 min (Miner *et al.*, 1990). This was not blocked by an $\alpha_2$-adrenoceptor antagonist which demonstrates that NPY does not work via an $\alpha$-adrenergic pathway.

### Growth hormone releasing factor (GRF, somatoliberin)

GRF (100 ng kg$^{-1}$) given intraventricularly stimulated intake of a concentrate food by about 25% only in the first hour after injection in sheep whereas with hay the stimulation of intake occurred later, from the 2nd to 8th hours (Riviere and Bueno, 1987). With both foods this was by increased rate of eating rather than a change in number of meals. When 10 times this dose was given intravenously (the minimum dose required to stimulate feeding) cerebroventricular administration of insulin (40 mU kg$^{-1}$) blocked the effect. The fact that GRF is effective at a much lower dose when given into the brain rather than peripherally suggests that it is acting centrally and the fact that its effects are blocked by insulin suggests it might be acting via growth hormone secretion, some of the metabolic effects of which are blocked by insulin.

### Steroid hormones

Oestrogen treatment, except at very low levels, depresses food intake (Chapter 9) and oestrogen receptors have been demonstrated in the hypothalamus of the rat. Crystals of oestradiol are effective in causing hypophagia in the rat particularly when implanted in the anterior and ventromedial hypothalamus, compared with other areas of the diencephalon (Wade and Zucker, 1970).

Following the demonstration that oestradiol infused intravenously into sheep and goats depresses intake (Forbes and Rook, 1970), small amounts were injected into the lateral ventricles of sheep (Forbes, 1974). A low dose (10 μg) led to a 60% increase in intake of a complete pelleted

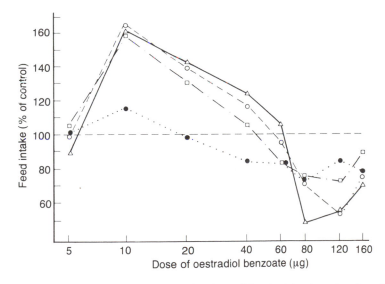

**Fig. 6.6.** Intake of a complete pelleted food by sheep following injection of various doses of oestradiol into the lateral ventricles (Forbes, 1974).

food during the 2-h period after injection, with little effect on daily intake; intake was progressively lower than this maximum as the dose increased and above 60 μg was lower than control (Fig. 6.6). The stimulating effect of 10 or 20 μg was blocked by simultaneous intraventricular injection with 1.25 or 1.88 mg progesterone.

## Ionic changes

The concentrations of several ions in the extracellular fluid are very important in controlling neural function. In laboratory animals it has been shown that ionized calcium salts injected into the cerebroventricles or hypothalamus stimulate feeding and it has been suggested that the calcium/sodium ratio controls body weight (Myers and Veale, 1971).

### Pigs

Baldwin *et al.* (1975) injected 12.5–50 μmol of calcium or magnesium ions into the lateral ventricles and found that food intake was increased by both, in a dose-related manner (Fig. 6.7).

### Sheep and goats

The sheep seems to be especially sensitive to ionic changes in the CSF but even so changes which are large enough to affect feeding are probably beyond the normal range.

Larsson (1954) showed that injection of several solutions, including hypertonic saline, into the lateral hypothalamus induced short-term hyperphagia in sheep and goats. Seoane and Baile (1973) injected solutions into the third ventricle of sheep in order to change the composition of the CSF in the region of the hypothalamus. Calcium increased voluntary intake during the 30 min after injection in a dose-related manner, Magnesium had a similar effect, and both were blocked by increasing concentrations of sodium or potassium. Calcium or magnesium (1 μmol in 1 μl) injected into the hypothalamus also stimulated intake (Seoane *et al.*, 1975) but the loci at which one was active did not necessarily respond to the other. Magnesium stimulation was not blocked by preinjection with several pharmacological blockers whereas the calcium effect was blocked by atropine. The intake-stimulating effect of pentobarbital injected into the ventricles was reduced by sodium chloride (Seoane *et al.*, 1988).

Olsson (1969) found that intraventricular injections of sodium or potassium into goats suppressed feeding whereas slow infusion of similar amounts over 30 min actually elicited feeding. Given that CSF

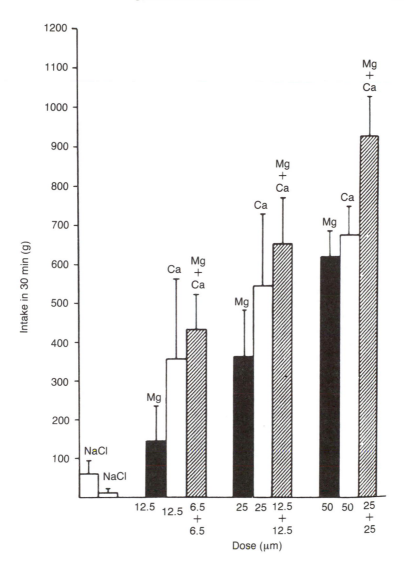

**Fig. 6.7.** Food eaten by growing pigs in the 30 min after injections into the lateral ventricles of calcium, magnesium or both. (From Baldwin *et al.*, 1975, reproduced with permission.)

is produced at around 0.5 ml min$^{-1}$, a slow infusion would result in a very much lower concentration being achieved than a single injection of the same amount and it may be that very low concentrations of these ions are stimulatory.

# Thermostatic Control

Brobeck (1948) said that 'animals eat to keep warm and quit eating to prevent hyperthermia' and as the anterior hypothalamus is the most important temperature sensor in the body it would be expected that heating or cooling of this part of the brain would affect heat loss and/or production.

Local cooling of the preoptic area and anterior hypothalamus stimulated feeding in satiated goats (Andersson and Larsson, 1961). Even if the animal was dehydrated to the point of aphagia, or heated until rectal temperature had risen by 1°C, hypothalamic cooling induced feeding. Warming the same area inhibited feeding and induced drinking; in one goat with lesions in the preoptic area food intake was normal even at body temperatures above 41°C. Although these observations support the thermostatic theory, measurements of hypothalamic temperature during feeding in the goat (Baile and Mayer, 1968b) showed no increase, whether during spontaneous feeding after a 20 h fast or during force-feeding. Infusion of acetate into the rumen, which suppressed feeding, also caused a 0.25°C reduction in hypothalamic temperature, so clearly does not act via a hypothermic mechanism. Although pentobarbital depressed hypothalamic temperature this occurred after the increase in feeding (see above) and was unlikely to be the mediator. Specific heating or cooling of the hypothalamus does not always have the expected effect, however, as no changes in voluntary intake were obtained by heating or cooling the hypothalamus of the pig (Carlisle and Ingram, 1973).

Ingram (1968) noted a positive relationship between hypothalamic temperature and food intake in pigs whereas Baile *et al.* (1968) found that hypothalamic temperature did not change with intraruminal feeding of goats as the thermostatic theory would envisage. Although increased hypothalamic temperature was observed during eating in sheep by Dinius *et al.* (1970) there was the same increase with force-feeding or sham-feeding. The temperature rise was, therefore, related to excitement rather than to ingestion and had usually subsided before the end of the meal and it appeared that thermostasis was not the main controller of food intake.

The thermostatic theory is true in the sense that mammals and birds maintain a relatively constant body temperature and that heat production is proportional to the weight of food eaten; too little food will, eventually, result in a shortfall in heat production although body reserves will normally be mobilized to prevent undue hypothermia. Overeating, on the other hand, will increase heat production and heat loss mechanisms are activated to prevent hyperthermia. It is only under conditions where heat loss cannot increase further that voluntary intake falls to prevent hyperthermia.

Thus, intake is controlled to supply energy for heat production in addition to energy for other purposes. If further evidence of the fallibility of the thermostatic theory were needed, it can be found in the observation that the lactating animal produces more heat than the non-lactating animal but also eats more food.

## CNS Sensitivity to Metabolites and Hormones

A question of considerable significance in the control of intake and metabolism is how the brain, which is well insulated from marked short-term fluctuations in nutrient flow, is informed of the energy status of the body. The evidence for direct effects of blood metabolites on the brain is sparse, but new hope of finding the missing link came from the observation that infusion of insulin into the lateral ventricles of baboons at physiological rates over many days causes lower food intake and body weight (Woods *et al.*, 1979). Insulin in the cerebrospinal fluid has a much longer half-life than it does in plasma but reflects plasma insulin in the long term. As insulin is secreted in increasing amounts with increasing fat deposition this might be how the brain is made aware of fatness as well as nutrient status.

Parts of the brain are sensitive to the direct effects of glucose and/ or insulin. Glucose-sensitive neurons in the lateral hypothalamus decrease their firing rate in the presence, locally, of glucose. These same neurons appear to be linked with glucose-sensitive receptors in the liver as most of these neurons in the lateral hypothalamus decreased their rate of firing when glucose was infused into the hepatic portal vein (Shimizu *et al.*, 1983). So far as feeding is concerned, the important receptors in the brain are probably not glucose-specific as infusions of mannose and 3-D-hydroxybutyrate (both of which can be utilized by the brain), as well as glucose, depressed food intake in hypoglycaemic rats (Stricker *et al.*, 1977).

Although there is incontrovertible evidence that the hypothalamus is intimately involved in the control of feeding, recent studies of the hindbrain, reviewed by Grill (1986) and Ritter and Edwards (1986), demonstrate that the area postrema and the nucleus of the solitary tract are sensitive to glucose and capable of exerting an influence on diet selection. Reciprocal connections exist between the hypothalamus and the caudal hindbrain which presumably form part of the neural circuitry which controls feeding.

Rats with forebrain–hindbrain transection still suck at a normal frequency when tube-fed into the mouth (Grill, 1986). Sucrose given into the stomach of such animals depressed the amount of sucrose accepted into mouth and CCK also suppresses intake as normal. Therefore the caudal brainstem integrates metabolic stimuli and can preform the important function of modifying feeding behaviour according to nutrient demands.

*Poultry*

The voluntary intake of chickens was depressed by the intraventricular injection of glucose (Matei-Vladescu *et al.*, 1977) but Robinzon and Snapir (1983) found this to be true only when the birds were satiated. Smith and Szper (1976) implanted gold thioglucose at several sites in the brain of chickens but found no effect on feeding behaviour; they concluded from this that there is no glucostatic control of food intake in birds.

*Pigs*

Parrott and Baldwin (1978) trained pigs aged 3–4 months to operant conditioning for 8 g reinforcements of food on a fixed schedule ratio of 5 and then injected 4 mmol of glucose, xylose or 2-D-Deoxyglucose (2DG) into the lateral ventricles. All three compounds stimulated drinking presumably because of osmotic effects on the brain. Food intake was only stimulated by 2DG (Fig. 6.8) which blocks the uptake of glucose into cells which supports the concept of glucopaenia outlined above.

*Sheep*

Infusion of glucose or acetate into the lateral ventricles of goats has no effect on feeding (Baile and Mahoney, 1967); in sheep 0.45 ml of a 320 g $l^{-1}$ solution of glucose had no effect whereas in calves this treatment caused a significant increase in intake (Peterson *et al.*, 1972). 2-Deoxy-D-glucose (2DG) stimulated sheep to eat more when infused into the third ventricle, but so did xylose and the results suggested an osmotic effect rather than a specific response to the 2DG (Seoane and Baile, 1972a). The absence of a direct negative effect on feeding of metabolites in the brain of ruminants suggests that the various types of visceral receptors referred to in Chapter 3 are of greater importance in the control of food intake.

There is strong evidence for an effect of insulin on the CNS which is part of the system for controlling body fat content (Chapter 9). Foster *et al.* (1991) gave 6-day intracerebroventricular infusions of insulin to sheep at what was thought to be a physiological rate (123 ng $kg^{-1}$ body weight $day^{-1}$) which depressed food intake by 40% and plasma insulin

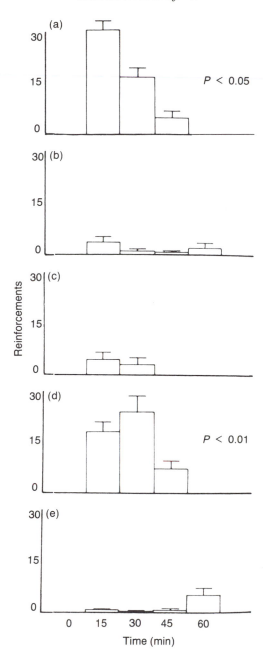

**Fig. 6.8.** Reinforcements of food obtained by young pigs after injection of (a) calcium chloride (positive control), (b) glucose, (c) xylose or (d) 2DG or (e) saline (negative control) into the lateral ventricles. (From Parrott and Baldwin, 1978, reproduced with permission.)

to about half that of controls. However, this treatment increased the concentration of insulin in CSF by 10–100-fold which suggested a supraphysiological rate of infusion so it is still not known whether insulin transferred from the plasma to the CSF is involved in the normal control of food intake.

## Possibilities of Pharmacological Manipulation of Food Intake

Tranquillizer drugs, given in the food or by injection, stimulate food intake and have been studied for their possible use as commercial intake stimulants.

Elfazepam, a benzodiazepine tranquillizer, stimulates food intake when included in the diet of cattle (Dinius and Baile, 1977). Both elfazepam and 9-aza-cannabinol injections depress rumen contraction rate in sheep (Della-Fera et al., 1977), delay rumen emptying, cause an increase in the digestibility of the diet and reduce the amount of time spent eating without affecting the number of meals per day (Krabill et al., 1978). Although it was initially assumed that elfazepam had its effects directly on the digestive tract, it was later concluded that it acts by central-nervous-system-elicited inhibition of gastrointestinal motility and rate of digesta passage. Abomasal secretion was significantly reduced whereas food intake during the three hours after injection was stimulated threefold (Van den Broek et al., 1979).

Effects of cyproheptadine on food intake and feeding behaviour of sheep were studied by Duquette and Muir (1979) in view of the stimulant effects of this antihistamine drug on appetite in man. They injected 0.25–1.0 mg kg$^{-1}$ intramuscularly and observed significant increases in the weight of food eaten during three hours after injection although daily intake was unaffected; the increase was achieved by a greater frequency of meals during the 3-h period. There are no reports in the literature of incorporation of cyproheptadine in the food to see whether the stimulus to eat is maintained over long periods, but given daily by mouth to chickens it resulted in significant increases in food intake and weight gain (Injidi and Forbes, 1987).

## Conclusions

Although lesioning studies helped to identify possible important control sites within the brain, they have been largely superseded by less invasive techniques. Finding that lesions of the VMH increase feed intake and deducing that this part of the brain is the 'satiety centre' is akin to hammering a nail into a portable radio, observing that this causes it to emit a loud whistle, and concluding that the nail had penetrated the 'antiwhistling centre' of the radio. The organization of the brain is not in discrete centres, but in circuits, each involving millions of neurons and interacting with other circuits and with other parts of the body.

Although other techniques for studying brain function in relation to feeding are less crude than lesioning, it is often difficult to decide whether what they are showing are artefacts due to the type of chemical injected, its dose, or leakage into other parts of the brain. Le Magnen (1992) warned: 'It is interesting to observe that almost all compounds, intraventricularly or locally infused in either deprived or satiated animals, augmented or inhibited food intake.' Just because a substance affects feeding when injected into the brain does not mean that it plays a significant role in normal circumstances.

The variety of substances found in the brain and the diversity of sites at which exposure to these substances, their analogues and antagonists affects feeding, means that this chapter is something of a catalogue. If any conclusion can be drawn it is that the PVN seems to be of paramount importance.

The results of experiments involving electrical and chemical stimulation give only glimpses into what might eventually become a well-described system of connections within the brain. Up to the present time there has been little work on the changes which take place in the brain which might be correlated with feeding behaviour. Changes have been seen in the firing rate of neurons in the lateral hypothalamus of rats in response to the carbohydrate status of their environment and Maddison and Baldwin (1983), recording from single neurons in the brain of the conscious sheep, found responses in the lateral hypothalamus to the sight of food and in the ventrobasal thalamus to tactile stimulation of the mouth and face.

Many of the responses made by animals to food are learned (Chapter 12) and the plasticity of the brain in the young animal means that it is possible for different neurons using different transmitter substances to be used for the same purpose in different individuals. It seems to me that we are likely to make as much progress in understanding the development and functioning of the CNS involvement in feeding by neural network modelling as by injecting yet more chemicals into the brain.

# 7 INTEGRATIVE THEORIES OF FOOD INTAKE CONTROL

- Energostasis
- Sensory factors
- Integration of multiple feedbacks
- Interactions between factors affecting food intake
- Maximizing efficiency
- Maximizing comfort
- Quantitative integration by means of mathematical models
- Conclusions

This chapter describes some of the theories which have been put forward to explain the control of intake in birds and mammals. In many cases they are developments of simpler hypotheses described briefly in Chapter 1 which postulated that feeding is controlled by a single factor, usually acting in a negative feedback manner. Stomach distension (Chapter 3), hypothalamic temperature (Chapter 6), blood glucose concentration (Chapter 5), body fat stores (Chapter 8) and plasma amino acids (Chapter 5) have all, in their turn, been proposed as the factor whereby intake is controlled to match requirements. However, none of these theories outlined so far can explain how intake is controlled under all circumstances. Balch and Campling (1962), having reviewed the control of voluntary food intake in non-ruminants, concluded that '... food intake is unlikely to be regulated by any single mechanism and ..., through the central nervous system, oropharyngeal sensations, gastric contractions and distension, changes in heat production and changes in the levels of circulating metabolites, may severally be implicated'.

# Energostasis

Several of the single-factor theories have in common the idea that some function of energy intake or storage is monitored by the brain which then controls intake in order to preserve the constancy of a bodily function (glucose concentration or utilization, deep body temperature, body fat stores). It is clear that any attempt at formulating a more complex hypothesis must rely on energy as the principal commodity. So far as we know the body cannot measure energy *per se*, although several recent theories imply monitoring of energy flows.

Le Magnen (1976), realizing the limitations of the 'classical' theories, has accumulated evidence to support the concept that the energy supply to some tissues is monitored and used to control food intake. He showed that during the day the rat has a lower metabolic rate than at night and speculated that this might be the cause, rather than the result, of the reduced frequency of meals during the day, compared with the night. Booth (1979) has coined the term 'cytischemetric' to indicate that the rate of use or supply of energy by cells is critical.

Le Magnen and Devos (1984) have concluded that the amount of food eaten from the onset to the termination of a meal, or meal size, is mainly determined by the peripheral, i.e. oral and gastrointestinal, action of ingested foods. Meal to meal intervals, and therefore the meal frequency, are mainly dependent on postabsorptive and metabolic factors. Another way of putting this is to say that meal termination is not finely controlled as it seems to be caused by numerous factors acting in concert, many of which are not directly related to the eventual nutrient yield of the meal. However, the products of the meal in question can be more accurately monitored during the subsequent intermeal interval and used to determine the onset of the next meal. The same idea is expressed by Sticker and McCann (1985): 'when eating, increasing gastric fill and increasing hepatic delivery of calories both serve to reduce the likelihood that animals will continue to feed. Once they stop eating ... they will remain satiated despite an empty stomach so long as the liver continues to get utilizable calories from the intestines.'

# Sensory Factors

Intake is not controlled solely by internal factors, however. It has been proposed that the hedonic properties of food influence the amount eaten and rats offered a choice of several highly palatable foods (cafeteria feeding) ate at least 30% more than similar rats offered the standard laboratory pellets and, as a result, gained proportionately more weight (Armitage *et al.*, 1983). (It must be recognized, however, that several of the foods typically used in cafeteria feeding are high in fat and low in protein, characteristics which tend to increase intake even in single foods.) The extra fat might be expected to feed back to the brain to depress voluntary intake and maintain a constant body weight and fat content (Chapter 9). If this does not occur the positive effects of the highly palatable food may be counteracting the signals generated by the extra fat. Wirtshafter and Davis (1977b) have formulated the idea of a 'settling point' for body weight which is a balance between negative feedbacks from the viscera and positive effects of palatability:

$$W = GS/(1 + GH) \tag{7.1}$$

where *W* is the body weight, *G* is the forward gain of the system, *H* is the feedback gain and *S* is the input. Although this relationship suggests a geometric combination of the factors, which will be challenged below, the general concept appears to be worthy of further development.

Not only do the hedonic properties of food affect its acceptability, they also enable the animal to characterize a food so that if ingestion of a particular food is followed by unpleasant consequences it can be avoided in the future; thus we have the concept of 'feed-forward' in addition to that of 'feedback' (Chapter 12).

## Integration of Multiple Feedbacks

To suppress feeding completely (cause satiety?) it is necessary to infuse not just a supply of energy, but also fat and protein (Nicolaidis and Rowland, 1976) and it is abundantly clear that satiety is not induced by a single mediator acting on a single group of receptors in a single target organ. Any experimental treatment given on its own must usually be applied at a level far above that achieved in the normal animal in order to prevent feeding completely. We therefore either have to reject such factors as stomach distension, concentration of glucose or other metabolites and osmolality and seek some completely different way of explaining how animals control their food intake, or we have to explore the likelihood that the various signals reaching the central nervous system from visceral and other receptors are integrated.

Although the discussion of 'modern' theories of the control of intake started off with energostasis, it is necessary to include other factors, particularly the physical fill of the digestive tract and the sensory characteristics of the food. There are many ways in which these signals might be combined in order to generate the final outcome in terms of feeding; two possibilities are that they are either added or multiplied.

Consider one set of receptors sensitive to stretch in the stomach wall, and another set of chemoreceptors in the liver, both responding to increases in stimulation during and after a meal. The signal from the stretch receptors will be $S \times N_S$, where $S$ is the degree of stretch and $N_S$ is the number of receptors. Similarly, the signal from the chemoreceptors will be $C \times N_C$, where $C$ is the concentration of the chemical(s) to which the liver receptors are exposed and $N_C$ is the number of such receptors. Geometric combination of the two signals would give:

$$IS = (S \times N_S) \times (C \times N_C) \tag{7.2}$$

where $IS$ is the strength of the integrated signal. However, should either of the families of receptors not be stimulated (as may occur with a highly concentrated food which does not stretch the gut wall, or a totally indigestible 'food' which does not yield any nutrients to stimulate the liver) and $S$ or $C$ are therefore zero, then the combined signal will be zero:

$$IS = (0 \times N_S) \times (C \times N_C) = 0 \tag{7.3}$$

or

$$IS = (S \times N_S) \times (0 \times N_C) = 0 \tag{7.4}$$

and intake will be uncontrolled. This led to an alternative possibility: that the effects on intake of stimulation of different groups of receptors are additive:

$$IS = (S \times N_S) + (C \times N_C) \tag{7.5}$$

Experimental evidence for additivity of feedback signals in support of this equation is presented below.

Booth (1978) found it necessary, in order to prevent excessively large meals, to include distension as well as energy feedback in his rat model in an additive manner, equating distension with joules and adding this to the genuine energy signal. This is in contrast to the models of Forbes (1977a, b, 1980) in which feeding was stopped by energy supply or gut fill, whichever was first to reach a critical level. There is sufficient evidence to be able to conclude now that some feedback signals combine additively in their effects on intake, rather than being mutually exclusive.

### Evidence for additivity

Hinton *et al.* (1986) examined a combination of putative intake controlling agents by using doses of glucagon (100 µg kg$^{-1}$), CCK (0.15 µg kg$^{-1}$)

or bombesin (0.75 mg kg$^{-1}$) which did not quite affect meal size of a liquid diet when given alone, but combined to depress meal size by 19–40%; this suggests a synergistic and not just an additive effect of low doses although higher doses had additive effects.

## Poultry

Shurlock and Forbes (1981a) showed that distension of the crop of chickens with wet food, or with hypertonic solutions, depressed intake during the following three hours. They also showed (Shurlock and Forbes, 1981b) that slow infusion of glucose solutions into the hepatic portal vein depressed intake in a dose-related manner and that the effects of various combinations of loading the crop with glucose solution and infusion of glucose into the portal vein on 3-h intake were additive.

Not only are the effects of the same nutrient administered into different sites additive, but also different nutrients given into the same site. A mixture of amino acids depressed intake much more when infused into the portal vein than into the jugular vein (Shurlock and Forbes, 1984). Several combinations of amino acid mixture and glucose given into the portal vein had similar effects on food intake during the 3-h infusion. Similarly, lysine and glucose infusions into the portal vein have additive effects (Rusby and Forbes, 1987); whereas the birds ate 71 g during the 3-h infusion of saline, intakes were depressed to 54 and 61 g with 300 mg lysine and 1260 mg glucose, respectively. When both metabolites were given together the intake was 46 g which is almost exactly the sum of the depressions caused by the two given separately (Fig 3.5).

## Cattle

With lactating cows Mbanya *et al.* (1993) showed that when distension of the rumen by a balloon (10.0 l), infusion of acetate (9.0 mol 3 h$^{-1}$) into the rumen and infusion of propionate (4.0 mol 3 h$^{-1}$) into the rumen, all at levels which had a small and non-significant effect on silage intake, were given together, there were additive effects in most cases, to give a significant depression in intake (Fig. 7.1). The only exception to the general observation of additivity was when sodium acetate infusion was combined with sodium propionate infusion. Although it is possible that this is a chance finding, it can also be explained in terms of an imbalance of nutrients. Infusion of a single metabolite, such as acetate, upsets the normal balance of volatile fatty acids which makes the animal feel uncomfortable. A simultaneous infusion of propionate, in a ratio with acetate similar to that normally produced by fermenta-

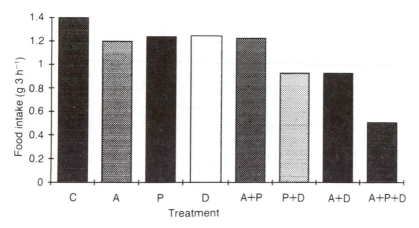

**Fig. 7.1.** Intake of silage DM by dairy cows given distension of the rumen (D, 10.0 l for 3 h), intraruminal infusion of acetate (A, 9.0 mol 3 h⁻¹) and propionate (P, 4.9 mol 3 h⁻¹) either separately or in combination. C is the control. (Mbanya *et al.*, 1993.)

tion, corrects the imbalance, making the animal more comfortable and therefore not depressing intake.

*Sheep*

Equivalent experiments with sheep have given similar results. When Adams and Forbes (1981) infused sodium propionate solution at 0.6 mmol min⁻¹ into the hepatic portal vein and sodium acetate into the rumen at 2 mmol min⁻¹ for 3 h the effects on the intake of a complete pelleted food during a 3-h treatment period were additive (Fig. 7.2), as were the effects of ruminal acetate infusion and balloon distension (1 l).

If one negative feedback factor is administered experimentally at a rate which initially completely suppresses feeding, it is to be expected that eventually, when other negative factors have declined to low levels due to an abnormally long period without food, the exogenous treatment will no longer be sufficient to prevent feeding. Infusion of sodium propionate into the hepatic portal vein of sheep at 1.2 mmol min⁻¹ for 3 h prevents feeding for the whole of this period (Anil and Forbes, 1980a). When infusion continued for longer periods small meals started to occur after about 6 h of treatment and were then more frequent than on control days (P.M. Driver and J.M. Forbes, unpublished results). Although intake was significantly depressed during 7 h of infusion, the fact that eating did resume agrees with the general theory of additivity. If one set of receptors is denervated and the brain is no longer aware of the extent of stimulation by negative feedback

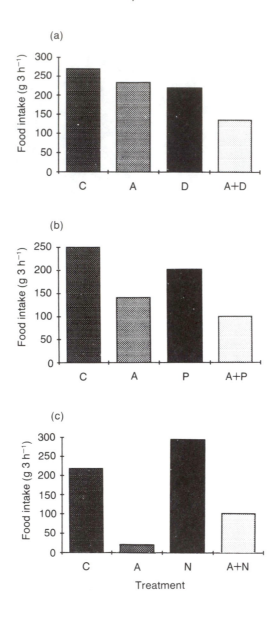

**Fig. 7.2.** Additive effects of two treatments on the intake of a pelleted food by sheep during a 3 h period: (a) acetate infused into the rumen (2 mmol min⁻¹) and distension (D) of the rumen (1 litre) (Adams and Forbes, 1981); (b) acetate (A) infused into the rumen (2 mmol min⁻¹) and propionate (P) infused into the hepatic portal vein (0.6 mmol min⁻¹); (c) acetate infused into the rumen (4 mmol min⁻¹) and noradrenaline (N) injected into the lateral ventricles (524 nmol) (Aydintug and Forbes, 1985).

factors, the animal might be expected to continue feeding for a longer time during each meal than before the denervation. Because of these large meals, levels of all feedback signals will rise to higher levels and for longer than usual which will lead to a longer interval before the next meal occurs. This happens when the liver is denervated in rabbits (Rezek *et al.*, 1975), sheep (Anil and Forbes, 1980a) and chickens (Rusby *et al.*, 1987).

There is general agreement, then, that small experimentally induced changes in several signals that might be involved in food intake act together to reduce food intake. The sum of such small changes which occur during a spontaneous meal might be sufficient to be satiating. The considerable complexity of the system is only likely to be understood by constructing mathematical simulations to test hypotheses; simple systems which use energy as their currency have been developed by Toates and Booth (1974) and Forbes (1980) but further sophistication should now be possible with the continued development of our ideas about the control of intake; the model of Poppi *et al.* (1994), detailed below, is an example of such an approach.

So far, our examples of additivity have been for signals which inhibit feeding. Aydintug and Forbes (1985) studied combinations of noradrenaline injected into the lateral ventricles of sheep (a potent stimulus to feeding, Chapter 6) with infusions of acetate into the rumen; additivity is, once again, quite clear: whereas noradrenaline stimulated intake (292 g vs. 217 g 3 $h^{-1}$ for control) and acetate inhibited feeding (18 g 3 $h^{-1}$), noradrenaline partly reversed the effect of acetate when both were given together (98 g 3 $h^{-1}$), i.e. almost exact additivity (Fig. 7.2).

The concept of additivity is also useful in understanding situations, such as lactation, where there is a very high rate of utilization of metabolites, leading to the understimulation of chemoreceptors. The animal can therefore suffer a greater degree of distension before the total of the negative feedback signals reaches the level at which feeding is switched off. Egan (1970) added casein to a straw diet or infused casein into the duodenum and saw increased voluntary intake by sheep. The volume of rumen contents was increased and Egan suggested that there is a mechanism which allows greater fill when protein nutrition is improved. He also saw the possibility that concentrate intake might be regulated by rumen volume being 'set' at a lower level than for forages; these ideas do not now seem so speculative as they did in 1970.

It may be, therefore, that additivity is a general phenomenon involving many factors which affect food intake, not simply the negative feedbacks from the viscera, and that intake and body weight are the net result of the effects of these many factors. This theory helps to resolve the conceptual difficulty of coping with the many factors which affect intake and may be involved in its control. No longer do we have to take the pessimistic view, expressed by an eminent animal scientist, that 'The problem in research in intake regulation is the establishment of evidence for or against *mutually exclusive* alternative hypotheses'. For such a view to be valid it would be necessary to assume that a feedback signal, say stomach distension, which was controlling intake with a poor-quality food, suddenly disappeared (or was suddenly ignored by the central nervous system (CNS)) when the quality of the food was improved so as to bring it into the 'metabolic' range. It seems highly unlikely that this would be the case.

## Interactions between Factors Affecting Food Intake

In many cases it is possible to speculate on the mechanisms of action of a particular stimulus but almost always the question remains as to whether the factor in question plays a significant role in the normal control of intake. Some of these difficulties can be overcome by a hypothesis that negative feedback signals are interpreted by the CNS in an additive manner (see above) but reliable unconfounded numerical relationships between stimulus and response are difficult to generate. We should be able to develop functions relating strength of stimulus to firing rate of visceral afferent fibres from experiments with anaesthetized animals but progress is slow in understanding how these signals are then interpreted by the CNS.

None of the pathways discussed in earlier chapters can account for the control of intake by itself. For example, in order to suppress feeding totally by infusion of glucose into the hepatic portal vein it is necessary to give quantities greatly in excess of those normally flowing in the portal vein, even after a very large meal. Thus, if all of the pathways described above are involved in controlling intake, their signals must be integrated by the appropriate circuits in the brain. Presumably these signals which fluctuate rapidly in relation to meals are added to a more constant signal coming from adipose tissue and a relatively small change in the strength of the signal from adipose tissue will, in the long term, play a significant part in controlling intake.

Food intake is also affected by positive signals, such as the sight or sound of other animals eating, and the delivery of fresh food. These are presumably added to the negative signals coming from the visceral receptors to determine whether or not feeding should occur.

Maximal stimulation of one population of receptors, perhaps causing pain, may saturate the control system and prevent other stimuli having additive effects on feeding. Grovum (1979) found that distension of the reticulum with 800 ml of water in a balloon depressed intake to a marked extent but that simultaneous abomasal distension had no further effect. This result might be explained by the likelihood that mechanoreceptors in the reticulum were grossly affected by a balloon of such large size in relation to the capacity of that viscus, especially as the reticular wall is relatively inelastic; our own work (Adams and Forbes, 1981) similarly showed lack of additivity when supraphysiological levels of stimulation were applied.

## Maximizing Efficiency

Dissatisfied with the concepts of distension and chemical feedback as controllers of intake in ruminants, Ketelaars and Tolkamp (1992a, b; Tolkamp and Ketelaars, 1992) have explored theoretically the costs and benefits of food consumption and proposed that intake is controlled to optimize the ratio of oxygen consumed to net energy made available. They give several examples of animals behaving in a way which minimizes the ratio of oxygen consumed:work done, showing that, for example, horses prefer to walk, trot or gallop at speeds at which they are most efficient. Using data collated by the Agricultural Research Council (ARC, 1980), they seek to demonstrate that ruminants eat that amount of food per day at which net energy production per mole of oxygen is maximized (Tolkamp and Ketelaars, 1992). Figure 7.3 shows the relationships between the efficiency of obtaining net energy by oxidation (ratio of net energy intake (NEI):oxygen consumption) and the level of food intake (ratio of net energy intake:net energy required for maintenance) for foods of several metabolizabilities which, according to the equations of ARC (1980), reach maximum values at points at which animals are predicted to consume each food voluntarily. For example, a food with a metabolizability ($q$) of 0.55 shows a peak of NEI/ $O_2$-consumption at the same level of intake of the food (1.4 × maintenance) that sheep consume voluntarily.

However, it is dangerous to extrapolate the relationship shown in Fig. 7.3 beyond the voluntary intake of the animal because by definition this cannot be supported by data. What happens to the efficiency above the level of voluntary intake has not been established and could only be studied by force-feeding to levels greater than *ad libitum* intake. Intragastric feeding, bypassing the mouth, does not result in the cephalic phase of insulin secretion, thus leading to reduced storage of absorbed nutrients in fat and muscle, i.e. inefficient utilization of nutrients. In attempting to answer the question: How can oxygen utilization be measured? Ketelaars and Tolkamp (1992b) suggest that intracellular pH is capable of being monitored and is, in

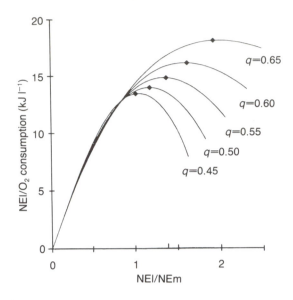

**Fig. 7.3.** The efficiency of oxygen utilization (NEI/$O_2$-consumption) as a function of NEI for roughages of metabolizabilities from 0.45 to 0.65. Diamond symbols on curves depict values corresponding to the average observed voluntary intake of such feed by sheep. (Tolkamp and Ketelaars, 1992, using equations from ARC, 1980).

part at least, influenced by oxygen consumption. However, intracellular pH is influenced by numerous other factors and would be an unreliable indicator of oxygen consumption. Even if the latter could be measured, why should animals seek to be optimally efficient? Presumably through evolution gross inefficiency has been avoided but there is no more evidence that animals want to be efficient than that they want to be comfortable. Although such a novel approach is refreshing, there is too little evidence on which to accept their claims at the present time.

## Maximizing Comfort

Knowing that animals learn to associate discomfort induced by ingestion of toxic or imbalanced foods with the sensory properties of those foods (Chapter 12) it seems reasonable to propose that animals eat to optimize their comfort. It is, as we know, uncomfortable to have an insufficient supply of nutrients, so we eat to reduce the discomfort of hunger. It is also uncomfortable, and sometimes painful, to eat too much food or to eat poisonous materials, so we avoid eating too much, and avoid eating poisonous foods. Thus, by eating for maximum comfort we integrate positive and negative signals but then rely to a great extent on what we have learned to be the consequences, in terms of comfort, of eating foods on previous occasions.

Although there are some experimental data on which to base theories of energetic efficiency, theories based on comfort have to rely on human experience and such animal feelings as can be deducted from learned associations, preferences and operant conditioning. Science progresses by dissatisfaction with current explanations leading to new or modified theories and then to experiments to demonstrate or otherwise the validity of these theories. The challenge now is to develop experimental methodologies to measure animals' comfort ratings.

# Quantitative Integration by Means of Mathematical Models

In a complex situation it is often helpful to construct a model to study the likely consequences of integrating the various parts of the system in a quantitative manner.

## Models of meal patterns

Figure 7.4 shows a hydraulic model of the control of feeding in which food energy is represented by water. It is based on the models for rats and human beings (Booth, 1978; Booth and Mather, 1978) and the model for sheep (Forbes, 1980).

An open tap simulates the ready availability of food, the funnel full of sand is the delay between ingestion and absorption and the small beaker which transfers water from tap to funnel takes the part of eating. Water accumulating in the reservoir represents repletion of a body pool of available energy which is depleted to support metabolism, as shown by the drain tap at the bottom. There is a reference point on the side of the reservoir which is used by the control system to determine when 'eating' should take place; when the water level is low beakers-full are transferred from tap to funnel. Because of the delay introduced by the sand in the funnel, eating will result in a build-up in the sand which will ensure a prolonged phase of satiation after each meal as the accumulated water slowly seeps into the reservoir. Thus the model generates a meal-taking pattern rather than continuous nibbling. It would be quite simple to construct such a model but it is more convenient and flexible in practice to translate such a concept into a

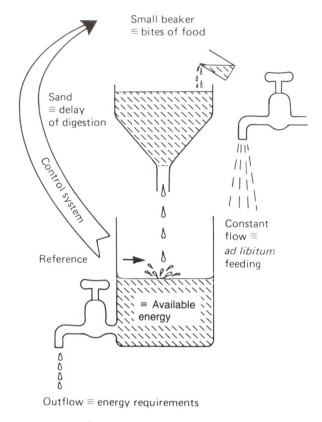

**Fig. 7.4.** Hydraulic model of feeding; see text for explanation (after Forbes, 1980).

computer program. Toates and Booth (1974) constructed such a quantitative simulation model of the rat on the plan outlined above in which
typical data on metabolic rate, rate of eating and rate of flow of digesta
from the stomach were put together in a computer program. When this
was run with parameters such that (i) food intake resulted in supply of
energy to tissues after a realistic time delay, (ii) feeding was switched
on when energy supply fell below rate of utilization and (iii) feeding
was switched off when energy absorbed exceeded requirements, meal
patterns were generated which closely resembled the observed behaviour, under a variety of conditions.

Simulations of feeding in rats with lesions in the ventromedial
hypothalamus were made by increasing the rate of fat deposition and
this increased the energy requirements. The size of meals which the
model predicted was unnaturally high; Toates and Booth (1974)
realized that stomach distension would prevent the occurrence of such

large meals and incorporated an upper limit to gastric distension into the model; this successfully mimicked actual feeding patterns of ventromedial hypothalamically lesioned rats. The model has since been refined and a human version has been produced (Booth and Mather, 1978) which incorporates learned responses and positive feed-forward, as well as negative feedback loops.

A ruminant model has been proposed, based on the premises of the rat model outlined above (Forbes, 1980). Although it incorporates more detail concerning rates of absorption of energy and rates of passage of food residues it is basically similar to the rat model in that it assumes that feeding is switched off and on by the relative rates of supply of and demand for energy or by gut fill. The requirements for metabolizable energy (ME) for maintenance of a 50 kg sheep were taken as 7.3 MJ day$^{-1}$, increased by 0.84 kJ min$^{-1}$ during eating and decreased by 10% during the hours of darkness; additions to ME requirements can be made to simulate growth, different mature body sizes, pregnancy, lactation or environmental temperatures below the critical tempera-ture. The food is characterized as the soluble (230 g kg$^{-1}$ for a good quality hay), insoluble digestible (420 g kg$^{-1}$) and the indigestible (350 g kg$^{-1}$) fractions. The soluble fraction is available for fermentation immediately after being eaten, according to a logistic function.

$$\text{ABS} = \frac{1}{1 + (1/e^{B\log_{10}t + A})} \qquad (7.6)$$

in which ABS is the proportion of the soluble fraction of a bite of food absorbed at time $t$ after ingestion and $A$ and $B$ are constants. This logistic curve gives an increase in absorption to a peak and a gradual fall to zero.

The insoluble digestible fraction starts fermentation after a lag period (6 h for a medium quality hay) and then digests according to the following equation:

$$\text{DIGRES} = \frac{D_0}{e^{(k_2 + k_3)\,(t - t_D)}} \qquad (7.7)$$

In which DIGRES is the remaining residue at time $t$ after the end of the lag period, $t_D$; $D_0$ is the original weight of insoluble digestible matter in the bite of food; $k_2$ is the rate of digestion and $k_3$ the rate of passage (Mertens, 1973). The sum of these two yields for the digesta from previous meals is the rate of absorption of energy at each iteration of the model.

The indigestible fraction starts to leave the tract after a lag period (13 h) according to the following:

$$\text{UNDIGRES} = \frac{U}{e^{k_3(t - t_U)}} \tag{7.8}$$

where UNDIGRES is the proportion of the indigestible matter of the bite remaining at time $t$ after the lag period $t_U$. The remaining indigestible fraction and the proportion of the insoluble digestible fraction of previous meals remaining at each iteration contribute the bulk of digesta which, when it reaches the maximum volume allowed for the rumen, terminates eating; the capacity of the rumen is reduced by competition for abdominal space from abdominal fat and/or the pregnant uterus. Feeding starts when the flow of energy-yielding substrates absorbed from the digestive tract falls below the rate of utilization by the tissues and stops when either the rate of absorption exceeds the rate of utilization or the rumen becomes full. Thus, the

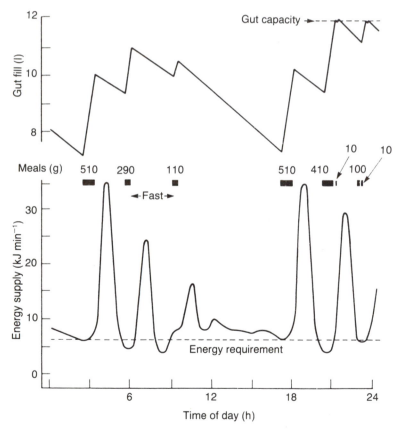

**Fig. 7.5.** Predictions of meals, stomach fill, energy absorption and fat deposition over a 24 h period from the sheep model of Forbes (1980).

model generates meals of various sizes and intervals which add up to realistic daily intakes, without being given any inputs concerning food intake, meal sizes and intervals, or rates of fat deposition, when run for several days. Figure 7.5 shows the predictions of rate of absorption of energy, gut fill and meals over a 24 h period for a mature sheep offered a food with a dry matter (DM) digestibility of 650 g kg$^{-1}$. It can be seen that six meals are predicted, the first four terminated by energy flow, the last two by gut-fill. The model needs to be refined to incorporate the additivity of feedback signals discussed above, but generally behaves in a similar manner to real animals under a wide range of circumstances.

With foods of high digestibility the rates of digestion and passage are rapid enough to allow high daily intakes and rates of fattening. With poorly digestible foods, or sparse pastures that can only be eaten at a slow rate, daily intakes are low and fat is mobilized to support the more important processes.

When the model was run with parameters appropriate for a cow there was reasonable agreement with reality (Forbes, 1983) but whereas this is not proof that the basic assumptions in the model are correct, it encourages the further development of the ideas incorporated in the model or suggested by its predictions.

These models assume that energy flow is monitored in animals, probably as the sum of several signals relating to concentrations and rates of uptake or release of metabolites, as discussed in Chapters 3–5. Their construction depends on several parameters which cannot be measured on the farm, so less-detailed approaches have been explored which do not attempt to model such short-term changes in metabolism as to be capable of simulating natural meal patterns. Some use an iteration interval of one day whereas others use a shorter time-scale, such as one hour.

### Within-day steady-state models

In the model of Illius and Gordon (1991) it is assumed that intake is limited by the capacity of the tract and can thus be predicted from the size of the animal and the dynamics of breakdown and passage of food particles, which are calculated in a manner similar to that of Mertens (1977; see above). However, no account is taken of any metabolic factors that might be involved. The model is run with three equally spaced meals per day until it reaches a semi-steady state; the number of meals per day is then increased until the mean daytime digesta load reaches 21 g DM kg$^{-1}$ body weight, the level specified by the interspecific mean digesta load found from the literature. Predictions of forage intake were highly correlated with observed values ($r = 0.78$) and were found to be particularly sensitive to changes in the model of the permitted average DM contents of the rumen, the digestible cell wall content of the forage and the rate of passage of particles out of the rumen.

Fisher *et al.* (1987) observed that previous models had used only the physically limited intake or, when the metabolically controlled intake was included, whichever was the lower was used as the predicted level of intake. They proceeded, therefore, to incorporate both factors simultaneously to take into account the likelihood (see above) that the factors that control intake do so in concert rather than separately. On the one hand they use Mertens and Ely's (1979) simulation of digestion and passage as a basis for the physical limit; fibre was classified into three particle size classes, each with different digestibility classes and a maximum rumen DM fill of 1.9% of body weight was assumed. On the other hand they assumed the optimal flow of nutrients to be that absorbed on a food of 650 g kg$^{-1}$DM digestibility, this being approximately the point above which intake appears to be controlled metabolically (Dinius and Baumgardt, 1970). Rate of intake ($I$) was assumed to be based on the ratio of current rumen contents to maximum contents ($D$) and the ratio of current nutrient flow to optimal flow ($C$) according to the equation

$$I_{t+1} = I_t DC^{aD^b} \tag{7.9}$$

in which the exponent $a$ limited the chemostatic effect relative to distension and the exponent $b$ gave an increased chemostatic effect at low levels of distension. When $a$ and $b$ were set to zero to eliminate the chemostatic feedback, intake increased with increasing digestibility (decreasing non-digestible fat (NDF) content) in a curvilinear manner right up to the highest digestibility, as expected (Fig. 7.6a). Setting $a$ to 0.2 and $b$ to 5 reduced the increase in intake per unit increase in digestibility and gave reduced intakes at very high digestibilities. Whereas rumen fill was constant when no chemostatic feedbacks were included, it decreased with increasing diet quality when such feedbacks were used (Fig. 7.6b). Daily intake declined with increasing NDF content and increased with increasing energy demand by the animal, although no quantitative information on the latter point is presented by Fisher *et al.* (1987).

In the model of Poppi *et al.* (1994) six potential limits to intake are calculated and whichever gives the lowest predicted intake is assumed to be the limiting factor; no attempt is made to integrate or add these limiting factors. Nevertheless there are several interesting ideas in this model. The six factors are:

**1.** Rate of eating; this is of importance as it is likely that there is an amount of time per day above which the animal will not eat, which is

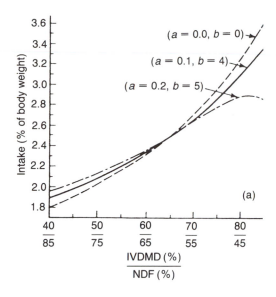

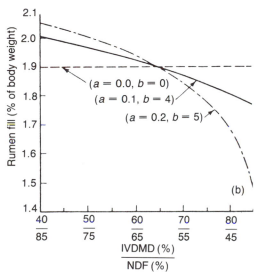

**Fig. 7.6.** Model predictions of (a) DM intake and (b) rumen DM contents, for a range of forage digestibilities and three sets of values for *a* and *b* in equation 7.9 (Fisher *et al.*, 1987).

thought to be 12–13 h day$^{-1}$ for ruminants. However, motivation to eat, and thus maximum time per day spent eating, is likely to be flexible and to depend on demand for nutrients.

**2.** Faecal output; Kahn and Spedding (1984) have found faecal output for steers for forage-based diets to be 9.6 g DM kg body weight$^{-1}$ day$^{-1}$. In practice the rumen is likely to be the limiting part of the digestive tract but this cannot be predicted from faecal output unless digesta flow is known.

**3.** Rumen turnover; this essentially is the rate at which the cell wall is digested and its particles leave the rumen.

**4.** Nutrient requirements; this is expressed as the potential for protein deposition and is acknowledged as being a difficult area in view of the fact that the level of food intake to some extent affects the rate of growth, milk yield, etc., and thus the 'nutrient requirements'.

**5.** Heat dissipation; there is a physical limit to the rate at which heat can be lost, depending on environmental factors such as air temperature, wind speed and humidity. Heat produced in excess of the capacity to lose it results in a rise in body temperature and a defensive reduction in voluntary intake.

**6.** Metabolism; a common factor is fluxes of ATP; ATP must be degraded with imbalanced diets and an upper limit can be set for this metabolism in order to limit intake.

As the authors did not consider that there is a good concept of how the short-term effects on intake, which might be additive, are used in the long term, they used the most limiting factor at any moment in time to predict intake. Seven diets were chosen to be representative; values for nutrient absorption were obtained from the literature and the model solved for the equations predicting the strength of each of the six limiting factors. For a steer of 100 kg empty live weight and starting with 15.4 kg of protein and 4.4 kg fat in the body, initial pool sizes were: ATP, 292 mol; $C_2$ equivalents, 5.8 mol; $C_6$ equivalents, 23.8 mol. Rates of eating of 3–30 g min$^{-1}$ were used, from the literature. Maximum capacity of the rumen was set at 13.8 g cell wall kg$^{-1}$ body weight and maximum faecal output was set at 9.6 g day$^{-1}$ kg body weight$^{-1}$. Particles can leave the rumen when 80% has been digested. Literature values were used for NDF content and rates of digestion of NDF and the genetic potential for protein deposition was set at 298 g day$^{-1}$ (AFRC, 1980). Duodenal absorption of protein from the different foods was used to estimate how much food could be eaten before excess limited intake, assuming a value of 80% for efficiency of utilization of amino acids. An upper limit of 1100 kJ kgwt$^{0.75}$ day$^{-1}$ at 20°C was used for heat dissipation; heat production is calculated from the inefficiency of utilization of ME, calculated from the ATP utilization and energy retained as fat and protein. The rate of ATP degradation is speculative, but was subjected to sensitivity analysis. A standard value of 45 mol ATP degradation day$^{-1}$ was taken, arrived at by iteration of the model. In general, there was good agreement between the model's predictions and the literature values, but predicted intakes were usually somewhat higher. Substrate cycling was a limiting factor for all foods whereas rate of eating did not pose a limit with any of the diets used, but is probably important in grazing animals. The assumption of a constant maximum fill of NDF may be wrong in view of the likelihood that different signals are interpreted additively by the CNS (see above). Fractional digestion rate is not sufficiently well documented and as digestion approaches its plateau, small differences in the rate of digestion will make big differences to the time taken to reach that point and therefore the residence time. The fact that rumen fill needs to be set lower than the assumed maximum supports the concept that animals often do not utilize their full rumen capacity. Substrate cycling limits intake in many of the simulations, implying that nutrient imbalances are often limiting intake. Where two or more factors are almost equally limiting, removal of one may not increase intake and lead to the conclusion that it is not important; however, we have established above that it is highly unlikely that various signals are used in an exclusive manner but that they are integrated, perhaps additively. If this is true then the model of Poppi *et al.* (1994) should be modified along the lines of the modifications suggested above for that of Forbes (1980).

This type of model, based on a time interval of less than one day but more than a few minutes, is particularly useful as it allows integration of voluntary intake into well-developed models of digestion and metabolism. It does not, however, allow meal patterns to be studied or simulated in a realistic way.

### Models of daily intake

The approaches adopted above do not allow for time lags in responses of intake to change in nutrient requirements. Monteiro (1972) proposed a model in which the voluntary intake of lactating cows responded to energy output with a finite lag period. He then subjected data collected from Friesian and Jersey cows to an iterative least squares procedure in order to estimate the lag parameters. Best fit of the data was obtained with a lag parameter whose value implies that it takes 100 days for the response in intake to reach 95% of the change in output. There is no evidence from cattle to support such a long lag and the rapid response of intake to changes in output in man (Edholm *et al.*, 1955) and rats (Adolph, 1947) suggest that such a slow response is unlikely. Although there was a good fit between the pattern of observed and predicted

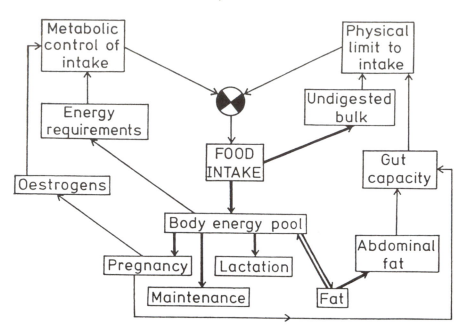

**Fig. 7.7.** Schematic diagram of a model of daily intake by sheep (Forbes, 1977a). The sectored circle indicates a comparator which uses whichever level of intake (physical or metabolic) is the lower.

intakes during lactation, prediction of milk yield was not accurate. Thus, Monteiro's approach to the problem of predicting voluntary intake by dairy cows has not been widely adopted.

Bywater (1984) followed Monteiro's approach but used energy rather than weight as the currency of his model. Intake was limited either by rumen capacity or by current ME requirements, as defined by a lag equation based on that of Monteiro (1972). Predictions of Bywater's model are higher than reality during the first part of lactation as a result of using long lag times on the basis of data on milk yield, rumen capacity and food intake from Tulloh (1966).

A less-sophisticated approach incorporating energostasis and physical limitation in a model of ruminant intake has involved assumptions that sheep (Forbes, 1977a) and lactating cows (Forbes, 1977b) will eat daily sufficient metabolizable energy to meet the animal's requirements for maintenance, production and fattening, unless physical limitations intervene. Figure 7.7 shows the flow diagram for the adult sheep model. The daily intake of food supplies energy to the body pool which is utilized for maintenance, pregnancy, lactation and fattening. Food intake also leads to stomach distension and this is compared with the abdominal space available (taking the size of the uterus and abdominal fat into account) to determine a physical limit to feeding. If the physically limited intake is less than the metabolically controlled intake then the former value is used and the shortfall in energy supply made up by fat mobilization. An important principle in this model is that fat deposition is seen to be driving food intake in that it is assumed that the sheep tries to deposit 100 g to fat per day if the quality of the food is good enough to avoid physical limitation of intake. Of course, if intake is so limited then fat deposition cannot reach this target and may even be mobilized if intake is very low. The deposition or mobilization of fat increases or reduces the volume of abdominal fat which, in turn, reduces or increases the space available for the rumen and hence for food intake.

This type of model produces a much steeper increase in daily intake in the period immediately after parturition than that seen in ewes or cows. The sharp rise is due to the sudden reduction in the volume of the uterus which releases the animal from physical limitation of intake and allows it to satisfy its greatly increased energy requirements for lactation. To cope with this anomaly the model was provided with a limit to the rate at which intake could increase but this is artificial as we do not know what are the physiological reasons for the unexpectedly slow increase in intake in early lactation (Chapter 9).

## Conclusions

Many theories of the control of voluntary intake have concentrated on single factors such as gastric distension, blood glucose concentration, body temperature or fat stores. In ruminants distension of the rumen and infusion of short-chain fatty acids have additive effects on intake but this has not been properly incorporated into models of intake by ruminants, although it is a feature of the early rat models.

More recent theories of intake control have included those in which the efficiency of utilization of oxygen for net energy production is maximized and this may in some way be coupled to feelings of metabolic 'comfort' which animals presumably seek to maximize.

Mathematical models help us to understand the relative importance of different factors affecting and controlling intake. Although typically such models work with an iteration interval of at least one hour, those which attempt to simulate the minute-by-minute events underlying meal-taking have generated realistic predictions of daily intake and body weight change. Models are only as good as the concepts and data from which they are built but play a vital part in the advancement of our understanding of what controls food intake.

# 8 GROWTH AND FATTENING

- Growth
- Fatness and food intake
- Conclusions

Changes in voluntary food intake occur during growth and fattening which, to a large extent, meet the changing nutrient requirements for protein and lipid synthesis. If food intake cannot meet these requirements then the rate of growth will decrease and/or body stores will be depleted. Hence the reduction in growth of young pigs when the feed is diluted so as to depress digestible energy intake or the slow rate of fattening of cattle offered only feeds of low energy content. It cannot be said in these cases that requirements control intake or that intake controls production; they are interdependent.

## Growth

An animal can only attain its potential growth rate when sufficient high quality food is available. In practice, however, both in the laboratory and on the farm, several factors may restrict intake and prevent the young animal achieving its potential rate of growth.

For mammals it is convenient to discuss pre- and postweaning growth periods separately as weaning is often abrupt and imposed before the young have begun to eat large quantities of solid food.

## The young chick

For the first 2 days after hatching chicks are not dependent on eating food as they have sufficient reserves from the yolk sac (Rogers, 1989). During this time they peck at small round objects and quickly learn which are food. They seem to have some innate knowledge, however, as beak-trimmed chicks, which cannot pick up food, show the same initial preference for grains over pebbles as intact birds. They do not maintain this preference, however, as the pecking is not reinforced by ingestion. Social hierarchy develops within the first three weeks, but chicks incubated in the dark, which randomizes the side of the brain responsible for feed location and selection (normally the left brain; right eye), develop a more flexible group structure than those incubated in light. Rogers (1989) has suggested that by incubating in the dark there may be a weaker pecking order with fewer low-dominant chicks which die from starvation.

Bate (1992) exposed young turkeys to maternal feeding calls from hatching or to brooding calls before hatching and feeding calls after but there was no effect on mortality although sound stimulation 'enhanced feeding behaviour'.

## Preweaning in mammals

Once the young has recovered from the acute affects of birth its activities are totally directed to teat-seeking, which are actively encouraged by the dam. Young nose around the underside of the dam and will persist for an hour or two if not rewarded. Foals suck within 15–30 min of birth and thereafter take milk about once an hour. By 6 months of age this has declined to about 10 times per day (Fraser and Broom, 1990). Calves sometimes do not succeed in obtaining milk from their mothers for over 6 h after birth but thereafter suck about 10 times per day. Most lambs have found the teats within 2 h and may then take milk as often as 50 times in the next 24 h. However, by four weeks of age they are only suckled about six times per day.

### Natural rearing

The mother's milk is the major source of nutrients during early life, with the exception of the calf in the dairy herd. Within a species both the composition of this milk and the quantity available may be limiting factors. Where the mother does not have enough teats for all the progeny, the weakest of the littler will receive only that left by the others and often die or have to be reared artificially. This often occurs in pigs when the litter is greater than about 14 and in sheep when three or more lambs are born.

Even when individuals receive a fair share, the total amount of milk produced may not supply the full nutrient requirements of the young. There is a negative correlation between litter size and growth rate of the individual in the litter (e.g. Widdowson and McCance, 1960). Supplementation of the diet with a highly palatable feed in such a way that the mother cannot steal it (creep feeding) is common practice for young pigs and lambs. The high energy requirements of the rapid relative growth rate of young animals might be expected to predispose them to eat solid food avidly when milk supply was insufficient but creep feeds must be highly palatable and low in fibre to encourage maximum intake.

## Pigs

Fraser and Rushen (1992) monitored milk intake by weighing piglets every 10 min for the first 4 h of life. There was little synchrony in the first hour but after that all tended to suck at the same time. Piglets soon establish a 'teat order' and thereafter always suck from 'their' teat. Whatever the potential intake, actual intake depends on the milk yield of the dam which is affected by nutrition, mastitis and metritis. Litter size is obviously an important factor.

The piglet takes enough of its mother's milk to supply about four times maintenance, depending on genetic potential for protein and fat deposition (which can be very variable); the faster the piglet's growth, the higher its intake (Fowler and Gill, 1989). In one study, creep-fed piglets each ate only 78 g of a high protein food in the first 3 weeks (Lightfoot *et al.*, 1987) or 89 g for those on a low protein food. In another observation with 39 piglets, intake of creep feed varied from 13 to 1911 g pig$^{-1}$ 3 weeks$^{-1}$ (Pajor *et al.*, 1991). In the second and third week of lactation, intake of creep feed by piglets is around 20 g pig$^{-1}$ day$^{-1}$ but this increases rapidly in the fourth week (Aherne *et al.*, 1982).

The young pig has some control over food intake; for example, loading the stomach with hypertonic saline or water, or giving nutrient loads, all depressed subsequent voluntary intake (Houpt *et al.*, 1977). Dilution of a milk substitute containing 4.68 MJ l$^{-1}$ so that it contained 2.38 MJ l$^{-1}$ caused a 36% increase in the intake by piglets which was not quite sufficient to prevent a reduction of growth rate (Wangsness and Soroka, 1978). Although this suggests that young piglets have a mechanism for matching intake with requirements, albeit imperfect, piglets of less than one week old did not respond to insulin injections (which increase energy uptake and increase intake in adult pigs) indicating an immaturity in the integration of feeding responses at that early age (Houpt *et al.*, 1977).

Ease of access to creep feed is a factor affecting the intake of food by suckling piglets. If there is insufficient space for all the piglets in a litter to eat at once, some will not eat at all. Appleby *et al.* (1992b) gave some litters access to a single two-space feeder and provided others with four similar feeders from 21 days of age until weaning at 28 days. With the more restricted system, at least four pigs in each litter did not use the feeder at all, whereas with the more liberal treatment less than one pig per litter on average did not eat creep feed. Those that did not eat tended to have had higher birth weights and growth rates to 21 days, suggesting that they were satisfied with the milk from the sow and were not highly motivated to eat solid food. Perhaps for this reason they had low growth rates from weaning to day 42 but their growth overall up to 42 days was no different from that of those piglets which ate creep feed. The authors suggest that low food intake before weaning is a predictor but not a cause of poor growth after weaning.

Three-week-old piglets have a strong preference for sucrose, glucose, lactose and fructose (Houpt and Houpt, 1976), but the thresholds of discrimination are higher than in adult pigs (Kennedy and Baldwin, 1972).

## Artificial rearing

Milk is the primary product of the dairy cow and in modern intensive dairy management it is too expensive to feed to calves. After access to the mother's colostrum for a day or so, the calf is separated from its mother and fed on reconstituted artificial milk from a bucket or automatic feeder until it is weaned at about 5–6 weeks of age. The quality and quantity of milk offered can both be controlled. Some adjustment of voluntary liquid intake occurs in response to changes in milk concentration in an attempt to maintain a constant dry matter (DM) intake, but this fails if the milk is too dilute (e.g. Pettyjohn *et al.,* 1963). Older calves can compensate better for dilution (Ternouth *et al.,* 1978a). DM intake from milk substitute declines when its dry matter concentration is less than about $100 \, \mathrm{g} \, \mathrm{DM} \, \mathrm{l}^{-1}$ and increases, especially in older calves, when the DM content is above about $200 \, \mathrm{g} \, \mathrm{l}^{-1}$.

Twice-a-day feeding of milk substitute leads to higher voluntary intake than offering one feed per day, although as the calves become accustomed to taking very large amounts of liquid in one meal so intake rises (Ternouth *et al.,* 1978b). The temperature of the milk on offer is not a very important determinant of intake, although cold milk (6–15°C) tends to be taken in greater quantities than warm (38°C) (Roy, 1980).

When 4-month-old calves were offered dry food the intake of this varied inversely with the DM content of the milk (Ternouth *et al.,*

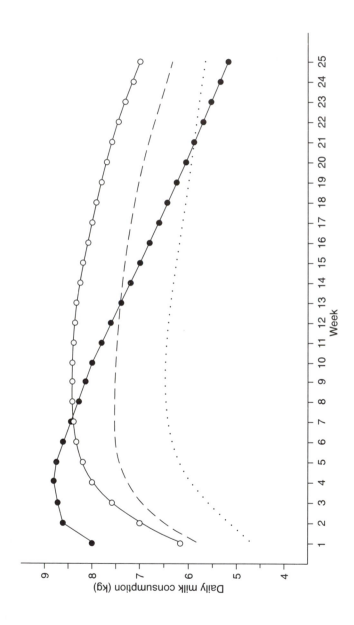

**Fig. 8.1.** Consumption of milk by Angus (... 1984, − 1985), Charolais (○) and Nalore (●)-sired calves from 1 to 25 weeks of age (Mezzadra et al., 1989)

1978b) whereas in lambs at grass, solid food intake was also inversely proportional to the allowance of milk (Hodge, 1966). Hodgson (1971c) found the following highly significant relationship between the intake of dried grass (GDMI, g kgLW$^{-1}$) and the amount of milk substitute offered (MS, g DM kgLW$^{-1}$) with 3-week-old calves:

$$GDMI = 7.5 - 0.26MS \qquad (8.1)$$

Calves of different genetic types have been found to show different patterns of milk consumption when suckled by dams of the same type (Mezzadra *et al.*, 1989). Charolais-cross calves consistently took more milk than Angus-cross in one year, whereas calves sired by Nalore bulls (an Argentinian *Bos indicus* breed) not only took more than Angus-cross calves, but had a completely different shape of curve, starting with very high intakes but declining more rapidly than the Angus (Fig. 8.1). It was suggested that *Bos indicus* calves reduce their dependency on milk at an earlier age than those of *Bos taurus* breeds, perhaps because of the shorter period of the year when good forage is available to support milk production.

*Lambs*
The intake of milk substitute by lambs separated from their mothers a few hours after birth increases rapidly to reach about 2.5 l day$^{-1}$ at 5 weeks of age, by which time their body weight is 10 kg (Bermudez *et al.*, 1984) (Fig. 8.3).

## Postweaning

Weaning is followed by much agitation and calling for the mother which overcomes hunger for several hours, especially if the dry food on offer is unfamiliar. The young animal may have difficulty in learning how to locate water and to drink from an unnatural container and this will further delay the onset of eating.

*Acute effects of weaning*

Although solid food is eaten in small quantities by the young of many species they are not usually eating enough to support full growth at weaning. A fall in body weight therefore occurs which is more severe the younger the animal at weaning. Hunger stimulates a rapid increase in food and water intake (perhaps the latter is critical) and weight gains are resumed within a few days.

*Pigs*

By weaning the piglet requires the equivalent of about 475 g of good food per day but in practice it is several days before it reaches this level of intake; in the first few days it usually manages less than maintenance. In one observation (Riley, 1989) the mean intake on days 1–3 after weaning was only 71 g day$^{-1}$, on days 4–7, 120 g, and on days 8–35, 518 g day$^{-1}$. Continuous availability encourages a higher intake than meal-feeding and those fed a meal every 2 h ate more than those given meals every 4 or 6 h (Bark *et al.*, 1986).

Water intake is important; it took a week before water intake reached that taken in milk before weaning. For the first time, the animal must separately satisfy its hunger and thirst. Behavioural problems such as navel sucking can occur, presumably due to a desire for the same comfort as provided by sucking the sow's teat. There was very low water intake on the first day after weaning, but a big increase on day 2, suggesting that the animals had difficulty finding or using the drinkers immediately after weaning (Barber *et al.*, 1989).

If solid food intake can be encouraged during the milk feeding period then the check at weaning will be less severe; highly palatable, sweet concentrate feeds encourage high intakes. Sucrose is sweet, provides energy and is commonly included in early-weaning rations. Soluble saccharin also enhances intake of starter feeds by early-weaned pigs but insoluble saccharin is less effective (Aldringer *et al.*, 1959; Kare *et al.*, 1965). Moist food is eaten in greater quantities than dry food (Braude and Rowell, 1967).

Attempts to familiarize piglets with food and drink before weaning have had variable effects on performance after weaning. Exposure to recordings of sow's chanting, to vanilla odour and to flashing lights before offering food to condition eating, had no effect on daily intake even though the anticipatory response was usually elicited (Thikey, 1985). Perhaps putting newly weaned pigs with experienced pigs would speed their learning about food and water but this might also encourage fighting and the spread of disease. Antibiotics in the feed often increase intake after weaning, due to suppression of pathogens and by sparing nutrients from microbial degradation. Copper sulphate has similar effects. The inclusion of organic acids such as citric acid in the food sometimes improves intake (e.g. Henry *et al.*, 1985), perhaps because stomach pH is elevated in stressed piglets, but the results are variable.

Early weaned piglets are susceptible to cold environments and to slippery floors and difficult access to feeders and drinkers. Attempts to improve intake with flavouring agents have usually shown no effect – flavoured foods which were preferred in a choice test were not eaten in any greater amounts when given as the sole food (Aumaitre, 1980).

However, McLaughlin *et al.* (1983) preference tested 129 flavours and found one with a cheese aroma which did increase intake in a sustained manner when no choice was available. This is unusual and unexplained as a change in the sensory properties of a food without any change in its nutritional value usually only results in a temporary change in intake.

Many things such as heat-damaged or putrefied proteins depress intake as do fungal toxins generated by contamination of cereal grains. Rapeseed meal contains glucosinolates, saponins, sinapines and tannins, all of which depress intake, although it is not clear to what extent they do so simply by their affect on food flavour and to what extent by damage to the gut and toxic effects after absorption. From evidence presented in Chapter 12 it is likely that toxic effects become associated with the sensory properties of the food so that a learned aversion to toxic foods ensues, whatever their flavour.

*Calves*

Intake of solid food by calves increases as the daily allowance of milk decreases (Le Du *et al.*, 1976) – when given 36 g DM $kg^{-0.75}$ of milk, the intake of grass DM was 33 g $kg^{-0.75}$, whereas when only 6 g milk DM $kg^{-0.75}$ was given the calves consumed 101 g DM $kg^{-0.75}$.

Between 7 and 13 weeks of age the calf has an increasing ability to compensate for the addition of food to the rumen via a fistula and there is a similar improvement in compensation for removal of digesta (Hodgson, 1971b) (Fig. 8.2). These results support the gradual development of visceral control of voluntary intake in young animals.

The apparent rate of live weight gain may be as fast when calves are weaned early onto solid food as it is when milk feeding is continued, but this is in part due to the increased gut fill. Calves do not voluntarily consume as much solid food dry matter as they do from milk substitute until their live weight is about 80 kg (Roy, 1980). Voluntary intake rises to about 3.0 kg DM 100 $kg^{-1}$ live weight at about 120 kg which is similar to the maximum level of intake seen in lactating cows.

The intake of long hay, but not of pelleted feeds, was enhanced by giving calves prior experience of the feed (Hodgson, 1971a). Intake increases as the digestibility of the food increases, implying physical limitation. As the calf gets older it can utilize roughage better and the intake of concentrates may be metabolically controlled, with a negative relationship between intake and digestibility. McCullough (1969) offered various diets with different concentrate:roughage ratios to calves. The all-concentrate feed was consumed in greatest quantities up to live weights of 136 kg; at heavier weights the intake of the 80:20 ration was highest. Kang and Leibholtz (1973) found that the maximum

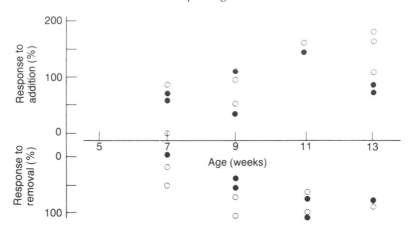

**Fig. 8.2.** Changes in the voluntary intake of chopped (○) or ground and pelleted (●) dried grass by calves in response to addition of food to, or removal of digesta from, the rumen via a fistula. (From Hodgson, 1971b, reproduced with permission.)

food intake of calves aged 5–11 weeks occurred when the diet contained 190 g straw kg$^{-1}$.

Hodgson (1973) found that the weights of the caecum plus colon contents at slaughter were similar in calves which had been offered feeds of different quality and suggested that the capacity of the large intestine might be limiting intake.

### Lambs

Faichney (1992) observed that Merino lambs, given access to solid feed from about 3 weeks of age while with their mothers, ate little for the first 10 days, but from 4 weeks of age intake increased, with large day-to-day variations, to over 50 g day$^{-1}$ kg$^{-0.75}$. There was little effect of weaning but the steady increase continued to reach a plateau at 16 weeks, at about 95 g kg$^{-0.75}$.

Bermudez *et al.* (1984) abruptly weaned artificially reared lambs at 5 weeks of age and offered concentrates, forage and water *ad libitum*. The lambs which were heavier at weaning, through taking more milk, suffered a greater setback when milk was withdrawn, as they had taken less solid food before weaning and took longer to establish an adequate intake of dry food. Within a few days of weaning the lambs were eating sufficient to resume their preweaning growth rate (Fig. 8.3).

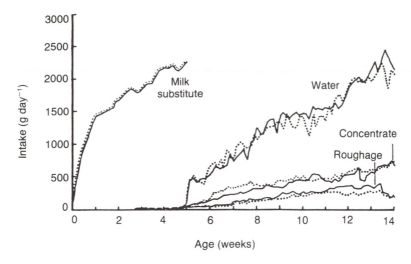

**Fig. 8.3.** Intakes of milk substitute, water, concentrates (—— high quality, … low quality) and forage by lambs from birth to 14 weeks (Bermudez *et al.*, 1984).

## Weaning to maturity

Once the stress of weaning is over the individual grows at a rate characteristic of the species, unless it is exposed to shortage of food, environmental stress or disease. There have been many attempts to describe the sigmoid growth curve mathematically. Suffice it to say that the daily weight gain accelerates for a period, followed by deceleration to an eventual asymptotic mature size, although fat deposition may lead to further increases in live weight.

As the animal grows feeding frequency usually decreases while meal size increases. For example, pigs fed *ad libitum* ate 10 meals per day soon after weaning, declining to three per day when adulthood was reached (Auffray and Marcilloux, 1980).

The voluntary intake of a nutritionally adequate feed increases as an animal grows, but is not maintained at the same proportion of live weight. It has been commonly assumed that intake is proportional to metabolic live weight (weight$^{-0.75}$) because comparison of mature animals of various species shows this to be an appropriate relationship, both for metabolic rate (Brody, 1945) and for voluntary food intake (Blaxter, 1962). Cole *et al.* (1967) found that the best exponent for the pig was 0.68, whereas the ARC (1981) preferred 0.51, which is far from 0.73. Re-analysis of several sets of data show that voluntary intake is related to live weight raised to a power close to 0.6 for an animal as it grows (Forbes, 1971), as distinct from a comparison of mature animals of different weights. As beef cattle grow from about 250 to 550 kg live weight, their voluntary intake of a silage-based complete feed is approximately constant when expressed per kg live weight$^{0.60}$, rather than per kg of live weight or live weight$^{0.73}$ (Forbes, 1982a).

## Poultry

As the broiler grows its daily food intake increases; the increase is not in direct proportion to body weight, however, nor to metabolic body weight (body weight to the power 0.73), but rather to a lower power such as 0.6 (Forbes, 1986a) or 0.66 (Hurwitz *et al.*, 1978). In a thermoneutral environment the energy requirement of the bird can be stated as the sum of the requirement for maintenance and that for growth.

$$\text{MER} = 8.0 \, \text{LW}^{0.66} + 8.6 \, \text{WG} \tag{8.2}$$

where MER is the metabolizable energy requirement (kJ day$^{-1}$), LW is the body weight (g) and WG is the weight gain (g day$^{-1}$) (Hurwitz *et al.*, 1978). This must be an oversimplification, however, as the composition of the weight gain changes as the bird grows – going from predominantly protein in the early stages to greater proportions of fat as the

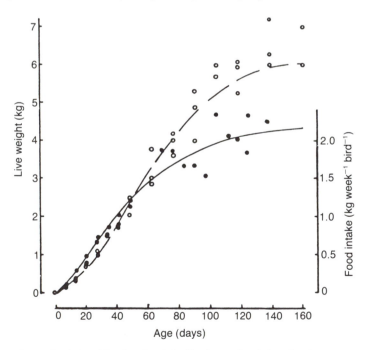

**Fig. 8.4.** Body weights (O) and food intakes (●) of broiler cockerels from hatching to 160 days. (From Prescott *et al.*, 1985, reproduced with permission.)

bird approaches maturity. Each successive gram of weight gain will therefore require a greater input of food in view of the greater energy content and lower water content of adipose tissue compared to non-fat tissues, and also the increasing mass of body tissue to be maintained.

Figure 8.4 shows food intake and both weight changes during growth of broiler chickens to maturity (Prescott *et al.*, 1985). Relative to body weight, intake is higher during the rapid early phase of growth, reaching an asymptote of 300 g bird$^{-1}$ day$^{-1}$ for mature birds weighing about 6 kg. Similar information for ostriches, now being farmed in several countries for meat, leather and feathers, is provided by Degen *et al.* (1991).

## Pigs

Castrated males eat 7–16% more than entire boars whereas gilts eat up to 7% more than entire boars (Cole and Chadd, 1989). However, Smith *et al.* (1991) found that the higher intake by gilts than boars only lasted up to about 60 kg live weight, after which they ate less. These differences are related to different propensities to grow and fatten due to the presence or absence of sex steroid hormones.

## Cattle

When the intake of growing cattle is plotted against their metabolic weight (body weight$^{0.73}$) there is a steady decline with increasing weight. Weight has to be raised to a lower power, close to 0.6, in order to get a constant value as the animal grows (Forbes, 1971, 1982b). This value was found to vary with breed and conditions: for Friesian cattle on pelleted diets (Pickard *et al.*, 1969, Fig. 8.5) 0.58; for Hereford cattle on a similar diet in Kenya (Rogerson *et al.*, 1968) 0.50; for groups of cattle fed on silage-based complete feeds (Beranger and Micol, 1980) 0.6. Karue *et al.* (1973) found that nine diets of different energy concentrations were eaten by growing zebu cattle in proportion to live weight$^{0.79}$; however, for individual feeds, as the concentration of cell wall constituents fell from 710 to 610 to 540 g kg DM$^{-1}$ the exponent changed from 0.87 to 0.69 to 0.56. This suggests that the intake of poor quality roughages, which is limited primarily by physical constraints, is related directly to body weight whereas more concentrated diets are eaten in relation to metabolic requirements. Re-analysis of the data collected from the literature for the chapter on voluntary food intake in the ARC (1980) publication on the nutrient requirements of ruminant livestock did not confirm this view, however, because although the best fit for all the data was:

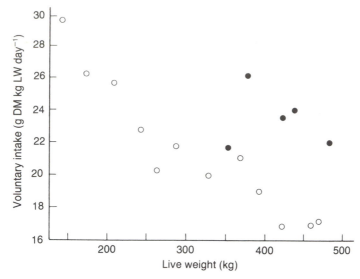

**Fig. 8.5.** Voluntary intake of a cereal-based food by growing cattle (O, fed *ad libitum* throughout; ● undergoing compensatory growth) (Pickard *et al.*, 1969).

$$DMI = 172.LW^{0.6} \tag{8.3}$$

when intakes of cattle offered complete feeds were included the equation was:

$$DMI = 98.LW^{0.75} \tag{8.4}$$

In this case physical limitation was probably not a limiting factor but the exponent was the same as that for interspecies comparisons. Colburn *et al.* (1968) found intake to be related to live weight$^{0.54}$ for Jersey steers growing from 150 to 490 kg.

Hodgson and Wilkinson (1967) measured the herbage intake of grazing Jersey calves, heifers and dry cows and found that intake was related to live weight$^{0.61}$. A similar exponent, 0.62, was fitted by Holmes *et al.* (1961) with young grazing cattle. Thus there is considerable evidence against expressing the voluntary intake of growing animals in terms of 'metabolic live weight', $W^{0.75}$, and Thonney *et al.* (1976) have suggested that it is more appropriate to include $W^b$ or log $W$ than $W^{0.75}$ in statistical models of heat production and body weight and this conclusion should also be applied to the analysis of relationships between food intake and body weight.

It is reasonable to assume that intake of complete diets was not limited primarily by physical restraint and that requirements for growth determined intake under the conditions in which these relationships were obtained. An increase in growth rate would therefore be expected to lead to an increase in voluntary intake and growth stimulants act primarily on growth with a secondary effect on voluntary intake. In one typical set of observations it was found that diethyl stilboestrol (DES) improved weight gains by 20% whereas intake increased by 6% (Oltjen *et al.*, 1965). Further discussion of growth stimulants will be found later in this chapter.

## Genetic effects

Undoubtedly, differences in food intake between different breeds of the same species are closely related to differences in potential to grow and fatten.

### Poultry

Selection of broilers for rapid growth is invariably accompanied by increased feed intake (Seigel *et al.*, 1984). It is possible that this increase in intake is due to a functional equivalent of hypothalamic lesioning because Burkhart *et al.* (1983) found that electrolytic lesions of the hypothalamus caused increased intake (and fattening) in broilers selected for low growth while having no effect in the high-growth line. However, another interpretation of these results is that the high-growth birds are already eating as much as their gut capacity will allow; this is supported by the results of Barbato *et al.* (1984) who found that it was much more difficult to force-feed broilers of a high-growth line than those selected for low rate of growth.

High-growth birds have higher thresholds for the detection of both sweet and bitter substances in the water (Barbato *et al.*, 1982). There was no difference in preference between the parent line and those selected for high or low growth at a quinine concentration of $0.25 \mathrm{~g~l}^{-1}$. As the concentration was increased, high-growth birds showed less aversion than those of other strains but by the time the concentration reached $3.0 \mathrm{~g~l}^{-1}$ there was once again no difference. For dextrose, there was no difference at 12.5 or $150 \mathrm{~g~l}^{-1}$ but high-growth birds showed less preference at intermediate concentrations. It can be concluded that selection for high growth renders birds less sensitive to taste.

Birds selected for high growth take longer than the low-growth strain to adjust their food intake when dextrose is included in the drinking water (Gidlewski *et al.*, 1982) suggesting that longer preference tests might be required to determine true preferences.

In addition to a line selected for high live weight gain, Pym and Nichols (1979) have selected other lines for maximum feed consumption and minimum feed conversion ratio and have also maintained a control, random-bred line. In the 12th generation the mean intake of high- and low-density diets from 5 to 9 weeks of age was 70 g day$^{-1}$ for the controls and 72 g day$^{-1}$ for the efficiency-selected line whereas for the gain- and intake-selected lines it was 100 and 109 g day$^{-1}$, respectively (S. Iskandar and R.A.E. Pym, personal communication). Whereas the control-, weight- and efficiency-line birds increased their intake when given the diluted diet, those selected for high feed intake did not and it was suggested, therefore, that these birds were eating to digestive capacity even with the nutrient-dense diet. This is supported by the fact that they had the most rapid rate of passage of digesta through the tract, the smallest gizzard and proventriculus and the shortest small intestine. The high-intake line also had the highest weight of abdominal fat pad and it is possible that this set a lower limit to gut capacity, as proposed for ruminants (see Chapters 4 and 10).

Selection of broilers for high or low fat-pad weight (R.A.E. Pym, personal communication) resulted in a 70% greater fat-pad weight after five generations. However, there was no difference between the intakes of the fat-line (100 g day$^{-1}$ from 4 to 8 weeks of age) and thin-line (97 g day$^{-1}$) birds and neither differed from the random-bred control line which ate 99 g day$^{-1}$. This shows that the physical size of the fat-pad does not directly affect intake. Selection for weight-gain alone or for weight-gain with a constraint on fatness resulted in higher intakes (108 g day$^{-1}$ in both cases).

Broiler chicks may eat no more per unit of body weight than do those of an egg-laying strain but convert food into live weight more efficiently (Savory, 1975), grow more quickly and therefore eat more than layer chicks at any given age.

## Pigs

The fact that the Duroc eats more than many other breeds of growing pig kept under the same American conditions (NRC, 1987) is presumably due to its faster growth but might be related to an ability to withstand heat stress more effectively.

'The selection of highly-productive pigs, in many cases, involves very little more than selecting those genes which promote eating' (Fraser and Broom, 1990). Selection for increased live weight gain over the last 250 years resulted in very fat animals with a high voluntary food intake. However, recent years have seen a demand for pig meat with a lower fat content and therefore selection for lean tissue deposition and against fat deposition to the extent that present-day pigs are sometimes thought to be eating too little, even when fed *ad libitum*. In a line selected for efficiency of production and carcass lean content, Ellis *et al.* (1979) found intakes of 78.8 kg in weeks 1–6 on test and 114.0 in weeks 7–12, compared to 85.5 and 117.0, respectively for a control, unselected line. Laswai *et al.* (1991) observed that modern pigs eat 16% less than predicted by the AFRC (1981), so great care needs to be exercised in formulating rations.

The pig is no longer to be thought of as a glutton! However, the pig, like any other animal, eats to supply its requirements and the cause of low intake is low potential for fattening.

There is important genetic variation in food intake between and within breeds. e.g. for the Pietrain it is 0.87 of that for the Large White (Webb, 1989). Within a breed, heritability of intake is about 0.3 and shows genetic correlations with growth rate (positive) and lean content (negative) but not with efficiency of utilization of food. The correlations between test station and commercial farm performance are low (0.25 for growth rate and 0.40 for backfat), so some of the genetic improvement must not be being expressed on farms, i.e. there are genotype × production system interactions. This may be due to test stations using individual feeding and some genes affecting social behaviour not being expressed in the test environment. It is less likely that different levels of feeding on test stations compared with commercial farms are responsible for the discrepancy, as genotype × feeding level interactions have not been conclusively demonstrated.

After seven generations of selection, with reduction in fatness being the major trait in the selection index, average daily food intake was reduced from 2.71 kg day$^{-1}$ in a control, random selection line, to 2.51 kg day$^{-1}$ (Wood, 1989). When selection of pigs was based on an index which included high live weight gain, low backfat thickness and efficient food conversion, voluntary food intake declined for 7 years but then plateaued (Smith *et al.*, 1991). The cumulative responses in intake after 11 years were −0.25 kg day$^{-1}$ for boars and −0.19 for gilts.

However, selection for efficiency is difficult as it involves measurement of intakes by individual pigs and, where it has been used, direct selection for efficiency has not always given an improvement. Selection for increased protein deposition and reduced backfat has usually led to improved efficiency, anyway, so breeders have not been worried about selecting for efficiency. Now equipment is available for monitoring individual food intakes (e.g. Bampton, 1991) and less emphasis is being placed on reduction of backfat. Thus, improvement in efficiency has recently become feasible and attractive but efficiency is a ratio of output to input and ratios have poor statistical properties so that selection responses can be erratic. An alternative is to select against high food intake but this leads to reduced performance.

Selection for efficiency and leanness on feeding *ad libitum* caused reduced voluntary intake; from years 2–4 to 6–8 of the Meat and Livestock Commission's Commercial Product Evaluation scheme,

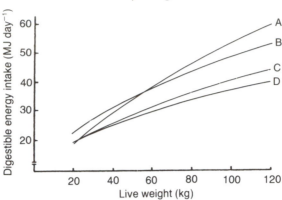

**Fig. 8.6.** Voluntary intakes of digestible energy by pigs growing from 20 to 120 kg body weight (compiled by Cole and Chadd, 1989). Data were published in 1967 (A), 1981 (B), 1987 (C) and 1988 (D) and show a reduction in intake at any given weight over the 20-year period.

voluntary intake fell 6% (Cole and Chadd, 1989). Paradoxically, when selection was done with restricted feeding, voluntary intake was found to be increased (McPhee, 1981). Figure 8.6 shows the increase in intake with body weight as pigs grow and how the intake at any given weight has fallen during the period from 1967 to 1988.

What is required is not low intake *per se* but low intake relative to performance, i.e. minimization of the difference between actual food intake and that predicted to be required for maintenance and production, known as Residual Food Consumption (RFC). Although RFC has a lower heritability (0.30–0.38) than food intake (0.45), it is better than for efficiency of food conversion (0.28) (Mrode and Kennedy, 1993). About half the variation in food intake is residual, the causes of which include food wastage, physical activity, digestibility, and efficiency of utilization for maintenance and/or growth. The use of RFI in selection programmes warrants further study.

Fat is now at about the right level in pigs, so the only way to improve efficiency is to increase lean tissue growth to reduce the maintenance cost per unit of production. In future, therefore, testing and selection should be made on *ad lib* feeding, penning in groups to allow expression of genes for behaviour under commercial conditions, and recording of individual intakes to measure genetic differences in maintenance which cannot be predicted either from growth rate or backfat.

The ability to feed *ad libitum* due to reduced voluntary intake accompanying selection for low fat deposition has enabled *ad lib* feeding systems to be used increasingly commercially with considerable saving in labour.

*Cattle*

Although intakes of cattle of various beef breeds are similar at the same body weight, those for Holsteins are usually higher, by some 8%, although this difference has disappeared by 450 kg (NRC, 1987). Perhaps the lower body fat content of growing Holsteins underlies this difference. Another difference is that beef calves are normally with their dams and can obtain milk up to 6 months of age whereas Holsteins are usually weaned from milk replacer at about 6 weeks and thus have had a longer time to adapt to solid food by the age the comparisons were made. Higher growth potential is likely to be the most important reason.

In a comparison of 1-year-old cattle of 25 breeds Taylor *et al.* (1986) found a close relationship between the logarithm of daily food intake and the logarithm of body weight. The regression coefficient of 0.42, indicating that intake was proportional to body weight$^{0.42}$, is much smaller than intrabreed coefficients, which lay between 0.61 and 0.82, indicating that intake cannot be predicted from body weight alone, without a knowledge of the animal's breed.

*Sheep*

Merino sheep selected for high weaning weight had higher food intake than a strain selected for low weight at weaning, which to some extent persisted even when intake was expressed on a per kilogram basis (Thompson *et al.*, 1985).

### Compensatory growth

Following a period of reduced growth, caused by restriction of feed or illness or environmental stress, animals grow at a faster rate than unrestricted animals of the same age (Wilson and Osbourn, 1960). This phenomenon is called compensatory growth and is due to increased voluntary food intake, increased weight of gut contents and improved efficiency of conversion. The latter may be due to reduced maintenance requirements. Whether the increased intake is a result of or a cause of the increased growth is not easy to answer; restriction will have reduced the fat content of the body which will tend to increase appetite (see below).

*Poultry*

Osbourn and Wilson (1960) demonstrated a compensatory increase in food intake by cockerels following restriction. However, more recent work with broiler chickens, in which restriction was to 85% of *ad libitum*, was not followed by an increase in intake when *ad libitum* access was restored (Yalda and Forbes, 1990). It must be noted that during restriction the protein content of the food was increased to maintain the same protein intake as controls and protein deposition was not reduced. It may be that compensation for a period of restriction is due to the low body protein for the animals' age, rather than to reduced body fat.

## Pigs

Restriction of pigs of 25–50 kg live weight to half of the *ad libitum* level of feed was followed by increased intakes when free access was given, to the extent of 15% above unrestricted controls (Cole *et al.*, 1968).

## Cattle

Ruminants are often subjected to periods of underfeeding, both in the wild and in practical animal husbandry. Therefore, many studies of compensatory growth in ruminants have been undertaken and Moran and Holmes (1978) have reviewed the results of trials with cattle and concluded that compensatory growth is largely dependent on compensatory increases in voluntary intake. Wanyoike and Holmes (1981) observed a significantly higher herbage intake by cattle which had been fed at a low level during the previous winter compared to those fed at a high level

The unexpectedly low heat production of adequately fed ruminants after a period of restriction may occur as a result of reduced thyroid hormone secretion (Fox *et al.*, 1974).

## Sheep

In sheep, Allden (1968) found that lambs recovered from a period of restricted feeding if subsequently fed *ad libitum*. Four-month-old wether sheep were held at a weight of 20 kg for either 4 or 6 months and then offered free access to a good quality feed. During the re-feeding period the wethers had a higher food intake and lower heat production than the controls which had been fed *ad libitum* throughout (Graham and Searle, 1975). The increased voluntary intake which occurs during compensatory growth was found to be unrelated to the metabolizable energy content of the diet by Lee (1974) although compensation was better on a high quality feed than one of poor quality (Moran, 1976).

From a review of the literature, Bassett (1960) concluded that the longer the period of restricted feeding, the greater the food intake when *ad libitum* feeding was resumed. His experimental results showed that gut fill was very high – as much as 25% of body weight – in compensating lambs, compared with 15% in controls offered free access to food throughout. Although this difference could be due to the greater availability of abdominal capacity in the restricted lambs, which were thinner, it is more likely that the increased rate of utilization of nutrients was the primary stimulus to higher intake which in turn resulted in a higher volume of rumen contents. The high intake during compensatory growth is not likely to be caused by low thyroid secretion rate *per se*, however, because treatment of sheep with exogenous thyroxine stimulates voluntary intake even though body reserves may be mobilized to support the higher metabolic rate (e.g. Lambourne, 1964). Figure 8.5 shows the decline in relative intake of a complete feed by growing cattle and the higher intake of animals which had suffered a period of restriction before introduction to the experiment (Pickard *et al.*, 1969).

*Between-species differences*

As with differences between breeds and between individuals, it is likely that differences in food intake between species can be accounted for by differences in potential to grow and fatten, by differences in gut capacity and/or differences in the types of foods eaten.

There have been numerous reports suggesting that alpacas eat less than sheep per unit of body weight. Using faecal output and digestibility of mature males weighing 42 kg, herbage intake was estimated by Reiner *et al.* (1987) to be 1.6 and 1.8 kg organic matter per day in the wet and dry seasons, respectively, when the crude protein contents were 81 and 126 g kg$^{-1}$, respectively. These are similar to intakes of sheep of similar weight.

## Growth manipulation

*Antibiotics*

*Pigs*
Several antibiotics may be included in pig diets. These often increase efficiency of digestion but also consistently increase voluntary food intake to a small extent in experiments in which *ad libitum* feeding was practised (e.g. Thrasher *et al.*, 1970 with carbadox; Costain and Lloyd, 1962 with zinc bacitracin; Barber *et al.*, 1978 with virginiamycin).

*Cattle*

Monensin and similar feed additives modify rumen fermentation to increase the production of propionate and reduce methane production. They are widely used commercially as they improve food conversion efficiency. In beef cattle there is either no increase in weight gain and reduced voluntary food intake or increased gain with no change in intake (e.g. Raun *et al.,* 1976). Beef cows produce milk more efficiently, forage intake being depressed from 9.6 to 8.3 and 7.7 kg day$^{-1}$ by the inclusion of 50 to 200 mg day$^{-1}$ of monensin in the food, with no consistent effect on weight change (Lemenager *et al.,* 1978). In a second trial by the same authors, weight gains were improved and milk yields were not affected, even though the amount of time spent grazing was decreased by the inclusion of monensin in the concentrate supplement. Baile *et al.* (1979) suggested that the decrease in intake which occurs when monensin is included in concentrated feeds for cattle is due to an aversion to some sensory cue associated with the malaise resulting from the change in rumen fermentation.

*Anabolic steroids*

*Poultry*

Oestrogens have been used commercially to stimulate weight gains; their effect, unlike that in ruminant animals, is primarily to stimulate feed intake and, in the absence of marked stimulation of true growth, the rate of fat deposition (e.g. Hill *et al.,* 1958). Even in force-fed broilers, oestrogen treatment significantly increased the weight of feed consumed voluntarily (Polin and Wolford, 1977). The use of steroidal growth promoters has now been banned in the EU.

*Pigs*

Voluntary intake decreased during treatment with 2.2 mg DES and 2.2 mg methyl testosterone, from 2.81 and 2.41 kg day$^{-1}$ in castrated males and from 2.42 to 2.35 kg day$^{-1}$ in gilts (Jordan *et al.,* 1965). To what extent this reduction was due to direct effects of the oestrogens on intake, and to what extent to reduced fat deposition induced by the steroid, is not clear. Anabolic agents of this type are not used commercially because of the risk of residues in meat and because the growth stimulation is less than in ruminants where intake is not depressed.

The use of uncastrated boars for meat production is increasing since the rate of lean meat production is increased and the propensity to fatten is sufficiently low that they can be fed *ad libitum* (see above).

*Cattle*

After the discovery in the early 1950s that DES, a synthetic oestrogen, had anabolic properties and was orally active in ruminants its use was widely adopted in the USA. Voluntary intake is increased in response to increased weight gain due to greater secretion of growth hormone which, by stimulating growth, increases the rate of utilization of metabolites. DES was withdrawn in the early 1970s because of fears concerning its safety to human consumers of meat. In the UK another synthetic oestrogen, hexoestrol, was used because it is not orally active and is therefore potentially safer, but this has also been banned.

Natural oestrogens, which have very similar biological effects to DES and hexoestrol but a much shorter half-life, were then used on an extensive scale; they stimulate growth in castrated or intact male ruminants and food intake is increased (Davis *et al.*, 1984).

Androgens stimulate growth by means other than growth hormone, probably by a direct effect on muscle. Trenbolone acetate was widely used as it stimulates growth without including undesirable male characteristics. It is likely that the effect of androgens on intake (e.g. O'Mary *et al.*, 1952) is due to the increased demand for nutrients, although a more direct effect was suggested by the results of Heitzman and Walker (1973) who reported a large and rapid increase in voluntary intake in ketotic cows treated with 60 to 120 mg trenbolone acetate.

*Sheep*

Voluntary intake by sheep of a 0.5 hay:0.5 concentrate feed was increased by DES from 1.43 to 1.50 kg day$^{-1}$ (Andrews and Beeson, 1953). This increase in intake is the response to increased weight gain rather than its cause. Restricting treated animals to the same weight of feed as controls does not completely prevent the increase in weight gain and carcass weight.

*Growth hormone*

There was a dose-related decrease in carcass fatness in lambs treated with growth hormone (GH) but live weight gain and food intake from 10 to 22 weeks of age were not significantly different although intake tended to decline with increasing dose, from 0.025 to 0.25 mg kg$^{-1}$day$^{-1}$ (Johnsson *et al.*, 1987).

*Somatoliberin*

Somatoliberin, otherwise known as growth hormone releasing factor, given intracerebroventricularly in sheep at a dose of 100 ng kg$^{-1}$, stimulated intake of concentrates only in the first hour but the intake of hay after a delay of 1 h (Riviere and Bueno, 1987). Insulin blocked this effect which suggests that it was due to release of GH whose effects on adipose tissue are blocked by insulin.

### Immunization against somatostatin

Somatostatin is a hypothalamic factor which reduces the secretion of GH by the anterior pituitary and immunization of sheep against it has been found to stimulate growth under some conditions. However, in an experiment in which food intake was measured (Zainurt *et al.*, 1991) there was no difference in plasma GH level, growth, feed intake or feeding behaviour, despite high antisomatostatin titres.

### Cortisol

Corticosteroids, whose secretion increases during stress, are catabolic in laboratory animals but have stimulated weight gains and food intake in several experiments with sheep. Bassett (1963) gave 25–75 mg cortisol per day intramuscularly to sheep for three weeks which resulted in plasma levels similar to those seen during stress. Intake and weight gains were increased, especially when intake was otherwise low because of seasonal factors. Doses of 25 mg given three times per week had no effect on the voluntary food intake of lambs but 100 or 300 mg stimulated intake from 934 to 1170 g day$^{-1}$ of alfalfa and from 1107 to 1306 g day$^{-1}$ of a 0.5 alfalfa:0.5 barley ration (Spurlock and Clegg, 1962). Cortisol tended to reduce the amount of protein in the carcass but increased the amount of fat significantly.

Ellington *et al.* (1967) combined cortisone treatment with DES to see whether the higher intake due to the former could be combined with the greater protein deposition induced by the latter. Control sheep ate 1.65 kg day$^{-1}$ of the pelleted diet whereas those implanted in the ear with 3 mg DES had a mean intake of 1.72 kg day$^{-1}$. Those given 100 mg of cortisone three times per week had a daily intake of 1.97 kg, but intake was slightly lower than this when both treatments were administered (1.89 kg day$^{-1}$). Withdrawal of the cortisone treatment 2 weeks before slaughter to reduce fat deposition also reduced the mean intake to 1.65 kg day$^{-1}$.

With cattle similar results have been obtained; Carroll *et al.* (1963) subcutaneously injected 1 g of cortisone acetate three times per week and found that voluntary intake was increased significantly from 12.1 to 13.9 kg day$^{-1}$ with an increase in carcass fat.

## β-Agonists

β-Adrenergic agonists were originally investigated for their ability to reduce fat deposition but were also found to stimulate muscle growth. Ricks *et al.* (1984) found that 10 mg day$^{-1}$ of the β-agonist clenbuterol in the feed for steers significantly altered carcass composition without affecting voluntary intake. Overdosing with 500 mg day$^{-1}$ to study the toxic effects depressed intake.

## Cyproheptadine

Cyproheptadine, a pharmacological antagonist to serotonin, stimulates food intake and growth rate in children and rats. Oral administration of 0.64–1.92 mg kg$^{-1}$ live weight day$^{-1}$ to growing cockerels caused a dose-dependent increase in daily food intake (Injidi and Forbes, 1987) but there was no improvement in feed conversion efficiency and it is unlikely that such treatment would be useful commercially.

## Maturity

### Poultry

Broiler breeder stock become very fat if allowed to eat *ad libitum* and, in practice, have to be fed at a severely restricted level if reduced reproductive rate is to be avoided (Chapter 9).

### Pigs

There are discrepancies as to whether intake actually declines in growing pigs once they have reached around 100 kg live weight. Ewan (1983) found a plateau but no decline whereas Siebrits and Kemm (1982) observed a decline once their South African pigs had reached 70 kg. Mahan and Gerber (1984) found a slight decline from 100 kg and Giles *et al.* (1981) reported a decline from 60 kg. In gilts there was a decline of 21 g feed per day as they grew from 125 to 180 kg (Friend, 1973) which might have been due to the onset of oestrus during this time.

### Sheep

Ewes lose their teeth from the age of about 6 years which can reduce rate of eating, especially of hard foods such as swedes. This is only likely to affect the intake of foods which are eaten very slowly, however, and Dove and Milne (1991) found almost no difference in intake of long herbage between ewes with full and broken mouths even though live weight gain and body condition score were lower for those ewes with poorer teeth. Newton and Jackson (1983) observed a positive relationship among old ewes between the number of incisors and intake of short grass and hay, but not with long grass.

## Fatness and Food Intake

### Relationships between body fat and intake

Most adults of many species maintain a more-or-less constant body weight despite changes in food quality and climate. Perhaps Kennedy (1953) was the first to propose that it was primarily by a control of body fat content that body weight was maintained – thus the lipostatic theory. It was not until the work of Liebelt *et al.* (1965) that evidence was found for the defence of fat rather than any other component. Surgical removal of part of the inguinal fat organ was followed by hyperphagia and a return to the preoperative level of fat and body weight. However, partial lipectomy of rats (Faust *et al.*, 1977; Gavin *et al.*, 1984) has not resulted in any compensatory increase in food intake or fat deposition, suggesting that it is not total fat mass but perhaps adipocyte size which exerts a control on intake.

The statement that body fat content is held constant by changes in energy intake (and/or output) cannot now be regarded as sacrosanct. Incorporation of fat in a diet for rats, for example, gives a reduction in intake, but not sufficient to maintain a constant level of digestible energy intake which remains slightly higher than with the standard food with the result that the animals gain weight slowly (e.g. Jacobs, 1967). Similar phenomena are also observed in chickens and pigs (see Chapter 10). Perhaps it is due to the improvement in the palatability of the food; certainly offering rats a wide choice of foods which they find attractive (cafeteria feeding) results in considerable overeating and weight gain, although such foods are often high in fat content.

On the other hand a theory of metabolic efficiency, heat production or comfort might account for these observations as dietary fat is used efficiently for body fat deposition so diets high in fat do not involve as much metabolic work and/or discomfort as carbohydrate diets for body fat deposition.

The influence of fatness on intake of those species which have been selected genetically for rapid weight gain, e.g. pigs, cattle, sheep, broiler chickens, seems to be less than in other species, e.g. rats, goats, laying hens, which have not been so selected.

## Poultry

Force feeding of chickens, at a level which caused great increases in the fat stores, was followed by complete absence of voluntary feeding for up to 10 days and even 23 days after the cessation of force feeding the birds had not recovered their pre-experimental level of intake (Lepkovsky and Furuta, 1971). Plasma triglyceride concentrations were elevated during the period of force feeding. In similar work Polin and Wolford (1973) showed that force feeding an amount equivalent to half the previous daily intake depressed voluntary intake to about 63% (i.e. 13% overeating). In birds of a laying strain force-fed with up to 150% of the *ad libitum* intake food intake was depressed to a few grams per day (Fig. 8.7) and there was a great increase in body fatness, including that of the liver (Nir *et al.*, 1974); this is not surprising as the liver is the major site of fat synthesis in chickens. These results do not necessarily show that excessive fatness *per se* depresses voluntary intake. Smith and Baranowski-Kish (1979), on the other hand, have argued that Polin and Wolford's results support the lipostatic theory because there was a decrease in voluntary intake in response to force feeding. In the

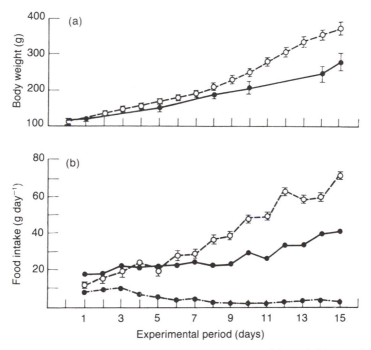

**Fig. 8.7.** Body weights and total intakes of *ad libitum* (O--O) and force-fed (●—●) chicks. ●--·-● shows the *ad libitum* intakes of the force-fed birds. (From Nir *et al.*, 1974; reproduced with permission.)

absence of any data on metabolic changes induced by force feeding this is only a demonstration that there is a control over food intake in chickens, however imperfect.

More recently Yalda and Forbes (1991) have shown that force feeding of growing broiler chickens the same amount as the voluntary intake of control birds, divided into five meals spread throughout the day, did not completely suppress feeding, which continued at 30% of control to give a total daily intake considerably higher than normal. This resulted in a great increase in fat deposition so it was surprising that, when force feeding was terminated, voluntary intake *increased* to 122% of control and only slowly declined to the control level over the next few weeks. Apparently the over-provision of nutrients during force feeding had stimulated the rate of fat deposition and this had got the body into such a metabolic state that the high demand for nutrients generated a high voluntary intake.

Reduction of body fat by a period of restricted feeding of young broilers of 4 to 7 weeks of age was not followed by significant overeating when *ad libitum* access to food was reinstated (Yalda and Forbes, 1990); in this case the protein content of the food was increased for the restricted birds so that muscle and bone growth were not stunted. Mild restriction (130 g day$^{-1}$) of older broilers from 18 to 47 weeks of age, without increasing the protein concentration of the food, was followed by hyperphagia (180 g day$^{-1}$) for 2 weeks before a steady rate (160 g day$^{-1}$) was achieved (March *et al.*, 1982). Probably the increased intake was a response to reduced protein deposition during the period of restriction.

A problem with these manipulations is that a period of abnormal nutrition is involved to which control birds are not subjected. This was overcome by partial lipectomy involving surgical removal of the abdominal fat-pad of chickens by Maurice *et al.* (1983) and Taylor and Forbes (1988). Table 8.1 shows that both lipectomized and sham-operated birds recovered their preoperative food intakes quite rapidly, ate similar amounts of food and gained at similar rates; when slaughtered at 14-weeks of age the lipectomized birds were lighter than the controls by an amount (154 g) very similar to the weight of fat removed at surgery (190 g). The conclusion drawn is that broilers of this age do not compensate for removal of fat by increasing their food intake. However, there might be a difference between: (i) birds which have had all their various fat depots depleted by a period of underfeeding, which can be repleted when *ad libitum* feeding is reintroduced; and (ii) those in which one fat depot is surgically removed thus preventing any more deposition at that site – the remaining depots might be depositing fat at the maximum rate throughout and there would be no possibility for them to increase their rate of synthesis after removal of the fat-pad.

**Table 8.1.** Effect of surgical removal of the abdominal fat-pad of 10-week-old female broiler chickens on weight gain, feed intake and fat-pad weight (gram ± standard error) (Taylor and Forbes, 1988).

|  | Sham-operated | Lipectomized | Difference |
|---|---|---|---|
| Body weight gain |  |  |  |
| during 3 weeks before operation | 758 ± 25 | 802 ± 61 | n.s. |
| during 4 weeks after operation | 1100 ± 49 | 1153 ± 94 | n.s. |
| Total feed intake |  |  |  |
| during 3 weeks before operation | 3631 ± 225 | 3658 ± 141 | n.s. |
| during 4 weeks after operation | 5455 ± 170 | 5400 ± 313 | n.s. |
| Live weight before slaughter | 4271 ± 101 | 4117 ± 154 | n.s. |
| Carcass weight including fat-pad | 3656 ± 91 | 3496 ± 135 | n.s. |
| Fat-pad at operation | – | 85 ± 6 |  |
| Fat-pad at slaughter | 190 ± 12 | – |  |

n.s., Not significant.

The abdominal fat-pad may not be truly representative of fat in general as it has a later maturity than other fat depots (J. Wiseman, personal communication). It is clear that the food intake of chickens is not closely controlled by the amount of fat in the body.

## Pigs

Domestic pigs may become grossly overweight, as if the feedbacks from fat are reduced or ignored by the brain. It might thus be suggested that the lipostatic theory does not apply and that intake is limited by the maximum rate of fat synthesis above which precursors will accumulate and prevent higher levels of food intake. Perhaps selection for rapid weight gain (with little regard for composition at a time when fat was more acceptable to the consumer) was a selection against negative feedback from fat to the central nervous system. Selection against fat deposition in recent years has been accompanied by reduced voluntary intake (see above).

## Cattle

European domesticated breeds of cattle become very fat if offered free access to high quality feeds, but eventually reach a plateau. Monteiro (1972) fed non-pregnant mature cows *ad libitum* on a pelleted food. Friesians were still gaining weight at about 1 kg day$^{-1}$ when they weighed 700 kg, whereas Jerseys showed signs of a plateau at about 430 kg. Bines *et al.* (1969) fed cows at two levels to bring them into either fat or thin condition. Subsequently when straw was offered alone mean intakes were similar for both groups but thin cows ate 31% more hay or 23% more concentrates than fat ones despite the fact that the fat cows were heavier. The weight of rumen contents was greater in the thin cows than in the fat cows when offered hay and it was thought that rumen capacity was limiting hay intake. The higher intake of concentrates by the thin animals was attributed to their greater capacity for lipogenesis.

*Sheep*

Food intake by sheep in generally inversely related to the proportion of fat in the body. Ewes with a body condition score of 3.0 or greater (on a 0–5 scale) had lower intakes of ryegrass/white clover swards in the autumn than did thinner ewes (Gunn *et al.*, 1991). Working with Scottish Blackface ewes, Foot (1972) observed a close inverse correlation between intake of dried grass pellets and condition score (Fig. 8.8).

Blaxter *et al.* (1982) kept sheep on an *ad libitum* feeding regime for up to 4 years from the age of 4 months. There was no difference between the level of intake per animal between 12 months of age and 3.5 years of age. Blaxter and Gill (1979) had concluded from these same data that 'voluntary food intake is established early in life and this determines the ultimate body size sheep attain on a particular diet', because asymptotic body weight was positively related to food intake. In a similar experiment Thompson and Parks (1983) offered a pelleted ration to Merino and Dorset Horn rams and wethers. Intake increased

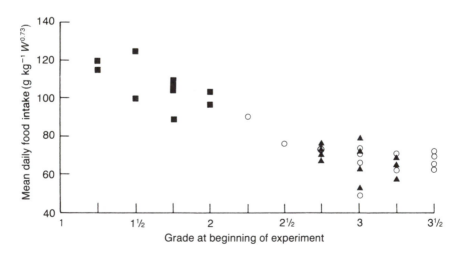

**Fig. 8.8.** Relationship between fatness of Blackface ewes and their intake of dried grass pellets. (From Foot, 1972, reproduced with permission.)

to approximately 50 weeks of age then declined contrary to the pattern seen by Blaxter *et al.* (1982).

Wild and undomesticated ruminants do not become permanently obese but show an annual cycle of fluctuating body weight and fatness (Forbes, 1982b).

## Mechanisms for effects of body fat

### Physical constraints

The underlying reason for the inverse relationship between fatness and voluntary intake in ruminants may be one of competition between abdominal fat and rumen for abdominal space and there have been several reports of negative correlations between the volume of abdominal fat and that of rumen contents.

### Cattle

Karkeek (1845) noted that '... in proportion as an animal [cattle] fattened, so in proportion did the organs which are chiefly concerned with nutrition become diminished in size ... it is rather a remarkable coincidence that the fatter an animal becomes at this period [later stages of fattening], the less food it consumes'. Makela (1956) measured the volume of rumen contents in cows after slaughter and found it to be negatively related to the volume of abdominal fat and further depressed in advanced pregnancy. A negative relationship between the weight of spring herbage eaten and the weight of internal fat at slaughter was found in cattle which had been wintered on different planes of nutrition (Tayler, 1959).

### Sheep

In pregnant ewes slaughtered at various stages of pregnancy it was noted that the volume of rumen contents and the voluntary intake of hay was inversely proportional to the volume of 'incompressible abdominal contents' and that abdominal fat was a significant cause of variation in this (Forbes, 1968) (Chapter 9). If physical limitation were the sole reason for the reciprocal relationship between fatness and intake then fat would not depress intake when highly digestible feeds were given but the work of Orr (1977) showed that intake was lower in fat animals even when a highly digestible diet was fed.

### Metabolic constraints

The continuous turnover of adipose tissue involves the release of fatty acids, glycerol and ketones. Glycerol levels in blood do not increase during a meal so that any involvement in the control of intake is more likely to be as a long-term signal of adiposity, added to the immediate signals of the nutrient value of food being eaten or recently eaten. Wirtshafter and Davis (1977a) showed that exogenous glycerol depressed intake and suggested that glycerol might be a factor linking adiposity with intake as adipose tissue is continually releasing fatty acids and glycerol. However, it might simply be oxidation in the liver that is responsible for the intake-depressing effect of exogenous glycerol. The effect of glycerol on feeding was prevented when a high protein diet was given, which would reduce the rate of glycerol oxidation in the liver.

The metabolic mechanisms of effects of fatness on intake have been reviewed by Scharrer and Langhans (1990). Inhibition of fatty acid utilization with mercaptoacetate reduced the latency to eat without affecting meal size, thus implicating fatty acid oxidation in the maintenance of satiety after a meal.

A net synthesis of lipids and deposition in adipose tissue is a drain on nutrients, particularly glucose and fatty acids, from the blood which will cause a compensatory increase in food intake. However, there must be an upper limit to the rate and amount of fat deposition and when either of these limits is approached the uptake of nutrients for fat synthesis will be reduced and food intake will decline.

Because of its importance in controlling fat deposition, insulin has received quite a lot of attention in studies on relationships between body fatness and voluntary food intake. In particular, insulin resistance increases with increasing body fatness.

*Poultry*
One of the effects of fat in the diet of mammals is to slow the rate of emptying of the stomach and this has been confirmed in hens (Mateos *et al.*, 1982) but not in young broilers (Golian and Polin, 1984). If a reduction in rate of passage does occur it might in turn depress feed intake by a stomach distension mechanism. In view of the discussion above, there is clearly a lot of scope for studies on the involvement of lipids in the mechanisms which control intake in the chicken.

*Cattle*
McCann and Reimers (1985) found that plasma insulin was higher in obese (condition score, 4.) than lean (score, 3.2) heifers and that there was a bigger insulin response to glucose in the obese, especially during oestrus.

*Sheep and goats*

There must be a positive relationship between intake and rate of fat deposition, other factors being equal and Mears and Mendel (1974) concluded from an experiment with young lambs that intake was stimulated in animals with greater numbers of adipocytes, due to the faster removal of metabolites from the circulating pool – 'the amount of glucose removed from the glucose pool could be the feed-back signal which results in a high long-term food intake'. It is in older animals that the established size of the fat depots affects intake in a negative manner.

Adipose tissue is continually undergoing lipolysis and lipogenesis and plasma free fatty acid levels are approximately proportional to body fat stores. Intravenous infusion of long-chain fatty acids depresses feed intake in sheep (Vandermeerschen-Doize and Paquay, 1984) but this is not likely to represent a simple feedback loop because high free fatty acid levels also occur in underfed animals which, if offered free access to food, eat more than well-fed animals. However, a well-fed animal has high plasma insulin levels whereas an underfed one has a low rate of insulin secretion. Perhaps fatty acids are only satiating in the presence of high insulin concentrations in plasma.

McCann *et al.* (1992) fed adult Dorset ewes in lean condition a pelleted hay-grain food and observed a doubling of body weight over 42 weeks from 47 to 97 kg and the lipid content of the carcass increased from 25 to 49%. Between weeks 5 and 20, intakes were at the maximum allowed (3.0 kg day$^{-1}$) but then fell steadily to about 1.2 kg at 42 weeks. Once they had reached the static phase of obesity, intake per unit body weight was the same as required for maintenance by lean sheep. Plasma insulin rose from 50 to 249 pmol l$^{-1}$ by week 30. At around week 25 thyroid hormones rose significantly, plasma free fatty acid levels rose and voluntary intake started to decline, changes which might have been related to changes in morphology and/or humoral signals emanating from adipocytes. The high insulin levels coupled with high plasma glucose showed that insulin resistance had occurred. Heparin, which activates lipoprotein lipase and increases plasma fatty acid levels, depressed food intake, but whether or not the observed increase in plasma free fatty acid levels is an intermediary is not known (Seoane *et al.*, 1972b).

In order to examine the relationships between fatness and intake critically it is better to work with animals whose differences in fatness are imposed by the experimenter, rather than by natural differences in fatness. Donnelly *et al.* (1974) controlled the food intake of mature Merino wether sheep, initially weighing about 33 kg, until one group weighed 37 kg, another 30 kg and a third weighed 28 kg and found no effect on subsequent intake. Graham (1969), starting with sheep with an average weight of 50 kg, fed them differentially until 33% or 7% of their weight was fat. Subsequent dry matter intakes were 65 and 106 kg$^{-1}$ live weight$^{0.75}$ day$^{-1}$ so that fatness had a clear effect on intake in these animals, which were taken to more extreme levels of fatness than those of Donnelly *et al.* (1974).

Vandermeerschen-Doize *et al.* (1982) found that plasma insulin concentration increased steadily from 10 to 300 μU ml$^{-1}$ over a 35-week period of *ad libitum* feeding of sheep; by the end of this period body weight stabilized. De Jong (1981b) also found that insulin concentration increased in goats as they got fatter. This suggests that the declining intake was not simply due to a reduction in rumen capacity with increasing volume of abdominal fat; had this been the only cause then insulin levels would have been more likely to decrease due to a fall in plane of nutrition. Orr (1977) offered feeds of three qualities (8.4, 10.0 or 12.2 MJ metabolizable energy (ME) kg$^{-1}$ DM) to lean or fat mature sheep (52.2 or 83.2 kg live weight). In both lean and fat animals voluntary food intake compensated for differences in ME concentration although intake was significantly lower in the fat groups. Thus, the fat animals were still controlling their ME intake, but at a lower level than the lean sheep. These experiments show that in animals with equal propensity to fatten (assuming random allocation of animals to experimental groups) increasing fatness is associated with declining voluntary intake.

The only experiment with ruminants reporting surgical removal of fat is that of Joubert and Ueckerman (1971) who removed the tail of fat-tailed sheep, which weighed 1.9 kg in the undocked animals at slaughter. However, the subsequent weight gains were the same as those of unoperated control animals and there was no increase in body fat to compensate for the loss of the large tail deposit.

It can be concluded, therefore, that the effects of fat and fattening on food intake are complex and the mechanisms involved will be difficult to unravel.

## Conclusions

The higher the intake of milk by the sucking animal the lower its intake of dry food and this can increase the setback at weaning, when the withdrawal of the supply of milk stimulates the intake of solid food, encouraged by creep feeding before weaning. Artificially fed ruminants respond to dilution of the milk replacer by changes in intake in the appropriate direction but not usually to an extent sufficient to maintain the same intake of energy.

Food intake increases as animals grow, not in direct proportion to live weight but more usually in proportion to live weight raised to the power of 0.6. A period of restricted feeding is followed by higher voluntary intake and a tendency to catch up with the live weight of unrestricted controls.

Although fatness depresses the intake of farm animals, as it does in other species, the effect is less and as they approach maturity pigs, broiler chickens, cattle and lowland breeds of sheep become very fat if fed *ad libitum* on good quality diets. We must accept that the control of feed intake is very complex and not expect to be able to make simple statements about its interrelationships with body weight and fatness.

# 9 | REPRODUCTION AND LACTATION

- Oestrus
- Pregnancy
- Lactation
- The laying hen
- Conclusions

The changes in nutrient requirements which take place during pregnancy, lactation and egg-laying lead to changes in voluntary food intake but these are not always well balanced and unwanted increases or decreases in body fatness often arise.

A decrease in food intake is often observed at the time of oestrus, when oestrogen levels are high and progesterone is low. Pregnancy, during which progesterone secretion is high throughout, is accompanied by increased food intake although in sheep there is often a decline in the last few weeks. The onset of lactation at the time of parturition is almost always accompanied by a sharp increase in food intake but this lags behind the increase in nutrient requirements of lactation. Forbes (1986b) has reviewed the physiological changes which are associated with these changes in intake in ruminants.

## Oestrus

There are several changes occurring during female reproduction which are responsible for changes in voluntary intake. Oestrogens, which are associated with small increases in intake when used at low doses as growth promoters, depress intake when secreted in larger quantities

(50 µg day$^{-1}$ in the ewe) by the ovaries at oestrus or by the placenta in the last few weeks of pregnancy.

Although it is known that there are oestrogen receptors in the brain and it had been assumed that the primary effects of oestrogens on behaviour were through these receptors, Wade and Gray (1979) have assembled a wide range of evidence for the concept that gonadal steroids also have important effects on peripheral tissues and it is changes in the metabolic activity of these tissues which cause secondary changes in feeding behaviour (Forbes, 1980b).

## Pigs

During the week which included oestrus in sows the total food intake was found to be 4 kg lower than in each of the other 2 weeks of the cycle (Friend, 1973). The most likely reason for this is that blood oestrogen levels are high at oestrus.

## Cattle

In the cow total food intake sometimes declines at oestrus (Hurnik *et al.,* 1975), less time is spent eating (Putnam and Bond, 1971) and there also seems to be a change in the choice of food. J.H. Metz (personal communication) noticed that the intake of concentrates declined whereas that of hay increased at oestrus (cows usually eat about 20% of their intake as hay if it is available free choice with concentrates (Bines, 1979).

## Sheep and goats

Concentrate intake is often decreased for a day or two around oestrus and intake was depressed in a dose-dependent manner when oestradiol was infused intravenously into lactating goats

$$I = 1.3 - 0.008 \, E_2 \tag{9.1}$$

where *I* is intake of concentrates (kg day$^{-1}$) and $E_2$ is oestradiol dose (µg day$^{-1}$) (Forbes, 1986b) although there was no effect on hay intake. The concentrate intake of goats was further depressed at oestrus by an amount equivalent to that caused by 50 µg of oestradiol per day – approximately the rate of secretion of oestrogens by the ovary during oestrus (Forbes, 1986b) (Fig. 9.1).

The differential effect of oestrogens on the intakes of concentrates and forage is also illustrated by the results of an experiment in which oestradiol was infused into castrated male sheep (Forbes, 1972). When hay was offered intravenous infusions of oestradiol at up to 400 µg

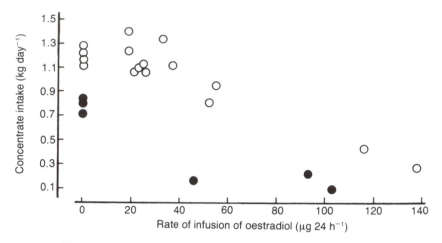

**Fig. 9.1** Effect of oestradiol infusion on food intake by a goat (Forbes, 1980b). When the animal was in oestrus (●) there was a further reduction in intake equivalent to approximately 50 μg oestradiol day$^{-1}$.

day$^{-1}$ had no consistent effect but when a complete pelleted diet was offered a 90 μg day$^{-1}$ infusion caused a lower food intake, followed by a significant increase in intake after treatment was stopped.

# Pregnancy

In rats and mice there is increased food intake during pregnancy which matches the high nutrient requirements of large litters of fetuses. On the day of parturition, intake is very low as the mother prepares her nest and enters the first stages of labour.

## Pigs

The pregnant sow tends to overeat and is usually fed at a restricted level to prevent overfatness. In an effort to develop a dilute food which could be given *ad libitum* to pregnant sows, Zoiopoulous *et al.* (1983) diluted a standard sow food with ground oat husks at 500 g kg$^{-1}$. The mean intake was 5.50 kg day$^{-1}$ which supported a pregnancy weight gain of 59 kg, which was considered excessive; the authors recommended trying an even more dilute food in order to restrict energy intake to provide for a weight gain of not more than 30 kg.

The possibility of using a food with high fibre content to restrict pregnant sows' intake was further investigated by Brouns *et al.* (1991).

Six foods were made to have equal digestible energy content, by including sugar beet pulp (650 g kg$^{-1}$), straw (360 g kg$^{-1}$), oat husk (370 g kg$^{-1}$), malt culms (460 g kg$^{-1}$), rice bran (610 g kg$^{-1}$) or wheat bran (670 g kg$^{-1}$) Five of these were eaten at 6–8 kg day$^{-1}$ with the sows gaining weight excessively but the food which included sugar beet pulp was only eaten at 2.3 kg day$^{-1}$ which gave a small weight loss. This prompted Brouns *et al.* (1992a) to study a food with 600 g kg$^{-1}$ of unmolassed sugar beet pulp and it was confirmed that this allowed sows to be fed *ad libitum* throughout pregnancy without becoming obese. They observed that low ranking sows were at a disadvantage when fed conventional food at a restricted level in a group, but not when fed *ad libitum* on the beet pulp-based food. The rate of eating of this food was much slower than of a conventional diet (Brouns *et al.,* 1992b). This group subsequently confirmed that the 600 g kg$^{-1}$ sugar beet pulp food can be fed *ad libitum* to gilts in their first pregnancy without excessive weight gain (Stewart *et al.,* 1993). Other fibrous materials such as malt draff also restrict intake by sows fed *ad libitum* (Edwards *et al.,* 1992). Such a feeding system reduces fighting among sows as well as preventing excessive weight gain and is therefore thought to be good for the animals' welfare.

Hutson (1992) studied the extent to which sows will work for food and nesting materials just before farrowing. Sows were trained to lift a lever to obtain straw, twigs, a portion of food or nothing. They lifted for food most frequently by a factor of 20–433 times demonstrating that motivation for food completely overshadows that for nesting materials. However, in two of the food-reinforced sows, the onset of nest building resulted in complete cessation of responding.

*Cattle*

Although pregnant ruminants may increase their voluntary intake in mid-pregnancy this increase is proportionately smaller than that which occurs in the rat or the pig. From the results of their experiments and a survey of the literature, Johnson *et al.* (1966) concluded '… it is safe to say that suggestions of increased appetite accompanying pregnancy in dairy cattle are entirely unfounded'. However, there is sometimes a modest increase in mid-pregnancy in heifers (Penzhorn and Meintjes, 1992).

There is often a noticeable decrease of intake in late pregnancy; Ingvartsen *et al.* (1992a) presented a comprehensive table of 20 groups of cows from nine publications which shows changes of voluntary intake in late pregnancy ranging from an increase of 0.2% week$^{-1}$ to a decline of 9.4% week$^{-1}$. In their own observations, heifers in the last 14 weeks of pregnancy reduced intake of a complete food by 1.53%

(0.17 kg) per week with an even higher rate of decline in the last two weeks.

Putnam and Bond (1971) noticed that in the last month of pregnancy cows spent less time eating than those in early pregnancy or non-pregnant cows. Cows in late pregnancy ate less hay than non-pregnant cows (Campling, 1966b) and the intake of hay by cows supplemented with 4.5 kg of concentrates per day also declined in the last 6 weeks of pregnancy (Curran *et al.*, 1967). Voluntary intake was also seen to decline during the last month of pregnancy in cows by Owen *et al.* (1968). There was a significant correlation between the decline in the last 6 weeks before parturition and the birth weight of the calf in the work of Lenkeit *et al.* (1966).

There can be no doubt, therefore, that in many situations cows reduce their intake in late pregnancy.

*Sheep*

With ewes fed on hay, small increases in intake in mid-pregnancy have been noted with grazing ewes (Owen and Ingleton 1963; Forbes, 1970). Hadjipieris and Holmes (1966) saw increased intake in mid-pregnancy in single-bearing ewes but not in those carrying twins.

In the last few weeks of pregnancy there is often a decline in intake which starts earlier and is steeper the larger the litter size. Intake of hay declined as the volume of the uterus increased (Fig. 9.2).

Figure 9.2 also shows falling intake in ewes in the last few weeks before parturition. Reid and Hinks (1962) and Owen and Ingleton (1963) found a decrease in voluntary herbage intake in late pregnancy, especially with twin-bearing ewes. Pregnant ewes failed to choose an adequate diet when offered a choice of protein concentrate, carbohydrate concentrate and hay (Gordon and Tribe, 1951); only one out of eight bore and reared lambs normally, demonstrating that the ewes did not choose a balanced diet even when suitable ingredients were offered *ad libitum*. Total intake again declined during the last 3 weeks of pregnancy.

Intakes of silage in the last 6 weeks of pregnancy by ewes with twins and multiples were 86 and 81% of those with singles, respectively (Orr and Treacher, 1989), similar to the figures for good hay. With poor quality hay or straw, however, the differences were much greater (63 and 71%, respectively), suggesting that the quality of the forage food has an influence on the severity of the decline.

The fact that forage intake usually falls in late pregnant ewes has prompted the practical use of concentrate supplements, given at increasing levels in the last 6 weeks before parturition. This has often been practised in experiments as well, leading to uncertainty about the

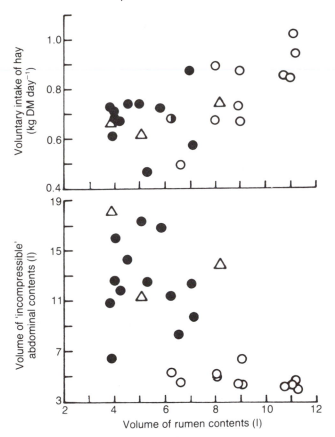

**Fig. 9.2.** Relationships between the volume of rumen contents and (a) the voluntary intake of hay during the 2 weeks before slaughter, and (b) the volume of 'incompressible' abdominal contents in ewes at various stages of pregnancy (Forbes, 1986b). (○) Non-pregnant, (●) single fetus, (△) twin fetuses.

cause of the decline. For example, Wylie and Chestnutt (1992) increased the rate of supplementation of silage from 400 to 600 to 800 g day$^{-1}$ over the last 6 weeks of pregnancy and observed that silage dry matter (DM) intake declined from 758 to 552 g day$^{-1}$ in those ewes which were fed the concentrates once per day, from 853 to 782 g day$^{-1}$ in those given the supplement twice or thrice per day, and from 996 to 876 g day$^{-1}$ in those animals for which the supplement was mixed with the silage. Similarly, Forbes *et al.* (1967) increased the level of supplementation and it is not possible to apportion the cause of the decline in silage intake between pregnancy and substitution for concentrates.

Fat ewes are particularly susceptible to declining voluntary intake in late pregnancy (Everitt, 1966; Foot and Greenhalgh, 1969) and there is a greater reduction in intake of a standard food in late pregnancy in ewes that have been fed at a high level, or on good quality silage, in mid pregnancy (Wilkinson and Chestnutt, 1988; Chestnutt, 1989).

## Causes of declining intake in late pregnancy in ruminants

It is quite possible that the commonly observed decrease in intake is due to the compression of the rumen by the growing uterus, exacerbated by abdominal fat. The displacement of the rumen by the growing conceptus is graphically illustrated by Forbes (1968) who killed sheep at several stages of pregnancy, froze the whole body, cut cross-sections of the abdomen and presented photographs of mid-abdominal sections. There was a negative relationship between the volume of rumen contents at slaughter ($RV$, l) and the volume of 'incompressible abdominal contents' (uterus plus abdominal fat, $IAC$, l) in ewes which had been fed on hay (Forbes, 1969a; Fig. 9.2):

$$RV = 10.4 - 0.39\,IAC \qquad (9.2)$$

Intake during the last 2 weeks before slaughter ($I$, kg day$^{-1}$) was positively related to volume of rumen contents at slaughter:

$$I = 0.50 + 0.03RV \qquad (9.3)$$

The decline in intake was proportionately less than that of rumen volume probably as a result of the increase in rate of passage (Graham and Williams, 1962).

Physical competition may not provide a complete explanation for the decline in intake in late pregnancy because there have been some observations of a decline when concentrates were the sole or main food (cows, Owen *et al.*, 1968; heifers, Aitken and Preston, 1964; ewes, Forbes, 1970). It is unlikely that physical factors would have been dominant in the control of intake in these circumstances. The decline in intake by cows in the last 3 weeks of pregnancy was steeper for high concentrate than for high forage rations (Coppock *et al.*, 1972) which does not support a purely physical theory for depression of intake. In view of the effects of oestrogens on food intake described above, and the fact that oestrogen secretion by the placenta increases in the last few weeks of pregnancy to rates similar to or greater than that at oestrus, it has been suggested that the late pregnancy decline in intake may be due entirely or partly to oestrogens (Forbes, 1971). Progesterone blocks many of the actions of oestrogens so Bargeloh *et al.* (1975) investigated the effect of progesterone on the decline of voluntary food intake in late pregnancy in cows. Progesterone (0.25 mg kg$^{-1}$ day$^{-1}$) was given subcutaneously for 15 days before the expected date of calving and treated cows ate 17.1 kg DM day$^{-1}$ in the last six days of pregnancy compared with 11.7 kg DM day$^{-1}$ for untreated controls. Pregnancy was prolonged in two out of the five treated cows so this type of treatment is unsuitable for practical use.

An imbalance between the nutrients required by the ewe and fetus(es) might be expected to reduce food intake. To see whether a shortage of amino acids and/or glucose was limiting intake in grass-fed pregnant ewes Barry and Manley (1986) infused glucose and casein into the abomasum. Voluntary intake 4 weeks before lambing was increased by the infusion from 0.6 to 0.85 MJ kg$^{-0.75}$. Intake of the infused animals then declined in the last 4 weeks whereas that of uninfused control groups increased towards parturition and the authors suggested that the higher level of intake in the infused animals rendered them more prone to the intake-depressing effects of pregnancy whereas the uninfused controls were still suffering from the imbalanced diet.

Other possible reasons for the decreased intake in late pregnancy, especially the very low levels in the last few days, include discomfort, preoccupation with seeking a suitable place for parturition, or other endocrine changes associated with parturition (e.g. corticosteroids, prostaglandins, oxytocin, relaxin). Whatever the cause, it seems that mixed feeding with forages supplemented by concentrates avoids too serious a decline in voluntary intake at a time when fetuses are very susceptible to undernutrition.

# Lactation

The females of many species can eat enough during lactation to support milk synthesis without having to call to any great extent on their body reserves, as long as good quality food is available *ad libitum*. In the rat, for example, voluntary intake of a standard laboratory food increases in direct proportion to the number of pups being suckled and the mother's body weight is maintained.

## Pigs

Sows eat their fetal membranes and may even eat still-born piglets.

The voluntary intake of lactating sows partly depends on the intake during pregnancy and on fatness at parturition. The fatter the sow at farrowing the less she eats during lactation (Mullan and Williams, 1989) and Salmon-Legagneur and Rerat (1962) observed a higher intake during lactation in sows which had been restricted to 0.5

of *ad libitum* during pregnancy than in those given as much as they could eat.

The pattern of intake during lactation follows that of milk yield, rising for the first 4 weeks and then declining (Friend, 1970) even though milk yield remains high. The decline might be caused by the increasing fatness which often occurs but this does not happen with modern genotypes which have a greatly reduced propensity to fatten compared with those of a decade or more ago (Chapter 8). According to Lynch (1989) there is no harm in feeding *ad libitum* right from farrowing.

When gilts had been given a low protein food ($90\,g\,kg^{-1}$) in pregnancy, they ate nearly 50% more in lactation if they were given a $180\,g$ crude protein (CP) $kg^{-1}$ food compared to those given a food containing $120\,gCP\,kg^{-1}$ (Mahan and Mangan, 1975), i.e. they were trying to regain the lost body protein. Those given a high protein food ($170\,g\,kg^{-1}$) in pregnancy ate only 5% more when given the higher protein food in lactation. The lower food intake during lactation following higher levels of feeding in pregnancy was due to reduce meal size rather than to changes in meal number (Dourmand, 1993).

Intake increases as the sow ages, to a maximum in about the sixth lactation. The increase with litter size is about $0.2\,kg\,piglet^{-1}$ but $0.5\,kg$ is required for each extra pig if growth is not to be stunted. This means that individual pigs in larger litters each get less milk and grow more slowly than those in smaller litters. O'Grady *et al.* (1985) found the following relationship between the voluntary intake of lactating sows (*VFI*, $g\,day^{-1}$) and parity (*P*), weight of conceptus at birth (*WC*, kg) and stage of lactation (*SL*, days):

$$VFI = 2192 + 297P - 22P^2 - 7WC + 15SL \qquad (9.4)$$

NRC (1987), summarizing results from many sources, reported an average food intake for sows during lactation of $5.17\,kg\,day^{-1}$, with gilts consuming 15% less. However, Lynch (1989) found that 10–12% of gilts and 3–4% of sows ate less than $3\,kg\,day^{-1}$. There are often fluctuations in intake during lactation (Dourmand, 1991) and Koketsu *et al.* (1992) found a consistent reduction between days 10 and 15 after parturition.

Given the large amount of heat produced by the very high rate of metabolism of lactating sows, it is not surprising that they are particularly susceptible to high environmental temperatures. Typically, a 1°C increase in temperature depresses intake by $0.1\,kg\,day^{-1}$.

*Cattle*

Cows eat their fetal membranes, sometimes before they are fully separated.

Voluntary intake usually increases rapidly after calving but Zamet *et al.* (1979) observed that this increase was slower for cows with abnormalities of various sorts, but only for those fed silage, rather than hay. This was not so severe with corn silage as it was with grass silage. Once the trauma of calving is over, voluntary intake increases but usually at a slower rate than necessary to support the rapidly increasing demands of the mammary gland.

Intake is invariably higher in lactating cows than during pregnancy, or in comparison with non-lactating cattle (Campling, 1966b). The nutrient requirements for lactation are up to five times the maintenance requirement. This high demand for nutrients may, by removing metabolites rapidly from the blood, reduce the level of stimulation of chemoreceptors so that physical limitation assumes greater importance than it does in similar, but non-lactating animals.

The limitation on intake assumes greatest importance with high-yielding dairy cows. The rapid increase in requirements during the first few weeks of lactation is not usually matched by such a rapid rise in voluntary intake and this lag is longer with forages (Owen *et al.*, 1968, 1969) and with heifers than with cows (Dulphy and Faverdin, 1987). Heifers are particularly susceptible to low intake of poor foods (Bines, 1985).

*Body condition*

Fat cows eat less than thinner ones in early lactation (Garnsworthy and Topps, 1982) and cows fed at maintenance level during the dry period ate 11% more during the first 16 weeks of lactation than those fed at 1.8 of maintenance (Lodge *et al.*, 1975). There was no difference in milk yield and the need to 'steam up' (give extra supplementary feeding) before calving was questioned. However, cows which have become very thin during lactation should be fed so as to build up some reserves during the dry period.

Neilson *et al.* (1983) found that silage intake varied inversely with body condition in groups of Friesian cows. Cows that were fatter at calving lost weight but milk yield was not affected. However, Land and Leaver (1980) observed that fatter cows ate less but gave more milk than thinner ones.

Cows which were thin at calving (condition score (CS) 2.15 or 2) had their intake of hay reduced by a high level of undegradable dietary protein (UDP) in the concentrate, whereas intake by fat cows (CS 3.15 or 3.5) was increased by such a supplement, compared with a concentrate low in UDP (Fig. 9.3; Garnsworthy and Jones, 1987; Jones and Garnsworthy, 1988). It is possible that the fat cows could utilize the additional protein by mobilizing fat to provide energy to balance the increased protein supply.

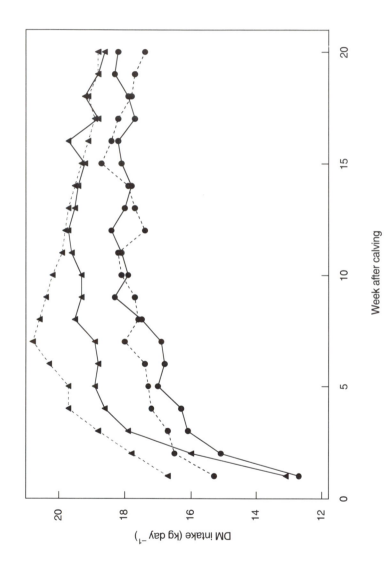

**Fig. 9.3.** Intake of hay by lactating cows which were (F, condition score 3.5) or thin (T, CS 2.0) at calving and supplemented with concentrates which were either high (H, 74 g kg DM$^{-1}$) or low (L, 45 g kg DM$^{-1}$) in undegradable protein (Garnsworthy and Jones, 1987). ●—●, FH; ●--●, FL; ▲—▲, TH; ▲--▲, TL.

Moreover, when given a high energy food (13.0 MJ kg DM$^{-1}$) thin cows ate more than fat cows and produced the same amount of milk (Jones and Garnsworthy, 1989) but when a poor quality food (9.8 MJ kg DM$^{-1}$) of the same crude protein content (180 g CP kg DM$^{-1}$) was given, intake was not affected by body condition with the result that thin cows produced significantly less milk; this was suggested to be due to physical limitation of intake but it is difficult to agree with this in view of the evidence that thin animals have a higher rumen capacity (Chapter 8).

The fat concentration of the diet (96 or 29 g kg DM$^{-1}$) had no effect on voluntary intake in lactation, nor was there any effect of body condition (Garnsworthy and Huggett, 1992). However, the higher fat diet decreased the loss of body condition in fat cows and increased milk yield in thin cows.

Level of feeding before calving did not affect intake in the work of Cowan *et al.* (1981) but a lactation diet containing 147 g CP kg DM$^{-1}$ gave higher intakes than one containing 111 g CP kg DM$^{-1}$. The increased intake with the higher-protein food was greater when it contained 40% forage than for a higher forage (60%) food.

### Heritability of food intake

There are large individual variations in intake of cows of similar milk yields which are consistent throughout lactation suggesting that efficiencies differ greatly between cows (Little *et al.*, 1991). At the Scottish Agricultural College, Edinburgh (Scottish Agricultural College, 1992), 293 lactations were studied to calculate heritabilities which were: milk yield, 0.20; fat and protein yield, 0.15; live weight, 0.34; DM intake, 0.52; efficiency, 0.13. This shows that responses in efficiency following selection for fat and protein yield will only be 47–74% as great as those selected directly for efficiency, i.e. if the selection objective is to improve efficiency then record intake. Genus, the largest cattle breeding company in the UK, is now recording intakes of its heifers in the multiple ovulation embryo transfer (MOET) scheme by the LUCIFIR system (Chapter 2).

### Bovine somatotropin (BST)

With the development of genetic engineering it has become possible to produce large quantities of bovine growth hormone, called bovine somatotropin (BST) which stimulates milk yield when administered to cows. The results of short-term trials indicated that this was not accompanied by increased food intake (Holcombe *et al.*, 1988); indeed initially there is a tendency for food intake to decrease (Peel *et al.*, 1981). It has been demonstrated that the energy for the extra milk comes initially from fat mobilization but that food intake starts to rise after

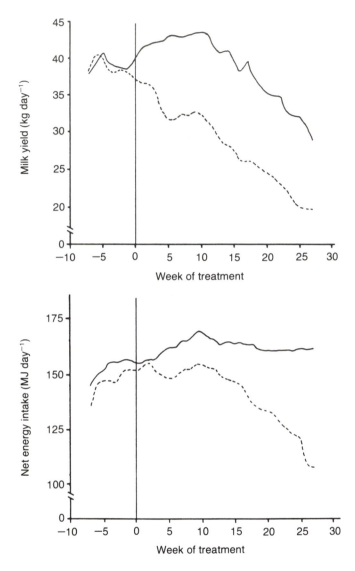

**Fig. 9.4.** Effect of recombinantly derived bovine growth hormone on milk yield and net energy intake. From 84 days post-partum (week 0) treated cows received a daily injection of 27 mg day$^{-1}$ for 26 weeks (Bauman *et al.*, 1984).

about 2 weeks of treatment and does not decline as rapidly as in untreated cows in mid-lactation (Bauman, 1984). Bauman *et al.* (1984) treated cows with bGH or BST for 188 days, starting 84 days after calving. Figure 9.4 shows that intake of a complete food remained higher than for control cows from about the fourth week of treatment. However, it must be noted that the quality of the food was adjusted according to the quality of milk produced so that the BST-treated cows, by producing more milk, were fed more digestible, higher-energy food than controls, which would be likely to result in increased intake (see Chapter 10). Further studies (Rijpkema *et al.*, 1987) also showed increased intake after the first few weeks of slow-release BST treatment, but again interpretation was confounded by the use of milk yield-related changes in diet composition. In another experiment, after 8 weeks of treatment control cows fed freshly cut grass individually ate 15.5 kg DM day$^{-1}$ whereas twins given 50 mg GH day$^{-1}$ ate 16.7 kg; in week 22 of treatment the intakes were, respectively, 15.4 and 17.5 kg DM day$^{-1}$ (Peel *et al.*, 1985).

*Sheep*

There have been relatively few studies of the voluntary intake of lactating ewes. After lambing there is a slow rise to a peak, trailing behind milk yield so that weight loss is common, particularly with poor quality foods. This lag is longer with forage diets than with concentrates (Forbes, 1971). Peak intake was seen by Hadjipieris and Holmes (1966) at weeks 4–6 of lactation. Clancy *et al.* (1976) showed that for a range of foods, lactating ewes ate more than wethers, even with diets low in digestible energy concentration where there was a positive relationship between digestibility and intake, implying physical limitation to intake.

Forbes (1969b) recorded the voluntary intake of hay and the milk yield during the first seven weeks of lactation in Speckle-faced Welsh ewes, 11 with single lambs and four with twins. Mean hay intake over the period of observation ($I$, kg DM day$^{-1}$) was positively related to milk yield ($MY$, kg day$^{-1}$) and live weight change ($LWC$, kg 42 days$^{-1}$):

$$I = 0.76 + 0.5MY + 0.03LWC \qquad (9.5)$$

The weight gain of the lambs from 2 to 7 weeks of age ($WG$, kg day$^{-1}$) was positively related to the hay intake of the ewe (kg day$^{-1}$):

$$WG = 0.17I + 0.05 \qquad (9.6)$$

Although lamb weight gain was probably dependent on milk yield, it is not certain whether milk yield determines intake or vice versa; almost certainly the two are interdependent.

Boucquier *et al.* (1987) found that intake of hay increased sharply in the first 2 weeks after lambing and reached a maximum in week 5 or 6. Surprisingly, intake was not related to the number of lambs being suckled, but was higher for mature ewes than for old ewes.

During lactation thin ewes eat more than fat ones, in proportion to the difference in rate of disappearance and extent of digestion of the food (Cowan *et al.*, 1980):

$$I = (54 - 1.2BF) / (MRT(1-DMD))$$                    (9.7)

where $I$ is the intake (kg DM day$^{-1}$), $MRT$ is the mean retention time of particles (h), $BF$ is body fat (kg) and $DMD$ is the DM digestibility. This might be taken as evidence to support the idea that low intake in early lactation is due to physical limitation but the fat effect could equally be a metabolic phenomenon.

Other reasons for the lag in intake might be slow metabolic adaptation to increased nutrient requirements and hypertrophy of the digestive tract and liver (Forbes, 1986b); there is no sound information on likely maximum rates of hypertrophy of these tissues.

Another possible reason for the slow increase of intake in early lactation is slow recovery from the effects of endocrine changes in late pregnancy. Although short exposure to small doses of oestrogens has a reversible effect on voluntary intake, more severe treatment can have long-lasting effects. When moderately fat ewes were injected with a high dose of 17β-oestradiol (10 mg) on two consecutive days there was a 60% decrease in intake of a pelleted diet which took at least 2 weeks to recover to pretreatment levels (J.M. Forbes, unpublished observations). Extremely high rates of oestrogen production which might have this sort of effect occur in the last few days of pregnancy. The results of Wright *et al.* (1990) suggest that the hypothalamus of cattle is very sensitive to oestradiol in the first few weeks of lactation.

Clearly further work is required to elucidate the usual lag between increasing nutrient demands and the increase in voluntary intake in early lactation; it is unlikely that the answer to this question will be a simple one.

## The Laying Hen

Laying birds eat more on egg-forming days than on non-egg-forming days (Bordas and Merat, 1976), presumably in response to the increased requirements for nutrients on egg-forming days. Mean egg production is correlated with food intake between groups of birds with different rates of production (Fig. 9.5) and high-producing birds gain less weight (Ivy and Gleves, 1976). Between individuals there is a positive correlation between food intake and shell thickness and between the weight of the egg and food intake on the same day (Bordas and Merat, 1976) but it is not clear which is cause and which is effect.

For 2–3 h before oviposition feeding activity is depressed as the

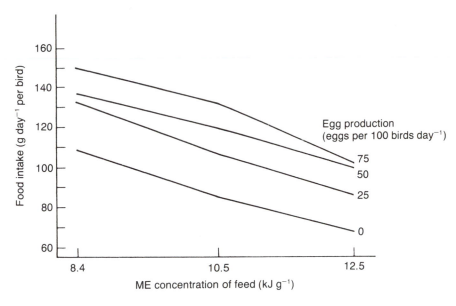

**Fig. 9.5.** Food intakes of hens at four levels of egg production offered foods of three energy concentrations (Ivy and Gleaves, 1976).

hen is occupied with pacing or setting (Wood-Gush and Horne, 1971). In broiler hens kept in continuous light, food intake is also lower during the hour or two before oviposition and intake increases markedly for a short period afterwards (Savory, 1977). Perhaps compression of the gastrointestinal tract by the egg inhibits feeding just before oviposition. There is also a depression about 32 h before oviposition, which is approximately the time of release of luteinizing hormone, and an increase around ovulation and for several hours after entry of the egg into the uterus; this latter change may be related to the demands for calcium for deposition of the shell (Chapter 14). The increase in food intake which occurs after ovulation is accompanied by increased intake of oyster shell (a source of calcium) and so is the peak 20–22 h later (Nys *et al.*, 1976).

Morris and Taylor (1967) found that, at normal environmental temperatures, hens ate 116.6 g on egg-forming days and 102.2 g on non-egg-forming days (Fig. 9.6). At 30°C, intakes were 100.9 g and 78.6 g, respectively. In a larger experiment with pullets, intakes were 125.1 g and 95.1 g. When intakes from 09.30 to 14.30 were examined it was seen that on egg-forming days it was 23.2 g and on non-egg-forming days it was 19.7 g. Intakes from 14.30 to 09.30 the next morning were 101.8 and 75.3 g, respectively, a true reflection of the effect of egg formation.

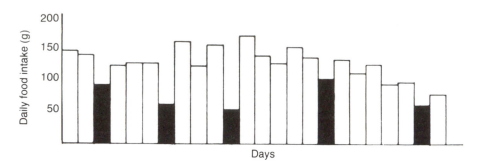

**Fig. 9.6.** Daily food intake of a laying hen in relation to egg formation (Morris and Taylor, 1967). (□) Egg-forming, (■) non-egg-forming.

These authors speculated that it is probably the increase in protein requirements to support the albumen deposition which is responsible for this effect of egg-laying on voluntary intake by the hen.

The concept of residual food consumption (RFC), discussed in Chapter 8 with regard to growing pigs, has also been developed for laying hens (Luiting, 1990). Factors related to RFC were fatness, behaviour pattern and metabolic heat loss. The heritability of RFC was estimated to be 0.37 and Katle and Nordli (1992) suggest using RFC from 25 to 29 weeks of age in cocks as a selection tool to improve conversion efficiency of laying hens. Katle (1992a) calculated that a breeding programme was 17% more efficient when RFC was included and concluded that it is better to record RFC in hens, but cheaper to do it for cocks.

Katle (1992b) recorded individual food intake during the first 5 weeks of life in pullets of high and low RFC lines and found moderate phenotypic correlations with RFC as adults, permitting the possibility of using food intake of young chicks as a selection criterion.

## Conclusions

Reproductive status can have a marked effect on food intake in the female. At oestrus, intake is often temporarily depressed by the oestrogens secreted by the ovaries but it is not clear the extent to which this is a direct effect on the brain and to what extent due to a change in metabolism in liver, muscle and adipose tissue. In sows intake increases in pregnancy which would, unless prevented by restriction of food allowance, result in gross deposition of fat. In the last few weeks of pregnancy there is often a decline in intake in ruminants, probably caused by competition for space in the abdomen and by the increasing oestrogen secretion by the placenta. On the day of parturition very little is eaten but then intake increases at the start of lactation. In cows and ewes this increase is not usually fast enough to keep pace with the increase in milk yield, as a result of which body reserves are mobilized. After the peak of lactation the level of voluntary intake stays high and reserves are replenished.

There is a rhythm of food intake in the laying hen which is related to the requirements for deposition of the components of the egg. It is not clear whether this is dependent on the changing requirements for different nutrients at different times of day, or on the changing hormone levels which accompany these fluctuating requirements. Hens eat less on days in which an egg is not being formed and over a longer period intake is proportional to the number of eggs layed.

# 10 DIET DIGESTIBILITY AND CONCENTRATION OF AVAILABLE ENERGY

- Poultry
- Pigs
- Ruminants
- Replacement of one food with another
- Conclusions

It has long been known that intake of simple-stomached animals increases if the diet is diluted with indigestible material and decreases when the energy content of the food is increased, for example by the incorporation of fat. However, this compensation is not perfect. For example, $250 \text{ g kg}^{-1}$ of fat in the diet of rats leads to slight but persistent overeating and gradual obesity (e.g. Jacobs, 1967) and excessive dilution of a mouse food with cellulose prevents complete compensation and results in a reduction in growth rate (Dalton, 1964).

In general, however, it is true to say that animals compensate for changes in the concentration of available energy in the food, unless the physical capacity of the stomachs (in the ruminant) restrict intake. Increasing the available energy concentration decreases the undigested bulk and vice versa, so it is not always easy to determine which factor(s) is important when comparing voluntary intake of different foods.

## Poultry

### Growing birds

Fat can be incorporated in the diet to increase the energy density.

In general it is thought that fats depress intake by a general energy-related effect because injection of small amounts of individual long-chain fatty acids (the major constituents of fat) intraperitoneally (Cave, 1978) or their inclusion in the food (Sunde, 1956; Renner and Hill, 1961) do not depress intake to a significant extent. Some short-and medium-chain fatty acids do depress intake, however, whether given intra-peritoneally (Cave, 1978) or in the diet (Cave, 1982). In the latter case propionic, but not acetic, acid was effective; caprylic and lauric acids gave a 5–6 g depression in daily food intake by 2–3-week-old broilers for each gram of the acid included per kilogram of diet. However, the modern broiler actually increases its intake when maize oil or tallow is incorporated in the food, presumably due to the improved palatability and the lack of complete control over digestible energy intake. Fats high in polyunsaturated fatty acids, such as cod liver oil and olive oil, depress intake by broilers, possibly due to deterioration or to toxic effects (J. Wiseman, personal communication). It is clearly inappropriate to refer to 'fat' in this context without specifying the type of triglycerides involved.

Growing Leghorn cockerels maintained the same weight gain as controls when given foods with 100 or 200 g kg$^{-1}$ kaolin by increasing their total food intake to regain the same intake of digestible dry matter (DM) (Savory, 1984). When 300 g kg$^{-1}$ kaolin was included they stopped gaining weight whereas with 400 g kg$^{-1}$ they lost weight because, although total food intake increased, it did not immediately do so sufficiently to maintain intake of digestible nutrients. Eventually, however, intake did increase but weight gains were still depressed, presumably because of the high cost of eating the greater amount of food.

## Laying hens

Laying hens adjust their food intake to satisfy their energy requirements when the energy concentration of the food is changed (Fig. 9.5; Powell *et al.*, 1972; Ivy and Gleaves, 1976; Jones *et al.*, 1976). Compensation is not always perfect, however, and Cherry (1979) found that hens given a diet high in metabolizable energy (ME; 12.5 MJ kg$^{-1}$) gained more weight than similar birds given a low ME diet (11.5 MJ kg$^{-1}$) for 112 days. He then switched foods and observed that it took some 12 days for a full reversal of daily food intake to occur. In a comprehensive experiment, de Groot (1972) showed that giving foods with ME concentrations (*MEC*s) ranging from 10.5 to 13.4 MJ kg$^{-1}$ caused partial compensation in intake but not sufficiently to maintain ME intake (*MEI*), egg weight or body weight gain. The economic optimum was around 11.7 MJ kg$^{-1}$ under the conditions of this experiment.

Morris (1968b) surveyed the literature available and found the following overall relationship between the voluntary *MEI* (*MEI*, kJ day$^{-1}$) by laying hens and the *MEC* of the food (kJ g$^{-1}$):

$$MEI = SMEI + ((2.28 \times SMEI) - 612.7) \times (MEC - 11.3) \qquad (10.1)$$

where *SMEI* is the intake of a standard food with a metabolizable energy concentration of 11.3 kJ g$^{-1}$ DM. The compensation in voluntary intake is not usually sufficient to prevent changes in ME intake, especially when intakes are low associated with low egg production at high temperatures.

Beh (1981) found that loading the crop of laying hens kept at 20°C with corn oil at 3 ml kg$^{-1}$ day$^{-1}$ caused an immediate compensation in voluntary intake so that *MEI* was maintained at the same level as before; cessation of treatment led to an equally rapid response. However, the same treatment applied to another group of hens kept in an environmental temperature of 32°C, where the pretreatment intake was lower than at 20°C, failed to affect intake.

# Pigs

As noted in Chapter 1, pigs tend to overeat and attempts to manipulate voluntary intake have concentrated on limiting the digestible energy (DE) intake while feeding *ad libitum* to save labour. (As detailed in Chapter 8, modern pig genotypes have much less propensity to fatten and *ad libitum* feeding of conventional foods to growing pigs is now widely practised in the UK.)

In many studies with pigs from weaning, energy density of the diet has not been shown to affect DE intake (NRC, 1987), i.e. there is complete compensation. Cole *et al.* (1967) offered diets ranging from 12.5 to 15.5 MJ DE kg$^{-1}$ DM to pigs weighing between 38 and 105 kg; DE intake was maintained. In a subsequent experiment (Cole *et al.*, 1969), in which a diet of 14.2 MJ DE kg$^{-1}$ was compared with one of 11.1 MJ kg$^{-1}$, voluntary intake was increased from 3.12 to 3.81 kg day$^{-1}$ on the more dilute diet but DE intake was depressed from 44.3 to 41.9 MJ day$^{-1}$ and live weight gain and carcass fatness were reduced.

Henry (1985) concluded from a broad review of the literature that as DE concentration increases DE intake also increases, whereas DM intake is reduced, resulting in pigs becoming fatter on more concentrated diets. Cole *et al.* (1972) also proposed that pigs ate for constant DE except when low energy diets limited intake physically, or very high density diets were eaten in greater quantities to avoid an underfilled stomach. It seems more likely, however, that the change in intake with DE content is smooth. Whether energy concentration was increased by

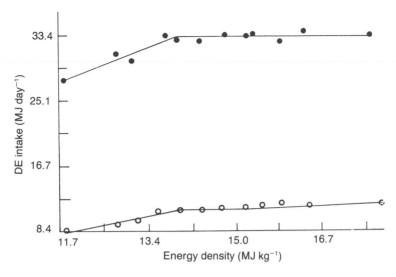

**Fig. 10.1.** Summary of the effects of the energy density of the food on voluntary intake by pigs growing from 5 to 30 kg (○) and from 30 to 100 kg (●) (NRC, 1987).

adding fat or starch, the effect on intake was similar (Cole and Chadd, 1989). However, growth decreased as the level of fat increased even though intakes were the same. This may be due to a poorer efficiency of utilization of the energy from high levels of fat for protein synthesis (Wiseman and Cole, 1987). Growing pigs maintained a constant digestible energy intake when the energy content of the food was increased from 14.0 to 17.5 MJ DE kg$^{-1}$by adding fat, but they failed to compensate fully for dilution to 12.5 MJ DE kg$^{-1}$ (Fowler *et al.*, 1981). Inclusion of fat is useful at higher environmental temperatures as it has a lower heat increment than carbohydrate or protein and therefore depresses intake less in hot climates.

Figure 10.1 is a compilation by NRC (1987) of data from numerous sources on the relationship between the energy density of the food and the digestible energy intake of growing pigs. Up to a density of about 14 MJ kg$^{-1}$DM there is a positive relationship but above that the intake of DE remains almost constant.

Although it has been shown that inclusion of inert fillers in the food of growing pigs reduces the intake of digestible energy, substantial dilution has to be made in order to depress DE intake sufficient to affect fattening significantly. Fillers such as sawdust are easy to obtain in small amounts, for experimental purposes, but if they were to be included in commercial rations the demand created would soon result in an increase in price. Lower grades of food, such as oat hulls, have been used to depress DE intake but compensation for such dilution occurs in older pigs, i.e. when the depression in DE intake is most required to prevent overfatness.

Owen and Ridgman (1967) used six foods with different levels of DE ranging from 10.3 to 14.1 MJ kg$^{-1}$; protein was kept in proportion to DE. From 27 to 50 kg body weight there was a slight increase in voluntary intake with decreasing nutrient concentration, this increase getting bigger as the pigs grew towards 118 kg. This led to big deficits in total digestible nutrients (TDN) intake with diluted diets and growth in the early stages but not such a big effect by the later stages.

Subsequently, Owen and Ridgman (1968) extended this work to investigate the ability of growing pigs to compensate for the effects of diet dilution when returned to conventional foods. Young pigs up to about 60 kg weight did not recover fully whereas older pigs did compensate by eating more, although it took some two weeks for this to occur. Once compensation has occurred, it takes a similar time to reverse when the diet is again changed. We should note, therefore, that the results of short-term experiments can be very misleading.

D.J.A. Cole (personal communication) has suggested that the modern pig may have changed genotypically in a similar way to the broiler where physiological control of intake seems to have given way to some extent to eating for bulk. The younger the animal, the greater its nutrient requirements per unit of body weight and the more important is stomach distension as a limit to food intake.

Maximum weight gains in weaner pigs, therefore, require a diet high in DE which can be achieved by adding fat. With the older pigs growing from 75 to 95 kg (Bosticco et al., 1975) inclusion of 60 g of fat kg$^{-1}$ depressed intake from 4.2 to 3.6 kg day$^{-1}$, but live weight gain increased from 640 to 650 g day$^{-1}$, suggesting that DE intake was probably increased despite the decreased food intake.

It can be concluded, therefore, that when the concentration of DE in the diet changes then pigs, like rats and mice, vary the level of voluntary intake in the appropriate direction to maintain digestible energy intake, but that compensation is not complete, giving increased DE intake with increased DE concentration in the food.

# Ruminants

## Preruminant

The preruminant calf or lamb compensates for dilution of its milk (Pettyjohn et al., 1963) although excessive dilution, necessitating high fluid intakes, causes loss of production (Chapter 8).

## Digestibility

It used to be thought that the response of the ruminant animal to changes in the digestibility of the food was entirely opposite to that of non-ruminants, a reasonable conclusion based on the evidence available up to the early 1960s, i.e. a positive correlation between intake of forages and their digestibility by ruminants (Balch and Campling, 1962; Baile and Forbes, 1974). There is a great deal of evidence that dilution of a forage-based diet depresses intake of ruminants, some of which will now be reviewed.

Diet density can be measured by physical means; Baile and Pfander (1967) adopted a standard procedure to measure density and found a high negative correlation ($r = -0.99$) between the bulk density of different foods over a range from 0.2 to 0.8 g ml$^{-1}$, and the weight eaten voluntarily by sheep.

In contrast to dilution with inert solid material, sheep (Davis, 1962) and cattle (Thomas *et al.*, 1961a) can compensate for dilution of forages with water because the free water is quickly absorbed. If, however, the water is trapped inside cells, as in fresh grass or silage, then intake is negatively correlated with water content (Chapter 16).

Crampton *et al.* (1960) realized the significance of intake in determining the nutritive value of forages whose value is proportional to the yield of digestible nutrients per unit weight multiplied by the weight eaten. Thus, nutritive value is proportional to the square of digestibility of foods whose intake is limited predominantly by physical factors and thus dependent on digestibility. For example, a food of 500 g kg$^{-1}$ DM digestibility might be eaten by cattle at a rate of 10 kg day$^{-1}$; another food of 600 g kg$^{-1}$DM digestibility would be eaten by the same animal at about 12 kg day$^{-1}$ thus increasing the intake of digestible DM from 5.0 to 7.2 kg day$^{-1}$. Crampton *et al.* (1960) also realized that between-animal variations in intake would obscure between-feed variations. They therefore used a standard food of alfalfa (lucerne) offered to each of their animals, against which the intake for the other forages could be compared. Unfortunately, since different batches of alfalfa vary in composition between experiments, comparisons are difficult. Moreover the use of whether sheep as the standard animal may not predict relative intakes for forages by dairy cows (INRA, 1979).

In the early 1960s, therefore, ruminants were thought to control their food intake by physical limitation. Then came several developments that suggested a role for metabolic control. Donefer *et al.* (1963) offered pelleted diets ranging from alfalfa hay alone to 40% hay, 60% concentrates and found that sheep controlled their intake to a constant intake of DE, i.e. DM intake falls as the concentration of DE increases.

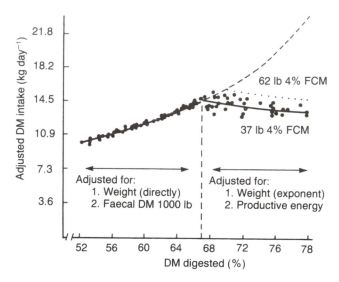

**Fig. 10.2.** Relationships between digestibility of the food and adjusted voluntary intake of lactating cows (Conrad *et al.*, 1964).

This implied metabolic rather than physical control of intake. Also around this time came a series of experiments in which it was shown that infusion of short chain fatty acids depressed intake (Chapter 5) which indicated the possible mechanisms of such metabolic control. Conrad *et al.* (1964) then published their analysis of a large volume of data obtained from routine digestion trials at the Ohio Research and Development Station. They described the voluntary intakes of lactating cows for a wide range of foods (Chapter 17; Fig. 10.2).

Their statistical analysis showed that when adjusted for body weight and faecal output food intake was positively related to the digestibility of dry matter below 67% and negatively related above 67% for cows of moderate milk yield (a mean of 17 kg day$^{-1}$). Although the validity of the multiplicative model can be disputed the general conclusion is important; with forages, intake is controlled primarily by physical means, whereas the intake of more concentrated diets is controlled mainly by the cows' energy requirements. The work of Conrad *et al.* (1964) has occasionally been misquoted as showing that physical limitation and metabolic control diverged at a fixed level of digestibility, 670 g kg$^{-1}$, but Conrad and his colleagues knew that there was no fixed point, since they reported that with higher yielding cows (averaging 28 kg milk day$^{-1}$) the point of inflexion in the graph of intake against digestibility was 700 g kg$^{-1}$. In general, the higher the energy requirements, the higher the digestibility above which intake is controlled metabolically.

In contrast to cereal-based foods of high digestibility, the intake of growing grass by ruminants continues to increase with increasing digestibility (Chapter 16). Curvilinearity is only a feature of data sets in which there are some milled foods and/or concentrates.

## Particle size

It has been found that the faster the rate of disappearance of food from the digestive tract, the lower is this point of inflexion. One way to reduce the time spent by food particles in the rumen is to offer forages in ground form. Inclusion of ground forages in complete foods for lactating cows allows digestible energy intake to be maintained, even up to 60% forage (Ronning and Laben, 1966), because the small particles of ground forage leave the rumen more quickly. Numerous experiments show that grinding leads to increased intake (Campling and Freer, 1966). Although digestibility is usually depressed, as there is faster rate of passage and thus less time for digestion, the yield of absorbable nutrients (intake × digestibility) is normally increased and animal performance is improved. The benefits of grinding are greatest with forages of low digestibility.

Among a range of forages Deswysen and Ellis (1990) observed the highest intake associated with the food which had the smallest particles leaving the rumen whereas P.J. Van Soest (personal communication) finds a high correlation between intake and the extent of digestion after 6 h of incubation.

## Relationships with dietary fibre

There are several types of fibre in most forages. Lignin is indigestible and so its content is inversely related to digestibility but it has no consistent relationship with voluntary intake. Cellulose and hemicellulose are degradable by the rumen microorganisms but the rate of digestion is variable and the time spent by a particle in the rumen also varies so there is no close relationship between a forage's content of these and the level of voluntary intake.

Van Soest (1967) has pioneered the cell-wall fraction of forages, as measured by the neutral detergent fibre (NDF) method, for predicting the physical fill created by food in the rumen. For a wide range of grasses, including many tropical species, Mertens (1973) found an almost constant intake of NDF:

$$I = 110 - 1716/(100 - CWC) \qquad (10.2)$$

where *I* is the voluntary intake (g DM kg live weight $(LW)^{0.75}$) by sheep and cell wall constituent (*CWC*) is the proportion of *CWC* in the DM (%). Osbourn *et al.* (1974) measured the intake by sheep of a standard reference forage and expressed intake of other forages relative to this and also obtained a negative relationship for sheep:

$$DMI = 95 - 7.3CWC \qquad (10.3)$$

Dulphy *et al.* (1980) found that for a 60 kg sheep a 10 g kg$^{-1}$ increase in the crude fibre content of forages gave a 38 g day$^{-1}$ decrease in food intake with 36% fewer meals, 4.1 min day$^{-1}$ less eating time and 6.6 min day$^{-1}$ increase in the time per day spent ruminating. Rumination time is not well correlated with the weight of food eaten but with the intake of NDF.

In legumes, the leaves are not structural so are low in lignin but the stems have a high content; for grasses there is only a small difference between leaf and stem although this gets bigger at higher environmental temperatures.

Although highly fibrous forages are eaten in lower amounts than those with low NDF content, there is a danger of feeding too little fibre which results in the lack of a 'mat' to trap particles in the rumen so that faecal particles are bigger! Sometimes grinding and pelleting increases faecal particle size because of this. There is also the risk of low milk-fat if the food is too low in fibre and the optimal NDF content of the whole ration for milk production is 360 g kg$^{-1}$, irrespective of the type of forage on offer (P.J. Van Soest, personal communication).

Although it is true that sheep show an approximately constant intake of NDF, cattle increase their intake of NDF as its content in food increases (P.J. Van Soest, personal communication). For any given level of NDF, sheep eat more DM kg$^{-0.73}$ than cattle because of the lower ratio of gut capacity per unit of metabolic rate in the smaller species.

Seoane (1982) found close relationships between the physicochemical characteristics of nine hays and their voluntary intake by growing male sheep:

$$DEI = 1659 + 1.38SOL - 3.18CF \qquad (10.4)$$

where *DEI* is digestible energy intake (kJ kg$^{-0.75}$), *SOL* is the initial solubility of the material (g kg$^{-1}$) and *CF* is crude fibre content (g kg$^{-1}$).

### Dilution with low quality food

*Cattle*

Reduction of digestibility by inclusion of up to 30% of straw in a compound food for growing cattle may be compensated for by an

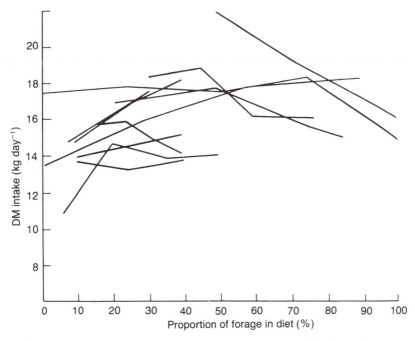

**Fig. 10.3.** Summary of the effects of the proportion of forage in the diet on the voluntary intake of lactating cows (Bines, 1979).

increase in intake (e.g. Lamming *et al.,* 1966), but not always sufficiently to maintain the same growth rate (e.g. Kay *et al.,* 1970).

Figure 10.3 is a summary of the relationships between intake by lactating cows and the proportion of forage in the diet (Bines, 1979). The general trend is that above and below approximately 0.5 forage in the diet there is a reduction in intake; the former is presumably due to physical limitation whereas the latter is due to metabolic control.

Polythene cubes (2 mm) included in a complete food at 40 or 75 g kg$^{-1}$ induced a compensatory increase in intake, whereas greater inclusion (up to 220 g kg$^{-1}$) resulted in a reduction in digestible energy intake (Carr and Jacobson, 1969). Similar results were obtained with steers by Boling *et al.* (1970).

*Sheep*

When lambs which had passed their stage of maximum growth were offered pelleted foods in which a barley/oats food was diluted with oat husks, to give a range of DM digestibilities of 600–780 g kg$^{-1}$, intake of digestible organic matter was constant and growth was unaffected

(Andrews and Kay, 1967). Because of the relatively low nutrient requirements of the sheep and the fast rate of passage of the residues of the ground, pelleted food, the point of inflexion of the intake/ digestibility curve was below 600.

Owen *et al.* (1969a) fed lambs on coarse or ground oat husks at 200, 400 or 600 g kg$^{-1}$ in meal or pelleted form with a barley-based concentrate. From 15 to 27 kg live weight intakes were constant or increased with increasing digestibility. From 28 to 40 kg, intakes of foods containing ground straw decreased with increasing digestibility giving evidence for metabolic control in older lambs when there was a fast rate of passage.

In several other experiments in which ground straw was used to dilute concentrate foods to give a range of digestibilities from 540 to 800 g kg$^{-1}$ there was complete compensation of voluntary intake by growing lambs (Montgomery and Baumgardt, 1965).

More inert diluents than straw also stimulated intake as long as the concentration of DE in the whole ration was at least 10.3 MJ kg$^{-1}$ DM in adult sheep or 10.4 MJ kg$^{-1}$ in growing lambs (Dinius and Baumgardt, 1970; Baumgardt and Peterson, 1971).

## Rate of digestion

Digestibility is the product of the retention time in the rumen and the degradation characteristics of the food concerned. The longer a portion of food stays in the rumen the closer it will come to being digested to the maximum extent possible, i.e. its potential digestibility, but factors such as level of feeding cause variations in residence time and therefore in actual digestibility. Hovell *et al.* (1986) found that the intakes of hays by sheep were closely related to initial solubility of diet and rate of disappearance from Dacron bags in rumen. Figure 10.4 shows the very close linear relationship between the potential degradability of the DM and the voluntary intake of four hays by sheep, which was much closer than the relationships of intake and digestibility or intake and rate of degradation, making rumen degradability a useful predictor of intake (Chapter 17).

Kibon and Ørskov (1993) used degradation characteristics of five browse plants to predict digestibility, voluntary intake and growth rate of goats. The highest correlations ($r^2 = 0.99$ for intake) were obtained with equations which included the digestion rate constant ($c$ from the equation $p=a+b(1-e^{ct})$), the soluble fraction of the food and the insoluble but fermentable fraction of the food. This very close fit allows extremely good prediction of intake and performance under conditions similar to those used in this experiment and this is a very promising way of predicting forage intake.

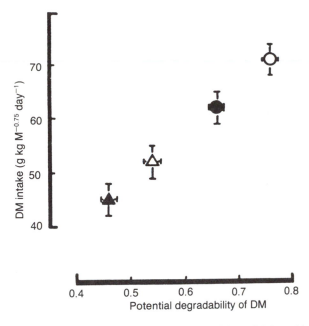

**Fig. 10.4.** Relationship between DM intake and potential degradability of four hays in sheep (Hovell *et al.*, 1986).

Rate of degradation of forages in the rumen is largely dependent on microbial activity, which produces gas. Blummel and Ørskov (1993) have shown that there is a high correlation (0.88) between total gas produced and food intake. As gas production *in vitro* is much easier to measure than degradation, this may provide a useful automated method of food analysis to predict food intake of forages.

Tropical breeds of cattle show a faster rate of passage for any given food than temperate breeds (Mann *et al.*, 1987) suggesting that the former are more useful where only poor quality foods are available. Goats show a lower digestibility (faster passage) than sheep when stall-fed but when given access to grazing they select better parts of plants and have the same digestibility as sheep (Huston *et al.*, 1988).

Increasing the level of incorporation of straw in complete foods for beef cattle reduced daily DM intake, except for ammonia-treated barley straw which increased DM intake as straw inclusion went from 350 to 450 g kg$^{-1}$ food (Ørskov *et al.*, 1991; Fig. 10.5). Ammonia treatment increased the rate of degradation of the insoluble fraction of the food in the rumen while having little effect on digestibility. The effect on intake was more closely related to the effect on degradability than digestibility.

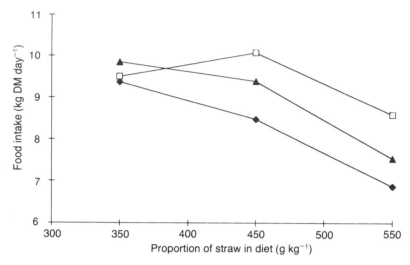

**Fig. 10.5.** Voluntary intake by beef cattle of complete foods containing untreated barley straw (◆), ammonia-treated barley straw (□) or ammonia-treated wheat straw (▲) at three levels (Orskov *et al.*, 1991).

### Feed processing

#### Pigs

Pelleting reduces food intake by weaners by 9% on average (Van Choubroek *et al.*, 1971) whereas at later stages of growth the effect is much less. However, it is difficult to know how much of this apparent reduction in intake is really a reduction in wastage.

#### Cattle

NRC (1984a) provide a comprehensive coverage of effects of food processing on intake and digestibility in ruminants. Increases in intake caused by grinding and pelleting are generally negatively related to forage quality (see above).

In order to see whether the hardness of high-density pellets of dried grass (1.3 g ml$^{-1}$) limited their intake, Tetlow and Wilkins (1977) introduced approximately one-third of the daily intake as wetted pellets into the rumen of young cattle through rumen fistulas. Voluntary intake was reduced by the amount of DM put into the rumen, showing that it was not chewing effort or lack of saliva which was limiting intake of the dry pellets.

Chopping increased intake of high-fibre hay by cows but not of better-quality hays (Susmel *et al.,* 1991). Whether this was due to a limit imposed by chewing or rumen capacity is not clear.

## Sheep

Sheep are much more sensitive to particle size than cattle (ARC, 1980). For cattle, unmilled and milled foods were eaten in similar amounts (87 vs. 90 g kg body weight$^{-0.75}$) whereas for sheep the intakes were 57 and 91.

The voluntary intake of dried grass pellets of two densities (1.24 and 1.14 g m$^{-1}$) were compared by Tetlow and Wilkins (1977). When fed alone there was no difference but when given for only 3 h day$^{-1}$, with hay on offer for the rest of the time, the lower-density pellets were eaten in greater amounts than those of higher density. However, the proportion of pellets gradually increased from 60% to 80% of total intake over a 42-day period.

When dried grass was ground to different degrees of fineness, with a binding agent incorporated to reduce dust, voluntary intake by cattle and sheep increased with decreasing particle size but the digestibility of organic matter was depressed resulting in unchanged intake of digestible organic matter (Wilkins *et al.,* 1972).

## Complete foods for ruminants

Knowledge of the relationships between intake and food characteristics can be utilized to manipulate the intake of ME and thus the level of growth or milk production. When nutrient requirements are relatively low a food of lower ME concentration can be offered, thus reducing the cost of feeding. A food consisting of concentrates and chopped or ground forage and presented in a form in which it is not possible for the animals to select one ingredient is often termed a *complete diet* (or *feed* or *food*). For any given level of animal performance there is an ME concentration which can be reflected in a forage:concentrate ratio which allows the ruminant animal to eat voluntarily the amount of food which contains ME appropriate to its requirements. Feeding of a complete food *ad libitum* may encourage a higher intake than conventional restricted feeding of concentrates with forage *ad libitum* and therefore gives the potential for better use of forages. Owen (1979) has presented a detailed account of the principles and practice of complete diet systems for cattle and sheep. Within a herd of dairy cows there is usually a wide range of milk yields and nutrient requirements, from the high yielding cow at the peak of lactation, which Owen suggests requires at least 50% concentrates, to the dry cow whose requirements can be met by good forage alone. It is implicit, therefore, that the herd must be grouped according to requirements and it is the complication of feeding and milking several groups of cows which has been largely responsible for the delay in the widespread adoption of the complete diet system for winter feeding on dairy farms in the UK.

In the USA, however, herds are often larger and fed on conserved foods at all times of the year, justifying expenditure on machinery for handling and mixing the diets. Everson *et al.* (1976) compared the production of cows fed on a complete food consisting of 60% forage:40% grain compared with others on a 50%:50% diet during the first 21 weeks of lactation, a 65%:35% food for the remainder of lactation and a 85%:15% food during the dry period. There was no difference between groups in milk yields or composition, although the fat content was higher in the cows on the complete diet of constant composition. The variable-composition system was closer to the animals' nutrients requirements and resulted in more rapid return to calving body weight, lower blood ketone values and earlier post-calving oestrus. A high concentrate diet in early lactation seems to be a good way to encourage high intake.

Inclusion of a high-energy ingredient such as fat has been used to increase energy intake in dairy cows. However, dietary fat seems to interfere with rumen fermentation and voluntary food intake is often depressed (e.g. Johnson and McLure, 1973) so that often no increase in metabolizable energy occurs.

The effects of changes in the DE concentration on intake of ruminants is therefore dependent on whether the animal is controlling its intake primarily by metabolic or physical means.

## Modification of rumen fermentation

Monensin is a commercially used food additive which modifies fermentation patterns in the rumen, giving increased propionate production and less methane. In beef cattle there is either no increase in weight gain and a reduction in voluntary food intake or increased weight gain with no effect on food intake, but in either case the efficiency of conversion is improved (e.g. Raun *et al.*, 1976). Beef cows also produce milk more efficiently, forage intake being depressed from 9.6 to 8.3 and 7.7 kg day$^{-1}$ by the inclusion in the diet of 50 or 200 mg monensin per day with no consistent effect on weight change (Lemenager *et al.*, 1978). In a second trial by the same authors weight gains were improved and milk yields were not affected, even though the amount of time spent grazing was decreased by the inclusion of monensin in the concentrate supplement. Baile *et al.* (1979b) suggested that the decrease in intake which occurs when rumensin (containing monensin sodium) is included in concentrate foods for cattle is due to an aversion to some sensory cue associated with malaise resulting from the changes in rumen fermentation.

Recently a yeast culture (Yea-Sacc) has become available for inclusion in the diet of ruminants. Mutsvangwa *et al.* (1992) found that DM intake of supplemented food by bulls was significantly greater than of unsupplemented food (5.55 vs. 5.32 kg DM day$^{-1}$) whereas total rumen VFA concentrations were also higher, but neither rate of weight gain nor efficiency of food conversion was improved.

# Replacement of One Food with Another

A major practical and theoretical problem for ruminant nutritionists is to be able to predict the effect, on the intake of one food available in unlimited quantities, of changing the quantity and/or quality of another food, given in restricted amounts. Although numerous empirical approaches have been made, the underlying theory is not often considered, perhaps due to lack of hypotheses to test, but more likely due to the great expense of performing the necessary research with cattle, which is where the main interest lies (Chapter 16).

Table 10.1 shows details of two foods: Food 1 is a forage and Food 2 is a concentrate. The animals' requirements for energy and protein and the limits to capacity to handle bulk and for heat loss are shown and the amounts of each food necessary to supply these requirements or limits. For example, the indigestible bulk of Food 2 is 0.2 kg kg$^{-1}$ DM and the capacity of the animal for bulk is 4 kg day$^{-1}$ so the animal can eat a maximum of 4/0.2, i.e. 20 kg day$^{-1}$ of Food 2 before it becomes physically full. However, the limit imposed by heat production and the energy and protein requirements are all below this so intake is restricted by one or more of these latter factors, rather than the bulk of the food. When these amounts are plotted for one food against the other

**Table 10.1.** Characteristics of two foods and the requirements or limits to intake of each one. From this can be calculated the intake of each food needed to meet a particular requirement or limit (see text for details).

| | Food 1 | Food 2 | Limit | Intake 1 | Intake 2 |
|---|---|---|---|---|---|
| Energy | 9.5 MJ ME kg$^{-1}$ | 12 MJ ME kg$^{-1}$ | 150 MJ day$^{-1}$ | 15.8 kg day$^{-1}$ | 12.5 kg day$^{-1}$ |
| Protein | 0.1 kg kg$^{-1}$ | 0.18 kg kg$^{-1}$ | 2.0 kg day$^{-1}$ | 20.0 kg day$^{-1}$ | 11.1 kg day$^{-1}$ |
| Indigestible bulk | 0.35 kg kg$^{-1}$ | 0.2 kg kg$^{-1}$ | 4.0 kg day$^{-1}$ | 11.4 kg day$^{-1}$ | 20.0 kg day$^{-1}$ |
| Heat | 8.0 MJ kg$^{-1}$ | 6.0 MJ kg$^{-1}$ | 100.0 MJ day$^{-1}$ | 12.5 kg day$^{-1}$ | 16.7 kg day$^{-1}$ |

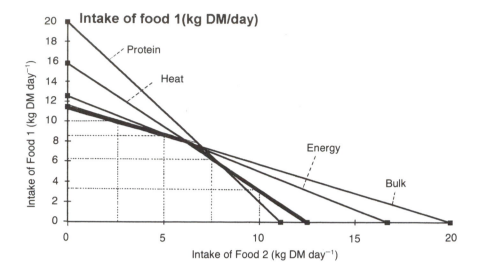

**Fig. 10.6.** Potential intakes of two foods according to calculated limitations of energy, protein, bulk and heat production (see text for explanation).

(Fig. 10.6) the factor most likely to control intake for any combination of the two foods can be seen and the substitution rate can be calculated. The thick line represents the factor most likely to be limiting the intake of Food 1 for any level of Food 2.

In this case Food 2 is likely to be given in restricted amounts and Food 1 *ad libitum* so vertical dotted lines have been drawn from allowances of Food 2 of 2.5, 5, 7.5 and 10 kg DM day$^{-1}$. From the point at which each of these lines meets the thicker prediction line a horizontal dotted line shows the predicted intake of Food 1 and it can be calculated from this that as the level of supplementation goes up from 0 to 10 kg day$^{-1}$ (indicated by dotted lines in Fig. 10.6) in steps of 2.5 kg, so the substitution rate increases from 0.28 to 0.32, 0.48 and 0.63.

Rather than indigestible bulk, CWC or degradation rate could be used to describe the quantitative physical limits to intake; the calculations would be very similar. As discussed in Chapter 7, it is likely that feedback signals are interpreted in an additive manner by the central nervous system whereas the above approach adopted in predicting substitution rates supposes, like the models of Forbes (1977b, 1980) and Poppi *et al.* (1994), that intake is controlled exclusively by whichever factor is the most important under a particular set of circumstances. Clearly there is further thought and work needed to refine these non-additive models as it seems inconceivable that one negative feedback factor is ignored as soon as it is overtaken by another in terms of their power to limit intake.

## Poultry

In an attempt to study the relative importance of energy/bulk and protein as controllers of food intake by broiler chicks Forbes and Catterall (1993) gave individually caged birds either 0.0, 10.3, 18.3, 27.1 or 38.3% of their total *ad libitum* intake as a high-protein food (HP, 280 g crude protein (CP) $kg^{-1}$; 13.9 kJ ME $g^{-1}$) and free access to a low-protein food (LP, 100 g CP $kg^{-1}$; 14.3 kJ ME $g^{-1}$). The intake of LP decreased almost exactly with the increase in allowance of HP resulting in no effect of treatment on the intake of DM or ME. Protein intake therefore increased markedly with increasing allowance of HP, giving increased carcass weight and reduced abdominal fat weight. Thus, there was no suggestion that protein played any part in the control of intake, in contrast to the situation with single foods, in which a marginal deficiency of protein leads to increased food intake (Boorman, 1979). Because the two foods were so similar in energy concentration it is not possible to separate bulk from energy as controllers of intake.

## Cattle

### Dairy cows

It is common practice to feed dairy cows predetermined amounts of compound food and forage *ad libitum*. The concentrate allowance is increased if forage intake is insufficient to meet the required level of production. However, increasing the concentrate input depresses forage intake to an extent which varies directly with the digestibility of the forage, among other factors. The decrease in forage DM intake for a unit increase in concentrate DM allowance is called the substitution rate and for dairy cows is usually in the range 0.4–0.8, i.e. despite the reduction in forage consumption the intake of digestible nutrients increases with supplementation.

Vadiveloo and Holmes (1979) found a mean substitution rate of 0.57 from 26 trials with lactating cows whereas Thomas (1987) found a mean substitution rate of 0.52±0.32 from 43 trials, with little curvilinearity, i.e. one increment of concentrates reduced forage intake by much the same amount as another. Sutton *et al.* (1992) offered 3, 6 or 9 kg of concentrates per day to lactating cows. The step from 3 to 6 kg had the bigger effect on DE intake and milk production, whereas the second step had the bigger effect on silage intake. Silage intakes were 12.8, 11.7 and 9.1 kg DM $day^{-1}$; intakes of DE were 211, 240 and 245 MJ $day^{-1}$; milk yields were 19.1, 24.3, 25.7 kg $day^{-1}$; live weight changes were 85, 159, 117 g day$^{-1}$, respectively, for the three levels of supplementation.

From a survey of the literature and the results of his own experiments Ostergaard (1979) concluded that the substitution rate increased as the level of concentrate allowance rose; he also found that substitution rate increased as lactation progressed, even at fixed levels of concentrate feeding.

A review of literature values by Bines (1985) strongly supports a positive relationship between forage quality and substitution rate. With growing heifers, Leaver (1973) found that with poor forages the substitution rate increased to 0.64 as forage digestibility increased but then remained steady with better forages, suggesting that physical constraints controlled substitution rate with poor to medium quality forages but that with good forages the control was primarily metabolic.

Increasing the level of supplementation with concentrates often causes a decline in the rate of digestion of forages in the rumen. It may be better, therefore, to use slowly fermenting concentrates which are high in cellulose, such as sugar beet pulp, rather than ones based on starchy materials such as barley (Thomas *et al.*, 1984) (Chapter 9).

In a total of eight trials at three centres, Faverdin *et al.* (1991) gave combinations of three levels of concentrate supplementation (L, M and H, with approximately 2 kg DM between each level), three types of forage (maize silage, grass silage, hay) and three types of concentrates (high starch, high digestible fibre, low digestible fibre). Each trial was of $3 \times 3$ Latin Square design, replicated three or four times, each period lasting one month. Substitution rates increased with increasing supplement level (Fig. 10.7) and on average were 0.47 between L and M and 0.67 between M and H; this agrees with the hypothesis set up in Fig. 10.6. For a given forage, the increase in the energy concentration of the concentrate gave an increase in substitution rate, mainly between L and M. The average substitution rate with maize silage was 0.7, with grass silage, 0.53 and for hay, 0.44. In mid-lactation, the higher the energy balance, the greater the substitution rate. There were highly significant relationships:

$$\text{Substitution rate} = 0.7 - 0.11 dMP \qquad (10.5)$$
$$\text{Substitution rate} = 0.50 + 0.14 EB \qquad (10.6)$$

where $dMP$ is change in milk production between levels H and L; $EB$ is energy balance in UFL (energy value for milk production).

Bath *et al.* (1974) gave lactating cows from 0.20 to 0.80 of their estimated net energy requirements as a concentrate food and offered a good hay *ad libitum*. The mean decrease in hay DM intake per kilogram of concentrates was 0.78. In contrast, Campling and Murdoch (1966) found no effect of supplementation on intake of poorer quality hay or

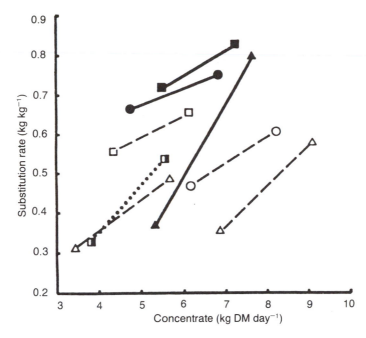

**Fig. 10.7.** Substitution rate (SR, kg kg$^{-1}$) at different levels of concentrate supplementation of dairy cows; each line is for a different forage/concentrate combination (Faverdin *et al.*, 1991).

silage with up to 6 kg of concentrate mixture per day whereas above this level the substitution rate was 0.2–0.4.

With lactating dairy cows, therefore, the mean substitution rate is around 0.5 but there is a positive relationship with the level of concentrates fed and with the quality of the forage.

*Beef cattle*

For growing cattle fed silage, substitution rate was curvilinear (Petchy and Broadbent, 1980). Barley was incrementally added to forages so that it formed between 0 and 90% of the diet for beef cattle; the addition was either by complete mixing or once daily as a separate food. As the proportion of barley (PB) increased, so did total DM intake, up to 40% inclusion, above which is decreased. For the complete foods:

$$\text{DM intake (kg day}^{-1}) = 6.63 + 6.91\text{PB} - 6.08\text{PB}^2 \qquad (10.7)$$

while for barley fed as a discrete meal once per day:

$$\text{DM intake (kg day}^{-1}) = 6.00 + 9.26\text{PB} - 10.57\text{PB}^2 \qquad (10.8)$$

The substitution rate was very low at low levels of incorporation of barley but then increased to very high levels when barley became the predominant component of the ration. The situation is complicated by the fact that the intake of barley varied with total intake, which declined at high levels of inclusion so that, between the 78 and 90% inclusion rates total intake fell and the concept of substitution is not very meaningful.

*Sheep*

Clearly there is a large influence on the intake of lactating ewes of the type of forage offered and the amount of concentrate supplement (Chapter 9). Orr and Treacher (1994) offered hay or grass silage *ad libitum* to ewes rearing twins with a supplement of 300, 650 or 1000 g of a barley-based concentrate per day. In one experiment in which hay (organic matter digestibility (OMD) 0.59) and silage (OMD 0.65) were compared, OM intakes and performance were similar but, whereas the substitution rate (the decline in forage DM intake per unit increase in concentrate DM allowance) was 0.09 for silage, it was 0.62 for hay; the former is a very low replacement rate whereas the latter is similar to that expected from similar work with dairy cows. In another experiment with three silages (OMD 0.56, 0.60, 0.67) substitution rates were not so low (0.29), and there was no significant difference between silages. In a third experiment with three hays (OMD 0.51, 0.59, 0.72) substitution rates were very similar to those for silages (0.30), again independent of hay quality. The lack of effect of forage quality on the decline in intake with increasing supplement level in the second and third experiments in this series is surprising in view of the findings with dairy cows.

### Methods of supplementation

At high levels of concentrate feeding many cows cannot consume their allowance in the milking parlour within the time it takes them to be milked which means that extra compound food may be offered outside the parlour and this must be rationed to prevent over-consumption. Automatic out-of-parlour feeders are now widely used on dairy farms; simple versions dispense a fixed weight of compound food to any cow which is wearing a metal chain around her neck (Broster *et al.,* 1982). More sophisticated equipment automatically identifies each animal from a collar-borne tag which transmits a unique signal and the equipment is programmed to allocate the amount of compound food appropriate to the milk yield and stage of lactation.

Efforts can be made to speed up the rate of eating in the parlour. Pelleting of the compound food increases the rate of eating and mixing with water to form a slurry causes an even greater acceleration. Clough (1972) observed that lactating cows ate loose meal at 323 g min$^{-1}$, pellets at 455 g min$^{-1}$ and slurry at 1670 g min$^{-1}$; similar rates were seen by Seidenglanz *et al.* (1974).

Flavouring agents, such as aniseed, are often included in dairy compound foods. These may encourage a faster rate of eating but the main reason for using them is to ensure that cows do not reject a new food when it is first offered.

# Conclusions

The content of digestible or metabolizable energy is probably the most important factor affecting voluntary intake in farm animals, from a commercial point of view. The cost of the food varies generally in relation to the energy content and providing the most economical diet demands a knowledge of the way in which dietary energy affects food intake.

Although there is compensation in the voluntary intake of poultry and pigs for changes in the DE content of foods, this is not sufficient to achieve an absolutely constant intake of DE; given high-energy diets poultry and pigs gain more weight than when given low-energy foods.

With ruminants there is a positive relationship between the digestibility of forages and the level of voluntary intake, due to physical limitation. Increasing the rate of degradation and/or outflow from the rumen increases the voluntary intake. With high-energy diets which are digested quickly this physical limit is not reached and the animal controls its intake to meet its energy requirements. In order to achieve the required level of production it is often necessary to supplement the forage with supplementary concentrates but this depresses forage intake to an extent that varies with the level of concentrate feeding and the quality of both foods.

# 11 SPECIFIC NUTRIENTS AFFECTING INTAKE

- Protein
- Amino acid deficiency and imbalance
- Minerals
- Vitamins
- Toxins in food
- Water deprivation
- Wet feeding
- Conclusions

Although the yield of available energy per kilogram of food is the major factor affecting its intake, the concentrations of specific nutrients such as protein, minerals and vitamins in the food are also of great importance. Although animals can usually tolerate mild over-provision of a nutrient, deficiency leads to disruption of normal metabolism causing ill-defined feelings of malaise. It is unclear whether there are direct inhibitory effects of impaired metabolic pathways on intake, or whether the animal learns that by eating more of the unbalanced food its condition deteriorates.

## Protein

Within the normal range of dietary protein contents voluntary intake is not affected by protein content. Intake is, however, depressed by diets of low or very high protein concentration. The lower critical content of protein in a food can be defined as that level below which voluntary intake is depressed, for any given class of livestock. Note that dietary 'protein' in this context can be replaced by non-protein nitrogen in the diet of ruminants, where the rumen microflora can use it for protein synthesis (see Appendix 1).

The decline in intake with very low protein foods leads eventually to death but if a greater demand for energy is created then intake increases and the total amount of protein consumed may once again be adequate for life. For example, rats on a low protein diet (10% casein) gained weight very slowly but ate more and gained more lean when forced to expend energy by exercise or low temperature (Meyer and Hargus, 1959). An excessive protein content in food, leading to increased heat production from deamination of the excess amino acids, may depress intake if heat dissipation becomes limiting and body temperature rises or if the products of deamination become marginally toxic.

Protein is more satiating than carbohydrate or fat. Geary (1979) observed a greater depression of voluntary intake when a protein hydrolysate was given via a gastric cannula (1.32 J of food energy J$^{-1}$ of infusate energy) than glucose (0.81 J J$^{-1}$) which is probably related to the fact that protein has a slower flow rate from the stomach and will give a prolonged period of intestinal stimulation.

*Poultry*

In studies with growing chicks Hill and Dansky (1954) found no difference in food intake or growth rate between foods containing 160, 180 or 200 g protein kg$^{-1}$. Comparing a 100 g kg$^{-1}$ with a 200 g protein kg$^{-1}$ diet, Tobin and Boorman (cited by Boorman, 1979) observed a somewhat higher daily intake of the low protein food. Boorman (1979) summarized the literature on the effects of protein content on the voluntary food intake of laying hens and found that there is some compensation for differences in protein concentration, but that this is not enough to maintain a constant protein intake. The situation is complicated by the fact that low protein intake leads to low growth rate and/or egg production leading to a decreased protein requirement.

Shariatmadari and Forbes (1993) offered growing broiler and layer cockerels foods containing 65, 115, 172, 225 or 280 g protein kg$^{-1}$ and found that food intake, although lower in all cases in layers than broilers, was unaffected by diet except the one with the lowest protein content. Live weight gain was maximal for foods with 172 g kg$^{-1}$ or more, i.e. the critical protein content for growth was higher than for food intake. Thus, the carcasses of those birds given the 115 and 172 g kg$^{-1}$ foods were fatter than those whose food was higher in protein content (Fig. 11.1).

Morris and Nurju (1990) gave foods with protein contents of from

167 to 251 g crude protein (CP) $kg^{-1}$ to growing broilers and layer chickens. Broilers grew three times faster than layer cockerels and optimal growth was attained on a food containing 251 g CP $kg^{-1}$ whereas layers only needed 188 g $kg^{-1}$. Broilers ate less than twice as much as layers and in both strains optimum conversion efficiency was attained with a food of 230 g CP $kg^{-1}$. Fat decreased from 87 to 29 g $kg^{-1}$ of whole body for layers and from 167 to 81 g $kg^{-1}$ in broilers as dietary protein increased.

When hens were given a high fat diet they showed signs of becoming protein-deficient and egg weight declined but during a spell of very cold weather when the temperature of the poultry house fell, food intake and egg quality returned to normal showing that sufficient protein was now being eaten (G.H. Smith, personal communication). This example indicates that intake of a single food is controlled so as to regulate energy intake rather than protein intake.

It should be possible to reduce gradually the protein content of the diet as the broiler grows and its amino acid requirements per gram of food decline. In practice a single change of diet is applied, at about 4 weeks after hatching, when the protein content is reduced from 220 to 190 g $kg^{-1}$.

## Pigs

Very low or very high protein content of a food reduces intake and the maximum dry matter (DM) intake is with a food whose protein and amino acid composition is close to that which gives maximum efficiency of growth when given at a restricted level (Cole and Chadd, 1989). The amino acid composition of the dietary protein is of particular importance in controlling the level of voluntary intake (see below).

As with poultry, so the food protein content below which voluntary intake by young pigs is depressed is lower than that for depression of growth (60 and 90 g protein $kg^{-1}$, respectively) (Robinson *et al.*, 1974).

Reduction of the protein content of the food to somewhat below the optimum for growth caused increased food intake (Kyriazakis *et al.*, 1991) but this was not seen when the food was of low energy content (Noblet and Henry, 1977). This compensation for the protein content of the food is not complete and is sometimes non-existent so that Henry (1985) concluded that protein and energy intake are regulated separately and that the mechanisms for both interact to determine the level of voluntary food intake.

It is likely that pigs offered *ad libitum* a food inadequate in protein still feel hungry as they increase their general activity, walking and rooting in straw in much the same way as they do when fed restricted

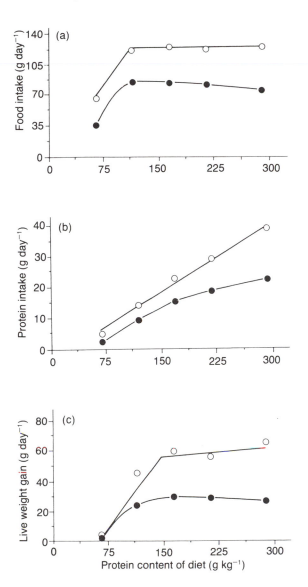

**Fig. 11.1.** The effect of dietary protein content on food intake, protein intake and live weight gain of chickens of layer (●) and broiler (○) strains from 4 to 9 weeks of age (Shariatmadari and Forbes, 1993).

amounts of a balanced diet (Jensen *et al.*, 1993). Rooting for straw declined with time, perhaps as the pigs learned that it did not provide much nutrition.

## Ruminants

As with other animals, low protein content of the food depresses voluntary intake, but the critical level is lower than in monogastric species because the ruminant animal supplements the dietary protein supply with urea in the saliva which can be used for protein synthesis by the rumen microorganisms. Mature sheep and cattle eat less when the crude protein content is below about 80–100 g kg$^{-1}$ DM (Blaxter and Wilson, 1963; Elliot and Topps, 1963) whereas lactating cows, where protein requirements are higher, need at least 120 g CP per kilogram of food (Bines, 1979). (CP is the nitrogen content multiplied by 6.25; this incorporates non-protein nitrogen but as this can be utilized by microorganisms in the rumen it is a useful expression of protein equivalent for the ruminant animal. See ARC (1980) for more details on the protein requirements of ruminants and Cottrell (1993) for a discussion of the importance of the proportion of protein which is degraded in the rumen.)

A low protein food can be supplemented with a high protein concentrate or with non-protein nitrogen in order to alleviate the nitrogen deficiency in the rumen and stimulate microbial activity. The intake of low protein forages is usually increased by such supplementation, i.e. a negative substitution rate (Chapter 10).

## Cattle

Supplementation of a low protein hay with low protein concentrates depressed the hay intake by cattle whereas high protein concentrates stimulated hay intake (Elliott, 1967). Straw intake by 13-month-old beef steers was significantly higher when 1.37 kg of a concentrate food containing 136 g CP kg$^{-1}$ was given, than when the same amount of supplement containing 89 g CP kg$^{-1}$ was given (Lyons *et al.*, 1970). There was no further increase with concentrates higher than 136 g CP kg$^{-1}$.

Alawa *et al.* (1986) found a significant positive relationship between the amount of rumen-degradable protein (RDP) given to pregnant beef cows:

$$I = 5.03 + 0.0035 RDPI \qquad (11.1)$$

and a similar relationship was found during lactation:

$$I = 4.71 + 0.0059 RDPI \qquad (11.2)$$

where $I$ is intake of forage (kg day$^{-1}$) and $RDPI$ is the daily intake of RDP (g day$^{-1}$).

Summarizing a series of six experiments with lactating beef cows Alawa *et al.* (1987) derived the following highly significant relationship between the amount of RDP supplied (*RDPI*, g day$^{-1}$) and straw intake (kg DM day$^{-1}$):

$$I = 5.52 + 0.0038RDPI \qquad (11.3)$$

although the relationship between straw intake and the total amount of crude protein supplied was not significant. They proposed that the first priority in supplementing straw-based diets for lactating cows should be high rumen degradability of the protein.

As well as providing nitrogen for the rumen microorganisms, the diet should also provide sufficient protein which escapes degradation in the rumen, to ensure that those amino acids which are not produced in sufficient quantities by the microorganisms are available to the host animal; such protein is called undegradable dietary protein (UDP) or 'by-pass' protein. In a comparison with lactating cows of supplements containing either 74 or 45 g kg$^{-1}$ DM of UDP, Garnsworthy and Jones (1987) observed that the higher level of UDP resulted in lower hay intake in thin animals but had no effect on intake in fatter animals, whose milk yield was increased.

In early lactation, intake by dairy cows can be increased by increasing the protein content of the food (Roffler and Thacker, 1983). Choung and Chamberlain (1992) found a tendency for increased intakes of silage by dairy cows given postruminal supplements of casein and of a soya-protein isolate with or without additional amino acids

In arid countries leguminous trees and shrubs are a useful source of supplementary protein and Muinga *et al.* (1992) found that intake of hay by lactating cows increased from 7.8 to 9.3 and 10.4 kg day$^{-1}$ due to giving supplements of 4 or 8 kg fresh weight of leucaena, respectively; live weight loss was reduced and milk yield was increased.

Supplementation of low protein forage with high protein concentrates is not always effective in increasing intake, however. For example, 2 kg of rolled barley did not affect straw intakes by yearling cattle nor were they affected when part of the barley was replaced with soya meal, fish meal, lucerne pellets, peas or urea to raise the overall protein content from 50 to 110 g kg$^{-1}$DM (Saghier and Campling, 1991).

*Sheep and goats*

Figure 11.2 shows the relationship between the CP content of the diet and intake by sheep, showing reduced intake of diets with less than 70 g protein kg$^{-1}$ (Milford and Minson, 1965).

Urea supplementation of straw increases its intake (Hemsley and Moir, 1963). In practice the basal food is often poor forage in which it is impossible to incorporate a supplement. Under these conditions urea is given in the form of a block in which it is mixed with cereals and

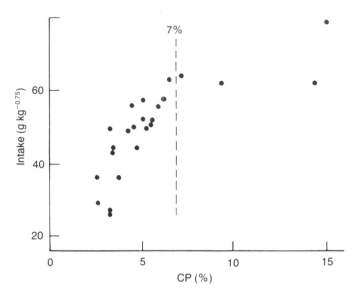

**Fig. 11.2.** Relationships between the crude protein content of tropical forages and daily intake by sheep (Milford and Minson, 1965).

molasses or in liquid form with molasses and salt. Although it is claimed that the continuous availability of this type of supplement ensures that all animals have a good chance to eat some. Ducker *et al.* (1981) found that 19% of hill ewes did not eat any.

Increasing the crude protein content of concentrates for lactating goats from 117 to 185 g kg$^{-1}$ increased hay intake and milk yield without affecting milk composition (Badamana *et al.*, 1990). In further work with a wider range of protein contents Badamana and Sutton (1992) concluded that the response above 182 g CP kg$^{-1}$ was too small to be worth while.

### Mechanisms for the effect of protein content on intake by ruminants

Protein deficiency in the ruminant reduces the activity of the rumen microflora and thus the rate of digestion of cellulose. It was therefore suspected that protein deficiency depresses voluntary intake by physical means but this is only part of the reason as clearly demonstrated by the experiments of Egan and Moir (1964). They compared the effects of duodenal infusion of casein, isonitrogenous amounts of urea, or phosphate (as control) into sheep on a low protein (41 g CP kg$^{-1}$) forage. Casein had a rapid effect and within a few hours intake was increased.

The effect of urea was delayed for 24 h, during which time there was an increase in rumen cellulolytic activity. Urea increased the digestibility of DM and accelerated the rate of digestion of cotton threads in the rumen, whereas casein had very small effects on digestibility and cellulose disappearance. Egan (1965b) concluded that casein alleviated a protein deficiency and thereby stimulated the rate of removal of metabolites by tissues and thus stimulated intake whereas urea acted primarily by increasing rates of digestion and passage after absorption from the intestines and secretion in saliva.

Longer periods of casein infusion gave persistent increases in intake (Egan, 1965a) even though digestibility decreased and the volume of rumen contents increased. Summarizing his work, Egan (1965b) found that:

$$DMI = 37.2 + 81.4N \tag{11.4}$$

where *DMI* is the dry matter intake (g kg body weight$^{-0.73}$ day$^{-1}$) and *N* is the nitrogen retention (g kg body weight$^{-0.73}$day$^{-1}$), and he concluded that '... differences in the level of *ad libitum* energy intake should be examined in relation to changes in the ability to utilise energy'.

## Amino Acid Deficiency and Imbalance

A food in which the essential amino acids are available in a ratio which is widely different from the animal's requirements for amino acids is as effective in depressing intake as a low protein food. Such an imbalance can be alleviated by supplementing the food with the deficient amino acid (or by infusion of this amino acid into the digestive tract or circulation). The review by Harper and Kumata (1970) covers the subject comprehensively for laboratory animals. The way in which the protein content of the diet is monitored by the animal is not fully understood but there are some clues as to the mechanisms of action of severe imbalance or deficiency of amino acids. It is likely that the primary effect of imbalance is on voluntary intake with a secondary effect on growth. Studies in the rat have shown that the imbalance is sensed in the brain, in a site(s) other than the ventromedial hypothalamus, probably the anterior prepyriform cortex and medial amygdala which have connections with the lateral hypothalamus (Rogers and Leung, 1973). It is likely that animals learn to associate eating an imbalanced food with the consequent feeling of malaise (Chapter 12).

Animals' ability to store amino acids in excess of immediate requirements is very limited so not only must the correct amounts of amino acids become available from the food, but they must also be available at the same time. Provision of an imbalanced mixture of amino acids slows growth and increases the oxidation of all but the most limiting amino acid thereby causing inefficient utilization of dietary protein as well as lower voluntary intake.

Although in theory it would be possible to control intake in situations where it is excessive, by altering the amino acid balance of the diet, it would be extremely difficult to maintain the desired amino acid composition in successive batches of the food in practice. The different sensitivities between individual animals to amino acid deficiency or excess would also reduce the effectiveness of this approach.

### Poultry

Amino acid imbalance depresses voluntary intake in poultry (Boorman, 1979). If the imbalance is severe there is a large fall in growth and intake. This can be induced by adding small amounts of one or a few amino acids to a balanced, low protein diet (Table 11.1).

Compared to a balanced food, a low protein food (deficiency of all amino acids) did not depress daily food intake by chicks, whereas deficiencies of individual amino acids caused a marked reduction in intake (Sughara *et al.*, 1969). Not only does a deficiency of an amino acid

**Table 11.1.** Food intake and growth responses to correction of amino acid balance by adding amino acid mixtures to the food for young chicks (From G. Tobin and K.N. Boorman, unpublished, quoted by Boorman, 1979.)

|  | | Diet | |
| --- | --- | --- | --- |
|  | Low protein $(100 \text{ g kg}^{-1})$ | Imbalanced $(200 \text{ g kg}^{-1})$ | Corrected $(200 \text{ g kg}^{-1})$ |
| *Experiment 1* | | | |
| Addition to control diet | None | 100 g kg$^{-1}$ mixture lacking histidine | 100 g kg$^{-1}$ of a balanced mixture |
| Food intake (g day$^{-1}$) | 20.4 | 12.1** | 19.5 |
| Growth rate (g day$^{-1}$) | 6.0 | 4.3** | 9.2** |
| *Experiment 2* | | | |
| Addition to control diet | None | 100 g kg$^{-1}$ mixture lacking lysine | 100 g kg$^{-1}$ of a balanced mixture |
| Food intake (g day$^{-1}$) | 24.2 | 13.7** | 20.8* |
| Growth rate (g day$^{-1}$) | 5.6 | 2.4** | 7.8** |

Means of six replicates of four birds each. Significant differences from control: *, $P < 0.05$; **, $P < 0.001$.

depress intake and performance, but an excess can also have this effect as shown by Latshaw (1993) who found optimum intake and growth by chicks when the diet contained 12.0 g lysine kg$^{-1}$. In addition to this there was reduced performance due to a small proportion of birds which developed leg problems, for unknown reasons.

To resolve the site of action of amino acid imbalances, Tobin and Boorman (1979) prepared young cockerels with indwelling catheters in the carotid artery and jugular vein. The birds were fed on a low protein diet (100 g kg$^{-1}$) which was imbalanced by the addition of a mixture of all the essential amino acids except histidine. Infusion of histidine into the carotid artery significantly increased intake whereas infusion into the jugular vein had no effect; this is direct evidence for an area of the brain being sensitive to the amino acid imbalance. In order to induce lysine imbalance cockerels were offered a diet with a low level of balanced protein (100 g kg$^{-1}$) and infused with lysine into the carotid artery or jugular vein at 100 mg h$^{-1}$. In both cases voluntary intake was severely depressed, from 40.4 to 11.6 g day$^{-1}$ with carotid infusion and from 48.4 to 26.6 with jugular infusion (Tobin and Boorman, 1979). The greater effect of the carotid infusion again strongly suggests that the sensitive area is in the brain.

The fact that imbalances of amino acids affect intake rapidly suggests that it is the primary way in which amino acid imbalance affects growth. Austic and Scott (1975) force fed chicks eating an imbalanced diet to the same level of intake as controls and obtained normal growth, demonstrating that the major effect of imbalance is on voluntary food intake.

However, others have noticed a deceleration of growth before a decrease in intake and put forward the idea that the drop in food intake seen under such circumstances is secondary to the reduction in growth rate (D'Mello and Lewis, 1970).

The results referred to above have been obtained using severe imbalances. If the imbalance is mild there may be a compensatory increase in food intake. Thus, G. Tobin and K.N. Boorman (cited by Boorman, 1979) showed increased intake by chickens when a supplement lacking histidine was added to a low protein food; this was, however, only a transitory effect. With growing birds there is some evidence of increased intake when the lysine content is slightly suboptimal (Lee *et al.*, 1971); the lysine content which gives maximum weight gain is higher than that giving maximum food intake, again pointing to increased intake in mild lysine deficiency (Boorman, 1979). A similar phenomenon also appears in the laying hen (Pilbrow and Morris, 1974). One practical consequence is that the dietary amino acid concentration required for optimum food conversion efficiency is higher than that for maximum production.

*Pigs*

Lysine is the first limiting amino acid for growing pigs. Increasing lysine supplementation from 4.3 to 9.1 g kg$^{-1}$ of the food increased intake from 1000 to 1400 g day$^{-1}$ with smaller increments at higher levels of supplementation (Baker *et al.,* 1975). Sparkes *et al.* (1981) included ten levels of lysine, from 5.5 to 12.7 g kg$^{-1}$, balanced for non-essential amino acids and isocaloric, in foods offered to boars, castrate male and female pigs. Voluntary intake was increased up to lysine contents of 9.1, 8.4 and 9.4 g kg$^{-1}$ DM, respectively, for the three groups.

When lysine was included in foods for growing pigs at levels from 6 to 30 g kg$^{-1}$, the maximum voluntary intake was with the food containing 10 g kg$^{-1}$, which is close to the optimum for growth according to work with restricted-fed pigs (Cole and Chadd, 1989). It was concluded that 'changing the level of a single amino acid to alter amino acid balance has a more drastic effect [on voluntary intake] than altering total protein'.

When pigs were given foods slightly deficient in lysine or threonine there was a slight increase in voluntary food intake (Henry, 1985). However, if the amino acid in question was present at below about 90% of requirements, food intake was depressed showing that the pig's ability to compensate for amino acid deficiency is quite limited, presumably by the consequences of eating more of the other compo-

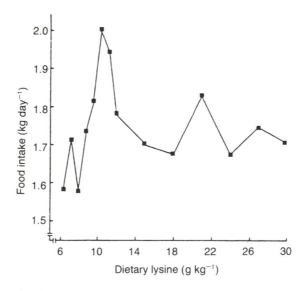

**Fig. 11.3.** Food intake of boars growing from 25 to 55 kg and given foods with different lysine contents (G.M. Sparkes, D.J.A. Cole and D. Lewis, unpublished observations).

nents of the diet, especially energy. Figure 11.3 shows the food intake response by growing boars to different levels of dietary lysine (G.M. Sparkes, D.J.A. Cole and D. Lewis, unpublished observations) and it can be seen that the highest intake is with a food containing just over 10 g lysine kg$^{-1}$, which is just below the optimum. At higher levels of lysine there is approximately constant food intake (apart from the anomalous point at 22 g lysine kg$^{-1}$) but when a toxic excess of an amino acid is included in the food there is a sharp reduction in intake (not shown on this graph).

Methionine supplementation also stimulated food intake, additively with the effects of lysine (Lunchick *et al.*, 1978). If threonine is limiting then voluntary intake is depressed (Robinson, 1975b).

If the environmental temperature is reduced to below the critical temperature and food intake is thereby stimulated to meet the increased requirements for energy, then the intake of a deficient amino acid is also increased and the deficiency is alleviated (Le Dividich and Noblet, 1982).

Henry *et al.* (1992) varied lysine and protein contents of food for growing pigs independently by offering foods with either 5.5 or 6.5 g kg$^{-1}$ lysine in foods containing 130 g CP kg$^{-1}$, a 156 g CP kg$^{-1}$ food with the same amino acid pattern as Food 1; or a 152 g CP kg$^{-1}$ food with glutamic acid added to Food 1 as a source of non-essential amino acids. At the same lysine content, increasing the protein content did not affect voluntary intake but reduced growth due to the increased load of catabolizing the excess protein. Increasing the protein supply with non-essential amino acids caused a fall in intake probably due to an inadequate supply of methionine and threonine in the basal food, as evidenced by the plasma amino acid pattern.

As with protein deficiency, pigs offered a diet deficient in tryptophan increased their explorative behaviour, compared to similar animals on a balanced diet (Meunier-Salaun *et al.*, 1991).

*Cattle*

High quality protein or single amino acids of dietary origin are degraded in the rumen so that it is necessary to infuse amino acids postruminally, or to feed them in a form in which they are protected from degradation in the rumen, to discover which are limiting growth or milk production. Methionine is usually the first limiting amino acid in ruminants but Steinacker *et al.* (1970) found no effect of abomasal infusion of methionine in steers on the intake of forage (120 g CP kg$^{-1}$).

*Sheep*

In a survey of the results of ten experiments in which postruminal amino acid supplementation was given to sheep on various types of food (Barry, 1976), voluntary intake was seen to be increased in seven cases and nitrogen retention or wool growth was increased in almost all instances. However, there was no effect in lambs offered a low-nitrogen purified diet (Schelling and Hatfield, 1968).

Intravenous infusion of methionine at $1\,g\;day^{-1}$ into sheep significantly increased the intake of a low protein straw (J. Twigg and J.M. Forbes, unpublished results). Removal of threonine or isoleucine from a milk substitute containing $80\,g$ protein $kg^{-1}$ halved voluntary intake by lambs (Rogers and Egan, 1975). There is thus some evidence that amino acid imbalance affects intake in sheep in a way similar to that in other species.

# Minerals

A deficiency of any of the essential minerals results in reduced food intake whereas an excess of many of the minerals causes toxic effects, including reduced intake. In most cases the role of each mineral in one or more metabolic pathways is known but the way in which a mineral deficiency or toxicity depresses voluntary intake is unclear. In Chapter 12 we discuss learned associations between the sensory properties of foods and their metabolic consequences and presumably animals learn to adjust their intake of a food to minimize the discomfort induced by that food. Chapter 14 includes a discussion of appetites for minerals.

## Arsenic

Toxic excesses of arsenic (Grimmett, 1939) depress food intake in ruminants.

## Calcium

There is an optimum dietary calcium content below or above which intake is depressed. When the contents of calcium and phosphorus of food for sows were increased from 6 and $5\,g\,kg^{-1}$ to 8 and $6\,g\,kg^{-1}$ there was an increase in voluntary food intake but this then decreased again when they were put up further to 9 and $7\,g\,kg^{-1}$ (Mahan and Fetter, 1982). Calcium deficiency causes depressed food intake in calves (Bechdel *et al.*, 1933).

## Cobalt

In adult ruminants deficiencies of cobalt have been reported to cause inappetence (NRC, 1957, 1963).

## Copper

Copper sulphate is used as a growth stimulant for pigs as it improves the efficiency of food conversion and has no effect on food intake up to an inclusion rate of about $1 g kg^{-1}$. At $2 g kg^{-1}$ or above intake is depressed but whether copper reduces palatability or is toxic at these concentrations is not known. In adult ruminants deficiencies of copper have been reported to cause inappetence (NRC, 1957, 1963) whereas an excess results in a haemolytic crisis and death.

## Fluorine

Toxic excesses of fluoride depress intake in ruminants (NRC, 1957, 1963).

## Magnesium

Voluntary intake of cattle introduced to a magnesium-free food fell to 32% of control by the fourth day; this was alleviated by inclusion of $10 mg$ magnesium $kg^{-1}$ live weight $day^{-1}$ in the food (Ammerman *et al.*, 1971). Cellulose digestibility was depressed by the magnesium deficiency, but not enough to account for the large decrease in voluntary intake.

## Manganese

In adult ruminants deficiencies of manganese depress intake (Maynard and Loosli, 1962).

## Molybdenum

Toxic excesses of molybdenum depress intake in ruminants (NRC, 1957, 1963).

## Potassium

In adult ruminants deficiencies of potassium have been reported to cause inappetence (Telle *et al.*, 1964).

## Selenium

Selenium deficiency in chickens depressed voluntary intake and when selenium was added to the food the birds started to eat more within three hours (Bunk and Combs, 1980). Toxic excesses of selenium depress intake in ruminants (Moxon and Rhian, 1943).

## Sodium

Sodium deficiency depresses intake by poultry; chicks offered a sodium-deficient food ate 11.7 g day$^{-1}$ compared with a daily intake of 15.7 g in those on a normal food containing 2.5 g sodium chloride kg$^{-1}$ (Summers *et al.*, 1967).

Diets high in salt can lead to sodium toxicity in pigs; they do not reduce their intake sufficiently to prevent this, suggesting that the excessive salt is not aversive.

Deficiencies of sodium cause inappetence in adult ruminants (NRC, 1957, 1963). Excessive salt also leads to reduced intake; addition of 30 g sodium kg$^{-1}$ to a sodium-adequate diet depressed the food intake of sheep without affecting plasma sodium concentrations (Moseley and Jones, 1974). However, plasma calcium and magnesium concentrations were depressed whereas calcium retention was increased, so it is not clear as to what actually depresses intake. Wilson (1966) saw no decrease in voluntary intake of Merino sheep until the sodium chloride content of the diet exceeded 100 g kg$^{-1}$ and sheep can tolerate up to 13 g l$^{-1}$ in their drinking water without serious effect on food intake (Pierce, 1962).

There was no effect on intake of 34 g Ca, 10 g P and 17 g Na day$^{-1}$, given twice per day by drench to sheep (van Houtert and Leng, 1991). Water intake and urine output were higher whereas DM digestibility, nitrogen retention and wool growth were reduced.

## Zinc

Food intake was reduced within one hour when adult hens were given 8 mg kg$^{-1}$ or more of dietary zinc (Gentle *et al.*, 1982). In adult ruminants deficiencies of zinc (Miller *et al.*, 1966) and toxic excesses (Ott *et al.* 1966) have been reported to cause inappetence.

# Vitamins

As with minerals, much is known about the metabolic roles of the vitamins and it is likely that animals learn to eat that amount of a food with a deficiency or excess of a nutrient which minimizes their overall feelings of discomfort (Chapter 12). Appetites for vitamins are discussed in Chapter 14.

### Vitamins A and D

In adult ruminants deficiencies of vitamin A or vitamin D cause inappetence (NRC, 1957, 1963).

### Folic acid

Folic acid supplementation of the diet reduced activity in pigs fed *ad libitum* and reduced nibbling of pen-mates in those restricted to 95% of *ad libitum* (Robert *et al.*, 1991).

### Riboflavin

Riboflavin deficiency causes depressed intake in calves (Wiese *et al.*, 1947).

### Ascorbic acid (vitamin C)

There is a decrease in food intake and growth when chicks are heat stressed and this is partly alleviated by supplementing the diet with about 200 ppm ascorbic acid (Kutlu and Forbes, 1993a). Supplementation of non-stressed chicks tends to reduce intake and the optimum level of supplementation can be assessed by appropriate choice feeding experiments (Chapter 14).

## Toxins in Food

### Pigs

Oil-seed rape meal is available in Europe in large quantities and is a good source of vegetable protein. However, it contains several toxic substances, including glucosinolates, sinapines and tannins. In a 4-week continuous feeding experiment, intakes and weight gains of growing pigs closely followed the acceptabilities established in an experiment in which they were not allowed to become accustomed to the effects of each food (Lee and Hill, 1983). Intake seemed to be more closely related to glucosinolate content than to contents of sinapines or tannins. However, gluosinolate level alone cannot be used as a predictor of intake and performance (Lambert *et al.*, 1992a).

*Cattle*

Heat/moisture treatment of rapeseed meal reduced its glucosinolate level and increased silage intake (Aronen and Vanhatalo, 1992). The improved performance could not be explained solely by the reduced rumen degradability so is likely to have been due to the increased intake. Stedman and Hill (1987) studied intake by calves and lambs of a range of types of rapeseed meal, with and without treatments designed to reduce the content of toxins but found no close relationship between intake and glucosinolate content. However, their tests lasted only one hour and learned associations between the sensory and toxic properties of each food might have influenced subsequent intake of these foods, even after extraction of toxins (Chapter 12).

*Sheep*

Barry and Manley (1984) found that binding tannins with PEG3350 increased intake from 0.48 to 0.69 MJ kg body weight$^{-0.75}$ day$^{-1}$ and increased digestibility. Whether this was the result of blocking the effects of tannins on the rumen microorganisms or on the intestine wall was not clear.

Fungal infestation of herbage has a negative effect on its intake. Although part of this effect might be due to the effects on the taste or smell of the grass, Aldrich *et al.* (1993) showed that a more important factor is the feeling of nausea generated in sheep after eating contaminated grass. They demonstrated that daily treatment of their sheep with an antiemetic (metoclopramide) increased intake of endophyte-infected tall fescue but had no effect on the intake of uninfected grass.

# Water Deprivation

Water is an essential nutrient, probably the most essential. In the early stages of water deficiency there is the discomfort of a dry mouth, later there is reduced secretion of digestive juices and ultimately a comprehensive disruption of bodily function. Not surprisingly, lack of water results in reduced food intake and eventually in complete anorexia. The voluntary intake of water is covered as 'water appetite' in Chapter 14.

*Poultry*

Intermittent water supply causes reduced food intake. When daily water allowance is restricted the reductions in voluntary food intake and growth rate which follow are proportional to the degree of restriction; as water supply was reduced from *ad libitum* to 50% of that level the daily food intake fell from 111 to 75 g day$^{-1}$ (Kellerup *et al.,* 1965).

## Cattle

By the fourth day of water deprivation the hay intake of cattle had fallen to 27% of control (Bianca, 1966). Cattle which normally ate 7.6 kg of food per day ate 4.2, 2.2, 0.9 and 0.5 kg on 4 successive days when water was removed (Weeth *et al.,* 1967). A reduction of 40% in the amount of water allowed to dairy cows over a period of 6 days resulted in declines of 16% in food intake and milk yield (Little *et al.,* 1976).

Although cows fed on silage took only a few drinks per day, most of these were large and associated with meals, often occurring in the middle of a meal (Forbes *et al.,* 1991). In this case the water trough was adjacent to the silage and it was convenient for cows to mix eating and drinking. If they had to walk some distance in order to drink they might either have forgone a drink and continued eating, but eaten less due to increased osmolality of rumen contents, or else gone to drink but not taken the trouble to walk all the way back to continue eating, as they were already partly satiated.

## Sheep

The food intake of sheep declined noticeably by the second day without water (Gordon, 1965). This was attributed to the difficulty of transporting the more viscous digesta through the digestive tract, but must also be due to the general feeling of malaise accompanying dehydration of the body.

A moderate reduction in water allowance (about 0.75 of *ad libitum*) does not affect the DM intake by sheep as urinary volume can be reduced to some extent without harm to the animal (English, 1966).

Ruminants in extensive agricultural systems sometimes have to walk extremely long distances to water. Squires and Wilson (1971) studied the effect on Border Leicester wether sheep of placing water and food pellets containing 15% sodium chloride different distances apart. As the distance increased from 1.6 to 5.6 km the number of drinks per day decreased and the food intake fell from around 70 to 45 g kg$^{-0.75}$ day$^{-1}$. The maximum distance walked by the wethers was 17.6 km day$^{-1}$.

# Wet Feeding

Wet mashes of food mixed with water were commonly given to backyard poultry and it is now common practice in Europe to feed growing pigs on wet foods. Some work with rats has shown improved DM intake and weight gain when the food is mixed with water.

*Poultry*

Foods with more water than is conventionally found in cereal-based mixtures have been examined for poultry feeding for two reasons: the utilization of wet by-products and the alleviation of heat stress. An example of the former is the incorporation of alfalfa juice to give DM contents of the food offered ranging from 900 to 680 g kg$^{-1}$ (Tsiagbe *et al.*, 1987). Chicks compensated for the added water and there was no effect on DM intake. Caldwell *et al.* (1986) showed that egg production was decreased when hens were fed diets over 300 g moisture kg$^{-1}$ by the addition of methane digester effluent; the suppression in performance was attributed to fungal growth. Laying hens fed a diet containing methane digester effluent to give 400 g moisture kg$^{-1}$ had egg production and food efficiency similar to those hens fed an air-dried control diet (Vandepopulier and Lyons, 1983). Thorne *et al.* (1989) developed an automated feeding system to deliver high moisture by-product diets with 50% added water to laying hens and found improvements in egg production, egg weight and food efficiency. On balance, there seems to be little benefit of feeding wet foods to poultry under normal husbandry conditions.

However, wet food can be useful in partially alleviating the reduction in food intake and performance under very hot climatic conditions. Tadtiyanant *et al.* (1988) found that feeding Leghorn hens a diet containing 50% added water under two environmental temperatures (21.1°C and 29.4°C) did not improve the performance but more recently Tadtiyanant *et al.* (1991) reported that giving hens food with 50% water added stimulated DM intake at 33.3°C by 38%. Abasiekong (1989) showed that offering broiler chickens a food with the addition of 33 or 50% water increased both food intake and body weight in the hot season (37°C); however, food intake and body weight were reduced significantly by wet feeding under normal temperatures (20°C). It appears, therefore, that the addition of an equal weight of water to food does not improve performance under the normal conditions of poultry husbandry.

It has been generally considered that dry pellets are better than wet mash for growing ducks (Elkin, 1986) but Roberts (1934) found moist mash to be better than dry pellets. However, the results were very variable, some birds were killed by rats and no proper statistical analysis was performed although it was claimed that there were 'probably significant differences' in some cases.

*Pigs*

It has become very common in intensive pig production throughout the world to feed growing pigs on liquid foods, the main advantage being that delivery can be automated. However, wet feeding can also have benefits for biological efficiency as indicated by a large-scale survey in Denmark (Danish National Committee for Pig Breeding and Production, 1986) which showed that on wet-feeding systems pigs ate 2.27 Scandinavian Feed Units day$^{-1}$ and gained 717 g day$^{-1}$ compared to dry-fed pigs which ate 2.03 SFU and gained 643 g. When 750 g of water was added per kilogram air-dry food to reduce DM content from 904 to 387 g kg$^{-1}$ food conversion efficiency in two experiments was improved significantly (Henry, 1968).

Partridge *et al.* (1992) gave foods with approximately equal weights of water and dry food mixed to weaner pigs. Food intake was always higher for those on the wet food, significantly so in most weeks, and as growth rate was improved there were no differences in conversion ratios.

Sows may also benefit from wet feeding as they ate more when fed from a trough with a water nipple in it, i.e. wet food (Moser, 1985).

# Conclusions

Foods containing a significantly lower concentration of an essential nutrient than required by the animal to which they are fed are eaten in smaller amounts than foods with an adequate content. This shows that when offered a single food animals are generally not able to respond to a deficiency by increasing their daily intake. A common feature of all deficiencies is that they interfere with normal metabolism and lead to feelings of metabolic unease and it seems likely that it is an innate response of animals to reduce their intake of a food which makes them feel unwell. In nature the animal could turn its attention to other sources of food but in intensive husbandry no such opportunity is available so the only option is for the animal to eat less in an attempt to relieve the metabolic discomfort.

A toxic excess of a substance in food causes reduced intake as does an imbalance, such as when a low protein food is supplemented with an individual amino acid, even with amounts which only bring its

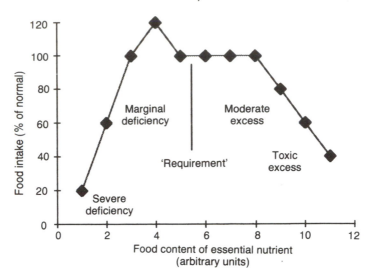

**Fig. 11.4.** Generalized diagram of the effects on voluntary intake of excesses and deficiencies of a nutrient in food.

concentration in the food to what would be normal for a high protein food.

Figure 11.4 is a general diagram of responses to changes in the content of an essential nutrient. For foods with a content of the nutrient just below the 'requirement' there is sometimes a modest increase in intake as the animal tries to maintain its intake of the nutrient in question. Below this and metabolic illness occurs with consequent depression in intake. For foods with a content which is above the 'requirement' there is little or no effect on intake until such a high content is reached that intake is depressed due to the toxic effects of the excess.

Water deprivation reduces the intake of food. Initially this is due to the unpleasantness of a dry mouth but ultimately the disturbance of metabolism will reduce feeding which is a major determinant of the need for water.

# 12 | LEARNING ABOUT FOOD: PREFERENCES

- Finding food; motivation; cognition
- Discrimination between foods
- 'Palatability'
- Learning
- Sensory-specific satiety
- Learning from other animals – social facilitation
- Competitive feeding: social inhibition and restricted access to food
- Prior experience of food
- Working for food: operant conditioning
- Conclusions

It has become abundantly clear in recent years that animals learn to associate the sensory properties of foods with the metabolic consequences of eating those foods. Nowhere is this more obvious than in the field of diet selection, to be covered in Chapter 13. In this chapter we first consider how foods are perceived by animals and how they learn about their nutritional value.

## Finding Food; Motivation; Cognition

Eating is continuous in very simple animals and the drive to eat must, therefore, be very primitive and powerful. It seems likely that higher animals have inherited this drive but that satiating factors have developed to temporarily override it. Sham feeding, in which the ingested food leaves the digestive tract via an oesophageal fistula before any gastric, intestinal or metabolic effects have occurred, is continuous in rats which have always been fed by gastric tube and have not learnt to associate the act of eating with eventual satiety (Mook *et al.*, 1993). This is in contrast to the results of other studies in which animals with gastric fistulas which were sometimes fed with the fistula closed so that they learned to stop eating after a certain amount of food had been eaten. Thus, where ingestion has not become associated with postingestional consequences the rat does not eat for nutrients but eats to satisfy a basic urge to ingest.

Motivation is a reversible brain state induced by internal and external signals which results in an increased tendency to perform a specific behaviour (Lawrence and Rushen, 1993). The tendency to seek food can be of similar intensity whether due to high level of hunger in the absence of food or low hunger in the presence of food. As an animal can only perform one behaviour at a time there must be a decision-making process to determine which activity the animal does at any given time. Models which are based simply on motivation to eat declining as ingestion takes place result in dithering output as the animal switches from one activity to another and back again. If a positive feedback is introduced then some semblance of real behaviour is seen. That is, feeding, once started, tends to reinforce itself until such time as satiating factors become dominant.

Learning can modulate the expression of motivational state. Animals are sensitive to a number of nutrients and can make appropriate choices, according to how they feel. Therefore, if a food is deficient or imbalanced for one or more essential nutrients, the animal is malnourished and feels ill which influences how much it eats. No animal offered a single food will have its requirements met exactly by the food for more than a very short part of its life.

If an animal learns that a food item is unpalatable and avoids it, does it forget the unpalatability by it not being reinforced? Do unreinforced encounters have a memory-jogging effect? Often animals sample from time to time foods to which they are averse, presumably so that they can be made aware of any change in its properties.

Non-primate species should not have their intelligence judged on the basis of their ability to form artificial associations between objects and rewards. Work on imprinting in chicks shows that natural stimuli are more effective than artificial ones (Johnson *et al.*, 1985). In general farm animals do not perform well on complex learning tasks involving the making of artificial associations but have no difficulty learning complex information about the natural environment.

## Poultry

Young chicks are reinforced by pecking at grains with a closed break (Rogers, 1989) and even those which do not ingest any grain learn to discriminate between grain and pebbles as quickly as those which are allowed to swallow it. Although beak-trimmed chicks showed the same initial preference for grains over pebbles they did not maintain this preference as it did not lead to the reinforcement of nutrient intake. This illustrates the point that, although there are inborn, innate preferences for some types of food, these preferences can only be maintained if they lead to nutrient intake.

Social hierarchy develops within the first three weeks, but chicks incubated in the dark, which randomizes the side of the brain responsible for food location and selection (normally the left brain; right eye), develop a more flexible group structure than those incubated in light. Rogers (1989) has suggested that by incubating in the dark, there may be less low dominant chicks which die from starvation.

*Sheep*

Sheep are thought to be colour-blind (Tribe and Gordon, 1949) although their eyes do possess cones (C.V. Ensor, unpublished observations). Temporary covering of the eyes does not interfere with the preference for herbage species by grazing sheep (Arnold, 1966a) suggesting that they use smell, taste and tactile stimuli to a great extent to discriminate between different plant species.

Sheep can discriminate between objects of different hue but this may be due to brightness rather than colour; there is uncertainty as to whether they can discriminate colour. In the study by Bazeley and Ensor (1989) the two hues were close in wavelength, i.e. colour, so the ability to differentiate between them was probably due to differences in brightness.

Sheep have all-round vision (290°C) although acuity is only good in the 40° field where the two eyes overlap, i.e. they can see food in front of them very clearly. Sheep, like cattle, goats and chickens, can make quite complex discrimination between shapes. Kendrick (1992) recorded electrical activity of single neurons in regions of the brain thought to be involved in feeding control. Cells in the lateral hypothalamus and zona incerta, responded to the sight, but not the smell of food, mostly only when food was moved towards the mouth. Sheep can also be trained to associate coloured non-food objects with food and cells in the zona incerta then respond to the sight of that object (Fig. 12.1). It takes 7–13 trials for the association to be established and only a couple of hours for it to be forgotten but it is well known that sheep retain preferences for certain foods for much longer than this. When the conditioned stimulus is a less artificial object, i.e. a novel food, learning is much quicker (one or two trials) and retention is much longer (months).

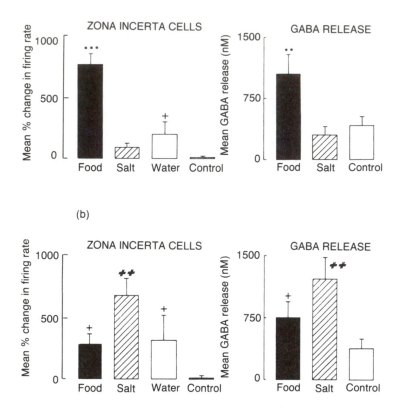

(b)

**Fig. 12.1.** Response in firing rate of neurons and release of gamma-aminobutyric acid (GABA) in the zona incerta of sheep to the sight of food, water and salt when the animals were (a) food-deprived for 12 h or (b) sodium deprived for 4–6 days (Kendrick, 1992).

The cells which respond to the sight of food only respond to palatable food, not to foods that the sheep will not eat. Probably these sites in the brain are associated with rewarding aspects of stimuli but not their negative aspects. Oats, which are highly palatable, cause stomach upsets when eaten in too great a quantity. Two sheep which had eaten too much rolled oats no longer responded as well in terms of increased firing rate of neurons as they had before this overeating. Cells which respond to food will respond to salt instead when the animal is made sodium deficient (Fig. 12.1). Similarly, release of gamma-aminobutyric acid (GABA) depends on what the animal's needs are. Cells which respond to the sight of food also respond to its ingestion; if an animal is not allowed to eat food, its continued presence in front of it does not continue to fire these cells. Cells which respond to food in solid form do not do so when the same food is liquefied.

Before parturition, firing rate increases most in response to foods and no cells respond to fetal fluid odours. After parturition, however, there is very little response to food odours but large responses to lamb odours, whether from the ewe's own lamb or from an alien lamb. Cells that are responsive to food sometimes fire in the absence of food; is this when the sheep is thinking about that food, i.e. when it is hungry?

## Discrimination between Foods

Without visual or taste cues animals cannot identify the appropriate diet. Visual perception is reviewed by Piggins (1992) whereas Perry (1992) discusses olfaction and taste, with particular respect to farm animals.

Wilcoxon *et al.* (1971) demonstrated that rats use taste more than vision as a cue for aversion to nauseating effects whereas quail use vision more than taste (Fig. 12.2).

### Vision

It has been reported that chicks prefer light-coloured foods, particularly pink (Hess and Gogel, 1954) but preferences for other colours can be induced simply by prior exposure to them. Colour is a strong cue for learned aversions (e.g. Martin *et al.*, 1977) and preferences (e.g. Kutlu and Forbes, 1993a) in birds.

Gillette *et al.* (1980) observed that chicks keep food in view while they approach it and eat but when they drink they do not appear to

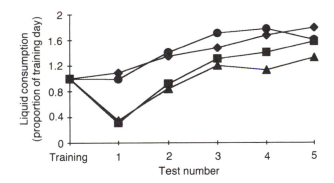

**Fig. 12.2.** Extinction curves for conditioned aversion to sour flavour or blue colour of water paired with injections of a nausea-inducing substance (Wilcoxon *et al.*, 1971). Rats took longer to extinguish the aversion to sour water whereas quail took longer to extinguish the aversion to blue water: ●, colour, rat; ■, colour, quail; ▲, taste, rat; ◆, taste, quail.

look at the drink. However, Gillette *et al.* used opaque drinkers whereas Wilcoxon *et al.* (1971) used transparent tubes in demonstrating that the colour of drink was a very good cue.

The preferred food colour is not necessarily the preferred trough colour; Hurnik *et al.* (1971) found that red was the most preferred trough colour but the least preferred food colour and it is possible that trough colour can be used as a cue for the quality of the food contained in it. Hurnik *et al.* (1974) subsequently exposed hens to different patterns and colours on the side of the feed trough facing them for one week each. The most complex pattern (blue, green, yellow and red) gave the highest food intake, by 27 g bird$^{-1}$ week$^{-1}$, with green/yellow next (+11 g) whereas yellow alone tended to *reduce* intake by 33 g of food bird$^{-1}$ week$^{-1}$ (the mean weekly intake was 784 g).

Bazely and Ensor (1989) found that none of their sheep learnt to discriminate between green and yellow of the same brightness but could differentiate between different brightnesses (41 or 77% reflectance). This does not discount the possibility that sheep have colour vision, but brightness might be important for grass as it is proportional to protein content of perennial ryegrass.

## Taste

Scott (1992) said that 'an animal's experience has a pronounced and enduring effect on behavioural reactions to taste stimuli'. In other words, the taste of food is used as a powerful cue with which to associate the nutritional properties of food. See Houpt and Wolski (1982) for a review of studies of taste thresholds and preferences in domestic animals.

For a review of the anatomy of taste receptors and the results of preference tests with pigs, chickens and ruminants, see Bell (1959).

Rats given a choice between fluid with 0.1–0.5% oil and without oil generally preferred the oily one (Ramirez, 1992). They prefer crude triolein to pure oil and show no preference for tristearin, which does not decompose as quickly as triolein. Rats trained to avoid a dilute suspension of triolein also avoided an aqueous extract of triolein and Ramirez proposed that rats use the smell and/or taste of decomposition products of fats to detect the presence of fats in foods.

The sensory properties of a food are as likely to encourage further feeding as they are to cause feeding to stop. Zeigler (1975) has shown that deafferentation of the buccal region in the pigeon, by section of the trigeminal nerves, leads to loss of interest in food although drinking and grooming were unaffected; clearly in this species the taste and texture of food in the mouth is an important reinforcer of feeding.

*Poultry*

The chicken has a good sense of taste (Gentle, 1971) but birds quickly become accustomed to aversive chemicals such as dimethyl anthraniline and many times the natural concentration in the food is required to depress food intake over long periods compared with the amount which is selected against when choice is given (Kare and Pick, 1960).

Some flavour preferences are very strong; chickens will not drink saccharin solutions but take readily to sucrose or glucose (Jacobs and Scott, 1957; Injidi, 1981).

Flavours as such, although initially able to influence intake and preference, soon lose this ability (Balog and Millar, 1989) if the birds learn that there is no nutritional implication of the different flavours.

A line of broiler chickens selected for high lean weight had lower preferences at any given concentration, for dextrose, and lower aversion for quinine, compared to low growth line (Barbato *et al.*, 1982) but it is not clear whether these differences are due to changed sensory abilities or changed nutrient requirements, compared to a slow-growing line.

*Pigs*

Baldwin (1976) has reviewed studies on taste preference in pigs. Young pigs are quite sensitive to taste and their preference for glucose or sucrose solutions increases with the logarithm of concentration in aqueous solution up to 0.1 M (Kennedy and Baldwin, 1972). The preference for saccharin solutions was not as marked and in other work was found to be very variable (Kare *et al.*, 1965). Aversion can develop to tastes associated with a feeling of illness (Houpt *et al.*, 1979).

Monosodium glutamate (MSG) was used to enhance the flavour of creep food and increased intake was observed from 18 days after birth but without increased body weight at weaning; however, the effect on intake was not seen when MSG was combined with a commercial flavour enhancer (Gatel and Guion, 1990). When MSG was added to the food after weaning, intake was increased by 10% and growth by 7% and there was more effect with lower-weight piglets. However, when the ambient temperature was low there was no effect of MSG on performance.

McLaughlin *et al.* (1983) studied weanling piglets put in a T-maze to assess preference to flavoured versus unflavoured foods (Table 12.1). Five flavours which were well preferred in these short tests (they did not belong to any one category as assessed by human taste) were used in sustained preference tests over 5 days and two of these were then tested for 5 weeks after weaning and resulted in significant

**Table 12.1.** Frequency of degree of preference or aversion of young pigs for different classes of flavour (McLaughlin *et al.*, 1983).

| Flavour group | No. of flavours | Preference | | | | Aversion | | |
|---|---|---|---|---|---|---|---|---|
| | | ext | sig | mild | none | mild | sig | ext |
| Buttery | 8 | 0 | 0 | 4 | 4 | 0 | 0 | 0 |
| Cheesy | 6 | 0 | 1 | 1 | 3 | 1 | 0 | 0 |
| Fatty | 4 | 0 | 0 | 1 | 2 | 1 | 0 | 0 |
| Fruity | 24 | 0 | 1 | 7 | 12 | 4 | 0 | 0 |
| Green | 10 | 0 | 0 | 4 | 5 | 1 | 0 | 0 |
| Meaty | 13 | 0 | 1 | 4 | 6 | 1 | 1 | 0 |
| Musty | 8 | 0 | 0 | 1 | 6 | 1 | 0 | 0 |
| Sweet | 23 | 0 | 1 | 4 | 15 | 2 | 1 | 0 |
| Total | 96 | 0 | 4 | 26 | 53 | 11 | 2 | 0 |

ext, Extremely; sig, significant.

improvement in performance in the first week after weaning. In a large-scale growth trial with over 1200 pigs, one flavour (cheesy) increased body weight gain, but only in the first week. It was concluded that some flavours might be useful in overcoming the stress of weaning.

Sugar and other flavouring ingredients are widely used in weaning and creep foods for young pigs to attract their interest in solid food and encourage high levels of intake before and immediately after weaning. Intake of food by weaned pigs can sometimes be stimulated by flavours (Campbell, 1976; King, 1979) but is not usually (Kornegay *et al.*, 1979; McLaughlin *et al.*, 1983).

### Cattle

Cattle are sensitive to bitter, sour, salty and sweet solutions (see review by Goatcher and Church, 1970), cattle being able to detect tastes with greater sensitivity than sheep.

Jackson *et al.* (1968) were able to modify the flavour of solutions of ammonium salts of short-chain fatty acids by adding molasses, sodium cyclamate or ethyl acetate so that cows drank more, but saccharin, vanilla or aniseed gave little or no improvement. The preference by heifers for a concentrate high in meat and bone meal increased when licorice, diary buds, milk buds or molasses were added (Arave *et al.*, 1989) whereas calves preferred a high quality food which included 2 ppm of MSG over a similar food without MSG (Waldern and Van Dyk, 1971).

When a flavour is added to the single food on offer there is sometimes a short-term increase in intake (e.g. adding sugar to food for calves) or rate of eating (e.g. masking the taste of rapeseed meal in concentrates for dairy cows; Frederick *et al.*, 1988). However, Weller and Phipps (1989) obtained a prolonged, 10% increase in silage intake with the addition of Simax 100 (a mixture of several flavours with a predominantly orange taste).

## Sheep and goats

Sheep and goats are sensitive to bitter, sour, salty and sweet solutions (see review by Goatcher and Church, 1970), goats being intermediate between cattle and sheep. However, preferences or aversions to tastes can be blocked by including 5–50 ppm of MSG in the solution (Mehren and Church, 1976).

The normal type of two-choice preference test confounds the sensory impressions of the foods or liquids offered with postingestive factors. By using sheep with oesophageal fistulas, Chapman and Grovum (1982) were able to determine the true palatability of various additions of sodium chloride or urea to hay. Sheep preferred hay containing up to 200 g kg$^{-1}$ of sodium chloride whereas Goatcher and Church (1970) found aversion to a 22 g l$^{-1}$ solution of salt in water due presumably to postabsorptive effects of sodium ions. Care must be taken in the interpretation of results from oesophageal fistulated sheep, however, as they lose much saliva through the fistula, become sodium deficient and might therefore prefer a higher concentration of sodium chloride than intact sheep. Urea was discriminated against at all levels of inclusion, from 10 to 80 g kg$^{-1}$.

Further work with oesophageal-fistulated sheep by Grovum and Chapman (1988) showed that 15–120 g kg$^{-1}$ sucrose in a pelleted food depressed intake in a dose-related manner. Although 6.25–25 g kg$^{-1}$ of hydrochloric acid had no effect, 50 g kg$^{-1}$ depressed intake by 50%. 50–200 g kg$^{-1}$ of common salt increased intake but not in a dose-related manner. 10–80 g kg$^{-1}$ urea depressed intake in one experiment whereas 5–40 g kg$^{-1}$ increased intake by 16 and 41% in two other experiments.

It has been demonstrated on several occasions that sheep prefer the taste of butyrate over several other compounds. Arnold *et al.* (1980) tested 32 chemicals found in plants for food preference by sheep and found that butyric acid increased preference but not total intake. Gherardi and Black (1991) obtained similar results, as did Buchanan-Smith (1990).

When foods containing 25 ml of 2M acetic acid kg$^{-1}$, 1 g kg$^{-1}$ of quinine or 20 g kg$^{-1}$ of sodium chloride were offered *ad libitum* to sheep, intake was less than the intake of untreated food; when carbocaine, a local anaesthetic, was added at 500 mg kg$^{-1}$ the intake of the acetic acid and quinine-treated foods returned to control levels (Baile and Martin, 1972). Carbocaine included in a concentrate food at 333 mg kg$^{-1}$ increased intake but it is not known whether this was an effect on taste or on rumen receptors. These tests were made over 2-day periods and it is unlikely that the effects would be long-lived. Baile (1975) reported that when phenobarbital was included in a 0.6 concen-trate:0.4 hay food at 1 g kg$^{-1}$ there was a 0.2 increase in voluntary food intake by sheep in a 2-day test; the frequency of meals was not affected and meal size was increased by accelerated rate of eating. Similar changes occurred with a 0.76 hay ration. However, this was over short periods and when phenobarbital was administered at 800 mg kg$^{-1}$ of food for 9 weeks to lambs there were no significant effects on live weight gain, carcass weight or conversion efficiency (Baile *et al.*, 1974a). Further work (Baile, 1975) with 800 mg of phenobarbital per kg of food resulted in significant improvement in carcass weight (20.0 vs. 18.9 kg) including a 0.12 increase in carcass energy content. Much of the increase which occurred in intake was in the first 4 weeks before tolerance developed and when the drug was withdrawn from the food of some animals there was a 0.20 decrease in voluntary intake. Because of the problems of tolerance and dependence there is little possibility of using this or similar drugs commercially and it is not known whether their primary effects are on taste receptors, on rumen receptors, or elsewhere in the body.

Jones and Forbes (1984) found that sheep which obviously dis-criminated against quinine-treated hay in a preliminary period ate equal amounts of treated and untreated hay in subsequent 5-day choice periods, thereby demonstrating adaptation as they learned that there were no harmful consequences to eating the quinine-flavoured food. Following a change in flavour, even without changes in nutritive value of food, sheep sample the food cautiously (Provenza *et al.*, 1993a).

## Olfaction

It is often said that poultry have no sense of smell because they are willing to eat grain contaminated with wild onion bulbs which other stock reject.

The importance of olfactory inputs to food intake in pigs has been investigated by Baldwin and Cooper (1979) who found olfactory bulbectomy to have no apparent effect, although it was difficult to confirm that the sense of smell had been removed because the pigs learnt very quickly to locate hidden food by exploration. Odour of a single food does not seem to influence the level of intake. Presumably, however, smell is used when selecting from a range of available foods.

Arnold (1970) found that the smell of food was an important determinant of food choice by sheep but Tribe (1949) thought that odour had little part to play in selection of plant species by grazing animals. Olfactory bulbectomy of individually penned sheep offered a complete pelleted food did not affect daily intake or meal pattern even though they had olfactory deficits (McLaughlin *et al.*, 1974); feeding was less intense, however, with more re-entries into the feeder during meals.

When given two bins of food, one tainted with odours of carnivore faeces, sheep took 95% of their intake from the uncontaminated pellets (Pfister *et al.*, 1990). There was no evidence of habituation and the sheep went as far away as possible from the odoriferous bins.

Bell and Sly (1983) observed that sodium-deficient cattle can detect sodium bicarbonate at a distance of up to 20 m if assisted by wind direction and that anosmic cattle took longer than controls to identify a salt solution from among an array of buckets of water. They thus deduced that cattle can smell salt solutions but could not explain how non-volatile salts can have a smell. Anosmic cattle can still taste salt, clearly demonstrating that the senses of smell and taste are separate.

## Texture of food

Hyde and Witherly (1993) propose that changes in texture, temperature and taste during a meal, or even a swallow, have a big impact on a food's palatability. They do not dispute that 'palatability' depends on context, including metabolic context. Memorable foods are more easily learned with regard to their eventual metabolic properties, compared with bland foods. Adding spices to foods enhances palatability, even if not at the first exposure, by making the food subsequently more identifiable. The authors propose the concept of 'dynamic contrast', which refers to the manner in which foods give changing sensations during chewing and swallowing. We should consider texture, in its various manifestations, as additional cues in characterizing a food, in conjunction with its sight, smell and taste. Memories of chewing pressures and number of chews/swallows help to recall how much food to eat for satiety (Miller and Teates, 1986).

Round and solid objects are pecked at more than angular and flat objects by newly hatched chicks (Fantz, 1957) but within 3 days they are pecking mainly at food (Hogan, 1973).

Pelleted forages are usually eaten in greater quantities than the same material in unpelleted form (Heaney *et al.*, 1963). Although much of this increase is attributable to the reduction in particle size associated with pelleting, some improvement in palatability is also involved (Van Niekerk *et al.*, 1973).

*Position of food*

In addition to the colour, shape and brightness, animals can also learn the position of the food if that is consistent between exposures. Gillingham and Bunnel (1989) offered three foods to deer in a small enclosure. Initially, apples were preferred to dairy pellets or alfalfa and when the foods were placed separately 5 m apart the deer searched for apples. When these were depleted a second food was accepted. When the food positions were changed, the animals' search paths were at first similar to those used successfully before the foods were moved, demonstrating a memory of successful paths to food.

Heifers learned more quickly than cows in which of two hoppers to find feed after two 10-min tests per day for 5 days (92% of heifers, 23% of primiparous cows and 54% of cows after their second calving) (Kovalcik and Kovalcik, 1986). After 6 weeks, tests were resumed and 77% of cows, but only 46% of heifers went straight to the correct feeder. The process of learning was quicker in heifers but they forgot sooner than did cows, which is in general agreement with learning at different ages in other species.

When cows have to push open a Calan door to obtain food they learn within about 24 h of 'their' door being changed.

# 'Palatability'

I do not believe that it is possible to define adequately the word 'palatability'. Although it might be described as the overall impression of the food given by all the animal's senses (Forbes, 1986a), it cannot be considered to be a quality of the food because it depends so heavily on the experience and metabolic status of the animals in question. There is no single way to measure palatability but Weingarten (1993) has listed several methods: (i) intake tests, which often give very different results depending on whether the two foods are offered simultaneously or sequentially; (ii) brief exposure tests with minimal ingestion; (iii) initial rate of eating on first exposure (lick analysis); (iv) oesophagostomy or stomach fistula tests; and (v) taste reactivity observations.

Forbes (1986a) stated that 'its importance in determining food intake is often underestimated', and went on to describe the ingenious method of separating how much of the difference between intakes of different diets is due to postingestional differences rather than to differences in palatability (Greenhalgh and Reid, 1967). Two foods of very different sensory and chemical properties were offered to sheep without involving any differences in the composition of the digesta. Either straw or dried grass was offered by mouth and equal weights of either one food or the other were introduced via the rumen fistula. When straw was given both by mouth and by fistula the total intake was 13.8 g kg$^{-0.73}$ day$^{-1}$ and the digestibility of organic matter (OMD) was 0.41; when dried grass was given by both routes intake was 59.4 g kg$^{-0.73}$ and OMD was 0.74. When equal amounts of the two foods were given, one by mouth and the other by fistula the digestibility was intermediate (0.55–0.57) but the voluntary intakes were very different – 23.5 when straw was given by mouth and 48.8 g kg$^{-0.73}$ when dried grass was given by mouth. This was said to demonstrate a powerful influence of palatability on voluntary intake. However, given the discussion above and in Chapter 13, it is quite possible that these sheep were eating according to learned rather than to innate preferences as they had experienced eating just hay or straw in some periods of the experiment.

An example of the lack of correlation between intake when a choice of foods is on offer and when they are given singly is the work of Forbes *et al.* (1967) in which pregnant ewes were offered one of three silages or else free choice of the three silages. Silage B was of poor quality but was eaten in quantities only slightly less than silages A or C by ewes which only had access to one food. However, the group that had access to all three ate equal amounts of silages A and C but very little of silage B.

Gherardi *et al.* (1991), studying the short- and long-term responses in intake of sheep to additions of chemicals thought to influence palatability, concluded that palatability effects are not important in determining the level at which a single forage is eaten, but can have marked effects on the relative intakes when two forages are on offer. Addition of butyrate plus MSG increased preference for a forage by sheep whereas magnesium oxide had the opposite effect.

## Learning

Selection of a food may be euphagic, i.e. implying nutritional wisdom, or hedyphagic, i.e. selection for pleasurable flavour. Because there will be some food items which have innately pleasant appearance or flavour but are nutritionally inadequate or even toxic, animals should not rely solely on inborn preferences to determine their food choice. Rather, they should sample a range of foods and, when they have learned which ones are nutritious, eat predominantly from those while sampling other foods occasionally to take advantage of any nutritious foods which may become newly available (Stephens and Krebs, 1986). The underlying process seems more likely to be a learned preference for an adequate food rather than a learned aversion for a deficient food, however, because birds tend to choose familiar diets even when they are made deficient, as against novel diets which might supply the missing nutrient.

## Learned aversion to food

It is known that when an unpleasant experience occurs around the time a novel food has been eaten, this food becomes aversive. For example, injections of lithium chloride, known to induce nauseous feelings, when paired with red food, induce aversion for that colour by chickens (Martin *et al.*, 1977). There can be a significant interval between the poisoning and the cue. In rats, the aversion becomes weaker as the cue is presented at increasing intervals, up to 6 h, after the injection of lithium chloride (LiCl) (Kalat and Rozin, 1971).

There are several unusual features concerning the conditioned aversion to food paired with abdominal discomfort: the aversion can develop after a single trial; it can occur even though there may be a long delay (several hours) between the unconditioned stimulus (US) and conditioned stimulus (CS); and tastes are much more effective than visual or aural cues, at least in mammals (Bernstein, 1994). Even rats which are under the influence of an anaesthetic when a painful stimulus (US) is given, learn to associate it with the food available when they are regaining consciousness (CS). It is important for food to be novel, with a strong taste and/or odour and these characteristics are often associated with high protein foods.

Neophobia is commonly observed in many species but animals on an imbalanced diet are more willing to test new foods than those on a well-balanced diet.

## Poultry

There is strong evidence that for birds the colour of food is a more effective CS than taste or odour. For example, Gillette *et al.* (1980) offered red food to chicks and then gave lithium chloride; aversion to red food ensued. Other animals failed to associate coloured water or flavoured food with LiCl. However, as far as drink is concerned, the flavour of water was a more important cue than its colour: chickens rapidly learn to associate sour flavour in water with illness.

Cholecystokinin (CCK) a gastrointestinal hormone implicated in satiety, when given at a high dose which is thought to be unpleasant (Savory, 1987), induced aversion to food of the colour with which the injection was paired (Covasa and Forbes, 1994a). Figure 12.3 shows the proportion of chicks which moved towards the colour of food which they had been conditioned to associate with discomfort following

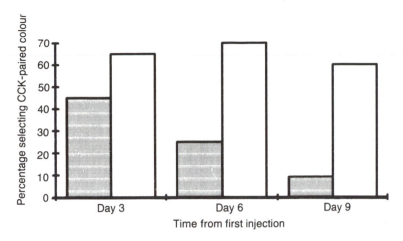

**Fig. 12.3.** Proportion (%) of intact (shaded) and vagotomized (unshaded) birds moving towards the colour of food which was paired with injections of CCK (Covasa and Forbes, 1994a).

intraperitoneal injection of CCK. After successive injections the aversion became stronger in intact birds but not vagotomized, showing that the discomfort was relayed to the central nervous system by the parasympathetic nervous system.

*Pigs*

Foods containing rape or soya were given to growing pigs each for only 24 h to avoid adaptation so that it was thought that only taste preferences were being measured (Lee and Hill, 1983). The lowest intake was of British-grown rape and the acceptability of this was not improved by molasses or sucrose; commercial flavouring agents increased intake of the rape-containing mixtures, but not to the level of the soya food.

*Cattle*

Provenza *et al.* (1992) has reviewed learned aversions to toxins in various types of foods with particular reference to ruminants. With variation of the concentration of a toxin in the food, food intake varies to maintain an approximately constant toxin intake. If the toxic effects of eating a food occur after a long delay, then this food is less likely to be aversive because the positively reinforcing effects of nutrients have occurred in the meantime. Zahorik and Houpt (1981) showed that cattle, sheep, ponies and goats learned to avoid a novel food which had been paired with poisoning as long as the food was presented alone and the consequences followed immediately after ingestion.

The rumen, by storing food for several hours, may act as a buffer between eating and its consequences and reduce the chance of a toxin being associated with its originating food (Thorhallsdottir *et al.*, 1987). Alternatively, the rumen may assist learning by elongating the time over which a toxin is available to the host animal (Zahorik and Houpt, 1981).

In two-choice tests heifers showed no preference or aversion for solutions of urea when they were restricted to prevent more than 0.35 g $kg^{-1}$ body weight being taken in any one test, i.e. an insufficient amount to cause toxic effects (Chalupa *et al.*, 1979). When they were given a food containing 25 g urea $kg^{-1}$ their daily intake was initially the same as that of control heifers fed a similar food containing soyabean meal but from the third day they ate significantly less. When the urea-containing food was replaced with the control food for 4 days and then offered again, in choice with the control food, there was significantly less eaten, i.e. they showed a mild aversion.

Heifers can be conditioned with LiCl to avoid eating larkspur but they lost this conditioning more quickly when kept with uncon-ditioned heifers than when not kept with such untrained animals (Ralphs and Olsen, 1990).

## Sheep

Sheep find LiCl, injected or in the food, to be unpleasant (Burritt and Provenza, 1990; du Toit *et al.*, 1991) and the degree of learned taste aversion varies closely with the dose. Strong aversion was shown with 150 mg $kg^{-1}$, similar to the dose which causes strong aversion in rats. Feeding neophobia was also increased in proportion to the last dose of LiCl used. When sheep and goats were given 2% LiCl in food they ate a maximum of around 39 mg $kg^{-1}$ for sheep and 27 mg $kg^{-1}$ for goats, levels not much higher than those causing mild discomfort in humans.

Thorhallsdottir *et al.* (1987) showed that when LiCl was put in food for lambs or ewes, they recognized these foods after 2 months without exposure. Sheep approached LiCl-paired foods very cautiously but always ate a little, although sometimes intake increased after a positive experience. Such continued sampling, even of toxic foods, is a charac-teristic of herbivorous foragers (Westoby, 1974). Even if sheep were deeply anaesthetized when given a LiCl injection, they still acquired an aversion to the food which was on offer when they recovered consciousness (Provenza *et al.*, 1994a).

The presence of bitter substances such as tannins, coumarins, isoflavones or alkaloids in food led to rejection (Arnold and Dudzinski, 1978) but it is unclear whether this is an innate aversion or one learned early in life.

Goatcher and Church (1970) got almost total rejection of a urea-containing food but the concentration of urea was high enough to cause illness and even death.

Antiemetic drugs attenuated the aversion to several cereals induced by LiCl (Provenza *et al.*, 1993a). Also, sheep receiving anti-emetic drugs ate more grain than those not receiving them; it thus appears that intake of cereal-based foods is limited by mild aversion to abdominal discomfort induced by overeating.

To see whether a learned aversion to a flavour in one food was transferred to another food with the same flavour, Launchbaugh and Provenza (1993) made lambs averse to ground rice flavoured with cinnamon, then they offered wheat flavoured with cinnamon. Those animals which had been rendered averse to the flavour of cinnamon only ate 3% as cinnamon-flavoured wheat when given it in choice with unflavoured wheat, whereas controls ate 45%. Aversion conditioned with the smell, rather than the taste, of cinnamon only lasted one test; odour alone is not a very effective unconditional stimulus.

Launchbaugh *et al.* (1993) offered lambs food with high, medium or low contents of LiCl; when all were subsequently offered the medium-LiCl food, those previously on the high-LiCl food ate more whereas those previously on low-LiCl ate less. In another experiment, lambs were given barley with either a sweet taste (saccharin) or a bitter taste (aluminium sulphate), then injected with LiCl 1 h later. Then, when offered a choice between barley with high or low concentration of the same flavour, they chose predominantly that with the low concentration of the flavour. These experiments show that sheep can clearly detect different concentrations of a flavour and prefer a lower concentration when that flavour is associated with unpleasant consequences.

Sheep find a food aversive only when discomfort is felt soon after ingesting that food. Provenza *et al.* (1993a) gave sheep 150 mg kg$^{-1}$ LiCl either at the time of offering oat chaff or 1 or 2 h later; only those given LiCl at the time of offering the chaff developed an aversion for that food. In another experiment sheep were given LiCl-containing pellets from 08.00–08.20 and then oat chaff from 08.20–10.30. The pellets became aversive as the lithium concentration in rumen increased very quickly during ingestion. When LiCl was administered slowly (by gelatine capsule), aversion developed to oat chaff as the rumen lithium concentration peaked at 1 h after eating the pellets, i.e. at the time chaff was being eaten.

*Learned preference for food*

The previous section has shown that animals can learn to associate the sensory properties of a food with malaise caused by that food. Equally, animals can learn to prefer foods which are metabolically satisfying. Thus, Tordoff and Friedman (1986) paired infusions of glucose into rats with one flavour of food and infusions of saline with another flavour. In rats with jugular catheters there was no subsequent preference for either flavour whereas the animals with portal vein catheters, in which glucose infusion depressed intake, subsequently showed preference for the flavour which had been paired with glucose infusion. Thus, not only was infusion of glucose at physiological rates not aversive, it actually formed the basis for the acquisition of a learned food preference. Tordoff and Friedman (1986) point out that reports which found no effect of hepatic portal infusion of glucose might not have controlled for previous experience in the test situation.

CCK, given at doses which significantly depress intake induce a food aversion but very low doses can induce a preference (Perez and Sclafani, 1991).

*Poultry*

Chicks show a significant preference for food of the colour which was paired with ascorbic acid supplementation when the requirement for ascorbic acid was increased by heat stress (Kutlu and Forbes, 1993b). Otherwise, when kept in thermoneutral temperatures, at which they can synthesize sufficient ascorbic acid, they preferred the colour of unsupplemented food.

# Sensory-specific Satiety

If rats 'satiated' with glucose solution are then offered normal food or powdered glucose they immediately eat significant amounts (Mook *et al.*, 1983) showing that satiety for one food is not absolute satiety. When a novel food is offered to rats they start to eat immediately without the transient decline in blood glucose that precedes a spontaneous meal of a familiar food (Campfield and Smith, 1986).

A corollary of sensory-specific satiety is that animals choose to eat a variety of foods when none of them is aversive. For example, Newman *et al.* (1992) found that, although it is widely held that sheep actively select clover rather than grass, they actually selected the one which they had not recently been eating. Highly palatable roughages are able to override to some extent the satiety signals due to rumen fill and digesta texture (Baumont *et al.*, 1990b)

Another example (Ramos and Tennessen, 1993) is from steers given either hay or silage for 18 days, or the two offered in succession. Total intake was not affected but when both foods were subsequently offered together, those animals which previously only had hay showed a proportional increase of 15% in the acceptance of silage whereas those which only had silage showed a 49% increase in the acceptance of hay.

# Learning from Other Animals – Social Facilitation

The food preferred by newly weaned rats is affected by their mothers' diet, possibly by transmission of flavours in milk and there is evidence of transmission of learned discrimination between foods from experienced to inexperienced rats.

*Poultry*

The sight and sound of the hen pecking and giving a low call stimulates newly hatched chicks to peck at food (Savory *et al.*, 1978). Bate (1992) exposed chicks to maternal feeding calls from hatching or to brooding calls before hatching and feeding calls after. Compared to unexposed controls there was no effect on mortality although sound stimulation was stated to 'enhance feeding behaviour'. Chicks can learn from each other but do not learn so well to get food if the demonstrator does not receive a reinforcement. To what extent is the demonstrator aware that it is teaching and does it modify its behaviour, e.g. by accentuation, when it realizes that it is a teacher?

Adult birds tend to feed in groups and visual, but not auditory, cues are important in the synchronization of feeding in individually caged birds (Hughes, 1971) although Clifton (1979) stated that feeding can be synchronized in the short term by sound alone. Grouped birds usually grow faster than those in individual cages (Savory, 1979). Although it had been assumed that this was due to higher food intake, Savory (1975) showed that there was no difference in intake and that, therefore, isolated birds were less efficient than those in groups.

*Pigs*

Farm animals are all gregarious species and even when penned separately, but within sight and sound of each other, tend to eat in synchrony. Weaned piglets penned close to suckling sows went to their feeder when they heard younger piglets sucking (Kilgour, 1978). There is synchrony of sucking within a litter of piglets and different litters in the same house tend to suck at the same time. Tape recordings of the sounds associated with nursing have been used with some success to increase the frequency of nursing and to improve weight gains (Stone *et al.*, 1974). Young pigs also accept a food more readily if it has the flavour of their mothers' milk (Campbell, 1976).

Within a group, feeding is stimulated by the sight of other pigs eating so there should be enough space for all pigs in a pen to eat at once; by the time they reach 90 kg they require about 350 mm of trough length per animal (Hsia and Wood-Gush, 1983). Barriers separating the heads of pigs at feeding reduce the incidence of fighting.

Social facilitation of feeding is known to occur in pigs but any attempt to investigate whether or not this might affect daily food intake would be fraught with difficulties of interpretation as it would involve keeping some pigs in isolation which might be stressful and depress intake. It has until recently been commercial practice in Britain to feed pigs heavier than about 60 kg in individual feeders adjacent to the group pen to ensure that each animal gets its correct ration. The development of lean types of pig now allows *ad libitum* feeding without excessive fatness.

Cole *et al.* (1967) found that pigs penned in groups ate more than those housed separately. However, many reports show no effect of group size on voluntary intake whereas others have shown that increases in group size depress performance.

*Cattle*

Calves are social drinkers. If one calf was allowed to drink to completion and then another calf in the next pen was allowed to drink, the first one resumed drinking (Barton and Broom, 1985). Even when the second calf was muzzled and put in the same pen it tried to drink and stimulated the first to drink more. Thus it is sensible to provide plenty of teats so that all calves can drink together, in order to get maximum intake.

Social facilitation of feeding also occurs in adult cattle (Balch and Campling, 1962) and cows fed in groups ate 7% more of a complete food containing 0.6 silage than did individually stanchioned cows, although there was no effect on milk yield or composition (Coppock *et al.*, 1972); Phipps *et al.* (1983) obtained similar results. Konggaard and Krohn (1978) examined the effects of separating first-lactation cows from older cows. In three herds the heifers spent more time eating when they were mixed with older cows (263 vs. 240 min day$^{-1}$), had more eating periods (6.7 vs. 5.3 periods day$^{-1}$) and, in the one herd in which silage intake was recorded, ate more food (9.3 vs. 7.7 kg DM day$^{-1}$).

Social interactions do not necessarily facilitate feeding, however, especially if there is insufficient feeding space for all animals in a group to eat at the same time. Trough space can be a limiting factor and less than 0.2 m per cow is likely to reduce intake (Friend *et al.*, 1977). Metz (1983) discusses the behavioural effects of competition for food in cattle.

## Sheep

Nolte and Provenza (1992b) demonstrated that lambs show preference for a food with a flavour they experienced in their mother's milk or even *in utero*. Lambs quickly learn to differentiate between their mother and other ewes, the former offering herself for sucking (positive reinforcement), the latter butting and moving away to generate aversion (Matthews and Kilgour, 1980).

Lambs also retain dietary preferences learned by observation from their mothers, for up to 3 years, without having eaten the food in the intervening time (Green *et al.*, 1984). Provided they are at least 7 weeks old, lambs could learn as well from either their mothers or from other adults, as demonstrated by the observations of Lynch and Bell (1987). On two commercial farms, ewes and lambs were given grain on 3

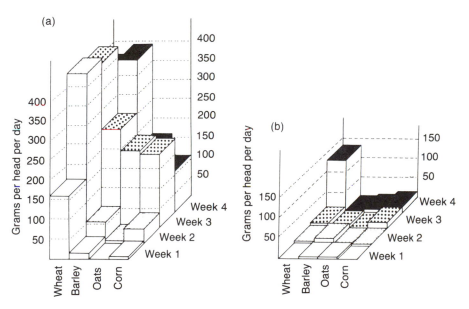

**Fig. 12.4.** Intakes of wheat, barley, oats and maize by sheep which (a) had or (b) had not had previous experience of wheat (Mottershead *et al.*, 1985).

consecutive days; 18 months later, 140 of these lambs and 140 naive lambs were offered grain; all of the experienced ones ate by end of day 3, whereas less than 10% of others ate by this time. Thus, the simple strategy of giving ewes grain for a few days just before their lambs are weaned will have a very big beneficial effect if and when these lambs have to be given grain. A limitation is that the same grain must be given as Mottershead *et al.* (1985) have shown that sheep trained to one grain behave naively when offered another (Fig. 12.4). Those which had no previous experience of wheat ate very little of any grain (wheat, barley, oats, maize) in the first 3 weeks of offering whereas those which had already had some wheat experience ate wheat from the first day of offering but did not take the other grains as readily even though they eventually ate more of them than did the totally untrained animals

Even when sight, hearing and smell are removed, learning is rapid. Sheep introduced to wheat in the presence of experienced sheep started to eat much more quickly than those penned with other inexperienced sheep (Chapple *et al.*, 1987a). In another experiment, sheep had their sight, hearing or olfaction, or a combination, temporarily impaired; only impairment of all three senses resulted in slower learning so there is no overriding role for any one sense in the learning process.

When supplementary food is offered in drought conditions in Australia, sometimes sheep fail to eat it and suffer undernutrition or even die (Chapple and Lynch, 1986). In order to see the extent to which prior experience would alleviate the problem, lambs were offered wheat with their mothers for 5 days for a few minutes each day in one of weeks 1 to 7 of age. When at a much later date they were offered wheat those which had been given it when 3 weeks or older ate more than those without prior exposure or those exposed in the first 2 weeks of life. Other work showed that lambs given wheat for 5 days subsequently ate much more than those only given it for 2 days. Weaner sheep which had never seen wheat ate almost none for the first 11 days, after which their intake increased rapidly. There is also a fear of unfamiliar troughs, with a reduction in the time taken to eat wheat if it was fed in troughs from which the sheep had previously obtained hay (Chapple *et al.*, 1987a). Sheep must overcome the fear of the trough, the fear of the food and then learn how to prehend, chew and swallow grains.

Lynch *et al.* (1983) gave lambs, varying from newborn to 9 weeks of age, wheat for an hour a day for up to 45 days in the absence of adults whereas other lambs were offered it in the company of their dams. When offered wheat 2 weeks after weaning those which had seen adults eat it immediately ate whereas the others did not. Even early weaned lambs which had access to wheat for 24 h per day did not eat it after weaning. Subsequently these animals were tested after 6, 12, 24 or 36 months and those which ate readily at 12 weeks still did so after 3 years. Those exposed to wheat without their mothers before weaning, did, however, eat wheat when offered it after 24 months, during a drought, whereas naive controls did not.

In a further demonstration of the power of observing adults eat, Lobato *et al.* (1980) found that preweaning exposure to molasses–urea blocks had a greater influence on subsequent acceptance than post-weaning exposure.

Odoi and Owen (1993) penned lambs in pairs or singly with or without sight of other lambs. There was no effect of visibility on intake but the paired animals ate more than those kept singly.

In a more specific experiment Provenza *et al.* (1993b) offered ewes a novel food (elm leaves) followed by LiCl or saline and some of their lambs were conditioned similarly. When lambs were offered a choice, those which were averse themselves, or whose mother was averse, took fewer bites of elm than controls, whereas there was no difference due to treatment on the number of bites of poplar, which had not been paired with a toxin and which they had previously eaten readily. It was concluded that the toxin was more effective than the mother in determining preferences as those lambs that received LiCl themselves avoided elm whether their mother had it or not.

## Competitive Feeding: Social Inhibition and Restricted Access to Food

The presence of competition for feeding space exerts a major influence on feeding behaviour, rate of eating being increased when there are more animals per feeder. In some studies, but not others, social dominance was found to be correlated with food intake, growth, milk production or egg production; this is especially true where there are not enough feeding spaces for all animals to eat at once (Syme and Syme, 1979).

Even with a well-balanced food available *ad libitum*, intake might be insufficient. Many farm species show social synchrony of feeding and it is possible that some individuals cannot get to the trough during these feeding periods, sometimes being excluded by dominant members of the group. In many cases the deprived animals compensate by increasing their feeding rate (Kenwright and Forbes, 1993; Young and Lawrence, 1994).

Where animals have to be vigilant for predators, then a larger group size might allow each individual to devote more time to grazing.

*Pigs*

Pigs in groups, took fewer meals, ate faster, and ate less per day than pigs penned individually (De Haer and Merks, 1992). Nielsen *et al.* (1993) agree except that daily intake was not affected in their work. The effect on meal number was most obvious with groups of 20 pigs, compared with 5, 10 or 15.

Competition is also affected by the amount of food obtained during each press of a panel. With feeders set to dispense either 1.4, 2.7 or 5.3. g per response, apparent food intakes by growing pigs (10 to one single-space feeder) were 1.97, 2.14 and 2.21 kg day$^{-1}$ resulting in growth rates of 727, 797 and 845 g day$^{-1}$ and improved conversion efficiency (Walker and Warren, 1992). Feeding times were 110, 78 and 87 min day$^{-1}$ with 52, 46 and 42 entries day$^{-1}$. Pigs worked for longer at the low setting which generated more queuing at the entrance to the feeder. There were fewer aggressive contacts when two feeders were provided but no difference in food efficiency or growth rate, compared to a single feeder (Morrow and Walker, 1991).

Hunter *et al.* (1988) found that, by and large, the social dominance order in a group of sows was the same as the feeding order to obtain a restricted amount of food from an automatic feeder. Feeding by some of the lower animals was disrupted by return visits by more dominant sows and experience was a major factor in determining the social hierarchy.

When a barrier was provided within a pen of young pigs, to allow the weaker pigs to escape from the more dominant ones, there was better performance in those subject to aggression (Waran and Broom, 1992).

Petherick *et al.* (1989) reported no effect of group size (6, 18 or 36 pigs with the same area per pig) on food intake or growth of young pigs.

When weaner pigs from several litters are mixed there is a short period of stress until a dominance order has been established but this does not appear to affect voluntary intake (Sherritt *et al.*, 1974). Intake of pigs in mixed-sex groups (gilts and castrated males) were lower by 0.018 compared with the mean for single-sex groups; although this is a small effect it was obtained from experiments with a total of 3200 animals (Ollivier, 1978) and may have biological and economic significance.

*Cattle*

When heifers were kept with older cows they lost weight whereas similar heifers fed separately gained weight, due to limited space at food troughs and dominance of older cows (Wagnon, 1965). Similarly, calves at the lower end of the dominance order ate fewer concentrates and gained weight more slowly (Broom, 1982). It is better to provide a feeding space for each individual rather than just one long trough. A barrier which separates the heads of adjacently feeding animals is better than one which just separates the bodies but a complete head and body barrier is best in allowing subordinate animals to eat (Bouissou, 1970).

Miller and Wood-Gush (1991) observed that feeding by dairy cows was more synchronized when they were grazing in summer than when in yard in winter because, even though each cow had her own Callan door, there were a lot of displacements usually by a low ranking cow being displaced by a higher ranking one. Also, Phipps *et al.* (1983) noted that group-fed cows had a higher intake of a complete food than those fed individually through Callan doors.

Reducing the width of a silage-feeding face reduced intake by young cattle (Leaver and Yarrow, 1980).

As with pigs, social relationships among cows during idling are very closely correlated with those at feeding (Kabuga, 1992a). Low ranking cows ate less frequently, whereas middle-ranking ones were ejected most frequently from feeders. Presumably the lowest learned not to eat when others were eating whereas ones in the middle did not find replacement as aversive. The frequency of agonistic interactions was 1.4 times higher during feeding periods (especially the first 30 min) than during idling periods whereas amicable behaviours were more frequent during idling (Kabuga, 1992a).

Rutter *et al.* (1987) used raw meal data from the LUCIFIR system to test the hypothesis that if one cow replaced another cow at a feeding position within one minute more times than the second cow replaced the first, then the former was dominant. A matrix of the frequency of competitive replacements was used to generate a social dominance order for a group of 12 cows and this was found to be almost identical to the social dominance order derived from visual observations of the outcome of all interactions by cows, i.e. it is possible to estimate an animal's position in the 'pecking order' from its feeding behaviour.

Cattle ate faster when there was only one stall for a group of animals than when free access to troughs was allowed (Striklin and Gonyou, 1981). However, diurnal pattern of eating did not differ between the two situations and dominant cattle did not prevent submissive ones from gaining access to the single feeder.

Wierenga and Hopster (1986) observed that dairy cows spend a lot of time visiting concentrate food dispensers and that the majority of visits are unrewarded, disrupting activity of the rest of herd. When they fitted cows with remote-controlled miniature beepers near the ear to tell them when they could get food there was a dramatic reduction in the number of unrewarded visits and consequently less disruption.

Calves (Warnick *et al.*, 1977) and beef cattle (Kidwell *et al.*, 1954) eat less if penned alone than if kept in a group; isolated rearing of calves reduces intake even more than individual crates.

Bulls are affected by diversions such as heifers or rain (Hinch *et al.*, 1982). Stags in rut with access to hinds in oestrus eat almost nothing and therefore show an even more pronounced fall in body condition in the autumn than do hinds, or stags kept in controlled conditions.

In an automatic intake-recording system Mason and Shelford (1990) found that mean forage dry matter intakes by cows were 11.4, 11.2 and 10.2 kg as the number of cows per station increased from 1 to 1.5 to 2.12. However, using a LUCIFIR system, H.F. Elizade and C.S. Mayne (unpublished results) did not find that silage intake by cows was significantly depressed until the number of animals per feed station exceeded five.

*Sheep*

In hill sheep given blocks of supplementary food, younger ewes have been seen to consume less than older ewes as a result of social competition (Lawrence and Wood-Gush, 1988), probably because the former kept together as a group, separate from the rest of the flock. Ewes of 2- and 3-years-old approached the feed blocks but were prevented from eating most of the time by the 4-year-old ewes. Thus, social behaviour limits the usefulness of supplementary feeding by causing wide variations in the intake between individual ewes.

Penning *et al.* (1993) tested the hypothesis that the amount of time spent grazing by sheep would be positively related to group size using groups of 1–10, 12 and 15. Grazing time did increase with group size, presumably due to the individual's need to be less vigilant when in a larger group:

$$GT = 629 - 311 \times \exp[-0.46GS] \tag{12.1}$$

where $GT$ is grazing time (min 24 h$^{-1}$) and $GS$ is group size, but there was no increase above a group size of about four. Grass height did not decrease for one to three sheep whereas bigger groups stocked at the same density did reduce grass height, i.e. small groups ate less as well as spending less time grazing. However, this may have been due to social facilitation in larger groups and it is clear that it is very difficult to design a good experiment to test hypotheses about group size under grazing conditions. There is no doubt that grazing studies with single sheep give poor predictions of the behaviour and intake of groups of sheep.

The common observation that sheep tend to feed at the same time as each other is corroborated by Webster *et al.* (1972), who showed that isolated lambs ate less than those in groups. Foot and Russel (1978) found lower intakes when sheep were kept in individual metabolism cages. The size of the group does not seem to affect daily intake, however. Forbes *et al.* (1972) found that ewes in adjacent individual pens ate 1.57 kg day$^{-1}$ whereas those kept in groups of six ate 1.58 kg day$^{-1}$. Foot *et al.* (1973) found that the intake of a concentrate supplement by ewes was related to their position in the social order of the group rather than to their nutrient requirements.

## Prior Experience of Food

Once sheep have eaten more than 10 g of supplement per day they will subsequently eat it readily even if they have not seen it for 3 years (Green *et al.*, 1984).

Sheep moved from two native pastures to high-quality pasture selected a food with significantly lower nitrogen content than sheep reared from birth on that pasture (Langlands, 1969). This was true even after the introduced sheep had been on the good pasture for 3 months.

Experience of eating a particular food is helpful, as shown by Flores *et al.* (1989b). Sheep reared on grass were more dextrous and had a higher biting rate for grass than those experienced in harvesting shrubs. Conversely those used to eating shrubs did so more efficiently than those with only grass experience. Goats with experience of browsing blackbrush ate faster and more by breaking twigs off than inexperienced goats (Ortega-Reyes and Provenza, 1993).

Lambs with experience of grazing the serviceberry shrub later grazed it more efficiently when it was sparse than did naive lambs whereas there was no such difference in the rate of eating of other foods (Flores *et al.*, 1989a).

Ramos and Tennessen (1992) exposed lambs to white clover or ryegrass pastures either at 14 weeks of age (before weaning) or 19 weeks of age (at weaning). At 4 weeks after weaning they were put on paddocks with alternating strips of the two in balanced pairs and the ryegrass-experienced lambs grazed ryegrass for 92% longer ($P < 0.01$) than controls whereas the clover-experienced lambs spent a significantly higher proportion of their time grazing clover than the ryegrass-trained lambs (69 vs. 45%). There was no effect of age at exposure.

# Working for Food: Operant Conditioning

When animals are trained to press a bar to obtain food and the number of presses required to initiate a meal is varied, increasing the effort required to start a meal causes a reduction in the number of meals but an increased meal size so as to maintain total intake and body weight (Collier, 1985). This shows that feeding is not absolutely dependent on metabolic factors but on the interaction of numerous factors.

Once animals are accustomed to working for their food they like to do so; Markowitz (1982) noted that ostriches preferred to peck at a button for peanuts than to obtain them 'free'. When a bag was accidentally dropped in the pen, they ate a few and then returned to the peanut dispenser. Similarly, rats trained to run down an alleyway to get food pellets continued to do so even if they had to wade through piles of pellets to get to the goal box (Stolz and Lott, 1964).

*Poultry*

In laying hens, daily food intake stayed the same up to a fixed ratio of reinforcements:responses of 160 (FR160) (Savory, 1989) but the total time spent feeding and meal frequency were negatively related to FR, whereas intermeal interval, meal size and rate of eating within meals were positively related to FR. It appeared that randomness in meal taking declined at higher FRs and FR20 seems the most appropriate to use in experiments in which it is desired to get birds to eat only when they feel hungry (Fig. 2.2).

Pre- and postprandial correlations are generally higher when animals have to expend some energy to get food. As the cost rose from 1 to 5000 pecks to gain access, so the number of meals fell from about 20 to 1 per day and meal size rose from being very small to over 200 g (Kaufman and Collier, 1983). Daily food intake remained approximately constant up to about 500 pecks per meal but rate of eating increased more or less continuously with FR. Unfortunately there was confounding between the FR imposed and the age/weight of birds so the observed reduction in daily intake at higher ratios might just have been due to a slowing of growth as birds were about 3 kg at this stage, and were growing only slowly.

Petherick and Rutter (1990) trained hens to push a weighted door to get food. When deprived of food for 12 h they took significantly longer to gain access to food by applying the required force × time than when deprived for 43 h, due to longer pauses between attempts to open the door. It is not necessary to construct special equipment in order to quantify animals' motivation to eat. For example, Petherick *et al.* (1992) trained hens to run down a 14.4 m alley for food. The speed with which

they ran was significantly increased by increasing lengths of deprivation but not between deprivation periods (0.29, 0.62, 0.65, 0.57 m s$^{-1}$ for
deprivation periods of 0, 6, 12 or 18 h, respectively).

Dawkins and Beardsley (1986) warn that an animal may not always
be able to learn an operant response, even though it is highly motivated
for the reward as they unexpectedly did not find that hens were
prepared to work for litter on the floor.

### Pigs

Hutson (1991) trained sows, fed at a commercial level of 2.3 kg per day,
to lift a lever to obtain reinforcements of 2.7 g of food on a 10:1 ratio.
After 1 h of responding, the FR was raised to 20 and so on. Extinction
(failure to respond sufficiently to obtain a reinforcement) occurred at
ratios which varied from 70 to 430 for different sows. For high FR
values, it was estimated that the energy cost of responding was greater
than the benefit gained from the food. Subsequently, Hutson (1992)
trained sows to lift a lever to obtain straw, twigs, nothing or a drop of
food. They responded for food most frequently by a factor of 20–433
times demonstrating that motivation for food completely overshadows
that for nesting materials. However, in two sows, the onset of nest
building just before parturition resulted in complete cessation of
responding.

An operant conditioning technique has also been used to determine whether pigs preferred whole or crushed cereals or pulses but no
significant preference emerged (Hutson and Wilson, 1984).

### Sheep

Sheep can quite easily be trained to respond for food (Hou *et al.*, 1991b).

## Conclusions

Animals are highly motivated to eat and drink and this motivation is
increased as metabolic demands increase. All the senses are used in the
identification of food and the absence of one sense does not, therefore,
result in a loss of selective or ingestive ability. Whereas mammals rely
primarily on taste to identify foods, birds use vision, and quickly learn
to associate the sensory properties of a food with the metabolic
consequences of eating that food.

Thus, the term 'palatability' is difficult to define as it depends not
only on the taste and appearance of the food, but also on the nutrient
requirements and history of the animal. For example, a food which is

initially preferred becomes aversive when its ingestion is coupled with injections of a toxic substance. Such learned aversions and preferences are long-lived and are likely to influence animals' behaviour for many years.

In addition to innate preferences/aversions and those learned by the animal from its own experience, it can also learn from conspecifics without itself ever having ingested the food in question. Thus, a mother can pass on information about food to her offspring before the young has itself started to eat solid food.

As will be made clear in Chapter 13, these learned associations form the basis of the ability of animals to make appropriate selections when a choice of foods is offered and may also play an important part in determining how much of a single food an animal eats, i.e. its voluntary food intake.

# 13 DIET SELECTION

- Theory of diet selection
- Evidence for diet selection
- Prerequisites for diet selection
- Social factors
- Mechanisms of diet selection
- Selection within a single food
- Limitations to diet selection
- Practical uses of diet selection
- Matching food composition with requirements
- Ruminant selection of leaf from stem
- Nutrient solutions
- Conclusions

In modern farming systems animals are typically presented with a single food. This is not a situation in which most species of birds and mammals have evolved and must be considered unnatural. The ancestors of our farm animals had the opportunity to select from a range of available foods and obviously were able to select a mixture which allowed them to grow and produce. It is possible that by eating at random from a variety of foods they obtained sufficient nutrients to survive but this would not be enough in some situations, e.g. when toxic food sources make up a significant part of what is available. It should be recognized that some species of animal have evolved to eat only a single food, i.e. they have an innate diet selection. However, many species eat a variety of foods and they need to learn the properties of these foods.

In the previous chapter we have seen the overwhelming evidence that animals can learn to associate the taste, smell or colour of a food with the feelings they experience when they eat that food. It was hinted that this is a powerful ability which allows animals to select from a range of foods to best meet their nutrient requirements, even if it is not of overriding importance in determining how much they eat if only one food is available. This chapter reviews the evidence for diet selection and shows how it might be exploited in farming practice, and Chapter 14 details appetites for specific nutrients. Chapters 12, 13 and 14 should be read in conjunction.

There are currently new opportunities in diet selection, both from scientific and commercial points of view. The realization that it is necessary for animals to be able to differentiate between foods with different nutrient compositions by colour, taste and/or position, and that they need to be taught to associate the sensory properties of foods with the metabolic consequences of eating them, has made it possible to envisage a learned appetite for each of the essential nutrients. Thus, there is now more certainty that if animals can be taught an appetite then this can be used in a choice-feeding situation to improve the balance between their nutrient requirements and their nutrient intake.

Most of the raw materials used in animal foods have concentrations of available energy within a fairly narrow range, from 9 to 13 MJ $kg^{-1}$ DM, whereas the content of nutrients, such as protein, minerals and vitamins, varies over a much wider range. An animal can control its energy intake by varying the amount of DM it consumes but can then only control its intake of nutrients independently of energy if it has access to two or more foods which differ in the content of the nutrient in question. Because of its quantitative importance, high cost and the polluting nature of its excretory products, protein has been widely studied in terms of diet selection. An appetite for protein seems to be very primitive in evolutionary terms as trained locusts eat more of a high protein food after preload of carbohydrate and *vice versa* (Simpson *et al.*, 1991).

Selection of a diet balanced for a particular nutrient, from among foods with deficiencies and excesses of that nutrient, constitutes an appetite and these are discussed in Chapter 14.

Some species of animal rely on a narrow range of foods for their sustenance and the recognition of these food sources is genetically predetermined. Other species will sample a wide range of potential foods and must learn by experience those which are palatable and nutritious. Newly hatched chicks, for example, peck at any small, round objects but within 3 days peck mainly at food (Hogan, 1973). Selection of a food may be euphagic, i.e. implying nutritional wisdom, or hedyphagic, i.e. selection for pleasurable flavour. Whereas deficiency of a nutrient for which there is a specific appetite will induce increased preference for a food which contains the nutrient, the reverse is not necessarily the case; that is, intake of a modestly greater amount of that nutrient than is necessary is not detrimental and may not induce a reduction in selection for a food containing it in high concentrations.

Taste and smell are the most important senses in feeding situations (Holder, 1991); visual and auditory cues are not normally part of the food experience and so are not conditioned as well in mammals, whereas the reverse is true for birds. Wilcoxon *et al.* (1971) used rats and quail which were given a sour-flavoured solution coloured blue while affected by a poison. Subsequently they were given either a blue solution or a sour one and, whereas rats primarily avoided drinking the flavoured solution, quail avoided the blue solution (Fig. 12.2).

# Theory of Diet Selection

The principles of diet selection have been outlined by Emmans (1991) and are illustrated in Fig. 13.1. When two nutrient properties of foods are considered the proportions of two foods necessary to meet an animal's requirements for both nutrients can be shown by a straight line (Fig. 13.1a). The two dimensions could be energy and protein. Foods A and B are both within the subspace representing adequacy and any mixture of the two would satisfy the animal's requirements; choice could therefore be random or according to the hedonic properties of the foods interacting with innate or learned preferences for colour, taste or other non-nutritional characteristics. Food C has too much protein and foods D and E too little protein. Offered a choice between (C and D) or (C and E) the animal could choose proportions of the two to make a balanced diet. Offered D and E it could not avoid under-eating protein.

In Fig. 13.1(b) the three dimensions are protein, energy and minerals. Foods C, D and E lie outside the adequate subspace but a line between C and D passes through this area so that an appropriate mixture of the two would be adequate; the line between C and E does not pass through the area so there is no mixture of these two which will be adequate. A choice between (A or B) and (C, D or E) requires that A or B is predominantly eaten if requirements are to be met. Thus, to test the hypothesis that animals make selections from two or more foods according to their nutrient requirements it is necessary for at least one of the foods to have a composition outside the adequate subspace.

Four nutrients are represented by the tetrahedron in Fig. 13.1(c) in which the four vertices represent energy, protein, calcium and phosphorus. There may be a few foodstuffs, such as A and B, which contain the right ratios of all four but it is more likely that two, three or four raw materials will be required to satisfy an animal's requirements.

This theory of what animals should eat is only realistic if we know

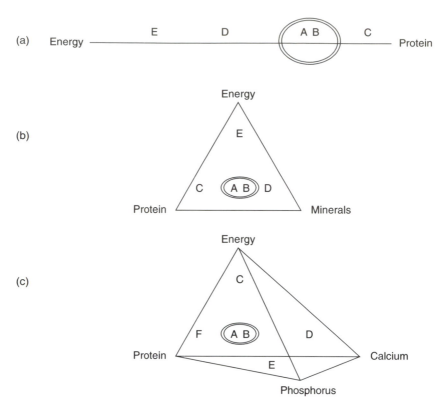

**Fig. 13.1.** Diagrammatic representation of mixtures of foods required to satisfy an animal's demands for nutrients: (a) two nutrients; (b) three nutrients; (c) four nutrients. The circled area is that in which the animal's requirements are satisfied. A–F are foods in positions which represent their content of the two, three or four nutrients. See text for details.

the requirements of the animal(s) in question. We can get an estimate of energy and protein requirements, for example, from results of experiments in other environments, i.e. standard textbooks or tables of nutrient requirements. However, to define the responses to nutrients under the conditions under which choice-feeding experiments are to be carried out it is preferable to conduct adequate experiments with single foods of a range of compositions but this is not often done. Further conclusions that animals are selecting foods with a nutritional purpose are strengthened if their requirements change with time and this change is reflected in appropriate adjustments to the proportions of different foods chosen. The change with time could be that naturally occurring during growth or an imposed change, such as one of temperature (see below).

# Evidence for Diet Selection

Considerable evidence has accumulated for the ability of laboratory animals to make directed selection from a choice of foods and in recent years such evidence has also become available for farm animals.

## Poultry

Kempster (1916) and Rugg (1925) observed that hens given a choice between foods could balance their own diets and produce more eggs than those fed a single food. It was confirmed in the 1930s that birds can select a balanced diet from among several imbalanced foods (Funk, 1932; Graham, 1932), and free-choice feeding has received continuous attention since. Laying hens, pullets, growing broilers and growing turkeys all show the ability to select an adequate diet from a choice of two or three foods which are individually inadequate (Forbes and Shariatmadari, 1994). In most cases the choice has been between one food which is clearly higher in protein content than required and the other lower in protein (these will be called HP and LP, respectively) but Ahmed (quoted by Rose and Kyriazakis, 1991) showed that broilers selected a diet from a range of nine different foodstuffs which provided nutrients in similar proportions to those normally recommended. On a commercial scale, choice feeding has given mixed results in layers though it has proved to be successful in broilers and growers (Cowan and Michie 1978). Conversely, Mastika and Cumming (1987) express the opinion that layers choose better than broilers because the broilers have so little time to learn how to make the appropriate choices.

## Pigs

There is considerable evidence for directed selection for protein and this is dealt with in more detail in Chapter 14. As an example, the work of Kyriazakis *et al.* (1990) included choices between two foods with different protein concentrations (Table 13.1). When one food contained more, and the other less, than the likely optimum protein level, then the pigs selected a mixture which gave almost identical overall protein contents of about 205 g crude protein (CP) kg$^{-1}$. When both foods had less protein than required (125 and 171 g CP kg$^{-1}$) more was eaten of the one with the higher protein level; it is, perhaps, surprising that they did not eat entirely or almost entirely from the higher protein food. When both foods provided too much protein, intake was almost all from the one with the lower protein content, suggesting a strong drive to avoid an excessive protein intake. As shown in Fig. 13.2 (Dalby *et al.*, 1994a) there is variation in the selection pattern between a low protein food

**Table 13.1.** Dietary choices of growing pigs offered high (HP) and low (LP) protein foods (Kyriazakis *et al.*, 1990).

| Choice between | | HP intake as proportion of total intake (g kg⁻¹) | CP content of selected diet (g CP kg⁻¹ FM) |
|---|---|---|---|
| LP (g CP kg⁻¹ DM) | HP (g CP kg⁻¹ DM) | | |
| 125 | 171 | 710 | 160 |
| 125 | 217 | 940 | 208 |
| 125 | 266 | 550 | 204 |
| 171 | 217 | 690 | 202 |
| 171 | 266 | 330 | 205 |
| 217 | 265 | 20 | 218 |

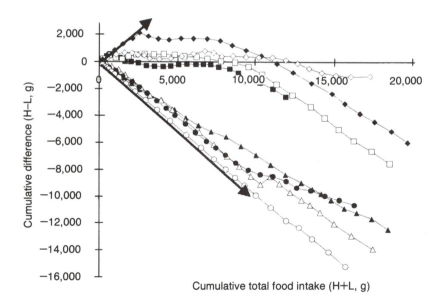

**Fig. 13.2.** Selection paths of eight pigs offered foods containing 155 (L) and 292 (H) g CP kg⁻¹ FM. The solid arrow rising at 45° represents intake of H only while that falling at 45° represents L; where a line is horizontal the pig was eating a 50:50 mixture of the two foods (Dalby *et al.*, 1994a).

(L) and one high in protein (H) by different animals: four pigs chose predominantly L throughout the 25-day experiment which started a few days after weaning at 3 weeks of age; three started by eating equal amounts of the two but from days 16–20 ate more L; one initially ate only H but on day 7 suddenly began to eat more L. It is not possible to determine from this type of experiment whether the lower protein intake by some individuals was a reflection of their lower potential for lean tissue deposition or due to a failure to select adequately.

Friend (1970) offered pregnant gilts a choice between cereal pellets and a protein concentrate. The proportion of cereal taken decreased as pregnancy progressed and the total dry matter intake declined during pregnancy, probably because growth decreased and fat deposition increased rather than because of the effects of pregnancy *per se*; without non-pregnant controls it is difficult to interpret these results.

### Sheep

Glimp (1971) observed that growing lambs switched from little discrimination among diets of different digestible energy concentrations when first introduced to them, to a preference for high energy foods as they learned the consequences of eating each one. However, Gordon and Tribe (1951) have demonstrated a case of a failure to select well, in pregnant ewes, and it is likely that the ewes were not given the opportunity to learn the nutritional properties of the range of foods offered. Cropper *et al.* (1985, 1986) and Hou *et al.* (1991a) have shown that sheep select proportions of low and high protein foods to give a protein intake matched to their presumed requirements for growth. The motivation for this is strong as sheep are willing to make at lest 30 responses in an operant conditioning situation to obtain a food reinforcement in order to obtain a 'balanced' diet (Hou *et al.*, 1991b).

## Prerequisites for Diet Selection

### The need for sensory differentiation

Clearly, it is necessary for animals to be able to differentiate between two or more foods if they are to select proportions in order to make up a balanced diet. If the nutrient in question is only required in trace amounts, and especially if it is colourless, it is necessary to give a cue by means, for example, of artificial flavouring and/or colouring. This is not usually a problem with foods differing markedly in protein content, for example, but is certainly necessary when a single amino acid is deficient in one food and in excess in the other.

## Training

In order for an appetite for a nutrient to develop it is necessary for animals to learn to associate the sensory properties of each food with its content of the nutrient in question. In many cases they will learn about two foods if they are introduced simultaneously but they may learn more quickly if each food is given in turn for a few days.

Kyriazakis *et al.* (1990) trained growing pigs to recognize the difference between HP and LP by offering them as single foods on alternate days for a week, before offering both in a choice-feeding situation. Shariatmadari and Forbes (1990a) adopted a similar method for chickens, but with half-day alternating periods on the basis that smaller animals, with a higher rate of turnover of nutrients, need shorter periods of exposure to learn the characteristics of different foods. It takes rats about 4 h to recognize a change in the protein content of the food (Harper, 1974) whereas hens take no more than 12 h (Chah and Moran, 1985).

Training birds by accustoming them to whole grains at an early age appears to confer benefits at the later stages of growth, in terms of ability to select foods to meet nutrient requirements. Broilers trained from 10–21 days after hatching by giving whole sorghum and protein pellets showed no difference in weight gain compared to complete-fed or untrained choice-fed birds, but the trained birds were significantly more efficient because the inexperienced choice-fed birds ate much more of the protein concentrate in the first 10 days of the experimental period than those with previous experience (Mastika and Cumming, 1987).

Covasa and Forbes (1993) found no effect on subsequent selection for whole wheat of time of access to wheat nor deprivation during the rearing phase but those birds which were given wheat alone for part of each day during rearing ate significantly more wheat during the growing phase. They had heavier proventriculus and gizzard than those which were given mixed wheat and starter crumbs during the rearing phase but growth and abdominal fat-pad weight were un-affected by treatment. Thus, it may be beneficial for subsequent diet selection to remove the standard food while offering whole grains to young chicks during the training period.

Dalby *et al.* (1994a) have shown that newly weaned pigs do not seem to benefit, in terms of subsequent ability to select between HP and LP, from a period of training such as that advocated by Kyriazakis *et al.* (1990). Whether they were given alternate exposure to each food for six days, given one for three days and the other for three days, or given free choice for six days, there was no difference in food intake or growth rate over the next 21 days of free choice feeding, compared with controls fed a single, adequate food throughout, but all choice-fed pigs ate significantly less protein than controls.

## Social Factors

It has been said that animals are more likely to learn about foods when they are in groups than in individual cages and there is evidence that rats can be taught to prefer a food by other rats which are accustomed to that food (Galef, 1989).

Most birds in a choice situation begin to eat from both foods on offer within a fairly short time, but there is often a minority which is slow, and there may be a few individuals who fail to select close to an appropriate diet. However, animals living together in a group tend to copy from each other and there is usually a leader which guides the others to the desired food. Individually caged broilers which did not voluntarily consume any wheat when given a choice with a standard grower food, immediately started to eat significant amounts when put in pairs, irrespective of whether the partner was formerly a wheat-eater or not (Covasa and Forbes, 1995). There were no differences in diet selection between broilers kept in groups of 20, 40 or 60 (Rose *et al.*, 1986).

Within 5 days of being given a choice between a calcium-deficient food and calcite broilers consumed enough calcium when kept in groups (Joshua and Mueller, 1979), However, individual caging inhibited this ability even when there was visual contact between birds but birds caged individually after learning to eat calcium in a group took an adequate amount of calcium.

Selection of herbage by cattle was not affected by grazing them with lambs, whereas there was a small effect on the lambs, those bonded to cattle grazing 7% more grass, 5% fewer forbs and 4% fewer shrubs than unbonded lambs (35% grass, 59% forbs, 5% shrubs) the proportions for cattle were 57, 35, 8%, respectively (Anderson, 1990).

Transfer of learned aversion from mother to offspring has been demonstrated in sheep. Ewes were allowed to eat *Amelanchier alnifolia* (a shrub) and trained, with lithium chloride, to avoid *Cercocapus montanus* (also a shrub) (Mirza and Provenza, 1992). After training, lambs aged either 6 or 12 weeks were put with their mothers for 5 min each day for 5 days in a small pen with both foods available. Trained ewes ate no *C. montanus* whereas control ewes took equal amounts of each. The lambs were then weaned and 7 days later tested, at which time trained lambs showed a tendency to prefer *A. alnifolia* (79% and 72% for lambs trained at 6 and 12 weeks, respectively) whereas lambs from control ewes showed no preference (49% and 53%).

Familiarity with straw has also been shown to increase its intake by lambs at a later date. Odoi and Owen (1992) offered some straw at pasture to 9–12-week-old lambs with their dams. After weaning the lambs were fed indoors on concentrates and straw and the intake of straw was higher in those previously exposed, especially in the first week, than those not exposed before weaning.

## Mechanisms of Diet Selection

Pathways are presumed to exist which transmit information concerning the metabolic effects of a food to the brain to allow development of learned associations with one or more sensory properties of the food. The simplest such pathway would be via the blood. For example, a low blood calcium level arising from eating a low calcium food might be sensed by the brain which would respond by increasing the intake of an alternative, high calcium food. Such a mechanism has been proposed for protein selection by Anderson (1979) who reported that an inverse relationship exists between the amount of protein consumed by self-selecting rats and their plasma concentration of tryptophan relative to the plasma concentration of large neutral amino acids (LNAA). It was also observed that the plasma tyrosine/phenylalanine ratio, and to a lesser extent the tyrosine/LNAA ratio, correlated directly with long-term energy intake in weanling rats. However, the significance of these relationships between plasma amino acid pattern and brain neurotransmitter concentration in the neuroregulation of feeding behaviour has been challenged, as adding either tryptophan or branched-chain amino acids to the diet has no effect on protein intake. This implied that in rats fed a single diet, the tryptophan/LNAA ratio was merely a reflection of dietary amino acid composition as modified by the animal's ability to catabolize amino acids, rather than a factor controlling food intake. Booth (1987) has criticized the tryptophan/LNAA theory as 'not even a scientific hypothesis'.

However, normal functioning of brain adrenergic and serotonergic systems has been related to the availability of dietary tyrosine and tryptophan respectively. Diets affect the plasma ratio of tyrosine to neutral amino acids, which in turn, influences brain tyrosine levels and consequent catecholamine synthesis. Similarly, dietary tryptophan affects brain 5-hydroxytryptamine (5-HT) levels in mammals. Fernstrom (1987) concluded, after a thorough review of the literature, that 'the available data do not sustain the [tryptophan/diet selection] hypothesis', at least as far as an appetite for carbohydrate is concerned.

Ackroff (1992) trained rats to work for protein, fat and carbohydrate, from separate dispensers. They were selective, composing a high fat, adequate protein diet and tended to alternate between protein and non-protein meals. Reductions in protein availability led to a proportional decrease in the intake of protein; the rats would rather change their diet than work harder for protein. Diet selection is thus a balance of internal and external demands. There seems to be no role for a carbohydrate appetite as carbohydrate is not required and fat is a more efficient source of energy.

Carbohydrate intake appears to be enhanced by hypothalamic injections of noradrenaline and neural peptide Y (NPY) and inhibited by 5-HT (Leibowitz *et al.*, 1991). There is a steady rise in hypothalamic NPY concentration from birth to puberty, at a time when protein intake increases. Fat intake is stimulated by galanin and aldosterone and inhibited by dopamine whereas protein intake is increased by opioids and growth hormone releasing factor. Intracerebroventricular corticotropin releasing factor (CRF) suppressed protein and fat intake in rats without affecting carbohydrate intake (Lin *et al.*, 1992). The fact that this effect was seen immediately after injection suggests that it was not due to the decrease in protein deposition caused by the corticosteroids released by increased adrenocorticotropic hormone under the influence of the CRF.

Given a choice between a tryptophan-deficient food and a control food, chickens preferred the latter but when the piriform cortex was separated from the rest of the brain they had difficulty in discriminating between the two foods (Firman and Keunzel, 1988). It is possible that the piriform cortex monitors amino acid levels, or that its separation disrupted the sense of smell (it is part of the olfactory system), or both of these. However, lesions of the nucleus taeniae, which is also a part of the olfactory system, did not affect the ability of birds to choose the right food.

### Nutrient infusions and preloads

In order to understand the link between metabolism and learning, numerous experiments have studied the effects of loading a substance or a certain type of food into the digestive tract or bloodstream of animals and observing the effects on diet selection.

### Poultry

Mechanisms of diet selection have been investigated in more detail by giving overnight-fasted broilers a meal of either HP or LP, to which they had previously been accustomed, and then offering both to choice. Whether the choice was given immediately after the initial meal or delayed for 1 h, significantly greater amounts of the opposite food were eaten (Shariatmadari and Forbes, 1990b). When the initial meal was given by tube into the crop there was no significant preference subsequently so it seems as if it is necessary for the bird to taste the food in order to predict its protein content according to its previous experience of the two foods. The independent control of energy and protein intakes was further demonstrated by Shariatmadari and Forbes (1992a) who force-fed broilers with 40 g of food containing 60, 135, 215 or 295 g CP kg$^{-1}$ daily for 10 days while given free access to foods with 60 and 295 g CP kg$^{-1}$. During the force-feeding period, the higher the protein content the greater the voluntary food intake but the proportion of HP was lower to give an almost constant level of protein intake across the treatments. After the cessation of force-feeding the birds which had been force-fed with the two highest levels of protein continued to have higher voluntary food intakes but with a lower proportion of HP, and deposited less protein in the carcass, than birds force-fed with lower-protein foods. This suggests that, although compensating only partly for the protein given by gavage during the force-feeding part of the experiment and thus ending this period with more carcass protein, the birds force-fed with the higher levels of protein then responded to their higher body protein content by voluntarily consuming less protein than those given low protein by tube.

It might be supposed from these results that birds which start to eat a meal from one food will tend to find the other food more attractive as the meal progresses. Indeed, 60% of the meals taken by broilers given free access to high and low protein foods are from both foods, i.e. there is a strong tendency to change foods during the meal (Shariatmadari and Forbes, 1992b). As metabolic receptors would not have had time to be significantly influenced by the food eaten earlier in the meal, this suggests that the choice of food is predominantly controlled by learned associations between the foods and their hedonic properties rather than by immediate feedbacks.

Even when the bird has learned that one food is nutritionally adequate it still samples other foods to ensure that a change in the quality of an extreme food does not go undetected and allow for novel foods to be sampled with relative safety. For example, broilers given two foods, one with a protein content higher than that needed to support maximum protein deposition, and another food with an even higher protein content, which ate predominantly from the former, still consumed a few grams of the higher protein food each day; similar behaviour is seen with low and very low protein foods (Shariatmadari and Forbes, 1990a).

*Sheep*

It might be expected in ruminant mammals that products of digestion in the rumen would affect diet selection. Azahan and Forbes (1992) infused sodium acetate or sodium chloride intraruminally in sheep and found large reductions in the intake of concentrates but no effect on hay intake. The effect was almost as great for chloride as it was for acetate so the major reason for the decreased intake was probably osmotic (Chapter 4).

## Selection within a Single Food

When grass or hay is offered in the long, unchopped form animals have the opportunity to select between stem and leaf. The proportion of leaf selected by sheep increases with amount of straw offered (Black and Kenney, 1984). Sheep given unchopped barley straw in sufficient amounts so as to leave uneaten 20, 30, 40, 50 or 70% of that on offer ate increasing amounts of leaf blade as the allowance increased, in a linear manner, at the expense of stem; leaf sheath was little affected (Bhargava *et al.*, 1988). Little stem was eaten until refusals were less than 40% of the amount offered and the dry matter (DM) digestibility of the whole diet increased from 594 to 638 g kg$^{-1}$ with increasing allowance from 20 to 70% excess.

## Limitations to Diet Selection

### Innately aversive compounds: toxins

Animals learn to ignore innately aversive cues (e.g. bitter tastes) if they are paired with essential nutrients, but such cues are usually associated with toxic substances, such as tannins. Rapeseed meal is an economically attractive source of protein but it is claimed that poor palatability prevents its use as more than a small proportion of the diet. Rapeseed meal, even the modern genotypes with low levels of glucosinolates, contains toxins, however, so the taste of rapeseed could be used as a cue to aversion even if the substance(s) being tasted was not itself toxic. Kyriazakis and Emmans (1992) showed that growing pigs given choices between 140 and 300 g kg$^{-1}$ protein foods with 0 or 180 g kg$^{-1}$ of rapeseed meal found both foods containing rape to be aversive, leading to over- or underconsumption of protein. Without rape, pigs chose 205 and 206 g CP kg$^{-1}$; when rape was in HP, the choice was 155 g kg$^{-1}$

whereas when it was in LP, they chose $271 g kg^{-1}$. In further studies, Kyriazakis and Emmans (1993) offered choices between a low protein food and one with added fishmeal, soyabean meal, low glucosinolate rapeseed meal or high glucosinolate rapeseed meal. In the first two cases the diet selected contained 193 and $190 g CP kg^{-1}$, respectively, i.e. close to that predicted, but when the high protein food contained rapeseed the protein contents of the selected diets were 177 and 161 g $CP kg^{-1}$, for low and high glucosinolate, respectively. When fishmeal and rapeseed meal foods of equal protein content were offered the preference was for the fishmeal-containing food, more so in the case of high than low glucosinolate rapeseed meal. Thus, the taste of rape is somewhat aversive and pigs eat excessive amounts of protein from other sources rather than taking a large amount of rapeseed meal.

Onibi *et al.* (1992) gave growing pigs choices between barley and soyabean meal, barley and rapeseed meal, barley and an equal mixture of soya and rape, compared to a complete single food. Growth was poorer in the choice treatments. The soyabean meal initially resulted in diarrhoea, but once this had gone there was a reduction in the ratio of protein:energy and good growth. Rapeseed meal reduced the intakes of foods containing it either alone or in mixture with soyabean meal whereas replacing rape with soya removed this constraint.

Young pigs given a choice of diets supplemented with rapeseed meal and soyabean meal initially selected 75% of that including soya but this increased to 95% as the pigs grew, presumably as they learned the goitrogenic effects of rape (Baidoo *et al.*, 1986).

These are examples of pigs preferring to avoid rapeseed meal, presumably because of its toxins, but ruminants sometimes continue to eat toxic plants, even after the toxic effects have become obvious. Provenza *et al.* (1992), reviewing this problem, state that not enough is known about affective and cognitive systems in herbivores.

### Neophobia

Although it was stated above that animals continue to sample even those foods which they have learned to be imbalanced, there are many examples of animals showing reluctance to sample novel foods. This is particularly true if the familiar food(s) is fairly well balanced with regard to nutrient composition. When rats were given just chow or chow and a single nutrient source for 4 days, and then given access to protein, carbohydrate and fat sources, those previously exposed to carbohydrate ate more carbohydrate and those exposed to fat ate more fat than the other groups (Reed *et al.*, 1992) and this led to loss of body weight. Those which had experienced protein ate more than those on carbohydrate or fat, but not more than controls. This persisted for at least 12 days. After a further 34 days more on chow alone the selection was much the same as before when they were offered a choice. The authors concluded that 'prior experience can be a more powerful influence than nutritional wisdom in determining the rat's food choice'. It must be borne in mind, however, that the rats initially given fat and carbohydrate had not been given a chance to learn the metabolic properties of casein, which is innately unpalatable to rats, anyway!

Lambs show a persistent preference for the type of shrub they had access to from 50 to 110 days of age (Nolte *et al.*, 1990) and similarly prefer either an onion- or garlic-flavoured complete food, whichever they experienced from 30 to 110 days of age (Nolte and Provenza, 1992a). Therefore, familiarity can influence food choice but is not likely to override strong nutritionally based preferences.

### Use of inappropriate foods

Another limitation of choice feeding is when both foods on offer are below the animal's requirements in terms of protein content. If LP contains considerably less than required and HP contains marginally too little protein then, rather than eat almost all of HP, as would be predicted from the majority of results presented above, there is considerable intake of LP leading to protein deficiency in broilers (Shariatmadari and Forbes, 1990b), laying hens (Holcombe *et al.*, 1976b) and growing pigs (Kyriazakis *et al.*, 1990). This is puzzling and suggests that animals do not feel very uncomfortable if they have a protein: energy ratio in their diet which does not quite provide for maximal lean tissue growth, whereas they try to avoid eating excessive protein presumably due to the toxic properties of deamination products of excess amino acids.

### Physical form of food

When offered to sheep in pairs, preference for a food was strongly related to rate of eating when offered alone (Kenney and Black, 1984). Reducing the length of straw from 30 to 10 mm increased the rate of eating from 5.5 to 12.4 g min$^{-1}$ and also the preference (Fig. 13.3). With rapidly eaten foods (over 24 g min$^{-1}$) there were no differences in preference associated with rate of eating.

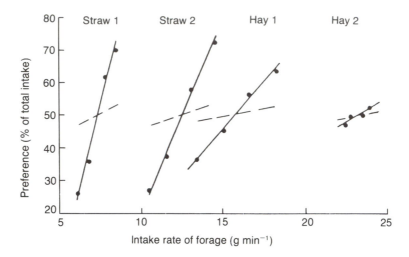

**Fig. 13.3.** Relationships between the preference shown for a particular mixture of long and short particles over a mixture of equal parts of long and short particles and intake rate of the particular mixture (Kenney and Black, 1984): – – – expected preference when sheep spend an equal time eating both forage mixtures.

## Practical Uses of Diet Selection

### *The potential advantages*

If animals do make nutritionally wise choices between foods there will be the following benefits:

**1.** Expensive determination and laborious calculations of nutrient requirements for use in food formulations could be avoided by offering a choice of two or more foods and allowing animals to choose a combination which will reflect their needs.
**2.** Separate sex feeding will be unnecessary. Within a mixed-sex, choice-feeding herd or flock the males and the females will be able to select different diets which reflect the different requirements of the sexes. Differences between individual animals and different strains with different growth potential will be compensated for.
**3.** Food changes will not be needed. Two foods, offered as a choice, could be used throughout the growing and finishing period. In addition, nutrient undersupply (with consequent loss in output) or nutrient oversupply (with no resulting benefit but increased cost) will be avoided since the diet selected by each individual will precisely meet its requirements. Changes in environmental temperature will be accommodated by the animals without the need for reformulation of the foods.

**4.** Excretion of nitrogenous and other waste will be reduced as individual animals select diets to meet their nutrient requirements. There is potential for a significant reduction in the pollutants generated by intensive animal units.

Of course research and development is needed to establish the optimum conditions for choice feeding, including the best training methods and the most appropriate cues.

## Poultry

### Whole-grain feeding

Wheat and barley are attractive ingredients for broiler foods in view of their low price but, because of their low protein content and imbalanced amino acid composition, they must be supplemented and this necessitates grinding and pelleting into a complete manufactured food. Whole grains of cereal can, however, be viewed as low protein foods which can be offered in free choice with high protein concentrate pellets but the extra expense of providing two feeding systems has prevented its large-scale adoption. It has recently been realized that there is no need to offer the two foods separately, as long as they are mixed in roughly the right proportions, they are visually different and they can be separately prehended by the birds. The concentrate is made by removing the cereal from a conventional formulation with added premix and calcium. (Note that it is not necessary to formulate a special high protein food to use as a balancer for wheat. Standard commercial foods are designed to provide sufficient protein for 95% of the birds, which means that the great majority are being over-provided.)

Advantages, in addition to those listed above, include the saving by not having to grind and pellet as much food and the fact that grain stores better whole, especially in hot humid areas. Trained birds change the ratio of intakes of the two foods within a few hours of a change in the energy content of the grain, or the protein content of the concentrate. Under heat stress, they decrease only their grain intake, but not that of concentrate. In the cool of the night they once again eat more grain and egg size is generally a bit better, especially in hot weather. Choice diets are cheaper but broilers take a bit longer to reach a given weight as they lose a day or two while they learn. They are less susceptible to coccidiosis and usually more efficient financially.

### Broilers

Performance of chicks given a choice between concentrate pellets and sorghum grains was about equal to that of pellet-fed controls but the choice-fed birds ate less protein and converted protein more efficiently

(Mastika and Cumming, 1981). Broilers given a choice of a cereal and a high protein concentrate performed just as well as controls, whether sorghum, wheat or both were the cereals and when both wheat and sorghum were on offer, they ate more sorghum than wheat (Cumming, 1983). It is appropriate to provide a small proportion of whole grains from an early age, to give the birds familiarity with their appearance and, hopefully, with their metabolic effects.

Many broiler producers in Northern Europe are now including whole grain in their foods. Adequate mixing takes place during the normal handling of the food through the augers, bins and feeders. Successive batches of food are ordered with increasing proportions of whole wheat to give a steady increase in the proportion of whole grain, calculated to meet the requirements of the average bird. Results in terms of growth rate and carcass quality are reported to be at least as good as with the commercial grower food fed on its own and in Scandinavia and other European countries it is now common practice to feed a starter food containing 240 g protein per kilogram throughout and add increasing amounts of wheat, up to 40%.

Although there are scientific grounds for controlling the proportion of whole grain more accurately to match the birds' potential and actual growth, and these are utilized in a comprehensive, computer-monitored and -controlled complete housing and feeding system (the Flockman system, Filmer, 1991), the expense of installing such a system seems unjustified at the moment in view of the good results being achieved with *ad hoc* methods.

## Laying hens

Lee *et al.* (1949) and Leeson and Summers (1983) reported reduced performance by laying hens with choice feeding. However, Robinson (1985) and Elwinger and Nilsson (1984) found production at least as good as conventional feeding, with higher egg weights, although there was a tendency for poorer shell strength and plumage with choice feeding (Al Bustany and Elwinger, 1988).

Cumming (1984) used three breeds of layer, half of the birds fed conventionally, the other half given a choice between whole wheat and protein concentrate from the first day of life. The choice-fed performed at least as well as those fed conventionally, being a little more efficient. In a smaller trial in which sorghum was the choice-fed grain, there were more large eggs than in the conventionally fed. Cumming emphasized the importance of experience of hens in choice feeding and advised exposing pullets during rearing to all the grains that they may be offered later in life. He also observed that water consumption has been found to be lower in choice-fed layers, and the droppings have tended to be dryer and to cone more readily under the cages. This may be due to the better gizzard development in choice-fed birds and requires further investigation.

The large-scale application of choice feeding of caged hens was studied by Tauson and Elwinger (1986) using two narrow flat-chain feeders, one distributing a mash concentrate, the other whole grain. In a semi-choice treatment the mash was given as a layer on top of the grain which was provided *ad libitum*. Two experiments with over 5000 birds showed greater egg size with choice and semi-choice feeding than conventionally fed controls, with no difference in the number of eggs laid. Egg shell quality and cracks tended to be worse in the choice treatments. Profit margin was higher over the two production cycles for both choice-fed groups than control and these authors concluded that choice feeding from flat feeders is feasible but that further studies are necessary before similar systems are used in practice.

A choice of whole grain/crushed peas and a concentrate was given to caged hens in a chain feeder and mechanized device for feeding restricted amounts of concentrates by Tauson *et al.* (1991). Choice- or semi-choice-fed hens produced significantly heavier eggs than those on a conventional mash diet and ate more food. The authors concluded that choice feeding may be economically beneficial to farmers with access to inexpensive cereals and peas.

Given a choice of pellets and wheat turkey hens ate 46% as wheat whereas males chose only 38% (McDonald and Emmans, 1980). There was no significant effect on body weight, but in early lay choice-fed pullets produced significantly fewer eggs; however, this was redressed to a large extent later in the laying period. Egg weights and hatchability were marginally lower on choice feeding. Farrell *et al.* (1989) have also obtained very variable results from hens given whole grain and protein balancer.

In summary, under commercial conditions laying hens usually performed well although efficiency is sometimes reduced (Rose and Kyriazakis, 1991). There is uncertainty about the optimum methods of training and feeding, however (Farrell *et al.*, 1989).

### Gizzard development and coccidiosis

Grit is not usually offered and poultry foods are low in fibre in current practice as a result of which the gizzard is small and the proventriculus may be dilated. This results in food passing very quickly through the stomachs and arriving in the duodenum in a particulate form in which penetration of digestive juices might be slow (Cumming, 1992). This might be conducive to coccidiosis and Cumming (1987) observed that a higher fibre food (62.5 g kg$^{-1}$) given to groups of cockerels from day-old to 4 weeks reduced the incidence of coccidiosis compared to a low fibre food (28.5 g kg$^{-1}$). All birds were dosed with coccidiosis oocysts and 7/50 died in low fibre group, three in high-fibre and none in a third, choice-fed group. The occyst outputs were 293, 96 and 6, respectively, at 6 days postinfection. It is also advantageous for gizzard development and coccidiosis prevention to offer limestone grit to ensure large particles which stay in the gizzard, rather than as powder incorporated in complete food (Cumming *et al.*, 1987). Gizzards were significantly heavier in choice-fed birds compared to those given a single complete food (Mastika and Cumming, 1985; Tauson and Elwinger, 1986).

When grit was available to broilers offered whole wheat and a high-protein food, they selected a higher proportion of whole wheat as presumably they were better able to grind it in the gizzard in which the grit is stored for this purpose (Amar-Sahbi, 1987) and when access to grit was later denied there was a reduction in the intake of the whole grain. Hijikuro and Takewasa (1981) observed that broilers prefer whole sorghum to flaked sorghum, suggesting that they like something which stimulates gizzard activity.

When the balancer food for broilers was given in mash form the birds selected more wheat if it was ground than whole whereas if the balancer was pelleted they selected more wheat when it was whole (Rose *et al.*, 1986). Presumably physical form influences gizzard development and pelleted food improves its ability to grind food and allows birds to make better use of whole wheat. Thus, they select more whole wheat when offered concentrate in the pelleted form rather than mash.

*Other cereal grains*
The high content of β-glucans in barley, which slow rate of food passage through the digestive tract, means that replacement of wheat with (cheaper) barley in a broiler food reduces intake (Cowan and Michie, 1977a). Rose and Njeru (1989) showed that treatment of ground barley with a β-glucanase increased the proportion selected by choice-fed broilers, presumably by overcoming the aversive properties of untreated barley.

*Ruminants*

Heifers offered a choice between grass and maize silages ate about 40:60 grass:maize although this varied widely between animals, from 25:75 to 66:34 (Weller and Phipps, 1985a). Intakes and milk yields were significantly higher in heifers offered the choice or just maize silage, compared to those on grass silage alone. Further work with cows (Weller and Phipps, 1985b) included the additional treatment of a 1:2 mixture of grass:maize silage and there was no maize silage-only treatment. For half the cows the grass silage was good quality, for the other half it was poor quality. Significantly more DM was eaten of the mixture, compared to just grass silage. The ratio of grass:maize silage in the free-choice treatments ranged from 30:70 to 77:23 for poor quality grass silage and from 48:52 to 81:19 when the grass silage was good quality, i.e. better grass silage gave a higher preference. Even with high quality grass silage, offering maize silage improved performance.

## Sequential feeding

One way to cope with the difficulties of providing two foods under commercial conditions would be to feed the two alternately. The length of time each food is offered will affect the outcome as there is limited storage for many nutrients in the animal's body.

If one food is eaten to satiety and another, contrasting, food is then offered animals usually eat again; this is known as sensory specific satiety.

### Poultry

Offering HP and LP to broilers for alternate half-days gave food intakes and growth very similar to birds fed the same two foods free-choice (Shariatmadari and Forbes, 1991) and it appears that alternate feeding would be an effective way of 'choice feeding'. Birds given HP and LP on alternate days had somewhat lower total intakes and significantly less fat in the carcass. When whole wheat and balancer were given to broilers during alternate 8 h periods, there was good selection; the higher the protein content of the balancer, the more wheat was eaten (Rose *et al.*, 1993).

Gous and DuPreez (1975) gave layer cockerels two foods which were individually poorly balanced but complementary in their amino acid composition, in alternating periods of 6 or 12 h. There were no significant differences in food intake or weight gain, either between the two alternating treatments, or compared with controls fed the two foods mixed together. Thus, the growing bird appears to have the ability to compensate for short periods on amino-acid-imbalanced foods.

Chicks offered a choice between high and low protein foods during the 12 h of daylight but a food with an adequate protein content at night adopted a nocturnal feeding pattern but did not completely eliminate daytime meals (Rovee-Collier *et al.*, 1982). Thus, although normally a diurnal feeder, if necessary the chick will eat at night in order to get a single, complete food. Chicks exposed to cold conditions at night ate more and selected a higher energy:protein ratio than

controls kept continuously in the warm and chicks kept in permanently cool conditions ate more food, with a higher energy:protein
ratio, than those put in the warm at night (Hayne *et al.*, 1986). The chick
has the ability, therefore, to compensate for changed nutrient requirements at one time of day by altering its diet selection at other times.

*Pigs*

Fowler *et al.* (1984) studied the effects of dietary novelty and frequency
of feeding on the food intake and performance of growing pigs. From
25 to 90 kg body weight they were offered nine foods in sequence or as
a mixture given nine times or twice per day. Initially the sequentially
fed groups ate more but at the end intakes were similar at 2.32, 2.35 and
2.33 kg day$^{-1}$ and live weight gains and food conversion efficiencies
were not different between groups.

# Matching Food Composition with Requirements

## Diet formulation

In commercial practice the protein content of food given to broilers is
reduced in a stepwise manner to match the changing needs of broilers
as they grow. Even if choice feeding is difficult to apply commercially
it has the potential to be used to define more precisely the changes in
requirements to allow more accurate formulation of rations. In particular, the optimum level of amino acids for birds of particular genotypes
at different stages of growth can be assessed more comprehensively by
diet selection experiments than by complex factorial experiments in
which different groups of birds are given all combinations of likely
amino acids at different states of growth (Forbes and Covasa, 1995).

Based on their results with choice-feeding, Sinurat and Balnave
(1986) recommended the optimum single foods to be given to birds
under different environmental temperatures, whereas Steinruck *et al.*
(1990b) have based recommendations on levels of methionine inclusion
in broiler foods on results from their diet selection experiments. Rose
and Abbas (1993) observed that cockerels selected different varieties of
wheat according to their nutritive value. This was well correlated with
the growth rate of broilers which were given foods containing 70% of
the wheats, providing a potentially useful method for evaluation of
nutritive value of wheats.

## New genotypes

If diet selection can be used to define more precisely the optimum content of protein, amino acids and any other essential nutrient, for existing genotypes, then it can also be used for novel genotypes, such as may be produced by genetic engineering techniques in the foreseeable future. Leaving aside the moral issues, there are likely to be immense technical problems with the feeding and management of animals whose potential for growth has been elevated considerably but whose ability to ingest, digest and metabolize the food to support such growth is unknown. Diet selection experiments are likely to lead more rapidly to a resolution of these problems than classical factorial experiments but the limits of diet selection as a technique for assessing optimal nutrition have yet to be defined and much more basic research is needed at this stage so that we are not to be taken unawares if, and when, novel genotypes are produced for commercial use.

New genotypes of crop plants can also be assessed as animal foods by diet selection techniques.

### Improved efficiency with diet selection

There is some indication that choice feeding improves the efficiency of utilization of protein. This may be due to the selection process itself or because of an excess of protein in the control food. Dove (1935) found that chicks given a food made up of proportions equivalent to those selected by his fastest growing choice-fed chickens did not grow as fast as did the selectors. Conversely, chicks fed a diet made up in proportions equivalent to those selected by his slowest growing chicks grew more rapidly than the slow growers.

# Ruminant Selection of Leaf from Stem

As indicated above, ruminants select leaves in preference to stems when given an excess of hay. Wahed *et al.* (1990) offered goats 50% more straw than they would eat and noted a significantly higher DM intake (18.9 g DM kg$^{-0.75}$day$^{-1}$) than those offered 20% more than *ad libitum* (14.4 g DM kg$^{-0.75}$ day$^{-1}$). Further work with goats and sheep confirmed this: offering 13, 57 or 70% excess increased straw intake from 15.5 to 22.8 and 26.2 g DM kg$^{-0.75}$ day$^{-1}$ and all refusals were of a lower digestibility than the food offered; estimated digestible organic matter intake (DOMI) values were 7.2, 12.8 and 14.5 g kg$^{-0.75}$ day$^{-1}$, i.e. very worthwhile increases in level of nutrition. The refused straw can be used as bedding or fuel.

In West Java, sheep are housed all year and given cut grass in excess of their requirements. Tanner *et al.* (1993) noted that the more grass offered to rams (25, 50 or 75 g DM kg$^{-1}$ live weight) the greater the intake (598, 922, 1019 g DM day$^{-1}$) and digestibility was also improved due to increased ability to select leaf (535, 599, 624 g kg$^{-1}$ DM).

### The need for roughage

Although foods with smaller particle sizes usually have a higher nutritive value, ruminants crave roughage and eat a significant amount of forage even in the presence of highly nutritious concentrates. Castle *et al.* (1979) offered dairy cows perennial ryegrass, with median chop lengths of 9.4, 17.4 and 72.0 mm. Voluntary food intake and milk yield increased as chop length decreased, whereas eating and ruminating times were reduced. Despite this apparent nutritional advantage of the short-chopped grass, cows given a choice of all three ate 16% of the long and 32% of the medium-length grass. Similarly, lambs offered two foods did not totally avoid the bulkier one (Cropper, 1987) and lactating goats (J.M. Forbes, unpublished results) and growing heifers (J.H.M. Metz, personal communication) took about 20% of their DM intake as hay when they also had free access to concentrates. Cooper and Kyriazakis (1993) offered foods with different nutrient densities but similar ME:CP ratios to growing lambs; all choice-fed lambs ate some of the poorer food and it was suggested that the better foods increased rumen osmolality or reduced pH to an uncomfortable extent.

Pulina *et al.* (1992) fed lactating ewes on mixtures of high-fibre pellets (F) mixed with conventional pellets (N) in ratios of 27:73, 42:58, 58:42 and 73:27. Although DM intake and milk yield were little affected, chewing time decreased with the decrease of F in the diet. The ewes showed some ability to choose between the two types of pellet and those with low inclusion of F increased their fibre intake by selecting for F, whereas those with high inclusion of F chose more of N so that the ratios of foods eaten were 33:67, 50:50, 50:50 and 68:32, for the four mixtures. There is thus ample evidence that ruminants do not eat for maximum efficiency, as implied by Tolkamp and Ketelaars (1992), but strive to maintain sufficient intake of long fibre to ensure proper rumen function.

## Nutrient Solutions

Almost all animals are choice-fed almost all of the time in that they are given food and water; water intake is covered in Chapter 14. Other nutrients can be included in the drinking water and the situation is then more obviously choice feeding.

Feeding a low energy food increased the preference by domestic chickens for a 100 g l$^{-1}$ solution of sucrose, compared with feeding a normal or a high energy food (Kare and Maller, 1967). In contrast, jungle fowl selected significantly more sugar solution than water irrespective of the energy and protein content of the foods, which were a 200g kg$^{-1}$ protein food diluted or enriched with 250 g kg$^{-1}$ of cellulose or corn oil. Jungle fowl have a low potential growth rate and therefore a low protein:energy requirement, and so choose to reduce the protein concentration of their diet by drinking sucrose solution.

The inclusion of 9% of glucose in the drinking water of cockerels of a laying strain did not reduce food intake but weight gains were not increased and it was suggested that the extra energy was mainly stored as fat (Injidi, 1981). In other experiments with broiler chickens intake was depressed by glucose solutions to maintain a constant total energy intake (Azahan and Forbes, 1989). To see whether the different response might be due to differences in the protein content of the food in relation to potential growth rate, either water or a 9% solution of glucose was offered to male broiler chicks fed on either low (150 g kg$^{-1}$) or adequate (195 g kg$^{-1}$) protein foods. Compared with those on tap water, those birds which had dextrose in the water ate significantly less

**Table 13.2.** Growth and feed intakes of broilers offered either water or glucose solution with two levels of protein in the feed (Azahan and Forbes, 1989). On the high protein food, glucose solution had no effect on food intake but allowed increased protein and fat deposition, whereas with the medium protein food, intake, protein and fat deposition were all depressed, presumably due to lack of protein to balance the increased energy intake from glucose.

| | Water | | Glucose (90 g l$^{-1}$) | | | |
|---|---|---|---|---|---|---|
| Feed protein (g kg$^{-1}$ DM) | 150 | 195 | 150 | 195 | s.e.d. | Sig. |
| Weight gain (g per 37 days) | 1588 | 2093 | 1375 | 2211 | 120 | P$\cdots$ |
| Total feed intake (g per 37 days) | 4500 | 4202 | 3636 | 4176 | 218 | G$\cdots$, G×P$\cdot\cdot$ |
| Total fluid intake (g per 37 days) | 7750 | 6034 | 6354 | 6994 | 517 | P×G$\cdots$ |
| Total energy intake (MJ per 37 days) | 78 | 77 | 71 | 86 | 4 | P$\cdot\cdot$, P×G$\cdot\cdot$ |
| Carcass protein DM (g) | 392 | 537 | 362 | 522 | 29 | P$\cdots$ |
| Carcass fat DM (g) | 300 | 341 | 247 | 473 | 41 | P$\cdots$, P×G$\cdots$ |

s.e.d., Standard error of deviation; Sig., significance; P, protein level of food; G, glucose level of drink; $\cdot\cdot$, $P < 0.01$; $\cdots$, $P < 0.001$.

food but there was a highly significant interaction between the effects of dietary protein level and type of fluid offered, glucose depressing intake on the medium protein food but stimulating it with the high-protein diet (Table 13.2). Fluid intake was generally closely related to food intake and did not differ between types of fluid on offer. It appears that chickens consider glucose solution to be a drink rather than a food (Shaobi and Forbes, 1985) and that having taken in extra energy, respond according to the new energy:protein ratio of the diet.

## Conclusions

The theory that animals can select from a choice of foods a diet which meets their requirements is difficult to prove, but it is clear that there are many situations in which they show considerable 'nutritional wisdom'. The most widely studied situation is one in which animals are offered two foods, with higher or lower protein contents than required in relation to the energy concentration of the diet. Manipulating the protein content of one or both foods is accompanied by diet selection to maintain a fairly constant protein intake; comparing animals with different protein:energy requirements also shows that protein and energy intakes are controlled independently.

In order that animals can select they must be able to differentiate between the foods. Mammals make most use of taste whereas birds use visual cues, although any animal can use a variety of cues, including the position of the foods in the environment. A training period, in which the foods are offered alternately, can be useful in ensuring that animals unambiguously associate each food with its nutritional value. Individuals can also learn about foods indirectly, from conspecifics, particularly the mother.

It is far from clear what internal mechanisms are involved in controlling diet selection; very few studies have been made in this area with farm animals.

There are two situations in which farm animals are offered choices in practice. One is grazing, which is covered in Chapter 16. The other is the apparently increasing practice of offering poultry a mixture of whole cereal and a pelleted balancer food, either in separate troughs or, more usually, in the same trough. However, there is little evidence to date that individual birds improve their diet by choosing disproportionate amount of the two foods.

Questions still to be answered include the following:

**1.** Is it better to offer a standard complete food in choice with whole grain or to formulate a higher protein balancer to complement the cereal?

**2.** Is the welfare of animals better served by offering them a choice of two or more foods?
**3.** To what extent can the principles and practice worked out for protein be extended to other nutrients? Under what conditions can success be achieved by offering a choice of three or more foods?

Further research and development are needed to establish the optimum conditions for diet selection, including the best training methods and the most appropriate cues.

# 14 APPETITES FOR SPECIFIC NUTRIENTS

- Regulation of protein intake
- Regulation of amino acid intake
- Appetites for minerals
- Appetites for vitamins
- Water intake
- Conclusions

Chapter 13 discussed the principles and practice of diet selection in farm animals, i.e. the ability to choose from two or more imbalanced foods a diet of adequate composition to meet the animals' nutrient requirements. It has been demonstrated that there needs to be learning of the metabolic effects of each food and association with some sensory property or properties of each food. This chapter examines evidence for appetites for many nutrients, giving the evidence where available. As protein was used to illustrate the principles of diet selection in Chapter 13 the next section should be read in conjunction with that earlier discussion.

## Regulation of Protein Intake

Interest in choice feeding has centred on foods with protein contents higher and lower than that required for optimum performance (HP and LP, respectively). Although there is a very wide range of protein content in readily available foodstuffs, from around 40 g kg$^{-1}$ for straw to 600 g kg$^{-1}$ for fishmeal, the range of usable energy contents is quite small, from 9 to 13 MJ ME kg$^{-1}$. Thus, selection from two foods is most likely to be on the basis of their protein content. Also, protein is an expensive dietary constituent and there is considerable interest in optimizing its dietary concentration in commercial practice.

It must be acknowledged that in most cases it is only an assumption that protein is the target of the animals' selection between HP and LP, as details of the content of minerals and vitamins are not always published. Thus, where whole grain is given in choice with a compound pellet, the latter will be higher in many minerals and vitamins as well as protein and it is possible that the results are clouded by an appetite for one or more of the trace constituents as well as, or instead of, an appetite for protein.

A learned hunger for protein has been demonstrated in rats by Baler *et al.* (1987) who paired injection of protein into the stomach with drinking a flavoured non-nutritive fluid; subsequently the rats showed a preference for that flavour.

*Growing chickens*

If a claim is made that birds are selecting an optimum diet from a choice of foods, it is necessary to demonstrate this by feeding other groups of birds in single-feed mixtures of the two foods used in the choice-feeding situation (Emmans, 1991). Shariatmadari and Forbes (1993) have done this for broilers and layer cockerels by using single foods with 65, 115, 165, 225 and 280 g protein kg$^{-1}$. For broilers, protein deposition increased with single foods up to 285 g kg$^{-1}$ whereas with layers deposition was maximized with the 225 g kg$^{-1}$ food. Broilers given a choice between foods with 65 and 280 g kg$^{-1}$ chose an average protein content of 189 g kg$^{-1}$ which gave them growth and carcass composition very close to that of the birds given a single food containing 225 g kg$^{-1}$ whereas the layers chose 167 g kg$^{-1}$ which gave them a performance close to that of birds given the 165 g kg$^{-1}$ food. This is evidence that growing chickens can approximate their protein requirements by taking appropriate amounts of HP and LP and, as they select a protein content somewhat lower than that which gives maximum growth, that they may utilize the protein more efficiently when choice-fed. Kaufman *et al.* (1978) also noted that young chicks given free access to HP and LP selected proportions which gave the same growth as controls but with a lower protein content in the selected diet.

To test the propositions illustrated in Fig. 13.1, Shariatmadari and Forbes (1993) offered pairs of food differing in protein content to broilers from 4 to 9 weeks of age. The results (Table 14.1) show that, where possible, the birds chose proportions of the two to give themselves a diet containing 180–220 g protein kg$^{-1}$. When both foods had protein contents below this range the birds ate predominantly

**Table 14.1.** Feed intakes of broiler chickens offered pairs of foods varying in protein content (Shariatmadari and Forbes, 1993). Protein intake, live weight gain, carcass weight and carcass composition of broiler chickens offered pairs of foods differing in protein content (Shariatmadari and Forbes, 1993).

| | | Mean food intake (g day⁻¹) on choice treatment | | | | |
|---|---|---|---|---|---|---|
| Feed | CP content (g kg⁻¹) | VLP–LP | VLP–AP | LP–AP | AP–HP | HP–VHP |
| VLP | 65 | 7.6 | 6.0 | | | |
| LP | 115 | 116.3 | | 35.6 | | |
| AP | 225 | | 121.4 | 95.1 | 126.7 | |
| HP | 280 | | | | 7.3 | 121.3 |
| VHP | 320 | | | | | 8.2 |

VLP, LP, AP, HP, VHP: very low, low, adequate, high and very high protein content foods.

from the higher one and when both foods had protein contents higher than this range they ate mostly from the lower. Thus, they were selecting a diet close to the optimum while still tasting the more extreme food from time to time to ensure that it was still unsuitable. When HP and LP were offered in alternate periods broilers still selected about 180 g protein kg⁻¹ of food, except when HP was offered in the morning and LP in the afternoon in which case they took somewhat less (Shariatmadari and Forbes, 1991).

Four foods of 195, 210, 227 and 242 g protein kg⁻¹ were offered simultaneously to male and female broilers from 2 to 8 weeks of age by Kaminska (1979). They ate most of the lowest protein food and this preference increased in the last 2 weeks; the mean protein content selected was 214 g kg⁻¹ up to week 6 but then it decreased to 210 and 207 in the last 2 weeks, results similar to those from broilers given only two foods by Shariatmadari and Forbes (1993). In a further experiment (B. Kaminska, personal communication) broilers were offered foods with ME contents of 11.6, 12.2, 13.0 and 13.8 MJ kg⁻¹. In this case they ate more of the higher energy diets, progressively as the experiment progressed. With a higher protein content there was even more preference for the high energy foods. It is clear from these experiments that broilers use diet selection to achieve their 'ideal' dietary energy:protein ratio.

Thus, an appetite for protein has been clearly demonstrated in growing chickens.

## Laying hens

Up to about 14 weeks of age the growing pullet requires protein only for feather development and a relatively slow rate of muscle deposition but around 15 weeks of age there is rapid development of the ovaries and oviduct which would be expected to increase protein demand and, thus, protein intake in a choice-feeding situation. This has been observed (Scott and Balnave, 1989) as a marked increase in the protein content of their diet about two weeks before the onset of lay in choice-fed pullets.

Laying hens are capable of choosing an appropriate protein intake when given the opportunity and showed a preference for HP which increased steadily during a 26-day observation period (Holcombe *et al.*, 1976b). However, when the choice was between foods which both had a protein content lower than that required, the initial increase in preference for the higher protein food for 17 days was followed by random choice.

Emmans (1977) gave laying hens aged 41–45 weeks a conventional food with a crude protein (CP) content of $172\,g\,CP\,kg^{-1}$, either as the sole food or with a choice of ground barley. There were no differences in egg production or total food intake. The choice-fed birds ate, on average, 84% of their intake as the compound food but this was affected by output: those with higher than average egg production ate more food, but this extra was estimated to be all from the compound food. Emmans was careful to point out that there were differences other than in protein content and quality between the layer mash and the barley, especially calcium, and that his results were not absolute proof of a protein appetite.

Pairs of foods containing 80/170, 110/170, 80/230 or $110/230\,g$ protein $kg^{-1}$ were offered as choices to laying hens by Steinruck and Kirchgessner (1992). There were no differences in egg output between any of the choice-fed groups compared with those on single foods of 170 or $230\,g\,CP\,kg^{-1}$, nor any significant differences in body weight gain. The dietary protein concentrations selected on the four choice treatments were 153, 152, 188 and $179\,g\,kg^{-1}$ respectively and this was claimed to demonstrate the ability of laying hens to select a protein intake corresponding to their requirements for optimal egg production but this ability was not very accurate.

HP ($351\,g$ protein and $8.12\,MJ\,ME\,kg^{-1}$) and LP ($79\,g$ protein and $13.30\,MJ\,ME\,kg^{-1}$) were offered to turkey hens by Emmerson *et al.* (1990). The choice-fed turkeys consumed 10% less food and 44% less protein than controls given a complete food with $181\,g$ protein and $11.23\,MJ\,ME\,kg^{-1}$, yet laid a similar number of eggs. Broodiness tended to be reduced by choice feeding but fertility and hatchability were increased (Emmerson *et al.*, 1991). Protein intake was again about 35% lower for choice-fed birds, giving an overall protein concentration of 110 g kg$^{-1}$ diet, i.e. considerably below NRC (1984b) recommendations.

These results show that good performance can be achieved with choice feeding by laying hens and turkeys.

*Pigs*

As described in Chapter 13, growing pigs choose between high and low protein foods in such a way as to meet their supposed requirements for growth, without overconsuming protein (Kyriazakis *et al.*, 1990).

As a further test of the theory that growing pigs can select for a protein intake which meets their growth requirements, Bradford and Gous (1991) offered pigs choices between pairs of foods containing 220/180, 220/140, 220/100, 180/100 or 140/100 g CP kg$^{-1}$. Compared to controls on a single 160 g kg$^{-1}$ food, choice-fed pigs grew leaner and more efficiently from 30 to 90 kg. The proportion of HP eaten fell as the pigs grew, except in the 140/100 choice, where they ate almost all from the 140 g kg$^{-1}$ food. Of course, the intake of protein might be controlled in order to obtain the appropriate amount of the first limiting amino acid and it was observed that the isoleucine content chosen was almost exactly what would be predicted, whereas lysine intake was higher than predicted, suggesting that isoleucine is the first limiting amino acid under the conditions used in that experiment. It will, therefore, be difficult to tell whether an appetite is for protein or for the most limiting amino acid.

There is variability in protein choice between batches of pigs reared in the same facilities as shown by Engelke *et al.* (1984) who fed corn and a protein supplement to growing pigs in complete and free-choice diets. In the first experiment, the pigs grew well and the proportion of protein supplement chosen declined as the pigs grew so that over the entire experiment the protein content of the chosen food was 136 g kg$^{-1}$ compared with 146 g kg$^{-1}$ for the complete food given to controls. In a second experiment, however, the choice-fed pigs ate a lot of supplement and consumed more protein than complete-diet-fed animals.

Synthetic foods with extremes of protein were used by Robinson (1974) who offered growing gilts a protein-free food and one fortified with casein. Each successive week the protein content of HP was increased, from 200 to 800 g kg$^{-1}$ in steps of 100. There was significant selection for the food containing protein up to a protein content of 600 g kg$^{-1}$, resulting in protein consumption greatly in excess of requirements. Foods containing 700 or 800 g protein kg$^{-1}$ were rejected. Even though the protein-free food was highly unpalatable and was avoided to a great extent, it was preferable to a very-high protein food which would exert considerable metabolic costs of deamination.

Although the mean ratio of HP:total food taken by pigs is close to that expected for optimum growth, there is considerable variation between animals, as illustrated by Fig. 13.2.

Henry (1968) concluded that rats and pigs show a variable appetite for protein which they can demonstrate separately from energy intake. Protein intake is regulated, in part, by requirements for protein deposition whereas energy intake is directly related to growth rate.

Jensen *et al.* (1993) offered female growing pigs 122, 206 or 240 g CP kg$^{-1}$ fresh food or choice between 122 and 240, and free access to straw. Those on L alone had lower live weight gain and food conversion efficiency and stood for longer, walked and rooted in straw more. They suggested that 'specific nutritional needs can increase the foraging motivation of growing pigs'. Choice group did not select well and grew a bit more slowly than M or H (due to positional, social and urination effects).

*Sheep*

Kyriazakis and Oldham (1993) gave growing sheep choices between two foods, one with a protein content above, and the other below, their presumed requirements and observed an apparently directed choice to achieve a dietary protein content of 131–133 g CP kg$^{-1}$ which was close to the protein content of a single food which gave optimal tissue protein deposition. When two foods with protein contents above requirements were offered the sheep consistently ate more of that with the lower content. However, when the choice was between a high protein food and one supplemented with urea, the HP food was preferred, giving an overall protein content of the diet of 173 g CP kg$^{-1}$, i.e. greater than required. The sheep preferred to eat too much protein than too much urea, presumably because of the more toxic effects of an excess of the latter.

Optimal growth by lambs was when they were fed on a single food containing 141 g CP kg$^{-1}$ dry matter (DM). When choice-fed sheep were given two foods, one clearly above this, the other clearly below, they chose a mixture close to 14 g kg$^{-1}$ and they performed as well as those on the optimal single food (Kyriazakis and Oldham, 1993). Individual sheep varied in the protein content they selected, presumably according to their requirements and the proportion of HP taken declined with time presumably due to decreasing requirements as fat deposition overtook that of protein in the body.

Pregnant ewes chose a significantly higher proportion of HP than did barren ewes when the metabolizable energy content of the foods was high but not when it was low (Cooper *et al.*, 1993).

Hou *et al.* (1991a) offered four foods containing 66, 123, 180 and 234 g CP kg$^{-1}$ DM in pairs to lambs and observed a tendency to choose 156 g kg$^{-1}$ when this was possible. This was thought to be close to the optimum protein content for growth in animals of this type.

It seems that lambs are able to differentiate between foods with different protein contents and to select between them according to their protein and energy requirements.

### Stage of growth and growth potential

As animals grow their relative requirements for protein and energy change and it is to be expected that their choice between foods with different protein or energy contents would change in parallel. Rats fed separate sources of carbohydrate, fat and protein ingest a precisely balanced diet to promote growth and reproduction (Leibowitz *et al.*, 1991).

### Poultry

As the bird grows its requirement for energy relative to protein increases, so that the concentration of protein required in the food declines with age (NRC, 1984). It would be expected that the ratio of HP:total would fall with age in choice-fed birds and this is often the case. Kaufman *et al.* (1978) observed the proportion of HP taken by chicks to fall from 0.25 at 15 days of age to 0.15 at 50 days, a decline in the protein content of the selected diet from 250 to 140 g kg$^{-1}$.

When HP and LP, offered as a choice to broilers, could provide a balanced diet there were significant decreases in the HP:total ratio as the birds grew, in line with the decrease in protein:energy requirements during this phase of growth (Shariatmadari and Forbes, 1991, 1993) (Fig. 14.1). However, when the two foods could not provide a balance there was little or no change in the ratio which was always very high or very low in these cases. Paradoxically, Summers and Leeson (1979) observed the choice of an increasing proportion of high protein food by pullets as they aged from 4 to 20 weeks.

Male turkeys offered HP and LP chose a diet containing 360 g protein kg$^{-1}$ from hatching to 4 weeks but thereafter the proportion of HP declined to give a protein:energy ratio similar to that recommended (Lesson and Summers, 1978b) which allowed them to produce good carcass finish and grades.

There is, after several decades of intensive selection, a very large difference in the potential for growth between chicks of layer and broiler strains. Because of the requirements of energy for maintenance,

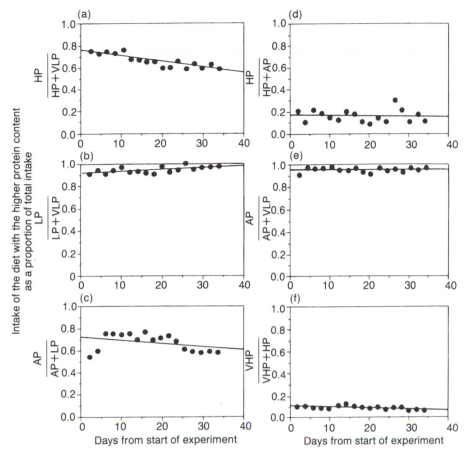

**Fig. 14.1.** The intake by growing broiler chickens of the food with the higher protein content of a pair of foods on offer, expressed as a proportion of total intake (Shariatmadari and Forbes, 1993). The protein contents of the foods were: VLP, 65; LP, 115; AP, 225; HP, 280; VHP, 320 g kg$^{-1}$ and the experiment started when the birds were 28 days of age.

slower growing birds require a lower protein:energy ratio in their food so would be expected to choose a lower HP:total than faster-growing birds.

Azahan and Forbes (1989) observed significantly higher intakes of HP than of LP by broilers to give an overall protein content in the diet selected of 205 g kg$^{-1}$ whereas layers ate similar amounts of HP and LP to give an overall content of 184 g protein kg$^{-1}$. Shariatmadari and Forbes (1993) also found a significantly lower HP:total intake in growing males of the layer strain than in broiler cockerels.

Leclercq and Guy (1991) selected broiler strains for fat or lean growth and offered a choice between HP (260 g protein kg$^{-1}$) and LP (145 g kg$^{-1}$). The mean protein content selected by the fat birds was 179 g kg$^{-1}$ whereas the lean selected 200 g kg$^{-1}$. Mature birds from a strain of broiler selected for high body weight ate more protein than a low-weight strain when given choice of HP and LP foods (Brody *et al.*, 1984) and birds of both strains ate less protein when given a choice of HP (467 g kg$^{-1}$) and LP (82 g kg$^{-1}$) than when given a complete food with a protein content of 188 g kg$^{-1}$. Low-weight birds increased their energy intake by 38–53% when given a choice of foods, compared to a single complete food, suggesting that the latter placed a considerable constraint on intake in birds of the low-weight strain, probably by having too high a protein content. These birds took considerable amounts of glucose solution when given the single, complete food, but much less when given a choice of HP and LP, showing that the complete food was providing too little energy (relative to its protein content) and that this imbalance depressed food intake.

Males have a higher growth potential and seem to be capable of responding to this by eating a higher proportion of the HP food than females. Whereas growing turkeys selected similar energy concentrations irrespective of gender the males, which have a higher growth potential, selected a higher concentration of protein than females (Lesson and Summers, 1978b); similar results were obtained with growing broilers (Rose and Lambie, 1986).

*Pigs*

As pigs grow the ratio of protein:energy required in the diet declines (ARC, 1981) and there is evidence that they select decreasing protein contents when offered HP and LP. Kyriazakis *et al.* (1990) noted that the protein content selected fell from about 250 to 180 g kg$^{-1}$ over an 18 day period starting at 15 kg live weight (Fig. 14.2).

Growing pigs were given a choice between two foods made from the cereal and protein components of a standard control food by Healy *et al.* (1993). The protein content of the chosen diet fell with age from 254 to 191 g protein kg$^{-1}$ over a 3-week period from 18 kg live weight. Similarly, boars given a choice of 119 and 222 g kg$^{-1}$ CP foods for 54 days chose a protein content which declined from 193 to 146 g kg$^{-1}$ and performance was as good as that of similar animals fed HP only (Kyriazakis *et al.*, 1993b).

Chinese Meishan pigs, of particular interest because of their great prolificacy, have low growth potential and a high rate of fat deposition. Given free choice between HP and LP, Large White cross animals chose 194 g protein kg$^{-1}$ whereas Meishans chose 144 g kg$^{-1}$ (Kyriazakis *et al.*, 1993c). The growth rates achieved by the choice-fed animals were not

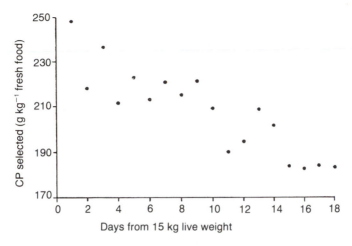

**Fig. 14.2.** The protein content of the diet selected by growing pigs given a choice of foods containing high and low protein concentrations (Kyriazakis *et al.*, 1990).

significantly different from the highest achieved on a single food (220 and 130 g protein kg$^{-1}$, respectively). These results agree with those of Vidal *et al.* (1992) who observed that Landrace/Large White crosses selected 188 g kg$^{-1}$ protein, whereas the Meishans chose 141 g kg$^{-1}$ and Meishan/Large White crosses chose 173 g kg$^{-1}$, in agreement with their protein:fat deposition rates.

Nutrient requirements for growth are influenced by previous nutritional history and Kyriazakis and Emmans (1991) have demonstrated that this is reflected in the choice pigs make for foods with different protein contents. Those previously given a single, low-protein food chose a diet containing 233 g CP kg$^{-1}$ when given a choice of HP and LP whereas those previously given a high protein food chose only 175 g CP kg$^{-1}$. By 33 kg body weight the two groups did not differ in carcass composition showing that the changes in composition induced by restriction in the first phase were compensated for by choice feeding in the second phase of the experiment. Males, with a higher growth potential, chose a diet higher in protein than females (228 vs. 181 g CP kg$^{-1}$).

*Environmental temperature*

Increasing the environmental temperature to above the thermoneutral range depressed food intake in animals given a single, complete food. If given a choice between HP and LP it might be expected that protein intake could be maintained while energy intake was reduced to relieve the heat stress. However, protein metabolism and growth are heat-producing processes and it is difficult to predict the outcome of choice-feeding at high temperatures. The experimental evidence is conflicting.

## Poultry

Several experiments have shown that increasing the environmental temperature tends to increase the protein concentration of the selected diet as energy intake falls, but this is not sufficient to prevent all of the temperature-induced reduction in performance, either in growing birds (Cowan and Michie, 1977b; Rose and Michie, 1986) or laying hens (Blake *et al.*, 1984). However, Sinurat and Balnave (1986) found no difference in the proportion of HP selected by broilers up to 44 days of age whether they were kept in a thermoneutral or heat-stressing environment while Brody *et al.* (1984), working with mature birds from high- and low-weight strains, found increasing temperature to have a proportionately greater depressing effect on protein intake than on energy intake, against expectations.

Broilers given a choice of protein concentrate and whole sorghum grains ate 30% more grain during the day under constant 20°C in the day with continuous illumination (Mastika and Cumming, 1985), i.e. the latter increased their HP:total ratio during the hot period. Similar results were obtained in a second experiment, in which the lights were on for 16 h day$^{-1}$ and choice-fed birds were more efficient than those on the complete food in the hot environment.

Under cold conditions (10°C) choice-fed broilers ate as much protein but more energy than at 20°C (Mastika and Cumming, 1987), a further demonstration of the ability of the broiler to control independently its energy and protein intakes according to changes in requirement.

Egg production was increased in a hot environment when a choice was given between a food high in ME and one high in protein, compared to a single low ME, high protein food (Balnave and Abdoellah, 1990) and it was concluded that hens eat to maintain an appropriate ratio of energy:protein, rather than separately for energy and protein.

## Pigs

Lactating sows were offered a choice of foods containing 100 and 320 g CP kg$^{-1}$ in environments of 20 or 30°C (Vidal *et al.*, 1991). Although sows at 30°C ate less food and produced less milk, they did not increase their HP:total food ration which was very variable, even within each temperature. They were only trained for 4 days first before the choice of foods was offered, which might not have been long enough for mature animals.

*Sheep*

Cropper and Poppi (1992) kept growing lambs in thermoneutral (12–20°C), cold (3–6) or hot (27–30) environments for 7 weeks and gave a choice of two foods containing 67 and 251 g protein kg$^{-1}$. There were no differences between those in the thermoneutral and cold environments which ate protein and energy at rates close to NRC recommendations and gave very high growth rates. Those in the hot environment increased their HP:LP ratio but reduced their total intake and growth rate. It was concluded that lambs change their selection in the appropriate direction when the environment is changed.

# Regulation of Amino Acid Intake

Diets which are imbalanced in the amino acids absorbed from the digestive tract lead to metabolic disturbances and a reduction in food intake which is directly proportional to the degree of amino acid deficiency or imbalance. The effect on intake may be due to the metabolic cost of deaminating the excess of those amino aids which cannot be utilized because of the deficiency, relative or absolute, of others. Sparrows even preferred a protein-free food to one with a severe imbalance of amino acids even though the total protein content of the latter was quite high (Murphy and King, 1989).

Appetites for individual amino acids can therefore be envisaged if the animal learns that one food contains too little of an amino acid for its requirements and another, too much, as long as there are discernible sensory differences between the two foods to act as cues. It may well be that the sparrows studied by Murphy and Pearcy (1993), which were offered foods deficient in valine and lysine or threonine and lysine, did not select a balanced diet because there were no obvious differences in appearance or taste between the foods.

*Poultry*

Newly hatched layer chicks offered a choice between a low lysine food and one with an excess of lysine ate some of the supplemented food but it was not enough to maintain a growth rate as high as the control group which were given a single adequate food (Newman and Sands, 1983). The two food containers were kept in the same place through the 21-day experiment but no colour cues were given and no separate training period was provided. In a second experiment a low lysine food was given in choice with L-lysine HCl but, although the birds ate some lysine it was not enough to support normal growth. In this case presumably the birds had no difficulty in differentiating the food from the pure lysine. When D-lysine HCl was offered as a choice with low lysine food the birds ate some of the former, suggesting the D-lysine triggers some recept mechanism even though D-lysine is unavailable for metabolism. Given a choice between L- and D-lysine, birds ate more of the L form. Thus, there is some evidence of nutritional wisdom but not sufficient to give a properly balanced diet.

Broilers made methionine-deficient by prior feeding on the low methionine food and then given a choice between a complete food and one with half the recommended methionine chose predominantly the former (Steinruck *et al.*, 1990a, b).

In laying hens a methionine-deficient diet depressed egg production from 85% to 67% whereas a choice between deficient and adequate diets resulted in a 58% choice of the adequate diet and egg production of 80% (Hughes, 1979). Selection for methionine therefore occurred, but not quite enough to prevent a decline in egg production.

## Pigs

Growing pigs selected a food with protein containing a balanced mixture of amino acids in strong preference (93%) to one with an imbalanced amino acid composition, whereas the preference for a balanced food paired with a protein-free food was not so marked (Devilat *et al.*, 1970); clearly the imbalanced diet was aversive. Robinson (1975a) found that it took approximately 24 h for pigs to recognize an imbalanced diet which is consistent with a learned aversion to a food which causes malaise.

Pigs preferred a protein-free food to a threonine-imbalanced one (Robinson, 1975b) and the imbalanced ration was clearly aversive (Robinson, 1974). Growing pigs selected a methionine-supplemented food in preference to an unsupplemented food containing $90 \, g \, kg^{-1}$ casein but this may have been due to the strong taste of the methionine rather than to a specific appetite (Robinson, 1975b). In the same report, there was no lasting selection for lysine-supplemented foods.

A 4% excess of methionine, tryptophan, arginine, lysine or threonine in the food for growing pigs led to reductions in weight gain of 52, 31, 28 16 and 5%, respectively and when given a choice of one of the imbalanced foods and the control food, there were strong preferences for the balanced food (Edmonds *et al.*, 1987). When choices were offered between foods with different excesses of amino acids, those with excess threonine, lysine or arginine were preferred to those with an equal excess of methionine or tryptophan. When given a choice between a protein-free food and one with an excess of tryptophan, they initially preferred the protein-free one, but by 12 days were eating more of the tryptophan-supplemented food.

Fairley *et al.* (1993) examined the possibility of a lysine appetite by offering growing pigs pairs of foods containing lysine at 25, 50, 109 and 141 g kg$^{-1}$ of digestible protein. Most of the pigs ate more than 85% of one food to give overall lysine contents of 126, 72, 99 and 79 for choices between 141/25, 141/50, 109/25, and 109/50, i.e. no consistent selection. However, the choice was for a more appropriate ratio in the first few days, probably due to only the position of the food being a cue. In another experiment, four different levels of threonine, 29, 35, 55 and 68, were used, with similar results as lysine. Although most pigs showed selection, they did not provide themselves with appropriate levels of lysine or threonine, according to current estimates. Dalby *et al.* (1994b) strengthened the cues by flavouring either the lysine-supplemented or unsupplemented food for choice-fed weaner pigs but still did not find evidence for selection for lysine.

Bradford and Gous (1992) also studied lysine appetite. In their first experiment foods containing 8.6, 11.7 or 17.4 g lysine kg$^{-1}$ were given singly and the 8.6 and 17.4 g kg$^{-1}$ foods were given as a choice to another group. The results supported the conclusion that the pigs chose for lysine but as lysine was confounded with protein content this could only be a tentative conclusion. In the second experiment, foods containing 14.7 g lysine kg$^{-1}$ were made, using either fishmeal, soyabean oil cake or sunflower/cottonseed/groundnut oil cake. These were fed alone or in choice with each other or with a low protein food (8.3 g lysine kg$^{-1}$). When they were offered as single foods, there were no significant differences in growth, but when given as choice the pigs preferred not to each much of the plant protein mixture. However, there was still no difference in daily food intake or growth. The question then arises as to whether the plant protein food contained an antinutritive factor or it was just unpalatable? The levels of the toxin gossypol were not high. With most of the food combinations in this second experiment, the lysine content chosen was 14.7 g kg$^{-1}$ or very close, except when the choice was between the food containing plant protein and one with a low protein content in which case only about 13% was eaten of the former, giving a lysine content of only 9.0 g kg$^{-1}$. Even though the three types of food had the same protein content, they were not eaten in equal amounts or at random, but for a remarkably constant lysine content, except where the plant protein was concerned.

# Appetites for Minerals

In order to demonstrate a specific appetite for an individual nutrient, rather than a particular type of food, deficiency of that nutrient is induced in the test animals and they are offered a choice between two similar foods, one of which is supplemented with the nutrient in question, whereas the other is not. A significant preference for the supplemented food demonstrates a specific appetite for the nutrient.

## Calcium

Rats increased their intake of calcium lactate after parathyroidectomy and decreased it when parathyroid implants were made thus demonstrating a specific calcium appetite (Richter and Eckert, 1937).

## Poultry

Perhaps the most widely recognized example of a specific appetite in farm species is the calcium appetite of the domestic chicken. Wood-Gush and Kare (1966) showed that calcium-deficient chickens preferred food containing calcium to a calcium-deficient food when the choice was given after 21 days of deprivation. Palatability is also involved, calcium lactate in food being selected for but calcium lactate in the water being avoided, even by deficient birds. Although this appetite for calcium developed slowly (2–4 days) in growing chickens, suggesting that it is learned (Hughes and Wood-Gush, 1971b), it develops very quickly (0.5 h) in laying hens where the calcium requirements are much higher. This has been used to support the suggestion that the calcium appetite in chickens is innate (Hughes, 1979) but it seems more likely that it is learned, given that most calcium salts are insoluble and therefore have little taste.

The higher food intake that is observed on days in which an egg is being formed might be due to the higher calcium requirement on those days, but might also be a response to amino acid or energy demand. Chah and Moran (1985) found differential intake of calcium and protein, however, as there was higher protein intake in the morning and higher calcium intake later in the day by hens producing at least 90% eggs and given choices of a high energy food, a high protein food and oyster shell flakes. Compared to controls given a complete food, there was no difference in egg production or body weight change but egg shells were thicker and the efficiency of utilization of nutrients appeared to be better in the choice-fed birds.

Given foods containing 8.9 or 3.5 g calcium kg$^{-1}$ and grit containing 380 g kg$^{-1}$, pullets chose diets which contained 11.8, 20.8 and 35.0 g

calcium kg$^{-1}$ during the growing, prelaying (medullary bone formation) and egg-laying phases, respectively, i.e. close to their requirements (Classen and Scott, 1982). Holcombe *et al.* (1975) had also found
that growing pullets self-regulated their calcium intake well, but laying
hens were not so good. When they switched containers for pullets
between left and right the birds gradually realized this and changed
their selection appropriately within about 3 days. The fact that this
change was not immediate suggests that the birds were using positional cues which they had learnt to associate with the calcium levels
of the two foods.

Clearly the animal must be able to distinguish between high and
low calcium foods by visual or taste cues, otherwise it cannot identify
the appropriate diet (Hughes and Wood-Gush, 1971b). What is the
reinforcement which leads to preference for a particular diet? It seems
unlikely to be a learned aversion for the deficient food because birds
tend to choose familiar foods even when they are deficient, as against
novel diets which might supply the missing nutrient. It is more likely,
therefore, that ingestion of calcium gives a feeling of well-being, which
becomes associated with that particular food.

In attempts to describe the mechanisms for control of calcium
appetite, Joshua (1976) gave several hormonal or chelating agents to
broilers but the preference for a high calcium diet only increased in the
case of parathyroid hormone; further work is clearly necessary.

Although voluntary intake declines around the onset of laying in
pullets their intake of oyster shell increases during this period (Meyer
*et al.,* 1970). Once in full lay, hens show a diurnal fluctuation in selection
for calcium, eating more limestone grit or oyster shell just before dark
(at a time when egg shell formation is proceeding) than earlier in the
day (Mongin and Sauveur, 1979). To separate the effects of egg
formation from those of photoperiod, hens were kept in continuous
light; there was still a consistent peak in calcium selection 6–10 h after
ovulation when calcium deposition in the shell is just about to start
which suggests an anticipation of need.

Hughes (1972) showed that calcium deposition is not a direct
stimulus to calcium intake, however. Shell formation was prevented by
placing a thread in the wall of the shell gland, but the peak in calcium
selection was still observed. Of the other events which occur during the
egg-laying cycle of the hen, oestradiol secretion is the most likely to be
involved in the diurnal changes in calcium selection. Oestradiol
treatment of cockerels causes an increase in calcium intake (Mongin
and Sauveur, 1979) and plasma oestradiol concentrations closely parallel differences in calcium intake on different days.

*Pigs*

Growing pigs offered a choice between water and a 25 g l$^{-1}$ solution of calcium lactate drank very little of the latter, even though they were on a low calcium diet. Even after parathyroidectomy, when plasma calcium concentration was significantly reduced, they did not choose calcium lactate and had to be revived with injections of calcium borogluconate (Pickard *et al.*, 1977). Intact pigs on a low calcium diet did, however, eat solid calcium carbonate but did not reduce the intake of this when calcium carbonate was added to their food at the rate of 5 g day$^{-1}$. Thus, if there is a calcium appetite in pigs it is not very specific. As calcium absorption is regulated according to the animal's requirements there is little need for mammals to have evolved a calcium appetite, or for a food containing an excess to become aversive.

*Ruminants*

It is widespread practice to offer ruminants access to mineral licks (blocks containing multiple minerals) on the assumption that they will regulate their mineral intake but this cannot be achieved when the block contains many minerals unless the composition is exactly in proportion to the animals' requirements, which is unlikely. D.W. Pickard (personal communication) has questioned the advisability of offering calcium salts *ad libitum* because absorption of calcium from the gut is regulated in mammals; a high intake of calcium leads to a lower rate of absorption and no change in total uptake from the gut. Pickard *et al.* (1978) observed wide differences in voluntary intake of dicalcium phosphate and calcium carbonate by pregnant cows fed a ration which was low in calcium and phosphate and it must be concluded that there is no evidence for a specific calcium appetite in cattle. This conclusion can also be drawn from the compilation of experimental results by Pamp *et al.* (1976), although some of the results they quote are suggestive of a selective intake of bone meal by cows.

In three experiments lambs failed to compensate fully for a calcium-deficient diet by eating sufficient of a high calcium supplement (Burghardi *et al.*, 1982). These authors state that '... required minerals should be provided in the diet rather than on a free choice basis'.

**Phosphorus**

*Chickens*

Laying hens choose diets with intermediate phosphorus contents (5–10 g kg$^{-1}$) and reject those with low (2 g kg$^{-1}$) or high (24 g kg$^{-1}$)

contents (Holcombe *et al.*, 1976a). When the calcium content was raised from 30 to 60 g kg$^{-1}$ the proportion eaten of a food containing 24 g phosphorus kg$^{-1}$ rose from 20 to 73% when the other food contained 10 g phosphorus kg$^{-1}$ which suggests homeostatic control of phosphorus intake to maintain a constant ratio to calcium. However, Hughes (1979) reports a failure to demonstrate a phosphorus appetite in laying hens. An excessively high dietary phosphorus content depresses intake probably because of the adverse effects of a low Ca:P ration on metabolism (Holcombe *et al.*, 1976a).

*Ruminants*

Phosphorus-deficient sheep and cattle will eat bones (Pamp *et al.*, 1976) but it is doubtful whether this is a true appetite for phosphorus because they do not specifically select a supplement containing a high level of phosphate. Grazing cattle and sheep failed to select a phosphorus supplement to correct a phosphorus deficiency induced by low phosphorus herbage (Gordon *et al.*, 1954). However, Merino sheep showed preference for phosphorus-fertilized plots of grass in the dry season (but not the wet season), even when the levels of phosphorus were higher than those giving maximum pasture growth (Ozanne and Howes, 1971). The major difference between the pastures was the phosphorus content but there was also a small but consistent fall in the phenol content as phosphorus increased so perhaps they were using this as a cue, or even as the primary stimulus. There was a close correlation between the extent a plot was defoliated (%) by grazing sheep and its phosphorus content (P, g kg$^{-1}$):

$$defoliation = 41 + 6.7P \qquad (14.1)$$

**Sodium**

*Poultry*

Several attempts by Hughes and his colleagues (Hughes, 1979) failed to demonstrate anything more than a weak sodium appetite in laying hens; even when a slight preference was shown for a higher sodium food it was not enough to prevent a reduction in egg production.

*Ruminants*

A specific sodium appetite has been demonstrated and studied by Denton and colleagues for many years. Housed sheep correct for sodium deficits very accurately when given sodium chloride solutions (see Denton, 1982), whereas on grazing they select plant species which are high in sodium. The increase in intake of sodium chloride solution when sheep were sodium-depleted by drainage of saliva via a parotid duct fistula was reversed by infusion of sodium salts into a lateral ventricle of the brain (Blair-West *et al.*, 1987), showing that the central nervous system is sensitive to sodium ions.

Sodium depletion of calves led to reduced food intake and the development of a relatively specific appetite for the sodium ion, calves responding more for sodium bicarbonate in an operant situation when they were more severely sodium depleted (Bell and Sly, 1979). The possibility that cattle can smell sodium salts was shown by Bell and Sly (1983) as they could detect sodium bicarbonate at up to 20 m distant, if assisted by wind direction. Anosmic cattle took longer than intact animals to identity a salt solution from among an array of buckets of water but it is not clear how non-volatile salts can have a smell.

Michell and Moss (1988) found no increase in the preference shown by ewes for salt when on a low salt diet during pregnancy or lactation, when salt requirements are known to be increased, but this increase in sodium demand is likely to be small relative to that induced by saliva drainage.

### Zinc

Hughes and Dewar (1971) observed that zinc-deficient chicks will consume more of a food containing 65 mg zinc $kg^{-1}$ than of one containing only 5 mg $kg^{-1}$. During the first 6 days after offering the zinc-supplemented food it was consumed at greater than twice the level of the low zinc diet by zinc-deficient bids. Control birds ate about 40% of the high zinc food for several days but this proportion gradually increased as they apparently became marginally zinc-deficient themselves.

## Appetites for Vitamins

### Thiamine (vitamin $B_1$)

Hughes and Wood-Gush (1971a) studied thiamine selection in chickens by inducing a functional deficiency with injections of oxythiamine hydrochloride, a metabolic antagonist of thiamine. When offered two foods, one deficient in thiamine, the other supplemented with 20 mg $kg^{-1}$, the depleted birds ate consistently more of the supplemented food than control birds, demonstrating a specific appetite for thiamine.

## Vitamin B$_6$

Broilers given a choice of vitamin B$_6$ sufficient and deficient foods at first ate too little of the former and showed signs of deficiency of the vitamin (Steinruck *et al.*, 1991). They then increased their relative intake of the supplemented food to re-establish normal growth and continued to eat proportions of the two foods which provided them with a balanced diet. Thus, they demonstrated a specific appetite for vitamin B$_6$ based on the learned consequences of eating the two foods.

## Ascorbic acid (vitamin C)

There have been several reports that the adverse effects of heat stress on food intake and performance are partially alleviated by supplementation of the diet with ascorbic acid (Kutlu and Forbes, 1993a). This is somewhat unexpected as it has been generally assumed that chickens could synthesize sufficient ascorbic acid and that dietary supplementation was unnecessary. To see whether the different requirements for ascorbic acid under temperate and hot conditions would be expressed as an appetite for ascorbic acid, Kutlu and Forbes (1993b) trained young chicks to differentiate a supplemented food from an unsupplemented one by means of colour and then gave them a choice of the two. Those birds kept in an unstressful environment ate a significantly lower proportion of the supplemented food than those maintained under mildly heat-stressing conditions. Figure 14.3 shows the ascorbic acid

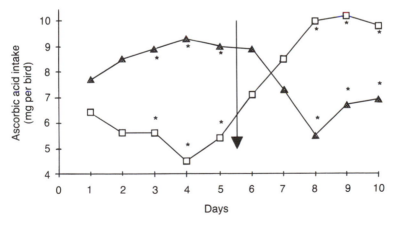

**Fig. 14.3.** Self-selected daily intakes of ascorbic acid by growing broiler chickens offered coloured foods which were unsupplemented and supplemented with ascorbic acid (Kutlu and Forbes, 1993c). Treatment ▲: birds in a heat-stressing environment for 5 days followed by a thermoneutral environment. Treatment □: thermoneutral, followed by hot environment. The vertical arrow shows the time at which the environments were changed.

intakes chosen by chicks under the two environmental conditions and the changes following reversal of the environments (Kutlu and Forbes, 1993c). It will be seen that following a change in environmental temperature the birds adjusted their ascorbic acid intake within three days; the voluntary intake of the vitamin in the thermoneutral environment was 5–6 mg day$^{-1}$ whereas under the hot conditions it was 9–10 mg day$^{-1}$ Clearly the colour-discrimination of the two foods had allowed the chicks to express their desire for an intake of ascorbic acid appropriate to their needs. If the two foods were offered without colour the birds ate at random.

# Water Intake

Water is the most important nutrient. If you doubt this statement then consider which nutrient, when removed form the diet, will cause illness and death most quickly. The fact that water is taken so much for granted in temperate countries is due to its ready availability and thus its low cost.

The voluntary intake of water is usually about twice the weight of DM eaten and, because many of the functions of water are related to the digestion and metabolism of food, water intake is closely related to food intake, both quantitatively and temporally. Simple-stomached animals usually drink before, during or after each meal of food whereas ruminants, with their great capacity for storing digesta with a high water content, often eat a meal without drinking and when they do drink, take a very large volume of water.

In addition to the water drunk by the animal it is also present in foods, especially fresh grass, silage and root crops, so it is not always necessary to provide drinking water. However, fresh water should always be available because animals which are ill reduce their DM intake and will then require water, especially if they are suffering from diarrhoea in which large amounts of water are lost in the faeces.

In addition to ingested water, the metabolism of substrates in the body yields water which provides a small but significant addition to the body's supply.

Water intake is depressed if water is difficult to obtain; a small degree of restriction is usually not harmful but in many areas of the world water is not expensive and is usually offered *ad libitum*. Prediction of water requirements and intake has not, therefore, received as much attention as has the prediction of food intake.

Water is required for wetting food in the mouth and stomachs; as a medium for digestive reactions in stomachs and intestines; as the major component of the body; as a medium for the excretion of soluble

material in the urine and for the secretion of sweat. Thus, its requirements are influenced by the amount and type of foods eaten and by the
environmental temperature.

Water intake is controlled by the hypothalamus and an increase in
the tonicity of cerebrospinal fluid is an important stimulus to drinking.

The control of water intake is a complex subject dealt with in detail
by Rolls and Rolls (1982). Andersson (1978) and Olsson and McKinley
(1980) have reviewed the subject for ruminants.

There is clearly a specific appetite for water and it is generally
assumed that the animal takes in as much water as is needed to meets
its requirements, although excessive water consumption can be
induced under some conditions, such as the schedule-induced polydipsia seen in pigs (Stephens *et al.*, 1983). There is relatively little cost to
the animal if it drinks too much water.

### Drinking behaviour

#### Poultry

Bailey (1990) has reviewed the water requirements of poultry and the
effects of water restriction. Chickens drink up to 40 times per day, but
make fewer visits to drink as they mature (Ross and Hurnik, 1983).

It is likely that poultry drink more than is strictly required because
when the water intake of chickens was restricted by adulteration with
quinine to about 75% of normal there was no effect on food intake and
only a small reduction in growth rate (Yeomans and Savory, 1989).

#### Pigs

Brooks and Carpenter (1990) carefully considered the theoretical and
practical aspects of the various requirements for water by growing and
finishing pigs and the routes by which the animal gains and loses,
water, including a complete water balance sheet for a pig. They
particularly consider wastage of water as introducing important errors
in assessment of the true water requirements of pigs. J. Barber (personal
communication) has found huge variation between water intakes by
pigs in different studies and thinks that much of this is due to
inaccurate water meters. Also there can be considerable wastage,
especially if there are many pigs per drinker and/or if fighting occurs.

Flow rate is important in determining how much pigs drink. A low
rate of delivery necessitates long drinking periods and pigs seem
unwilling to drink for more than a few seconds at a time. Barber *et al.*
(1989) found pigs to have a significantly lower food intake during the

3 weeks after weaning from drinkers with a flow rate of 175 ml min$^{-1}$, compared with 450 ml min$^{-1}$.

Lactating sows have a high requirement for water (Fraser *et al.*, 1990) and water quality has an important effect on intake.

## Cattle

Lactating cows fed a fixed amount of concentrates and silage *ad libitum* took about four drinks per day, even though silage was taken in 15 meals per day and concentrates in a further 2–4 allocations per day (Forbes *et al.*, 1991). Figure 2.4 shows the feeding and drinking pattern over a 24 h period for a cow yielding 25 kg of milk per day and eating 14 kg of silage DM. There were four drinks, ranging in size from 1 to 13 l and all in association with meals of silage.

## Sheep and goats

Cooper *et al.* (1991) showed that it is possible to induce goats to drink more than usual by adding vinegar or orange flavour to the water and that this reduced calcium and magnesium levels in urine, thereby reducing the risk of urolithiasis.

## Environmental temperature

Water intake by poultry is positively correlated with environmental temperature but the initial increase which accompanies a sudden rise in temperature is not sustained as the birds become acclimatized (e.g. Smith, 1972).

In pigs there is a rise in the ratio of water intake to dry matter intake between 20 and 30°C from 2.7 to 4.3 kg kg$^{-1}$ DM (Close *et al.*, 1971). Above 25°C this is mainly due to the decrease in food intake rather than an increase in water intake (Fuller, 1965). In cold weather, if the temperature of drinking water is warmer than that of the environment then pigs drink more whereas in hot weather they drink more if the water is cold (J. Barber, personal communication).

Above 0°C there is a positive relationship between environmental temperature and water intake in cattle (Winchester and Morris, 1965). Below freezing, however, the water intake of lactating cows increases, probably due to the increased metabolic rate (McDonald and Bell, 1958).

Sheep also drink more as temperature increases but, like cattle, also increase water intake per unit of DM eaten below about 0°C (Forbes, 1967; Fig. 14.4).

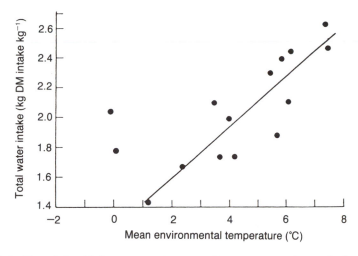

**Fig. 14.4.** The relationship between environmental temperature and water intake per unit DM intake in pregnant ewes (Forbes, 1967).

## Dry matter intake

The greater the DM intake, the greater the urinary excretion and the requirement for water. In addition, heat production is increased by increased food intake which leads to greater evaporative heat loss and thus to greater water intake.

Water intake by poultry increases with increasing food intake (e.g. Patrick and Ferrise, 1962), the best single predictor of water intake is DM intake (Hill, 1977) and drinking usually follows meals (Hill *et al.*, 1979). Fasted 4-week-old broilers drank about one-third of the normal daily intake of water (Bierer *et al.*, 1966).

Barber *et al.* (1991) identified two phases of drinking in growing pigs, one of which was closely associated with eating, the amount of water being about 89% of the weight of food eaten, whereas the other was drinking between meals which was fairly constant at $2.2 \, l \, day^{-1}$ (J.Barber, personal communication) (Table 14.2). The total weight of food and water intake was nearly 12% of body weight per day in each case and it was speculated that there might be a weight or volume limit to intake.

Yang *et al.* (1981) observed that restricting the food allowance for pigs to half the usual amount or complete fasting increased the volume of water consumed by up to sixfold. As discussed in Chapter 2, chronic hunger leads to oral activities such as bar-chewing and it is likely that the polydipsia of underfeeding is such a displacement activity. Stalled

**Table 14.2.** Effect of level of feeding on water intake by growing pigs (J. Barber, personal communication).

| Level of feeding (g kg$^{-1}$) | 80 | 90 | 100 | 110 |
|---|---|---|---|---|
| *TWI* (l day$^{-1}$) | 3.29 | 3.45 | 3.53 | 3.60 |
| Water/feed | 2.65 | 2.43 | 2.21 | 2.08 |
| Water consumed between feeds (l day$^{-1}$) | 2.18 | 2.19 | 2.15 | 2.19 |
| Water during meals (per feed) | 0.89 | 0.89 | 0.88 | 0.89 |

*TWI*, total water intake.

sows have been noted to stand with their snouts pressing nipple drinkers for up to an hour a day but without drinking.

Water intake increases in direct proportion to the intake of food DM eaten by cows (Winchester and Morris, 1956).

Total water intake (free water plus water in the food) is correlated with DM intake in sheep and goats. In observations on non-pregnant ewes of two breeds of very different type, fed on silage, hay or dried grass, the relationship (Forbes, 1967) was:

$$TWI = 3.86\,DMI - 0.99 \qquad\qquad (14.2)$$

where *TWI* is total water intake (l day$^{-1}$) and *DMI* is DM intake (kg day$^{-1}$). Similar observations were made by Calder *et al.* (1964).

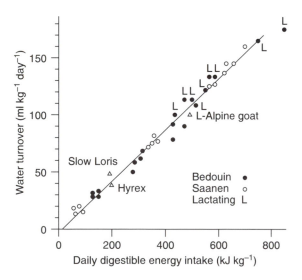

**Fig. 14.5.** Relationship between water turnover and intake of digestible energy for goats and other species (Silankove, 1989).

Silankove (1989) found a close relationship between water turnover and digestible energy intake in desert and temperate goats:

$$WT = -5.4 + 0.22\ DEI \tag{14.3}$$

Where $WT$ is water turnover (ml kg$^{-1}$ day$^{-1}$) and $DEI$ is digestible energy intake (kJ kg$^{-1}$ day$^{-1}$). This is shown in Fig. 14.5 which shows that the relationship holds good for a wide range of sizes and physiological states.

## Diet composition

Increasing the salt concentration or the protein level of the diet stimulates increased water intake in all species because of the increase in urine volume necessary for the excretion of the salt or urea.

Increases in the fat, protein, salt or potassium content of the food all lead to an increase in water intake by poultry (Hill *et al.*, 1979). Water intake in pigs is also increased by protein (especially unabsorbed protein) sodium, potassium and by some antibiotics (J.Barber, personal communication).

Pregnant gilts and sows given restricted amounts of food with different levels of fibre showed a significant reduction in the time spent drinking and in water intake with higher fibre foods (Robert *et al.*, 1993). This suggests that some drinking is a substitute for eating and that the longer time spent eating and chewing a high fibre food reduces the desire for further oral stimulation by drinking.

Water drinking was induced by intracerebroventricular infusion of hypertonic solutions in cattle but there was no effect on the intakes of food or sodium chloride (McKinley *et al.*, 1987). The effect of NaCl infusion was greater than those of mannitol or sucrose despite the fact that they caused very similar increases in osmolality of cerebrospinal fluid. When given intravenously, NaCl and mannitol had equal effects demonstrating that there are central NaCl receptors as well as osmo-receptors in cattle.

A dried grass diet was associated with a higher intake of water per unit of dry matter by sheep than hay presumably because of the higher ash and protein contents (Forbes, 1967). Increasing the intake of DM and/or CP increased water intake by sheep (Bass, 1982) and the diurnal distribution of water intake was directly related to feeding times.

In summer when other grasses are available as well as saltbush, sheep in Australia only drink once per day but in autumn only saltbush is available and they must drink twice per day (Squires, 1981). They then spend about 3 h per day walking to and from water. Where there is no saltbush, they normally only drink once every 2 to 3 days and only in very hot weather do they drink every day.

*Physiological state*

Inadequate water intake has sometimes been thought to be the reason for the postweaning growth check in piglets and flavouring the water has been found to be effective in overcoming this problem (Barber *et al.*, 1989).

Bermudez *et al.* (1984) also deduced that low water intake might be a cause of low food intake and loss of weight for a few days after weaning of lambs and suggested that ways should be sought to increase water intake, perhaps by offering it before weaning when lambs can sometimes drink considerable amounts (Penning *et al.*, 1980).

Water intake increases during pregnancy in the ewe in proportion to the number of fetuses carried (Forbes, 1967). Lactation stimulates water intake in ewes by more than the volume of water in the milk presumably because of the increased food intake and heat production of the lactating animal.

# Conclusions

Poultry and pigs can select a diet containing a ratio of protein to energy which is close to that providing for optimal growth. However, the presence of 'unpalatable' materials in one food induces higher than predicted intakes of the other and this is not clearly related to toxins in the former. Changes in the requirements for protein during growth are accompanied by reductions in the proportion taken of the high protein food and animals with a higher propensity to grow or produce eggs eat more protein than those with a greater potential to deposit fat.

There is considerable evidence that animals can select between foods according to their requirements for individual amino acids although the balance of amino acids in a food can have a profound effect on its selection.

Many minerals and vitamins have been shown to be capable of being selected as long as the animals are able to differentiate the deficient and sufficient foods by means of sight, taste or position.

Water intake is regulated largely by the intake of food and response to such factors as environmental temperature, pregnancy and lactation. Overconsumption of water is a common problem of intensive housing, especially when restricted feeding is practised.

Overall, therefore, it has been clearly demonstrated that appetites for essential nutrients can be developed. This depends on animals sensing their metabolic 'well-being' and associating this with the sensory properties of the foods on offer. The possibility of any appetites being innate seems remote although the salt appetite of sheep seems to be very accurate, even in untrained animals.

Faced with a wide range of plants, it may be important for grazing animals to avoid toxic species rather than select those which are nutritionally best balanced. If they eat several non-toxic species they are likely to take a diet which is not far removed from the optimal. However, the nutritional aspects of optimal foraging have been little studied and the limits to animals' ability to develop appetites for two or more nutrients simultaneously requires further research.

# 15 ENVIRONMENTAL FACTORS AFFECTING INTAKE

---

- Environmental temperature
- Photoperiod
- Exercise
- Feeder design
- Group size
- Frequency of offering food
- Disease
- Conclusions

This chapter considers intake responses to changes in temperature, photoperiod, the social environment, housing and feeding conditions and disease.

## Environmental Temperature

Unless otherwise stated the term environmental temperature will refer to the effective ambient temperature, which is the actual temperature modified by the effects of humidity, wind and rainfall. A continuum in the effects of temperature can be seen in the comparatively few experiments in which a wide range of environments have been studied.

Above the thermoneutral zone body temperature rises and so food intake decreases in order to reduce the heat production associated with feeding, digestion, absorption and metabolism and to prevent an excessive increase in body temperature. Below the thermoneutral zone heat production must increase in order to maintain body temperature and intake rises to provide substrates for this increased heat production.

*Poultry*

Feeding behaviour is erratic at very low temperatures and few data are available on the quantitative responses. Below an optimum temperature, which depends on the size and feathering of the birds, food intake increases and the efficiency of conversion into body weight gain declines; above this temperature, food intake and growth are depressed. For broilers in the later stages of growth this optimum temperature for efficiency was found to be 21°C (Deaton *et al.*, 1978). A similar temperature is optimum for growing pullets (Vo *et al.*, 1978) and for laying hens. Every degree increase between 25 and 34°C results in a 1–1.5 g day$^{-1}$ decline in food intake by laying hens; above 35°C the decline is greater (Davis *et al.*, 1973).

In broiler chicks there was lower food intake at 29 than at 21°C but the depression was similar with foods of between 140 and 230 g protein kg$^{-1}$ (Adams *et al.*, 1962) and weight gains were lower at 29°C and with low protein foods. Part of this depression in intake and growth can be reversed by supplementing the diet with ascorbic acid (vitamin C) (Kutlu and Forbes, 1993a). Plasma corticosterone is reduced during such treatment of broilers, water intake increases and body temperature falls. Birds can be trained to know the difference between supplemented and unsupplemented foods and are then able to select their desired intake of ascorbic acid (Chapter 14).

*Pigs*

The temperature above which voluntary intake is depressed varies with the size of the animal. Younger or thinner pigs have a greater surface-to-weight ratio and can more easily get rid of excess heat than older or fatter animals. Thus, at any given temperature above the thermoneutral zone, intake by heavy pigs is depressed relatively more than that of lighter pigs (NRC, 1981). In practice, there is a continuous decline in intake with increasing environmental temperature (Fig. 15.1).

*Growth*
After weaning daily food intake declines at 21 g/1°C increase in temperature between 5 and 20°C. From 20 to 25°C the fall was only 7.2 g/°C. Close (1989) re-analysed data from four experiments which yielded the equation:

$$MEI = 9.6 + 0.075ET + 0.52BW - 0.012ET \times BW \qquad (15.1)$$

where *MEI* is ME intake (MJ day$^{-1}$), *ET* is environmental temperature (°C) and *BW* is body weight (kg). Thus, ME intake increased by 0.16 MJ

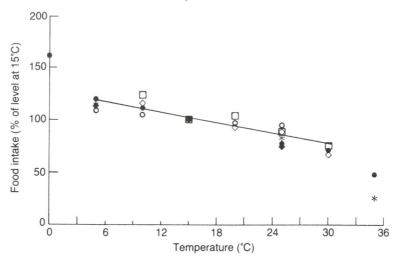

**Fig. 15.1.** Effects of environmental temperature on voluntary food intake by growing pigs, compiled by NRC (1987) from several sources.

day$^{-1}$ for each °C for pigs of 20 kg and by 1.12 MJ day$^{-1}$ for pigs of 100 kg.

Cool temperatures do not increase colostrum intake in newborn piglets as they become less vigorous and spend less time sucking. This means that it is difficult to arrange for optimum temperatures for both sow and piglets in the same house (Close, 1989). Once they get to about a week of age piglets do respond to cooler temperatures by taking more milk. Reduced nocturnal temperatures at night, when growing pigs have a lower body temperature, increased intake and growth by about 10%, but with no improvement in efficiency.

For growing–finishing pigs, intake decreases as environmental temperature rises from 5 to 20°C (Verstegen *et al.*, 1978) and overall, for temperatures of 5–30°C (NRC, 1987) the relationship is:

$$PCI15 = 126.3 - 1.65T \qquad (15.2)$$

where *PCI*15 is the percentage change from the level of intake at 15°C and *T* is environmental temperature.

The increase in intake under cold conditions does not usually prevent retardation of growth and so the proportion of food energy retained in the carcass is reduced. However, the increase in voluntary consumption is sometimes greater than that necessary to maintain weight gain and Holme and Coey (1967) found that cold-stressed growing pigs not only ate more than controls but also gained more weight. Suguhara *et al.* (1970) kept young (10–335 kg) pigs in environments of 7, 23 or 33°C with relative humidity maintained at 50% and found that the voluntary intakes were 1.61, 1.33 and 0.91 kg day$^{-1}$ with average daily gains of 0.64, 0.61 and 0.40 kg. As the critical temperature of such small pigs is around 30°C this represents a stimulating effect of a cold environment rather than a depressing effect of a hot environment. Jensen *et al.* (1969) found increased daily intakes and weight gains in older pigs kept in temperatures in the range of −23 to 15°C compared with a range of 16–24°C.

Rinaldo and Le Dividich (1991) found, for growing pigs:

$$\text{Intake (g day}^{-1}) = 1163 + 16.8T - 0.8T^2 \qquad (15.3)$$

i.e. for a 20 kg pig, there is an increase of about 1.5% in food intake for every degree decrease in environmental temperature within the 15–25°C range.

Constant cold stress does not change the normal nychthemeral distribution of food intake in growing pigs (Herpin *et al.*, 1987) but if it is only cold at night, then there is an increase in the proportion of food eaten at night (Rinaldo *et al.*, 1989).

Food intake of pigs kept chronically at 10°C stayed high for at least 24 h after moving to 25°C and there was a closer relationship with metabolic rate than with body temperature (Macari *et al.*, 1983). Plasma levels of thyroid hormones changed within a few hours after changes in environmental temperature but food intake took at least four days (Macari *et al.*, 1986). Transferring thyroidectomized pigs from hot to cool was accompanied by increased intake but not vice versa and they concluded that thyroid hormones, although not controlling intake directly, are responsible for the metabolic adaptations which affect intake.

*Sows*

Voluntary intake by lactating sows fell by 12% when environmental temperature increased from 21 to 27°C and by 25% when it was increased from 16 to 27°C. This led to a greater weight loss at the higher temperature (Lynch, 1989).

Temperature has a particularly great effect on lactating sows: weight loss of lactating sows increased as environmental temperature increased although the use of wet food and higher energy food have increased the daily intake of the sow (O'Grady and Lynch, 1978). As well as sows losing more weight, piglets grow more slowly at higher temperatures.

Diet can be manipulated to reduce the effects of high temperature and fat inclusion improves performance under hot conditions as it has a lower heat increment than carbohydrates. Sows ate more of a food containing 200 g CP kg$^{-1}$ than one containing 140 g kg$^{-1}$ at 16°C but less at 28°C (Lynch, 1989), presumably due to the high heat increment of protein metabolism.

## Ventilation

Ventilation rate can also affect growth and food intake in pigs. Morrison *et al.* (1976) found no difference between 6.9 and 11.5 air changes per hour (intakes of 2.37 and 2.42 kg day$^{-1}$) but a significant depression in food intake (2.24 kg) when the ventilation rate was very low. Mount *et al.* (1971) concluded that an increase from 10 to 56 cm s$^{-1}$ in air speed is equivalent to a 4°C fall in air temperature, in terms of its effects on pigs. However, huddling together at low effective temperatures will reduce the cooling effect and the results from individually penned pigs are not directly applicable to groups of pigs (Mount, 1968).

At high temperatures, evaporation is very important as a means of losing heat. At 22°C, increasing relative humidity from 50 to 95% has no effect on voluntary food intake or growth, but at 28 and 33°C, each 10% increase in humidity depressed intake by 36 g day$^{-1}$ (Morrison *et al.*, 1969). Localized cooling of the head increases intake by sows, especially at high temperatures (Stansbury *et al.*, 1987). McGlone *et al.* (1988) found that when snout cooling was provided, sows increased their intake from 3.99 to 4.86 kg day$^{-1}$ and reduced weight loss from 19.8 to 14.3 kg in 28 days. A water drip increased intake to 5.29 kg day$^{-1}$ and weight loss was 10.8 kg in 28 days whereas with both snout cooling and a water drip intake was 5.84 kg day$^{-1}$ and weight loss was 2.0 kg in 28 days.

## Cattle

Disruption of feeding behaviour occurs in cattle at very low temperatures (less than −10°C) especially in beef cattle, which are more susceptible to increased heat losses because their heat production is less than that of dairy cows. DM intake by grazing beef cattle increased when daily temperature increased or decreased from the mean of previous days but the magnitude of the response was only 0.0005% kg$^{-1}$ body weight day$^{-1}$ °C$^{-1}$ deviation (Bekverlin *et al.*, 1989). Grazing time decreased with deviations in effective temperature, whether higher or lower than the previous few days (0.01 h day$^{-1}$ °C$^{-1}$ deviation). Fluctuations in temperature in the range −16 to 8°C had minimal effect on intake or grazing behaviour and it was concluded that fluctuations within that range within a familiar environment were minimally stressful.

Adams *et al.* (1986) found that, for beef cows within a range of minimum daily temperatures from 0 to −35°C, grazing time (*GT* = h day$^{-1}$ spent eating) decreased in proportion with minimum daily temperature (*MDT*, °C):

$$GT = 9.32 + 0.16MDT \text{ for 3-year-old cows} \qquad (15.4)$$
$$GT = 9.02 + 0.009MDT \text{ for 6-year-old cows} \qquad (15.5)$$

with little effect of snow cover.

Increases in gut motility under cold exposure lead to increases in rate of passage which could be responsible for increases in food intake if physical constraints were limiting intake (Christopherson and Kennedy, 1983).

Under hot conditions, provision of shade increased intake, as evidenced by weight change and plasma free fatty acid levels (Silankove and Gutman, 1992). Unshaded cows increased their intake of poultry litter, compared with shaded cows, presumably in an attempt to reduce the heat increment of feeding, compared to fibrous herbage. Head cooling increased the food intake of cattle working on treadmills (Thomas and Pearson, 1986).

The acute effects of heat exposure may be more severe than the chronic effects on food intake; Johnson *et al.* (1961) exposed heifers to temperatures which increased from 18 to 29°C and found that growth was depressed during the 20-day period after the change, but not subsequently, even though the high temperature was maintained. This shows that prolonged exposure leads to acclimatization and that short-term observations can give misleading results (Hahn, 1981). One way in which cattle adapt to hot conditions is to eat at night, when it is cooler, which allows them to eat more than would be predicted from the results of experiments with continuous exposure to hot environments in a heat chamber (Maust *et al.*, 1972).

Although heat stress has a greater effect on the intake of *Bos taurus* than on *Bos indicus* cattle, the level of intake is generally higher in *B. taurus* (Colditz and Kellaway, 1972); at 17 and 38°C, respectively, Friesians ate 29 and 25 g kg$^{-1}$, Brahmans ate 24 and 22 g kg$^{-1}$ and first crosses between the two ate 29 and 28 g kg$^{-1}$ live weight.

As the proportion of concentrates in the diet is increased so the heat increment of feeding decreases; this can be used to alleviate heat stress to a limited extent. Martz *et al.* (1971) noted a faster peak in rumen volatile fatty acid concentrations after a large meal in steers at 35°C compared with 29°C or less and suggested that this accounted for the lower food intake and that foods which result in lower ruminal acetate production might be useful in hot areas.

In addition to the direct effects on animal, high environmental temperatures affect the growth of food plants. Typically there is an increase in the proportion of cell wall constituents (CWC) especially in tropical grasses, because of the faster maturation (Dirven and Deinum,

1977). The increased stem:leaf ratio, as well as depressing the nutritive value, will also reduce the palatability of the herbage.

*Sheep*

*Cold environments*
Below the critical temperature the animal has, by definition, to increase its rate of heat production in order to maintain its deep body temperature within the narrow range compatible with normal function. This increase in energy requirements would be expected to result in increased food intake and this is indeed so.

At a fixed level of feeding, sheep eat faster in a colder environment and there is an increase in rumen motility, a reduction in the volume of rumen contents and in the extent of digestion of cell wall constituents (Kennedy *et al.*, 1985).

Winfield *et al.* (1968) exposed pregnant ewes on a hillside in individual pens. Compared with similar animals kept indoors the exposed ewes ate significantly more of a complete pelleted food (45 vs. 38 g kg$^{-1}$ day$^{-1}$). This was sufficient for them to gain weight at the same rate and to produce lambs of the same birth weight.

Thyroxine secretion is increased by reducing the environmental temperature, and this might be responsible for increased voluntary food intake. Treatment of sheep with 1 mg thyroxine day$^{-1}$ increased food intake but weight gains were reduced (Ferguson, 1958); the increase in intake is due, presumably, to the greater energy required to support the increase in metabolic rate; 60 mg implants given subcutaneously at 3-month intervals also stimulated intake. Although body weight was lost in the first month, food intake was even higher in the second and third months after implantation as weight was regained (Lambourne, 1964). Again it is apparent that intake is responding to changes in energy expenditure.

*Shearing*
Shearing increases heat production in sheep and this is matched by increased food intake (about 25% at 13°C, Davey and Holmes, 1977). Wodzika (1963) noted that the increase in voluntary intake occurred about a week after shearing although heart rate increased at once; the rise in intake peaked at 50% above the preshearing level and was entirely due to a greater intake of concentrate pellets although hay was also available *ad libitum*. There was marked shivering during the week between shearing and the start of hyperphagia. Subsequently Wodzika (1964) showed that a 39% increase in intake by young ewes after shearing was not accompanied by any difference in live weight gains, compared with controls, suggesting that the increase in intake was a

response to the increased heat losses. During the few weeks after shearing, intake was inversely related to environmental temperature but by the seventh week the difference in voluntary intake between shorn and unshorn sheep had disappeared; presumably sufficient wool had grown to afford adequate protection by this time. Ternouth and Beattie (1970) reported a 15% increase in intake 2–3 weeks after shearing, followed by a fall during weeks 4 and 5 whereas Minson and Ternouth (1971) found little effect on the intake, already high, of a highly digestible lucerne food but a marked increase with low-intake poorly digestible forages. Shearing of housed pregnant ewes was followed by an increase in intake of 16 and 43% on two silage-based diets, 9% on swede-based diets but only 2% on a hay-based diet (Vipond *et al.*, 1987). The increase was greater in lighter ewes, presumably as they had less subcutaneous fat to compensate for the loss of the fleece.

These results from sheep show that, although the response takes at least a week, increased heat loss is compensated for by increased voluntary food intake to provide the necessary metabolizable energy. If heat production is already high then shearing does not bring the animal to below its critical temperature and intake is unaffected.

*Hot environments*

Sheep are also affected by high temperatures. Brink (1975) exposed shorn lambs, whose lower critical temperature was approximately 13°C to environments ranging from −5 to 35°C and found the following relationship.

$$DMI = 111.3 - 0.52T \tag{15.6}$$

where *DMI* was the dry matter intake (g kg live weight$^{-0.75}$) and *T* was the temperature (°C). The depression of intake at high temperatures is probably smaller with high-concentrate rations than with forages because the latter have a higher heat increment (Moose *et al.*, 1969).

As with cattle, acclimatization can overcome the acute effects of high temperatures and Silankove (1987) found no effect of a hot climate on food intake by sheep despite heat stress in these well-acclimatized sheep.

# Photoperiod

The most obvious difference between day and night as far as feeding is concerned is the ease with which animals can see their food. However, the regular sequence of dark and light in a 24 h cycle acts as a synchronizer to entrain diurnal rhythms in many biological functions which are not directly dependent on the presence of light or dark. In many cases it is not known whether rhythms of approximately 24 h are entrained in which case they should correctly be called circadian rather than diurnal rhythms. The need to consider time-of-day when studying the control of food intake, with particular reference to the rat, is discussed by Armstrong (1980).

## Poultry

Poultry do not normally eat during darkness. If daylength is short (less than 8 h) hunger overcomes the reluctance to eat at night and feeding occurs to a limited extent during darkness (Morris, 1968a). In continuous darkness intake is as high as in long daylengths indicating that lack of visual contact with food is not the only reason for the aphagia normally seen at night (Cherry and Barwick, 1962). If chickens are subjected to constant illumination, following experience of light–dark cycles, there is a residual rhythm of feeding although this does not remain at exactly 24 h (Duncan and Hughes, 1975). Chickens which have been in continuous light from hatching do not show such a rhythm unless some event such as servicing occurs sufficiently regularly for it to be used as a *zeitgeber* or synchronizing agent (Savory, 1976).

Within the light phase the rate of taking meals is not usually constant. There is often a peak at the beginning and/or at the end of the light phase (Savory, 1979). Laying hens tend to show this peak in the evening, presumably to fill up the crop for the night, whereas non-layers usually eat more in the morning. Whereas the evening peak might be related to the laying cycle in the hen, when it occurs in non-layers it implies anticipation of darkness; this is obviously possible when the light dims slowly at the end of the day but not when the lights go out abruptly. Birds which show a feeding peak before dusk eat more than other, similar, birds which have peak feeding activity shortly after dawn (Savory, 1976). Broiler fowl seldom show the pre-dusk peak unless the lights dim slowly and maximum intake is achieved by the use of 23 h lighting, by intermittent illumination or by simulated dusk. When the daylength is extended by adding 3 h, the evening feeding peak moves to 3 h later over a period of about 3 days. If the extra 3 h is added at the beginning rather than at the end of the day the evening peak does not move, showing that the hen can predict the time at which the lights will go out, rather than the length of the light phase; perhaps servicing at a fixed time of day acts as an indicator (Bhatti and Morris, 1978).

To determine whether domestic fowl can anticipate a period of food deprivation Petherick and Waddington (1991) individually housed pullets in a circadian-free environment. On days 17–47 half were shown a coloured card during the final hour of food availability, prior to food deprivation of 8 or 12 h. There was no indication subsequently of increased intake to fill the crop when the coloured card was shown. May and Lott (1992) found that broilers were able to anticipate withdrawal of food if this coincided with the onset of darkness, but not in continuous light. Continuously lit birds consumed more at the onset of a 12 h period of food availability whereas those with a dark period ate more towards the end of the light period. Thus, the ability to predict food unavailability depends specifically on a daily period of darkness and not just on a period of fasting.

When chickens are exposed to ahemeral cycles (lighting cycles other than 24 h) their feeding pattern shows signs of keeping to a cycle of approximately 24 h. Thus, Bhatti and Morris (1978) found that laying hens kept under 21 h cycles (12L:9D or 11L:10D) showed an 'evening' peak of feeding activity which continued into the early part of the night. Conversely hens in 30 h cycles (12L:18D or 20L:10D) ate considerably less in the last few hours of the light phase than would be expected (Fig. 15.2).

When the light phase is divided by a dark phase in the middle

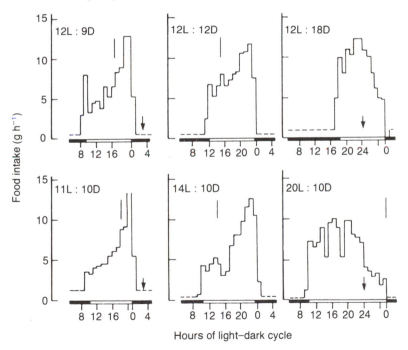

**Fig. 15.2.** Feeding patterns of laying hens under normal or ahemeral days (Bhatti and Morris, 1978). Vertical line is time of oviposition; arrow is 24 h after previous 'sunset'; solid abcissa is dark period.

(skeleton photoperiod, for example 2L:8D:2L:12D) some food is eaten during the 8D period, which the bird treats as 'day' rather than 'night' (Mongin *et al.*, 1978). Feeding, therefore, is not 'switched' on by light and off by darkness, but rather is related to a metabolic rhythm which is entrained by the pattern of lighting.

Giving chicks under different daylengths the same amount of food resulted in no effect on growth rate (Schutze *et al.*, 1960). Intermittent light flashes might, therefore, not be as good as continuous long days in stimulating growth in chickens as the total amount of light is less.

## Mechanisms

It has been established that the pineal gland is an important mediator of the effects of photoperiod on reproduction and growth, both in birds and mammals. The pineal receives information from the eyes via the superior cervical ganglion and influences other parts of the brain by the secretion of hormones, particularly melatonin. Melatonin given during the daytime might be expected to cause the cessation of feeding. Not only did this prove to be the case, but cockerels actually went to sleep for up to 3 h after intraperitoneal injection of 10 mg melatonin (Bermudez *et al.*, 1983). This dose is clearly unphysiological but, as much of the melatonin will be extracted by the liver and the remainder will be separated from the brain by the blood–brain barrier, the amounts entering the sensitive parts of the brain may be within the physiological range. At lower rates of injection there is dose-related hypophagia with drowsiness but not sleep.

If melatonin is responsible for the nocturnal aphagia in chickens, removal of the pineal gland, which is the major source of melatonin, would allow feeding to take place at night. This did occur, although the quantity eaten during the 12 h of darkness (4.4 g) was much less than that eaten during the daytime (Injidi and Forbes, 1983). Total daily intake was significantly higher than in sham-operated birds and growth was significantly faster. Thus the pineal plays a role in the circadian patterns of feeding, but is not the only factor.

As voluntary food intake is related to energy requirements the effect of melatonin may be to lower metabolic rate of the sleeping or drowsy bird. Measurement of oxygen consumption showed that it was significantly depressed within the first hour after injection (Bermudez *et al.*, 1983). Simultaneous injection of triiodothyronine ($T_3$, 200 µg, intramuscularly) blocked the effects of melatonin immediately but the stimulating effect on metabolism was not shown until 3 h later (Bermudez *et al.*, 1983); the effects of these hormones are, therefore, direct and not via effects on metabolic rate. As $T_3$ concentration in plasma is lower at night and melatonin injection depresses $T_3$ concentration, thyroid hormone metabolism may be involved in the diurnal cycle of food intake and metabolism.

## Pigs

Pigs which had free access to food and were observed for 24 h periods ate for at least twice as long per hour during the day compared to night. There was a peak of feeding activity in the late afternoon with 10 min spent eating per hour in that period of the day (J.H. Metz, personal communication). There are few reports in the literature of effects of photoperiod on the voluntary food intake or productivity of pigs although Stevenson *et al.* (1983) found increased intake if 16 h or more light per day was provided to lactating sows.

## Cattle

The overall feeding pattern is related to photoperiod, with larger, more frequent meals during the day, but this can be modified if the middle of the day is very hot when cattle eat more at night especially if the moon is bright (Dulphy *et al.*, 1980, Fig. 15.3).

In winter more time is spent eating during the hours of darkness

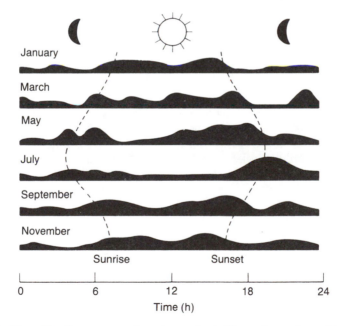

**Fig. 15.3.** Diurnal feeding patterns of grazing cattle at different times of year (Dulphy *et al.*, 1980).

since the days are too short to allow cattle to meet their requirements during the day (Waite *et al.*, 1951). Beef cattle in open feedlots spent 75% of their feeding time between 06.00 and 18.00. Reversal of lighting or lengthening the hours of light is accompanied by changes in feeding behaviour so that feeding takes place predominantly in the light period (Putnam *et al.*, 1965). In the work of Chase *et al.* (1976) fresh food was provided after each meal so that any circadian changes in food intake could not be caused by changes in the availability or palatability of the food. Their results show that meals occurred more frequently during the period from 08.00–20.00 with a peak around 08.00 (intermeal interval of about 80 min); during the early part of the night the intermeal interval averaged 180 min whereas from 24.00–06.00 it was about 300 min.

Although some studies under naturally fluctuating conditions have shown small increases in voluntary intake with increasing daylength (e.g. 0.32% $h^{-1}$, Ingvartsen *et al.*, 1992b), artificial extension of natural winter days has shown bigger effects. Peters *et al.* (1980) showed a significant increase in the voluntary intake of heifers given a complete food and provided with 16 h of light per day compared with those under natural winter daylengths in Michigan (5.20 vs. 4.80 kg $head^{-1}$ $day^{-1}$) or those under continuous light (4.86 kg $day^{-1}$). The effect on live weight gain preceded that on food intake, supporting the hypothesis that the effects of long photoperiod on food intake are due to the stimulation of growth and the increased energy requirements.

In dairy cows exposed to 16 h of fluorescent lighting per day, compared with those kept under natural lighting conditions from October to March (9–12 h $day^{-1}$), food intake was increased by 6% which approximately matched the requirements for the recorded increase in milk yield of 1.4 kg $day^{-1}$ (Peters *et al.*, 1981). Adjusted for parity and milk yield the food intakes were 17.4 and 16.4 kg dry matter (DM) $day^{-1}$. Although long days tended to increase food intake in the first experiment of Phillips and Schofield (1989), there was no apparent effect in a second experiment.

*Sheep*

Sheep kept in long days eat more than those in short days due to the stimulation of growth. Although growth is increased by long daylength even at restricted levels of feeding, the maximum response is obtained when the animal is allowed to fulfil its increased growth potential by *ad libitum* feeding. A 1 h 'flash' of light in the middle of long nights is as effective as long days (Schanbacher and Crouse, 1981; Fig. 15.4).

Meals are smaller and occur less frequently at night than during the day in housed growing lambs (e.g. Schanbacher and Crouse, 1981).

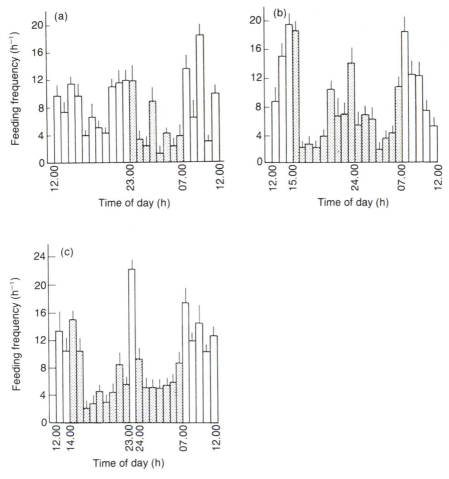

**Fig. 15.4.** Feeding patterns of ram lambs in (a) long days, (b) short days and (c) skeleton long days (Schanbacher and Crouse, 1981).

Figure 15.4 shows the number of meals taken during hourly intervals in 8 h and 16 h daylength and with a 1 h 'flash' in the middle of the night. In all treatments there was a lower feeding frequency during darkness, although there was more feeding in the middle of the long nights and a sharp peak during the 'flash'.

Since significant amounts of food are eaten at night there is no question of a block such as that caused by melatonin in chickens (200 or 400 µg melatonin injected into the lateral ventricles of sheep had no effect on feeding, Driver *et al.*, 1979). The metabolic rate of ruminants is lower at night (Toutain *et al.*, 1977) although not sufficiently to account for the large difference between daytime and night-time intake.

In the work of Hidari (1977) sheep fed *ad libitum* on hay showed higher intake during the day especially after fresh food has been offered. Rumen volatile fatty acid concentrations increased during the day and decreased at night so the animals were not eating in order to achieve constant conditions in the rumen, nor to achieve a constant metabolic rate. Although they do not sleep deeply, ruminants become less aware of their surroundings at night and may also be less aware of internal signals. Sheep trained to self-stimulate in the posterolateral hypothalamus showed reduced self-stimulation during the 12 h dark phase with a compensatory increase during the day so that the total activity was the same as for sheep kept in continuous lighting, under which there was no diurnal rhythm (Baldwin and Parrott, 1982).

Under conditions of natural lighting in latitudes where there is a marked annual rhythm in photoperiod, sheep show an annual cycle of daily food intake, with a peak a few weeks after the longest day and a nadir after the shortest day. Gordon (1964) observed this annual cycle in food intake and attributed it, probably wrongly, to ambient temperature. Tarttelin (1968) also recorded this in forage-fed ewes. Artificial manipulation of photoperiod showed that long days stimulate wool growth and that 0.75 of the variation in wool growth was associated with variation in food intake (Williams, 1964). Kay (1979) showed that the intake cycle is caused by changes in photoperiod rather than in temperature or food quality, by compressing the annual lighting cycle into 6 months (Fig. 15.5). It would appear that the intake, growth and fattening cycles have greater changes in unimproved breeds of sheep, such as the Soay, compared with improved breeds like the Suffolk. There is also a cycle of food intake in red deer and in white-tailed deer which is due to photoperiod and there is particular inappetence in stags during the rut (Kay, 1979).

Superior cervical ganglionectomy, which prevents fluctuations in pineal function, reduces but does not totally inhibit the cycle of appetite in Soay rams kept under six-month compressed annual cycles of lighting (Kay and Suttie, 1980). This annual cycle of food intake is associated with a parallel cycle of fasting metabolic rate in sheep (from 204 to 264 kJ $kg^{-0.75}$ $day^{-1}$; Baxter and Boyne, 1982) and in Soay rams the estimated maintenance requirements for metabolizable energy (ME) were 400 in midwinter and 530 kJ $kg^{-0.75}$ $day^{-1}$ in summer (Argo and Smith, 1983).

Exposure of growing lambs to fixed daylengths of either 8 or 16 h per day resulted in higher intake of a complete pelleted food in the longer photoperiod (Forbes *et al.*, 1979). However, neither the speed of onset nor the statistical significance of this increase was as great as the effects on growth rate and gut fill. The nutrient requirements of

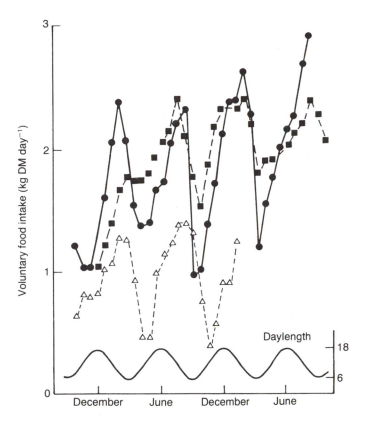

**Fig. 15.5.** Intake of balanced foods by stags (●), Suffolk rams (■) and Soay rams (△) subjected to an artificial 6-month pattern of lighting (Kay, 1979).

stimulated growth probably caused a secondary increase in food intake. This conclusion is supported since the effect of photoperiod on growth can still be seen in pair-fed lambs (Forbes *et al.*, 1981) although there was no change in mean retention time of stained particles (Schanbacher and Crouse, 1980) observed increased intake both in rams (1.56 to 1.77 kg day$^{-1}$) and wethers (1.45 to 1.63) in 16 h daylengths compared with 8 h, with parallel increases in weight gains. In a comprehensive experiment including short days, long days and a nocturnal 'flash', Schanbacher and Crouse (1981) saw significant increases in daily intake of a complete food with 16L:8D (1.83 kg day$^{-1}$) or 7L:9D:1L:7D (1.79 kg day$^{-12}$) as compared with 8L:16D (1.62 kg day$^{-1}$).

Occasionally environmental factors other than daylight can entrain a feeding rhythm. For example, sheep on North Ronaldsay, which eat mostly seaweed as they are restricted to the outer part of the island, exhibit a grazing pattern which is controlled by the tide (Patterson and Coleman, 1982).

*Deer*

Deer show a marked annual cycle of food intake and weight change and extended daylength gave a significant increase in intake and growth so that slaughter weight was reached 50 days earlier than controls (Davies and Wade, 1993). However, no changes in retention time or digestibility were observed in red deer which had large annual fluctuations in food intake (Milne *et al.*, 1978). Melatonin implants depressed voluntary food intake and rumen pool size as a proportion of rumen capacity (Domingue *et al.*, 1992) but opioids, which show a circennial rhythm in many species are probably not involved in the seasonal cycle of food intake in deer (Plotka *et al.*, 1986).

## Exercise

Enforced exercise reduced food intake and growth rate of pigs with no effect on backfat thickness (Morrison *et al.*, 1968); the reduced time spent eating could be due to either fatigue or stress.

Intake by cattle of rice straw supplemented with 18 and 27 g concentrates $kg^{-1}$ live weight was reduced by 11 and 14%, respectively, when oxen worked to increase their energy daily expenditure by 1.3–1.6-fold (Pearson and Lawrence, 1992). However, there was no depression due to exercise with a diet of hay which had higher ME but lower nitrogen content than the straw. On both diets there was a return to pre-work levels of intake in the week after exercise.

Matthewman *et al.* (1993) exercised Hereford × Friesian cows 5 days $week^{-1}$ for 3 weeks over 10.6 km $day^{-1}$ with 480 m $day^{-1}$ climbing with 4 kg $day^{-1}$ of supplement and barley straw *ad libitum*. There was no effect of exercise on straw intake but body weight was lost when exercising and gained when not. This confirms previous results that animals performing moderate work and given poor forage do not in the short term increase intake and that intake may even decrease when animals work.

Henning (1987) exercised sheep on a treadmill over 9 km $day^{-1}$ at 3 km $h^{-1}$ up a 10° gradient for 6 days. Intake of chopped hay was decreased from a pre-exercise level of 1347 to 1125 g organic matter $day^{-1}$ with little effect on rumen retention times.

In the short term, therefore, exercise tends to reduce intake rather than increase it in parallel with the increase in energy expenditure.

Long-term exercise must result in a compensatory increase in intake otherwise hard-working animals would die of underfeeding.

## Feeder Design

Shallow cages for poultry gave a feeding pattern more closely related to the birds' requirements (more first thing in the morning and just before dusk) than a deeper cage with the same floor-space per bird, which had less feeding space per bird (Hughes and Black, 1976). When the front of the battery cage was vertical bars, hens fed most frequently singly whereas with horizontal bars they fed usually in threes, i.e. closer to the birds' inclination to synchronize their feeding (Sherwin *et al.*, 1993).

Appleby *et al.* (1991) offered piglets creep food in a dirty feeder, a clean feeder with food supplied once a day, food provided three times a day, or three times the normal number of feeders. Intake was higher in this last situation than the other three, by 2.1 times at 3 weeks of age, and 1.4 times at 4 weeks, as a result of less competition for feeder access.

Petchey and Abdulkader (1991) observed no differences in intake or number of visits by cattle between four types of barrier but there was more waste at a post and rail barrier than at other types.

Goats have a greater vertical reach than sheep of the same body weight, so can eat food spread more widely behind any given type of barrier (Muhikambele *et al.*, 1993).

## Group Size

Group size and floor area per pig are important factors affecting stress. Increasing the area per animal, with groups of eight bacon pigs, from 0.56 to 1.19 m$^2$, resulted in an increase in food intake from 2.46 to 2.73 kg animal$^{-1}$ day$^{-1}$ (Bryant and Ewbank, 1974). There was a reduction in food intake when space was reduced from 0.25 to 0.17 m$^2$ pig$^{-1}$ (Lindvall, 1981) and a further 10% reduction if space was reduced to 0.13 m$^2$, although other work has failed to show such an effect (e.g. Heitman *et al.*, 1961).

Kornegay and Notter (1984) found that each 0.1 m$^2$ reduction in space was associated with a reduction in voluntary intake of 50 g day$^{-1}$. The optimum space allowance for intake was 0.4 m$^2$ for weaners, 0.6 for growing pigs and 1.0 for fattening pigs (NRC, 1987). As group size increased from three to six to twelve, food intake declined from 2.57 to 2.33 kg day$^{-1}$ with Duroc pigs weighing 35–50 kg even though the floor area per pig was maintained (Heitman *et al.*, 1961). To what extent this decline was due to reduced heat loss is not known.

As the space allowance for lambs was increased from 0.37 to 0.62 to 0.99 m$^2$/head, intake increased from 1.36 to 1.32 to 1.49 kg day$^{-1}$ with no effect on cortisol, adrenaline or noradrenaline (Horton *et al.*, 1990).

For group size, each additional pig in a pen of weaners reduced intake by 0.9%, whereas for growing and fattening pigs the reduction was 0.25 and 0.32%, respectively. Ammonia reduced intake by 3 g per 1 ppm increase but the levels of ammonia commonly found in practice had no detectable effect.

## Frequency of Offering Food

Lactating and dry cows, given an average of 7 kg of concentrates per day, did not change their silage intake or feeding pattern, irrespective of whether the concentrate was given in 2 or 22 feeds per day (Gill and Castle, 1983).

Blaxter *et al.* (1961) found no difference in daily intake whether forage feeds were offered to sheep two or four times per day; food was available at all times. However, Adams *et al.* (1983) noted increased food intake and fatter carcasses in lambs which were fed *ad libitum* with fresh food offered four times per day rather than once per day.

Concentrates were given to ewes, increasing from 400 to 600 to 800 over the last 6 weeks of pregnancy, once, twice or thrice daily or mixed with silage (Wylie and Chestnutt, 1992). In weeks 5–6 before lambing, silage intakes were 758 g DM day$^{-1}$ for once, 853 for twice/thrice and 996 for mixed, respectively. In 3–4 weeks before lambing, intakes were 655, 830 and 987 and in weeks 1–2 they were 552, 782 and 876 g DM day$^{-1}$. These improvements in silage intake are probably due to a more regular flow of nutrients from the concentrates to balance those coming from silage.

## Disease

Reduced voluntary food intake is one of the first sign of many diseases. Although in some cases this can be attributed to fever, many diseases do not increase body temperature and some other reason for the reduced intake must be sought. Pair-feeding experiments show that anorexia is not responsible for all of the loss of performance, e.g. chickens infected with *Eimeria* spp., sheep with *Strongylus matthei*.

As with other species, a reduction in food intake is one of the first signs of disease in poultry. Johnson and Reid (1971) studied the effect of various degrees of infection with *Eimeria mivati* (one of the coccidia) and found decreased weight gains and food intakes. Vaccination against Marek's disease had no effect on intake although it did lead to the production of more extra-sized eggs and a tendency to reduce mortality (Lee, 1978).

Anthelminthic (thiabendazole) treatment of lactating dairy cows naturally infected with roundworms had no significant effect on production or voluntary food intake, although cellulose digestion was improved by 10% (Fox *et al.*, 1985).

Infestation with helminths causes a primary depression of food intake in sheep (Dargie, 1980), possibly by the continuous stimulation by the parasites of receptors in the gut wall. The steady decline in intake, which occurs even with a constant level of infestation, is in parallel with the reduction in plasma protein concentration and it is possible that a deficiency of amino acids is responsible. Plasma levels of cholecystokinin (CCK) increase as intake falls during the course of infestations with *Trichostrongylus colubriformis* (Symons and Hennessy, 1981) and this is another factor which might be involved in the loss of appetite. Plasma levels of CCK are elevated during parasitic infections and, in view of the effects of CCK on food intake (Chapter 5), the possibility that this is involved in the anorexia of parasitism has been investigated. A central CCK blocker (Mederantil) given to sheep infected with *T. colubriformis* blocked the intake depression for about 2 h after injection but had little effect in non-infected controls (Dynes *et al.*, 1990). However, a peripheral CCK blocker (Loxiglumide) had no significant effect in either control or infected lambs (perhaps because the dose was too small or the experiment too short) and it was concluded that CCK produced by nematode infection acts centrally to inhibit food intake. Plasma gastrin levels are also increased in gastric parasitization and gastrin infusion into the hepatic portal vein depresses intake in sheep (Anil and Forbes, 1980b; Grovum, 1981). Further work is required to elucidate the possible role of gastrointestinal hormones in the anorexic effects of gut infection.

Pair-feeding experiments, to prevent the difference in food intake which would otherwise occur between infested and uninfested animals, show that there is still some loss of production probably as a result of the cost of plasma protein synthesis (Sykes and Coop, 1976, 1977). Holmes (1993) states that '... it is still not possible to construct accurate balance sheets of protein synthesis in parasitised animals ...' and '... the cardinal feature of such infections is the loss of considerable quantities of host protein into the gastrointestinal tract and consequent changes in protein synthesis in host tissues'. Animals on low nutrition, particularly when the food is low in protein content (Symons, 1985), are more susceptible to the hypophagic effects of parasites, so it is paradoxical that they eat less food. Infusion of 50 g protein per day into the duodenum of lambs infected with *Trichostrongylus colubriformis* resulted in a food intake depression that was less (22 vs. 32%) and worm burdens reduced, compared to non-infused controls (Bown *et al.*, 1989).

Kyriazakis *et al.* (1993a) offered lambs infected with *T. colubriformis* a choice of foods high and low in protein content (Chapter 14) and found that, relative to uninfected controls, they had reduced daily intake but increased the proportion of the food high in protein, to give approximately the same daily protein intake as the controls. The increased protein:energy ratio chosen by the infected lambs is presumed to be in response to the increased requirements for protein induced by the parasites.

A relatively low level of dosing with *Fasciola hepatica* (liver fluke) for 25 weeks caused a 15% decrease in intake in sheep (Sykes *et al.*, 1980) whereas large doses severely depressed intake (Hawkins and Morris, 1978).

Mice force-fed after *Listeria monocytogenes* infection had increased mortality compared with anorexics and it has been suggested that the purpose of the anorexia is to starve the infecting organisms or to stimulate the immune system. Holmes (1993) concludes that '… present explanations for anorexia in parasitic infections are so rudimentary that this is a most interesting and fruitful field for future study'.

Heavy external parasitic infestation can also depress intake (e.g. the tick *Boophilus microplus* on cattle; Seebeck *et al.*, 1971).

Metabolic diseases of ruminants such as acetonaemia (Kronfeld, 1970), ketosis (Krebs, 1966), lactacidosis (Dunlop and Hammond, 1965) and bloat (Clarke and Reid, 1970) are accompanied by hypophagia.

## Conclusions

Below the lower critical ambient temperature energy requirements increase and food intake normally increases in parallel. In very cold environments, especially with strong winds and heavy precipitation, animals seek shelter and intake may be reduced. In hot environments there is a specific negative effect on intake, with a decline in the level of production; the results of short-term experiments can be misleading, however, as acclimatization to hot weather usually gives opportunity for compensatory intake in the cool of the night. In reality there is an almost continuous negative relationship between environmental temperature and voluntary food intake.

Long daylight stimulates food intake. In poultry this is a primary effect as they do not normally eat at night but in ruminants it is secondary to the stimulation of growth.

Social facilitation encourages feeding in all farm species and animals usually eat more when kept in groups than when penned individually. However, if competition for limited feeding space is severe then feeding is disrupted (Chapter 2) and daily food intake can be reduced.

Other environmental effects on intake include the type of housing and the distances which have to be travelled to food and water in extensive situations.

Diseases of most type depress voluntary intake. They are likely to do so by causing abdominal discomfort or by disturbing nutrient requirements in such a way that the food on offer is no longer suitable to meet the new requirements. As discussed in earlier chapters, this is likely to reduce intake in order to lessen the imbalance.

# 16 THE INTAKE OF FRESH AND CONSERVED GRASS

- Grazing behaviour
- Diet selection at pasture
- Models of grazing behaviour and diet selection
- Herbage intake
- Factors affecting herbage intake
- Grassland management
- Conserved forages: silage
- Conclusions

Although many animal species eat grass, few are as well adapted as the ruminant with its symbiotic population of rumen microorganisms. Since ruminants can survive on fibrous plant material and need not compete directly with humanity for food this group of mammals occupies a central role in agriculture and will continue to do so worldwide for the foreseeable future. Optimum utilization of herbage depends on our ability to predict its feeding value, which determines to a large extent the level of voluntary intake. This chapter discusses methods of measuring herbage intake and factors which affect grazing behaviour and intake. In temperate areas, where there are distinct seasonal changes in weather, herbage growth occurs predominantly in the spring and summer, but not in winter, so that conservation of summer production as hay, dried grass and silage is necessary for maintenance of high levels of production. Intake of conserved forages is therefore also included in this chapter.

The coverage of this chapter is by no means exhaustive and the interested reader is referred to reviews by Hodgson (1985) and Mayne and Wright (1988) and to books by Morley (1986), Fraser (1985), Valentine (1990) and Hodgson (1990) on grazing intake and grazing behaviour. Books by McDonald *et al.* (1991) and Raymond *et al.* (1986) cover the basic and applied aspects of silage, respectively.

# Grazing Behaviour

As the intake of herbage over a day or any longer period is the product of the number of bites and bite size, it is necessary to consider grazing behaviour, its measurement and interpretation before proceeding to describe factors which influence daily intake.

Behavioural constraints are more likely to be important in the grazing situation than indoors. Not only are animals outdoors exposed to changes in weather, but have to seek their food before harvesting it. Where the mass of herbage per unit area is low then the amount of food taken per bite is small and the total amount of time which the animal can spend grazing each day is likely to become a limiting factor to intake. A thorough study and understanding of grazing behaviour is therefore of considerable practical, as well as theoretical, importance and much research effort has been devoted to monitoring and analysing grazing behaviour (Forbes, T.D.A., 1988).

The amount of time spent grazing is very variable, depending among other things on the quantity and quality of the available herbage and on the physiological state of the animal. Most grazing is during the hours of daylight, with more rumination at night. In very hot weather, however, more time is spent grazing during the cooler hours of the night.

## Monitoring grazing behaviour

In theory the intake of grass could be calculated by multiplying the grazing time by the bite frequency by the weight harvested in each size. The frequency of biting and the weight prehended per bite are difficult to measure absolutely, however, and should be looked upon as '... a means of explaining observed effects on herbage intake rather than as a means of estimating herbage intake itself' (Hodgson and Maxwell, 1981). Visual observation has been commonly used to monitor the number of bites and other parameters of grazing but is tedious, expensive and often inaccurate. Automation typically involves fitting a headband with detectors for jaw movement and head position; chewing with the head down is eating whereas chewing with the head up is rumination (Chambers *et al.*, 1981). This equipment is connected to a recorder mounted on the animal's back whose recording medium can either be changed at regular intervals or which can transmit the information telemetrically. Several automatic devices have been employed to record the time spent eating and the number of bites. The most widely used is the Kienzle Vibracorder (Kienzle Apparate GmbH, D-7730 Villingen, Germany) which includes a clockwork-driven disc which is scribed by a pendulum-operated pen. Electronic methods are now being used and radiotelemetry is becoming sufficiently well-developed to be of regular use in research. These methodologies are described and discussed by Hodgson (1982).

It has proved to be very difficult to automate the analysis of these records by computer, especially the difference between eating and ruminating, if a head-position switch is not used. Penning *et al.* (1984) have compared the automatic method and visual observation and found that the former gave more bites per minute during eating (78 vs. 67) but no differences during rumination. P.D. Penning (personal communication) reports steady improvement in the automatic analysis of chewing records.

## Cattle

Grazing cattle wrap their tongues around a bunch of grass and pull; this makes it impossible to graze shorter than about 10 mm. Several bites are taken, then chewed and swallowed. As herbage declines in height, bite mass decreases; peak grazing time and number of bites occur with about 1 tonne dry matter (DM) ha$^{-1}$ (Chacon and Stobbs, 1976). As the herbage becomes further defoliated, there is reduction in grazing time, number of bites and bite mass due to low leaf density. Cattle prefer to eat leaf rather than stem, so move on to another area when the benefit of staying in the same patch becomes less than the likely benefit of moving to another patch (see below). Leaf is more rapidly and readily digested, so takes less processing time and yields more nutrients per kilogram of intake and, usually, per minute of feeding time.

Krysl and Hess (1993) provide a comprehensive review of feeding behaviour in cattle with extensive data. They warn that 'Monitoring daily grazing behavior without measuring forage intake will not provide the meaningful insight needed to understand the complex interrelationships that exist in the grazing ruminant.'

## Sheep and goats

These small ruminants have narrower mouths and graze by biting grass between lower incisors and upper hard pad. They can therefore graze more selectively than cattle and goats are more selective grazers than sheep. They spend up to 13 h day$^{-1}$ grazing and can graze very close to the ground. Grazing in sheep is most intensive in the evening and Penning *et al.* (1991) observed that whereas 70–99% of grazing was

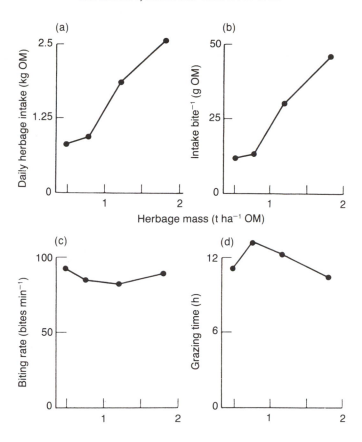

**Fig. 16.1.** The influence of variations in herbage mass on daily intake, intake per bite, biting rate and grazing time of ewes OM, organic matter. (From Bircham, 1981, cited by Hodgson and Maxwell, 1981.)

during daylight, 25–48% of the total was concentrated in the 4 h before sunset. A grazing time of more than about 9 h indicates that herbage mass is limiting intake and the animal is having to extend its grazing time to get enough food to eat. Bechet (1978) observed that lactating ewes in the spring spent 587 min day$^{-1}$ eating and 423 min ruminating; in the summer, after weaning, the times were 450 min eating and 382 min ruminating. Diet selection by sheep and cattle on the same pasture can be quite different; a detailed example is given by Grant *et al.* (1985). This is due to differences in the shape and size of the mouth (Gordon and Illius, 1988). Figure 16.1 gives examples of grazing behaviour parameters for ewes.

*The role of experience*

Arnold and Maller (1977) found that 3-year-old sheep without previous experience of grazing ate significantly less when put out to pasture than experienced grazers and even after 15 weeks of grazing were still eating more slowly. Experience of manipulating a plant influences subsequent behaviour; sheep reared on grass had a higher biting rate for grass and handled it more dextrously than those experienced in harvesting shrubs (Flores *et al.*, 1989b). Conversely those used to eating shrubs did so more efficiently than those with only grass experience (Chapter 12).

Goats grazing savannah with high plant diversity chose diets which varied according to the place of origin of each animal, even though they had been under common management for 4 years (Biquard and Biquard-Guyot, 1992). Diets chosen by successive cohorts reflected the pasture composition of the year of their birth, i.e. selection by groups of kids was partly learned or inherited from their parents and partly due to the plants available when they were young.

*Foraging strategy*

It is assumed that animals have, through natural selection, developed to harvest herbage efficiently, i.e. maximize intake for minimum feeding time, energy or risk of predation. Given a range of plant types, animals are expected to choose those with the highest content of energy (or other limiting nutrient); whether a type of plant, or a particular cluster of one type of plant, is selected is not an absolute property of that plant but depends on whether more highly ranked plants or clusters are available.

There is a body of theory called optimal foraging (Stephens and Krebs, 1986) which encompasses a variety of models, one of which is the marginal value theorem (Charnov *et al.*, 1976). The grazing environment is considered as a series of 'patches' of the same species of grass and this theory predicts the time spent in a patch to maximize intake rate subject to the constraints of travel time between patches and the form of the gain function which describes the cumulative gain from a patch. It is assumed that food is patchily distributed and that food availability within a patch decreases as a result of the forager's activity. The gain function (decrease in rate of eating as the patch becomes depleted) and travel time (distance between patches) are outside the control of the forager. The longer the travel time, the longer an animal should stay in a patch (Fig. 16.2). If patches vary in size or density, then an animal should continue to graze a patch until the gain equals the average for the environment. In order to test this hypothesis for sheep

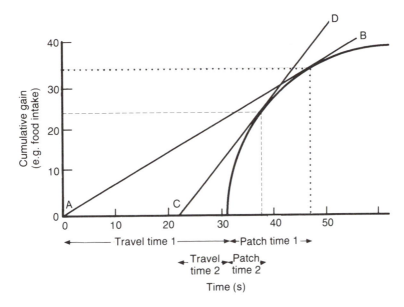

**Fig. 16.2.** Optimal foraging theory. The line A–B crosses the time axis at 0 s and is a tangent to the cumulative intake curve; where the travel time between patches is long (travel time 1) then the animal will have to stay in the patch for longer to achieve maximal intake, compared to a situation in which the travel time is less (travel time 2).

Bazely (1988) placed turves of good grass in a bare paddock and varied the travel times (by varying number of patches of good grass and/or by hobbling the sheep) between patches to see how well the theorem predicted residence times. Gain curves were obtained by feeding ryegrass swards in trays indoors; the line of best fit was a negative exponential, where the constants $K_1$ and $K_2$ were found to have typical values of 16.9 and −0.115, respectively. Although this relationship was significant, the points were quite scattered for some sheep. Nevertheless, it is clear that deceleration occurred. Observed patch residence times were frequently greater than predicted using the gain function derived indoors, especially for longer travel times. Although these experiments show that sheep increase their time in a patch when travel time increases they do not show that they maximize rate of eating and it seems that they stay longer than predicted to minimize the risk of not finding another patch quickly. Also, as other sheep were around, an animal may have stayed longer than predicted in a patch in case the next patch was occupied by another sheep.

# Diet Selection at Pasture

When two or more species of plant with different morphological and nutritional characteristics are available in the sward the animal has a more complex set of decisions to make. It is very difficult to monitor selective feeding behaviour in animals at pasture so studies have been carried out with small areas of pasture, either natural turves (e.g. Newman *et al.,* 1991) or built up from individual stems on a 'sward board' (e.g. Kenney and Black, 1984). These are offered to individually penned animals for short periods and may not give a good representation of the selection which animals would take if given larger amounts over longer periods of time. In the short tests sheep eat very quickly at the start of the bout and may be less selective than normal or only eat from the top layer of sward. If they have been fasted before the test, in order to ensure that they eat during the test, then their selection might not be representative. Thus, the information available from these short-term artificial tests and from longer-term observations made under more natural grazing conditions does not always give comparable results.

It is a widely held opinion that sheep prefer clover to grass, as they usually select a higher proportion of clover in the diet than is present in the grass:clover sward from which they are grazing (Newman *et al.,* 1992). This could be explained on the basis that sheep grow faster, produce more milk and can eat faster when grazing clover, compared to ryegrass. However, attempts to demonstrate ryegrass/clover preferences have yielded conflicting results. For example, Ramos and Tennessen (1992) put ryegrass- or clover-experienced weaned lambs on paddocks with alternating strips of the two and observed grazing behaviour. Those lambs with experience of white clover spent a significantly higher proportion of their time grazing clover than those with ryegrass experience (69 vs. 45%). On the other hand, Newman *et al.* (1992) showed that ewes previously grazed on a pure ryegrass sward showed a strong preference for turves of clover when given in free-choice with turves of ryegrass, and that clover-accustomed ewes preferred ryegrass. Thus, the nature of the test and the age of the animals are confounded and it is very difficult to draw firm conclusions. In subsequent work Parsons *et al.* (1994) monitored choices between clover and ryegrass for several days in ewes previously grazed on monocultures of either; whereas on the first day they showed a clear preference for the species of which they had not had recent experience, by the sixth day they had reverted to a preference for their background diet. Short-term neophilia was tempered by long-term conservatism. These examples demonstrate the plasticity of diet selection – it is necessary to know an animal's nutritional history and to be aware of all the details of the protocol in order to predict its behaviour when presented with a choice.

When there is plenty of herbage available the grazing animal is free to select the plant parts and species it prefers because of their acceptable taste, smell, feel or a combination of these. As well as selection between plant species there is also selection of leaves in preference to stems of the same plant (Ellis, 1978) and for green material in preference to brown. Reduction in the mass of herbage on offer induces the animal to eat a broader range of species or to graze to a lower level in the sward. Some plants will always be avoided; for example, even when little grass is available, sheep still avoid capeweed although sometimes they pull it up by the roots and then drop it (Broom and Arnold, 1986).

Even within a species of grass there can be large differences between a grazing animal's selection of different strains, e.g. up to 36% preference was recorded for one strain of *Phalaris arundinacea* (Roe and Mottershead, 1962). Clearly the special senses of the grazing animal are involved in this selection (Arnold, 1966a, b) and the odour of the herbage seems to be of particular importance (Arnold, 1970). It is,

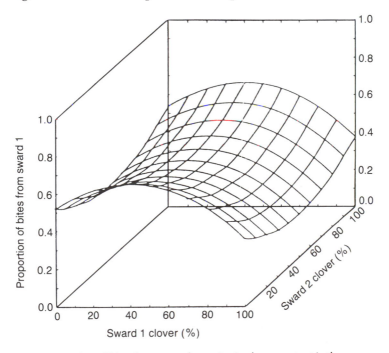

**Fig. 16.3.** Proportion of bites from swards varying in clover content in the presence of alternate swards varying in clover content and with the same pregrazing height (Illius *et al.,* 1992).

however, very difficult to know whether sensory or physiological factors are primarily affecting intake in any particular situation.

It is clear that sheep can select DM and nitrogen in significantly higher concentrations in the diet than that on offer (Curll *et al.*, 1985) but for what they are selecting is not clear. This ability is learned, as even after three months grazing a high-quality pasture, lambs which had been reared on that pasture were selecting food with a significantly higher nitrogen content than lambs reared on poor pastures (Langlands, 1969). Where animals have been shown to select a higher nitrogen content than the sward in general was this simply because the full depth of grass was cut for analysis whereas the animal only grazed the top layer?

The hypothesis that large herbivores seek to maximize intake rate was examined by Illius *et al.* (1992) who found that tall patches were selected in preference to short ones. Although these patches gave the highest rate of eating, there was no evidence that this was the reason they were selected. Patches with an intermediate clover content were preferred to ones with low or high clover (Fig. 16.3).

The results of Parsons *et al.* (1994) do not support the idea that sheep select the plant which gives the highest rate of eating because there was no difference in rate of eating between clover or grass even though there were distinct preferences. In further experimentation Newman *et al.* (1994) observed that clover was not eaten exclusively from a mixed pasture even though it was eaten at a faster rate than ryegrass, further refuting the concept that sheep always select for maximum rate of ingestion.

When sheep were given a choice of hay cut to different lengths, they chose short lengths which gave them the fastest rate of eating (Kenney and Black, 1984; Fig. 13.3). Sheep are colour-blind, but seem to be able to discriminate brightness. They spent more time grazing tall, bright patches than short, dull ones. When height and brightness were separated, sheep always preferred bright (i.e. dark green) patches, irrespective of height. There was a positive relationship between N content and colour density, but a negative relationship between water-soluble carbohydrate and colour densitometer reading. When light and dark green grasses were presented on trays, there was preference for dark on the first day but not thereafter (30 s trials). It can be concluded that sheep use the brightness of grass as an indicator of its nitrogen (protein) content and also that the results obtained from these short-term tests can vary as the sheep's experience grows.

Diet selection is affected by physiological state as Newman *et al.* (1994) observed that, not only did 24 h fasted sheep eat faster than unfasted animals, but also chose a lower ratio of clover to grass. They advised that it is necessary to be wary of extrapolating from short-term diet selection studies in which animals were pre-fasted as the animal's selection between foods is dependent on its nutritional state (Chapter 13 and 14).

After a 36 h fast cattle increased the time spent eating and intake on a ryegrass sward, but bite size was unaffected at 0.47 g DM (Greenwood and Demment, 1988). Although there was no effect on the neutral detergent fibre (NDF) content of the herbage eaten, mastication was lower after fasting (0.78 chews g $NDF^{-1}$) so larger particles were being swallowed which might reduce rate of digestion.

## Models of Grazing Behaviour and Diet Selection

There have been numerous attempts to describe the grazing situation in modelling terms and some of these are dealt with in Chapter 17.

In a comprehensive model, Demment and Greenwood (1988) integrated ingestive and food-processing behaviours to predict the combination of behaviours which gives the maximum rate of energy digestion per unit of time. In all simulations the optimal solution involved animals eating to maximum rumen fill but this is not surprising as no physiological limits were built into the model. Rather, the aim was to maximize digestible energy intake per unit of time.

Spahlinger and Hobbs (1992) have adapted the classical predator/prey modelling approach for the situation of grazing herbivores. They defined three processes of foraging: where the plant species being harvested is (i) dispersed and hidden, (ii) dispersed and apparent, and (iii) concentrated and apparent. They include the concepts that herbivores can handle (chew and swallow) the food just eaten while continuing the search for the next bite and that the animal does not only look ahead but also to each side, thereby foraging along a strip of the sward rather than just a single line. They point out that what is a discrete food item for a big herbivore (e.g. a bunch of grass) is a continuous patch for a small animal.

Thornley *et al.* (1994) have recently presented a cost–benefit model of grazing intake which is developed to cover diet selection in a ryegrass/clover sward. Working on the basis that animals seek to maximize the difference between the benefits and costs of eating, the model suggests that for grazing animals daily intake is not strictly limited by physiological or morphological constraints on the animals, such as gut fill or maximum rate of utilizing substrates, neither is it limited solely by sward factors, such as height of herbage or proportion of clover. Rather, the animals' behaviour is directed at optimizing the marginal efficiency of eating more food or selecting more clover.

However, these models take no account of learning, nor do they explicitly consider nutrients other than energy, although 20 years previously, Westoby (1974) had set out the foundations on which much of our thinking about diet selection is based, including long-term learning and the need to avoid toxins and select for nutrients. Publication of further work by Thornley and colleagues (quoted by Thornley *et al.*, 1994) promises some interesting developments.

# Herbage Intake

## *Measurement of intake at pasture*

It is difficult to measure the amount or quality of food eaten by animals which are unrestrained; the problems are similar to those of studies on intake in groups of housed animals which have been discussed in Chapter 2. It is, of course, possible to cut grass and to feed it to individually penned animals but this ignores the influence of factors such as sward height, social interactions or selective grazing, although observations made in this way may be relevant to zero-grazing (a farming system in which fresh grass is cut by machine and fed to housed or yarded animals). Chenost and Demarquilly (1982) have reviewed the techniques for measuring herbage intake by housed ruminants offered freshly cut grass whereas Wanyoike and Holmes (1981) have made a comparison of indirect methods of estimating feed intake on pasture.

The simplest method for measuring the intake of grass in the field is to cut sample areas of the field to a standard level before and after the animals have been allowed to graze. The difference in weight of grass, scaled up for the whole field, indicates the amount eaten. If, however, grazing has continued for several days a significant amount of grass growth will have occurred and must be assessed by protecting some areas from grazing with fencing or cages. Cutting and weighing methods can be used to calibrate simpler measurements such as visual estimation, measurements of height and density, use of a 'grassmeter' (Castle, 1976; a disc which is thrown on the sward and the height at which it settles is recorded) or the electrical capacitance of the sward. These methods are reviewed in more detail by Meijs *et al.* (1982). A disadvantage is that they only tell how much grass has been removed by all of the animals which have had access to the field and give no information on individual intakes or on feeding behaviour.

## *Weighing technique*

A simple technique for estimating herbage intake is to weigh animals before and after grazing. It is, of course, necessary to account for faecal and urinary loss and this can be done by collection using bags and harness. Evaporative losses must be calculated from those occurring during non-feeding, control periods. Penning and Hooper (1985) used a computer-logged balance to overcome the problems of sheep movements while being weighed and found a small bias in rate of eating of $-0.8$ g min$^{-1}$ compared with measurements using housed sheep. The results were similar to those obtained by the chromic oxide method but it is labour-intensive, disturbs the animals and does not provide information about short-term behavioural aspects of grazing.

*Indigestible markers*

In principle, estimates of (i) the faecal output of the animals and (ii) digestibility of the herbage that they consumed will allow intake to be calculated. Although sheep or cattle can be harnessed to allow total collection of faeces in bags, the harness and the weight of the bag might interfere with the animal's normal behaviour. Faecal output can be estimated indirectly by oral administration of a marker, such as chromic oxide, and collection of samples of faeces either by grab sampling from the rectum or by identification of voided faeces from individual animals by means of coloured plastic particles administered with the chromic oxide. The content of marker in the faeces is determined from representative samples. Other markers investigated include ruthenium and other rare earths (Le Du and Penning, 1982, have reviewed the methods) and $n$-alkanes (see below). Digestibility of cut samples of herbage is estimated by feeding to penned animals indoors and collection and analysis of faeces. It is thus an expensive method with plenty of scope for inaccuracy and error.

*Natural markers*

An alternative to an orally administered marker is the use of an indigestible fraction of the food, such as lignin. The major problem with this is that the composition of the herbage selected by the animal may not be the same as that of the herbage collected for analysis by the investigator. Oesophageally fistulated animals have been used to sample herbage but the possibility exists that the fistulated animal might not select grass of the same composition as that selected by the experimental animals, especially if they are of a different species or physiological state.

A further possibility for the estimation of faecal output is by the use of the relationship between digestible OM intake and faecal nitrogen concentration based on penned animals. Although this relationship is quite good between different levels of intake by similar

animals on similar pastures there are wide variations between different situations, necessitating calibration before each experiment; this
method is strictly a procedure for estimating dietary digestibility and
is not widely adopted for estimating intake. Chromic oxide dilution
remains the most widely used method for estimating faecal output but
it may well not be as ideal a marker as alkanes.

   *n*-Alkanes, natural constituents of most plant species, have been
used as undigested markers and the review by Dove and Mayes (1991)
is a useful summary of this recent development. Seed, leaf, stem of the
same grass plants have different patterns of alkanes which allow the
intakes of these plant fractions to be estimated separately (R. Simpson
and H. Dove, personal communication).

## Estimating diet digestibility

Once faecal output has been measured or estimated there remains the
problem of estimating the digestibility of the herbage consumed. The
most obvious way is to cut grass manually (or pluck it to simulate the
action of the ruminant's mouth) and feed it to other animals penned
individually for faecal collection. It would be better to use oesophageally fistulated animals to collect grass, however, as they will give
more realistic samples of the herbage actually grazed. The fistula is
normally plugged but the plug is removed for short periods at several
times of day to allow collection of extrusa in a bag tied around the neck.
Forbes and Beattie (1987) compared ingestive behaviour and diet
composition in oesophageal fistulated and non-fistulated cows and
sheep and, finding no consistent differences, concluded that results
from fistulated animals are valid for normal animals of the same
physiological type.

   The oesophageal extrusa is not suitable, either in quantity or
palatability, for feeding to other animals for assessment of its digestibility and is usually analysed by an *in vitro* technique or by suspension
in nylon bags in the stomach of rumen-fistulated animals. It is
obviously easier and less expensive to use sheep rather than cattle for
rumen fistulation and for the *in vivo* measurement of digestibility but
level of intake, species of animal and physiological state all affect
digestibility and it is doubtful whether application of results from
wether sheep fed at the maintenance level to lactating cows fed *ad
libitum* is valid.

   Le Du and Penning (1982) reviewed the methods outlined above
and Greenhalgh (1982) pointed out the pitfalls, discussed the expense
and difficulties and warned that they should only be used when
absolutely necessary.

# Factors Affecting Herbage Intake

## Sward factors

Hodgson (1982) has reviewed sward characteristics affecting selection and intake of herbage in detail and has further covered all aspects of grazing (Hodgson, 1990).

### Herbage mass, sward height and density

#### Cattle
Other factors being equal, herbage intake increases with increasing height or density of the sward because the amount taken per bite is increased (Stobbs, 1973). Animals rarely graze for more than 12 out of the 24 h so that very slow rates of eating caused by sparse pastures will lead to low intakes as shown by Greenhalgh *et al.* (1966) for dairy cows and by Leaver (1974) for young stock.

The rate of eating also slows when the animal is eating selectively as it does when leaves are fewer in sparse or old herbage. Green herbage is always selected in preference to brown.

#### Sheep
Black and Kenney (1984) prepared artificial swards which they could tailor to any required density and height of tiller. They showed that the density of tillers as well as their height regulated bite mass in sheep and Fig. 16.4 shows the effect of the number of tillers per square metre on grazing behaviour from which it can be seen that as tiller density increases so does the weight prehended at each bite, giving an increase in rate of eating.

Allden and Whittaker (1970) found tiller height to be closely related to the size of bite taken by sheep up to 100 mm, levelling out with taller swards. The amount of time spent grazing and the frequency of biting increase with shorter swards (Hancock, 1954; Freer, 1966).

In a critical examination of the long-term effects of herbage allowance on herbage intake, Penning *et al.* (1991a) varied the stocking rate to maintain a constant allowance of grass and observed consistent increases in intake from about 1.5 to about 2.5 kg organic matter (OM) day$^{-1}$ for increasing allowances from 40 to 160 g OM kg$^{-1}$ live weight. Thus, even when a great excess of herbage is available, intake is still limited by the ease with which it can be harvested by the grazing animal.

The herbage mass below which daily intake is depressed varies according to many factors, including the size of the animal, the stocking rate and the method of grazing management, e.g. strip grazed vs. set-

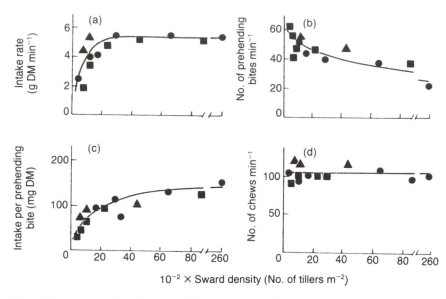

**Fig. 16.4.** Effect of tiller density on (a) rate of eating, (b) biting rate, (c) intake per bite and (d) chewing rate of sheep (Black and Kenney, 1984). Number of tillers per hole: ●, 3; ▲, 2; ■ 1.

stocked. For lambs Rayburn (1986) found that intake reached a maximum with a herbage mass of about 1.2 tonnes DM ha$^{-1}$ whereas for mature ewes Fig. 16.1 shows intake still increasing at herbage masses of 2 tonnes OM ha$^{-1}$.

### Digestibility

As with forages in general (Chapter 10) there is a positive relationship between digestibility of herbage dry matter and level of voluntary intake. The digestibility of young leaves of temperate pasture grasses is usually between 800 and 900 g kg$^{-1}$, falling to 700 g kg$^{-1}$ as senescence occurs. Stems have a high digestibility initially but this falls to around 500 g kg$^{-1}$ at maturity due to lignification. There is variation in the digestibility of herbage eaten according to the height above the ground because of changes in the proportion of leaves to stems. Minson (1982) reviewed the relationship between herbage digestibility and intake and found that it was in most cases linear, intake increasing even up to DM digestibilities of 800 g kg$^{-1}$. He noted that many factors affect this relationship, especially the rate of digestion and that no single laboratory measurement can be used to predict herbage intake satisfactorily.

Hodgson (1968) found that the linear equation

$$OMI = 30HOMD - 143.3 \qquad (16.1)$$

where *OMI* is organic matter intake (g kg live weight$^{-0.73}$) and *HOMD* is the digestibility of herbage organic matter (g kg$^{-1}$), held true for calves over a range of *HOMD* from 68 to 82%. Similar results were obtained by Hodgson *et al.* (1977), also with calves; the level of intake was greater for primary growth than for regrowth at any given level of digestibility, however (presumably due to the presence of some dying herbage in the latter or to differences in sward structure), again emphasizing that digestibility is not a sufficient predictor of intake. It is not clear why the intake/digestibility relationship is not curvilinear in a manner similar to that obtained with indoor feeding.

## Contamination of herbage

Application of animal waste slurry to pasture depresses grazing intake (Reid *et al.*, 1972) and cows prefer clean herbage if given any choice. The effect has almost disappeared by the second grazing after application of slurry (Broom *et al.*, 1975). Slurry should be spread on grassland which is to be cut for conservation, or animals should be stocked at a low density so as to give them the opportunity to graze the less heavily contaminated areas (Pain *et al.*, 1974).

Urine does not noticeably affect selection (Norman and Green, 1958) but areas around dung pats, up to twelve times the area of the pat itself, are avoided because of the smell (Greenhalgh and Reid, 1969). Under British conditions dung disappears in about 100 days. Although the immediate effect of faeces is to reduce the grazing area, the increased growth of grass due to the fertilizing effect more than offsets this in the long term (MacDiarmid and Watkin, 1972).

## Supplementation at pasture

The whole question of the extent to which forage intake is affected by concentrate supplementation is discussed in Chapter 10. Because growing herbage is usually highly digestible, the amount eaten by grazing ruminants is particularly susceptible to supplementation when concentrates are fed.

### Cattle

Marsh *et al.* (1971) found that total DM intake of cows was increased by only 0.46 kg and grazing time was reduced by 22 min for every kilogram of compound food eaten. Because of this displacement the increase in milk yield of dairy cows when pasture is supplemented is

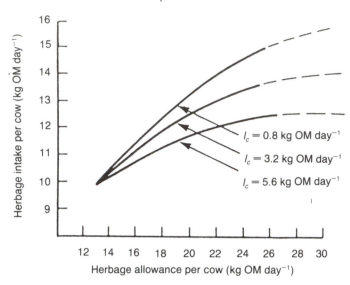

**Fig. 16.5.** Herbage intake by cows at a range of herbage allowances and three levels of supplementation (Meijs and Hoekstra, 1984).

often disappointing – the mean response is around 0.3 kg milk kg$^{-1}$ of concentrates (Leaver *et al.*, 1968). Extra feeding at grass can only be justified if the stocking rate is increased or where herbage mass and digestibility are low, i.e. in summer.

Increasing the mass of herbage available gave higher substitution rates with dairy cows (Meijs and Hoekstra, 1984, Fig. 16.5). This is to be expected as high herbage mass allows high herbage intake and the cow is therefore closer to its intake limits, whether they are primarily physical or metabolic, and more susceptible to the effects of supplementary concentrates.

Meijs (1986) supplemented grazing dairy cows with high (350 g kg$^{-1}$) vs. low (100 g kg$^{-1}$) starch concentrates. Grass intake was lower for the high-starch supplement (11.5 vs. 12.6 kg OM day$^{-1}$) and the substitution rates were 0.45 and 0.21, respectively. This agrees with results of supplementing silage with high or low starch concentrates (see below).

### Sheep

In a comprehensive experiment with lactating ewes Milne *et al.* (1981) found substitution rates (reduction in herbage OM intake per unit increase in concentrate OM input) of 0.70 and 0.93 with herbage masses of 500 or 750 kg OM ha$^{-1}$, respectively, when 480 g OM day$^{-1}$ of concentrates was given. Supplementation with 960 g OM day$^{-1}$ gave substitu-

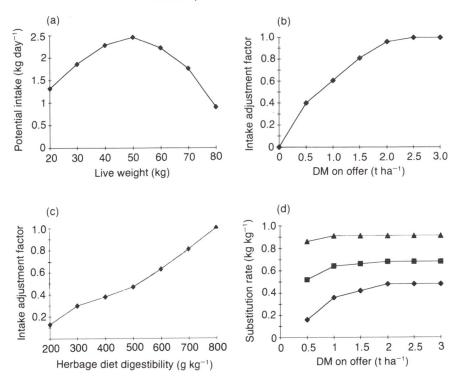

**Fig. 16.6.** Relationships used in the model of Orsini (1990) for (a) potential intake, (b) potential intake adjusted for total DM on offer, (c) potential intake adjusted for herbage digestibility and (d) substitution rate. Herbage diet digestibility: ▲, 650 g kg$^{-1}$; ■, 500 g kg$^{-1}$; ◆, 350 g kg$^{-1}$.

tion rates of 0.52 and 0.80 for the two levels of herbage on offer, which indicated that substitution rate falls with increasing level of supplementation. This is a surprising conclusion because the literature for cows fed conserved forages suggests the opposite trend (Chapter 10). Much lower substitution rates were found for grazing ewes by Penning *et al.* (1988) especially when the supplements were high in protein and might to some extent have been alleviating a protein deficiency.

From a survey of the literature Orsini (1990) concluded that, for grazing sheep, substitution rate increases with the total amount of herbage DM on offer and with the digestibility of the herbage (Fig. 16.6).

### Animal factors

In general, the effects of growth, fattening, pregnancy and lactation on herbage intake are similar to those reviewed in Chapters 8 and 9.

In addition, however, extra requirements for nutrients, particularly energy, may be imposed by wind and rain and by the increased muscular activity associated with biting and walking. The energy cost of eating is related to the time spent eating rather than to the weight of herbage eaten (sheep, Osuji, 1974; cattle, Adam *et al.*, 1984) so that sparse pasture imposes extra demands for energy.

Blaxter (1962) considered the influence of environmental effects on energy requirements. He has also calculated the cost of walking and climbing to be 2.5 J kg$^{-1}$ m$^{-1}$ for horizontal movement and 20 J kg$^{-1}$ m$^{-1}$ for vertical movement, from experiments involving sheep trained to exercise on treadmills. The energy cost of eating has been calculated by Osuji (1974) to be at least 40 J kg$^{-1}$ body weight min$^{-1}$ spent eating by sheep. The total of the extra expenditure of energy by a sheep grazing on sparse pasture is thus 25–50% above that of housed sheep and it has been observed that the voluntary intake of grazing animals is often greater than that of those kept indoors by about this margin.

*Nutrient requirements*

When plentiful amounts of high quality grass are available to lactating cows their voluntary intake changes in proportion to their milk yield (Huffman, 1959; Greenhalgh *et al.*, 1966). Similarly, lactation stimulates grazing intake in sheep (Arnold and Dudzinski, 1967) as does shearing in cold weather (Wheeler *et al.*, 1963; Chapter 15). With poorer or sparser grazing, however, correlations between intake and yield are more likely to be due to intake limiting milk secretion; the correlation may be similar but the causality is different.

As with housed sheep, voluntary intake of herbage declines as the animal becomes fat (Arnold *et al.*, 1964).

## Grassland Management

The way in which growing herbage is used in animal production is very much dictated by the level of intake achieved by the grazing animals. Although it is possible to increase intake by individual animals by decreasing the stocking rate this will not usually yield the maximum output of animal product per hectare. At the other extreme, maximum herbage consumption per unit area can be achieved by stocking the pasture very heavily, but the intake by individual animals is so low as to satisfy only their maintenance requirements, or less. This may, in the overall context of a production system, be satisfactory; for example a store period where animals have to wait for the growth of spring grass in order to obtain more than their maintenance requirements.

In practice, herbage mass is a good index for grazing management. An excellent review of grassland management under British conditions is the book edited by Holmes (1989) whereas that of Hacker (1982) is much broader in its scope. Hodgson (1990) covers the interface between science and practice.

A good example of a model of a grazing system is the 'Summer-Pack' model of Orsini (1990) in which herbage is described by up to five components with coefficients for sheep preference. The first component has a palatability of 1 and if another component has a higher preference it has a coefficient greater than 1 and vice versa. Green material has a rating of 15 relative to dry material. When herbage mass is low sheep cannot be as selective and preference tends towards 1 for all components as the amount of herbage on offer falls below 1500 kg ha$^{-1}$ (Fig. 16.6b). Intake increases with increasing herbage digestibility (Fig. 16.6c), with no levelling off at high digestibilities (see above). Potential intake is maximum at 50 kg live weight (Fig. 16.6a) as both small and fat sheep have lower intakes than those of average build (Chapter 8). Supplementary feeding has the effects shown in Fig. 16.6d, that is an increasing substitution rate as either the availability or the digestibility of herbage increases. The model behaves realistically and is proving useful in field situations in Australia.

## Conserved Forages: Silage

Conservation is necessary in much of the world where grass stops growing for part of the year due to coldness or drought. Traditionally the grass has been cut, left to lie in the field to dry and then stored under cover. The quality of the original grass is better retained if the drying is more rapid and avoids rain falling on the cut grass. Artificial grass drying has therefore been used in developed countries but the cost of fuel for drying is very high. It is possible to preserve grass by pickling rather than by drying; grass preserved in this way is called silage and is produced by compressing the grass within a few hours of cutting to exclude air and encourage the production of acids by naturally occurring anaerobic microorganisms. It is common to add acids at the time of ensiling and the addition of a culture of particularly effective organisms is also now widely used. Approximately 85% of the grass conserved in the UK is as silage (Milk Marketing Board, 1987) as the frequent rain makes hay-making a risky process.

In hay-making, artificial grass-drying and silage-making the grass undergoes processes which alter its physical and chemical properties. There have been relatively few direct comparisons of the voluntary intake of hay or silage with the grass from which it was made but it is generally recognized that conservation results in reduced intake. The possible reasons will be discussed.

Silage and hay made from the same grass and fed at the same level can usually be expected to support the same level of production (Murdoch and Rook, 1963) but the voluntary intake of silage is often less than of hay made from the same grass (e.g. Gordon *et al.*, 1961) although this is not such a problem with the better silage-making techniques now being used. Although the yield of grass for conservation is increased by cutting later in the summer, this is obtained at the expense of decreased digestibility. It is better to cut early and then take a second cut of the regrowth. The optimum strategy depends on the class of livestock to be fed on the conserved forage (Blaxter and Wilson, 1963).

When the grass has been cut it lies in the field, with periodical mechanical turning, until it is sufficiently dry to be baled and stored. In areas which are prone to rainfall during this period the grass becomes leached of some of its soluble constituents; its nutritive value is reduced and moulding may occur if the hay is not dry enough $(850 \, g \, DM \, kg^{-1})$.

Ensilage does not directly affect the digestibility, metabolizable energy concentration or efficiency of utilization of ME, but intake is often lower than that of the fresh crop. For sheep, a review of 87 silages (Demarquilly, 1973) showed a mean reduction of 33% (range 1–64%) of the intake of the fresh grass or legumes from which the silages were made. The reduction is greater with sheep than with cattle and greater with grass silages than with maize silages. ARC (1980) found average silage intakes by sheep to be only $46 \, g \, DW \, W^{-0.75}$, compared to 57 for long hay or 91 for ground hay feeds.

The physical effort required by the cow to pull silage directly from the clamp reduces the rate of eating compared with the same silage cut and fed in a trough (Bines, 1985).

### Dry matter content

In general there is a positive relationship between the DM content of silage and its intake by ruminants. Overnight wetting of a silage, which had an original DM content of $227 \, g \, kg^{-1}$, to $169 \, g \, kg^{-1}$ depressed its intake by sheep (Dodsworth and Campbell, 1953). However, adding water just before offering silage to young cattle did not affect daily intake compared with unwetted silage (Thomas *et al.*, 1961b); it is likely that water outside plant cells is absorbed very quickly from the rumen and does not contribute to the bulk of the food, whereas the volume of intracellular water does, until it is released. In the USA, Coppock (quoted by Wangsness and Muller, 1981) showed, from a wide range of data, that intake is positively related to dry matter content for alfalfa and corn silages. It follows that intake can be increased by wilting the grass before ensilage although there have been several instances of an accompanying drop in the yield of fat-corrected milk possibly because of adverse effects of fermentation. Castle (1983, p. 143) concludes that '... it is extremely doubtful whether there will be consistent benefits [of wilting] in terms of animal production'. This is in contrast to the conclusion of Osbourn (1976) that '... wilting must continue to be the only method available in practice to reduce this disadvantage of ensilage as a method of conservation'. It is likely that grass for silage is nowadays cut at an earlier stage of maturity than formerly and the effects of wilting are greater with silage of lower digestibility. The use of additives now improves the control of fermentation of wet silages (see below) and wilting is recommended more to reduce the volume of effluent than to improve the nutritive value of the silage.

An extreme form of wilting has been investigated by R. Simpson and H. Dove at the University of Melbourne (personal communication). Pasture is sprayed with half the normal level of glyphosate (a herbicide) 1 or 2 weeks before flowering. This stops growth but does not completely kill the grass and the soluble carbohydrate content remains elevated for at least 60 days whereas in untreated grass it declines after flowering. Intake and performance of animals fed on this grass are greatly increased compared with those on unwilted material.

### Fermentation pattern

The silage-making process ferments soluble carbohydrates to produce organic acids, predominantly lactic, but also significant amounts of acetic acid, and many nitrogenous compounds such as amines. These substances, and those additives which are incorporated to improve the silage, have been under suspicion as the cause of the lower intake of silage, compared to hay or grass, and have been infused into the rumen in a number of experiments. Infusing the rumen with nitrogenous constituents of maize silage extracts depressed intake of hay but no evidence that specific constituents could inhibit intake was found (Phillip *et al.*, 1981a). In further work (Buchanan-Smith and Phillip, 1986), sheep were infused intraruminally with isosmotic saline, organic acids or lucerne silage extracts, with or without additional acids and amines. Silage extracts depressed intake for 4 h after feeding which was at the end of the 4 h infusion. Various other additions depressed intake and it was concluded that soluble constituents in silage can inhibit intake but no single constituent is primarily responsible.

Clancy *et al.* (1977) compared the effects of rapid intraruminal infusion of silage juice with a mixture which contained the same volatile fatty acids, lactate, soluble carbohydrate, ammonia and nitrate, and was of the same pH and osmolality. The depression of hay intake with this mixture was only 40% of the depression with juice so that other factors such as amines must have contributed to the depressing effects of silage juice. Slower infusion of silage juice (2 l in 3.5 h) also depressed intake of hay or frozen grass compared with control (Smith and Clapperton, 1981).

Histamine is present in some silages in amounts which might depress rumen motility, but when given at 1 g day$^{-1}$ to sheep it did not affect their silage intake (Neumark, 1967). In the presence of formic acid, however, it was thought that sufficient histamine might sometimes be absorbed to cause a reduction in silage intake.

Poor ensilage conditions, which encourage a clostridial type of fermentation, yield a silage with particularly low intake characteristics. The products which depress intake appear to include ammonia and volatile fatty acids, particularly acetic (Tayler and Wilkins, 1976). Partial neutralization sometimes increases voluntary intake whereas addition of formic acid, which has sometimes been used as a preservative, depresses intake (McLeod *et al.*, 1970). Thomas and Chamberlain (1983) quote correlations between voluntary intake and several chemical components but point out that there are also intercorrelations between the various components; acid concentration, and ammonia nitrogen are negatively related to intake whereas the ratio of lactic acid:total acid is positively related. Cows can ingest up to 1 kg day$^{-1}$ of lactic acid in silage, but this amount added to hay did not depress intake to the same level as that of silage (Morgan and L'Estrange, 1977). It appears that no single constituent of silage is responsible for its low intake but it is possible that the additive effects of a number of substances might be important.

Attention has turned to the possibility that the peculiar composition of silage influences its acceptability to ruminants. Buchanan-Smith (1990) fed oesophageal-fistulated sheep on lucerne hay but fasted them for 5 h before offering silage with added solutions, with the oesophageal plugs removed to prevent the test foods entering the rumen. Acetate added alone depressed intake whereas a mixture of two amines and gamma-aminobutyric acid (GABA) stimulated intake at low levels, but had no effect at higher levels. The author suggested that the intake of silage with a high acetic content is limited by palatability. However, the animals were sham-fed both during training and experiments so that they had no chance to learn anything about associations between taste and metabolic properties of the various test foods. It will be necessary to train animals to make such associations before we can draw firm conclusions about the mechanisms responsible for low intakes of silage (Chapter 12).

*Physical limitation of silage intake*

Another possible reason for low silage intake is physical limitation, given the slower rate of rumen breakdown, relative to hay. However, Waldo *et al.* (1965b) noted that rumen dry and wet matter contents were less in heifers fed on silage than on hay and concluded that silage intake was not restricted by rumen capacity. The total contractile activity of the rumen and its organic matter content were significantly greater for hay (at equal levels of feeding to cattle) than silage and more time was spent ruminating on hay when both were fed once per day (Thiago *et al.*, 1992). Whereas hay offered once per day at a restricted level was all eaten in 2 h after offering, an equivalent amount of silage took about 10 h. Perhaps metabolic discomfort accompanies the slow rate of fermentation of silage and the animal learns to eat less and/or more slowly to avoid this.

Intake of silage does not always appear to be positively related to digestibility (Harris and Raymond, 1964), due to a small range of digestibilities observed in some comparisons and to confounding with other factors, but with a wider range of digestibilities there has been a positive correlation between digestibility and intake (Murdoch, 1965). The demonstration that water-filled bags in the rumen (16 l) depressed the intake of a high quality silage by 16% in dry cows confirms that physical fill of the rumen is important, while the fact that reducing the particle size by chopping or mincing increased voluntary intake by cows (Murdoch, 1965; Dulphy and Demarquilly, 1973) and beef cattle (Wilkinson *et al.*, 1978) supports this. Campling (1966a) concluded that silage particles stay in the rumen for longer than those of hay and there is more pseudo-rumination in silage-fed sheep and cattle than in those offered hay, suggesting that the slow breakdown of fibres is making it more difficult for the animals to regurgitate (Deswysen *et al.*, 1978). In addition to the possibility that rate of digestion is slow with silages, there is also evidence that rumen motility is depressed; infusion of lucerne silage juice intraruminally depressed rumen motility and rate of eating (Smith and Clapperton, 1981). Thus, chemicals in the silage, particularly amines (Thomas *et al.*, 1980a), might act through physical mechanisms.

With the fermentation of soluble carbohydrates, 10% of grass DM disappears during ensilage. This is equivalent to half the potential to generate adenosine triphosphate (ATP) in the rumen and results in a very poor energy supply for microbial growth even though there is plenty of energy for the animal itself. Microbial growth and activity are therefore restricted, with the consequence that rates of fermentation and particle breakdown of silage are lower than for materials with higher contents of soluble carbohydrates. The problem is to some extent overcome by supplying readily fermentable energy to the rumen, i.e. supplementation with concentrates.

## Additives

Several additives have been developed for commercial use in order to alleviate problems associated with undesirable fermentation. Formic acid reduces the production of volatile fatty acids and ammonia by acting as a sterilizing agent. Although it has been associated with decreased voluntary intakes, this can be avoided by supplementation with a high protein concentrate (McLeod *et al.*, 1970; Thomas *et al.*, 1980b). Formalin is also useful for lucerne (alfalfa) but not for grass and it depressed intake when used at greater than 10 l tonne$^{-1}$. In one trial treatment of a clover/ryegrass mixture with 4.8 l formalin and 1 l formic acid per tonne improved the preservation of the herbage and voluntary intake increased from 30 to 50 g kg$^{-0.75}$ day$^{-1}$ (Barry, 1975). Acetic acid (Hutchinson and Wilkins, 1971) or various nitrogen additives (ammonia, histamine, tryptamine, tyramine) have been tested, but with little advantage (Vetter and Von Glan, 1978). Because of the relationships between intake and pH, partial neutralization with bicarbonate before feeding has been investigated (Thomas and Chamberlain, 1983) and it is sometimes, but not always, effective in stimulating intake, especially with calves. Partial neutralization of silage depressed intake by cattle and had little effect in sheep (Farhan and Thomas, 1978); in both species, it increased water intake.

Propionic acid can control silage fermentation and increases the intake of maize silage (Hiber and Soejono, 1976) but it is more expensive than formic and is not likely to replace it. A mixture of salts of carboxylic acids (Maxgrass, BP Chemicals) has been developed which is applied at sufficiently high rates to grass before ensilage that fermentation is largely prevented. The increased soluble carbohydrate content, compared with conventionally made silage, enhances microbial activity in the rumen when the material is fed which results in higher levels of intake. For example, Maxgrass increased intake by beef cattle from 7.67 to 8.83 kg$^{-1}$ day$^{-1}$ with increased gain and efficiency and also less bale storage losses (Weddell, 1992). For lactating cows, additives of various types, including inoculants and formic acid, gave increases in silage intake equivalent to between 1.4 and 2.5 kg concentrates day$^{-1}$, the best response being with Maxgrass (Mayne, 1992).

Although somewhat variable results have been obtained with bacterial inoculants, they are capable of giving higher intakes than some acid additives, even when the chemical composition of the conserved grass is similar (Mayne, 1990). In a comparison of formic acid, sulphuric acid and a bacterial inoculation as additives in silage making, Mayne (1993) found a significant increase in intake (12%) due to formic acid for first regrowth but a smaller effect of inoculant (4.6%). Sulphuric acid tended to reduce intake of first regrowth and none of the treatments had significant effects with a second regrowth of grass.

## Protein

It has been suggested that, although the nitrogen content of grass silage implies an adequate protein content, some of the nitrogen is as non-protein nitrogen compounds whereas some is in proteins rendered indigestible during ensilage, particularly if overheating has occurred. The provision of a protein source which is largely undegraded in the rumen, but which yields amino acids in the intestines, has been proposed to alleviate this problem. Once again, the results have been variable, Sanderson *et al.* (1992) finding that although a fishmeal supplement increased silage intake by growing steers, the increase was only as great as the increase in live weight. For growing calves, soyabean meal did not affect silage intake or performance relative to fishmeal whereas maize gluten did not affect production in one experiment but did in the other (Steen, 1992). There was no effect of giving 2.5 kg DM day$^{-1}$ of a supplement containing 0, 200, 400 or 600 g kg$^{-1}$ of soyabean meal on the intake by young bulls of a silage containing 140 g crude protein (CP) kg$^{-1}$ DM (Steen, 1991).

Low nitrogen status is not always the reason for low intake, however, as duodenal infusion of casein in sheep offered grass silage *ad libitum* improved nitrogen retention with no effect on intake (Hutchinson *et al.*, 1971). Similarly, supplementation of grass silage for young cattle with isonitrogenous amounts of degradable (63 g groundnut meal kg$^{-1}$ DM) or undegradable (50 g fishmeal kg$^{-1}$ DM) protein resulted in no change in silage intake but an improvement in digestibility and in the nitrogen retention of the animals (Gill and England, 1984).

## Chop length

The intake of silage can be increased by chopping the grass at harvest which improves fermentation in the silo and increases the rate of passage through the digestive tract. In nine comparisons with sheep, mean intake was increased by 56% for silages harvested with a precision-chop machine rather than with a simple flail harvester. This was more effective than chopping just before feeding (McDonald *et al.*, 1991). Young beef cattle ate 66% more silage made from grass cut to 8 mm at harvest, compared with that cut to 33 mm and the finely chopped material was also more digestible (Wilkinson *et al.*, 1978).

Deswysen *et al.* (1978) compared grass silage chopped to either 53 or 18 mm before ensilage or to 18 mm just before feeding. Sheep offered the long silage had lower intakes and spent less time ruminating. Pseudo-rumination was significantly increased on the long silage, suggesting difficulty in regurgitating the long, slippery strands. There were no differences between silages chopped to 18 mm either at ensilage or just before feeding.

Cattle prefer unchopped to chopped silage (Duckworth and Shirlaw, 1958) and this may be because they get a larger amount of food per mouthful.

The intake of silage made from perennial ryegrass and the yield of milk by cows increased as chop length decreased (72.0, 17.4 and 9.4 mm) (Castle *et al.*, 1979). Eating and ruminating times reduced as chop length decreased but the mean retention time of food particles in the digestive tract was not affected.

## Clover silage

Clover is a good source of protein for ruminants and there have been a few studies of clover silage intake. A mixture of grass and white clover silages had a high intake by dairy cows (15.2 kg DM cow$^{-1}$ day$^{-1}$) but there were unusually high substitution rates of 0.76 for barley and 0.66 for barley + soyabean meal supplementation (Castle *et al.*, 1983). Thomas *et al.* (1985) found that for silages with similar digestibility, red clover silage gave higher food intake and milk yield by cows than ryegrass silage when fed with 7 kg DM day$^{-1}$ of a cereal/soyabean supplement. However, feeding clover silage in early lactation tended to be followed by reduced yields when grass silage was given later in lactation.

When lucerne was fed to sheep as hay or silage there was no difference in intake and no difference in response to intraruminal introduction of food (Etheridge *et al.*, 1993). Thus, any benefits of clover silage are not very large and it is probably better to ensile a clover/grass mixture than just clover.

## Corn silage

Maize silage has lower levels of acid than grass silage, typically, while having a similar pH. Lactic acid, in particular is about half and acetic perhaps two-thirds of that for grass silage. Maize silage has about 200 g kg$^{-1}$ DM of starch whereas grass silage has very little; as discussed above, a supply of rapidly fermentable carbohydrate is essential for normal microbial function in the rumen.

Because of low protein content of maize silage it is better to feed it with grass silage and/or a protein supplement. Mineral and vitamin supplementation must be adequate due to low levels of Ca, P and vitamin E in maize silage. The high starch content can cause acidosis especially if fed with starchy supplements such as cereals. For these reasons maize silage should not exceed about 75% of the total DM intake.

Compared to grass silage, cows fed maize silage, or a mixture, ate more DM and produced more milk (Weller and Phipps, 1985a). Even when high quality grass silage was available, offering maize silage as well improved the performance of dairy cows (Weller and Phipps, 1985b). Offering dairy cows one-third of the forage as maize silage, brewers' grains or fodder beet increased DM intake by about 1 kg day$^{-1}$, compared to grass silage alone (Phipps *et al.*, 1993).

In a comparison of maize silage only, maize silage and lucerne or maize silage, lucerne and wheat, intake of digestible OM was highest for maize silage alone even though the digestibility of this was the lowest of the three diets (Moran *et al.*, 1988).

## Concentrate supplementation of silage

Since silage cannot usually be eaten in sufficient amounts to satisfy the nutrient requirements for rapid growth or high milk yield some supplementary food is usually provided. Supplements which are high in readily fermentable carbohydrates may result in a reduced rate of cellulose digestion and therefore have a greater depressing effect on silage intake than might otherwise be predicted. Castle and Watson (1976) found a substitution rate of 0.51 for barley supplementation of grass silage for Ayrshire cows. If the supplement was given frequently in small amounts a more even pattern of fermentation was seen in the rumen, but this did not affect the substitution rate (Gill and Castle, 1983). Supplementation with dried grass cubes gave a substitution rate of 0.36, i.e. a smaller reduction in silage intake per unit of supplement compared to barley; molassed beet pulp, which also has a slower pattern of nutrient release than barley, gave a substitution of 0.4 (Castle and Watson, 1979). Similar conclusions have been drawn for sheep by Wernli and Wilkins (1971), for dairy cows by Jackson *et al.* (1991) and for young cattle by Tayler and Aston (1972). Although barley supplementation depresses silage intake more than dried grass supplementation the resulting level of production is often higher because of the higher digestibility of the barley, compared to typical dried grasses. Bulky supplements depress silage intake to a greater extent than do cereals or dried grass. For example, hay offered to cows depressed silage intake by 0.84 kg kg$^{-1}$ (Castle, 1983), to give a useful increase in total DM intake. Similarly, Miller *et al.* (1965) and Waldern (1972) found that lactating cows ate significantly more when both hay and silage were offered than when either was offered alone.

It is usually intended to feed silage *ad libitum*, but in practice this is not always achieved either because cows wait for fresh silage to be cut down from the face of the silo rather than pulling it off themselves or because they are purposely restricted to avoid wastage. When silage intake is reduced because of restricted access, increasing the level of supplementation does not reduce silage intake (Harb and Campling, 1983).

Waldo *et al.* (1965a) found that less nitrogen was retained by cattle when silage was fed than when hay was fed, but attributed this to the lower voluntary intake. However, recent experiments have revealed that supplements which provide greater amounts of protein result in smaller depressions of silage intake. The lower the nitrogen content of silage, the greater the beneficial effects of nitrogen supplements on intake (McDonald *et al.*, 1991). A supplement of dried lucerne was better in this respect than dried grass (Tayler and Gibbs, 1975), oilseed meals did not affect silage intake at all and soyabean meal resulted in an increase in the voluntary intake of silage in some cases (Castle and Watson, 1979). In practice, the provision of 'balancer' cubes high in protein and low in soluble carbohydrate appears to be of considerable benefit (Castle, 1983) and commercial concentrate supplements for dairy cows are now available tailored to the characteristics of the individual silage.

In a comparison of patterns of allocation of concentrates for silage-fed dairy cows Taylor and Leaver (1984) observed that feeding at a flat rate of 9 kg day$^{-1}$ was accompanied initially by a small increase,

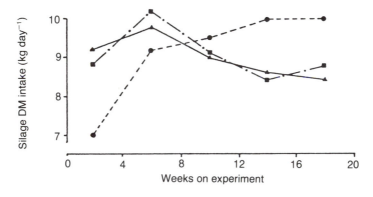

**Fig. 16.7.** Silage intakes of lactating cows fed at a fixed level (▲), a declining rate (●) or according to yield (■) (Taylor and Leaver, 1984).

followed by a progressive decline in silage intake as lactation progressed; feeding concentrates according to yield gave a similar pattern of silage intake over lactation. On the other hand, giving the same total amount of concentrates but reducing from 11 to 7 kg day$^{-1}$ as lactation progressed, resulted in a steady increase in silage intake (Fig. 16.7).

## Conclusions

Measurement of intake at pasture is more difficult than with housed ruminants and a variety of methods have been developed, many depending on marker dilution, particularly chromic oxide. Although it is quite easy to monitor the time spent grazing and the number of bites, this information is only of full value if the weight taken at each bite can be measured, and this is not possible with current methodology.

The most important factor affecting herbage intake is the height of herbage available, which is closely related to the mass of herbage available. Herbage intake is also affected by the stocking density as well as by the water content and composition of the grass. There are effects of previous experience and hunger status on the selection of preferred types and parts of plants.

The nutrient requirements of the grazing animal influence its potential intake in the same way as for dry feeds but there are complex interactions between the changing quantity and quality of the herbage and the changing nutrient requirements of the grazing animals; great skill and experience is required on the part of the grassland farmer in order to make optimum use of his pastures.

Grass and other types of plant are often conserved during the growing season for use as food at other times of the year. Hay, dried grass and silage are common forms of preserved herbage. The intake of silage is often seen to be lower than of hay made from the same sward, although this is not so much a problem now as it was in the past. Low DM content, slow rates of degradation, low pH, high ammonia, nutrient imbalance and unavailability of protein are all recognized as factors in the depression of silage intake but the relative importance of these in any given situation is hard to estimate. Intake of maize silage is usually higher than that of grass silage and a useful technique is to mix grass silage with either maize or clover silage to get maximum intakes by cows.

Supplementation of herbage or silage with concentrates depresses forage intake although in situations in which there is marginal protein deficiency, such as is often suspected with silages, high protein concentrates can sometimes lead to increased forage intake.

# 17 PREDICTION OF VOLUNTARY INTAKE

- Poultry
- Pigs
- Ruminants
- Conclusions

In order to optimize the utilization of food or to decide the optimum formulation of a ration to meet the animals' requirements under conditions of *ad libitum* feeding, it is necessary to be able to predict the level of voluntary intake of a food or foods by farm animals.

There are two general methods for prediction, regression analysis and mathematical modelling, but the division between them is not absolute. The first involves measurement of several parameters, including voluntary intake, followed by regression analysis to find the equation which best fits the data. For example, measurement of live ($LW$), daily gain ($LWG$), milk yield ($MY$) and voluntary intake ($I$) would yield an equation of the form:

$$I = a + bLW + cLWG + dMY \qquad (17.1)$$

which could be used to predict intake in other animals of the same type. Note that this equation is a 'model' insofar as live weight, live weight gain and milk yield might reasonably be expected to be causal factors in the determination of food intake. The regression approach was adopted by ARC (1980) in their summary of voluntary food intake of ruminant livestock. The most comprehensive review of the quantitative aspects of food intake with particular reference to farm animals has been made by NRC (1987), using predominantly North American data. The reader is referred to this for more detailed coverage of the prediction of food intake.

The second type of prediction method involves incorporation of more basic biological principles and functions which describe the relationships between factors likely to underlie the control of food intake. Such methods are likely to be less accurate at prediction but to be more general in their application. A dynamic model is one in which the predictions of one iteration are used as starting values for the next iteration, where time is incremented between successive iterations. Thus, equations which describe the relationship in ruminants between intake and digestible energy concentration (metabolic control) on the one hand, and intake and rumen capacity (physical control) on the other can be solved for animals of given live weight, fatness and energy requirement (e.g. Forbes, 1977a). Whichever intake was the lower would then be used to determine the level of weight gain (or loss) which will change body fatness and live weight for the next iteration, and so on. Such a model might well be constructed using two or more equations derived empirically, as described above. Some examples are given below.

## Poultry

Simpson and Raine (1981) proposed for broilers the equation:

$$I = A - B(e^{-1/\text{age}}) \tag{17.2}$$

where $I$ is the voluntary intake (g day$^{-1}$ kg$^{-0.67}$) and $A$ and $B$ constants related to the metabolizable energy (ME) content of the food and the environmental temperature. Since a change from one food or environment to another will not result in immediate compensation in voluntary intake, the authors introduced a variable (beta) which describes the rate at which the change in intake occurs after a change in conditions. Their equation thus becomes;

$$I = (A_{\text{old}} + (A_{\text{new}} - A_{\text{old}}) \, e^{\text{beta}/(x-x^*)} - (B_{\text{old}} + (B_{\text{new}} - B_{\text{old}}) \, e^{\text{beta}/(x-x^*)} \tag{17.3}$$

where $x$ is the current day and $x^*$ is the day on which the change was made. To solve this equation Simpson and Raine suggest a large-scale experiment with four levels of food ME concentration, four environmental temperatures plus several groups of broilers which, at different ages, are changed from one ME to another at a constant temperature and from one temperature to another at constant ME.

The intake of broiler chicks was measured from hatching to 210 days of age by Wilson and Emmans (1979). They derived the equation:

$$dF/dt = c(1-e^{-t/t^*})$$                                   (17.4)

where $F$ is food intake, $c$ is the mature weight, $t$ is age and $t^*\ln 2$ is the time for an increment of $(c-dF/dt)/2$.

Byerly (1979) reviewed the derivation of equations for predicting the voluntary intake of laying hens. For controlled environments, where the temperature range is not large, the following equation was found to be satisfactory for individually caged layers:

$$MEI = (3.14 - 0.031T)LW^{0.75} + 33WC + 9.6EM$$          (17.5)

where $MEI$ is the ME intake (kJ ME bird$^{-1}$ day$^{-1}$), $T$ is the ambient temperature (°C), $WC$ is the weight gain (g bird$^{-1}$ day$^{-1}$), $EM$ is the egg mass (g bird$^{-1}$day$^{-1}$) and $LW$ is the live weight (g).

Morris (1968b) surveyed the literature for experiments relating intake by hens to diet digestibility and derived the equation:

$$EI - Y11.3 + (0.000547)Y11.3 - 0.147(DIETE - 11.3)$$      (17.6)

in which $EI$ is energy intake (kJ bird$^{-1}$ day$^{-1}$), Y11.3 is the intake of a food with 11.3 MJ ME kg$^{-1}$ and $DIETE$ is the ME content of the food in question (MJ kg$^{-1}$).

According to NRC (1984):

$$MEI = W^{0.75}(173 - 1.95T) + 5.50WC + 2.07EE$$           (17.7)

where $MEI$ is ME intake (kJ day$^{-1}$), $T$ is ambient temperature (°C), $EE$ is egg production (g day$^{-1}$), $WC$ is change in weight (g day$^{-1}$).

In any predictions of food intake by poultry account must be taken of food wastage; this is impossible to eliminate completely, is difficult to measure and therefore difficult to predict. Summers (1974) suggests that overfilling the feeder can cause up to 6% wastage; cold environment, 10%; rodent infestation, 1%; parasites and disease, 7%; food spillage, 5%. NRC (1987) gives tables of intake for various combinations of food, animal and environment, with no explicit validation.

## Pigs

There was little interest in the prediction of voluntary food intake of pigs as long as the domestic pig had a very high propensity to deposit fat above a live weight of about 60 kg and was therefore fed at a restricted level to prevent excessive deposition. In recent years, however, intensive selection for leanness and the use of uncastrated boars which deposit little fat has meant that growing pigs can be fed *ad libitum*.

NRC (1987) summarizes data for intake of creep food by sucking piglets up to 35 days of age from various sources by the equation:

$$DEI = 46.8DAY - 634 \qquad (17.8)$$

where $DEI$ is digestible energy intake (kJ day$^{-1}$) and $DAY$ is age (days), i.e. intake of creep food is predicted to start at 13 days.

After weaning it can be expected that voluntary intake will be such as to meet the animal's energy requirements and therefore to be proportional to body weight and weight gain. Ewan (1983) found that the relationship between intake of digestible energy ($DEI$, kJ day$^{-1}$) and body weight ($LW$, kg) for pigs weighing between 5 and 20 kg to be:

$$DEI = 1931LW - 40.6LW^2 - 6.40 \qquad (17.9)$$

In an extension of this work, Ewan (1983) reported that, for pigs from 5 to 11 kg, his data fitted the equation:

$$DEI = 55017(1 - e^{-0.018LW}) \qquad (17.10)$$

Cole *et al.* (1967a) found the relationship between digestible energy intake and body weight of growing pigs between 30 and 100 kg to be:

$$DEI = 2410LW^{0.68} \qquad (17.11)$$

while ARC (1981) presents the equation:

$$DEI = 4700LW^{0.51} \qquad (17.12)$$

The values calculated from these two curves are, in fact, very similar within the normal range of weight.

De Vries and Kanis (1992) developed a growth model based on a linear-plateau relationship between protein deposition and food intake incorporating a minimum fat to protein deposition ratio and a maximum protein deposition rate. If capacity to eat was too low to realize maximum protein deposition, then increasing the intake capacity had a positive economic value whereas if it was too high it had a negative value, whereas previously, increased intake was always considered a bad thing. Kanis and de Vries (1992) used the model of de Vries and Kanis (1992) to simulate effects of various selection indexes and concluded that if intake capacity is too low, selection emphasis should be on this trait.

For lactating sows intake increases up to day 17 but then declines (NRC, 1987):

$$DEI = 56012 + 2491DAY - 7.19DAY^2 \qquad (17.13)$$

This prediction should be adjusted for environmental temperature:

$$\text{Percent change in } DEI = 0.0165(T_o - EAT) \qquad (17.14)$$

where $T_o$ is the optimal temperature and *EAT* is effective ambient temperature:

$$EAT = 0.065DBT + 0.35WBT \qquad (17.15)$$

where *DBT* is dry bulb temperature and *WBT* is wet bulb temperature (°C).

Kornegay and Notter (1984) have presented equations for predicting the effects of different space allowances for weanling, growing and finishing pigs, in relation to the intakes of animals with ample space. For optimal food intake, the space allowances were 0.4, 1.06 and 12.09 m²/animal, respectively. There is an effect of group size which is independent of space allowance, which Kornegay and Notter (1984) have quantified as a 0.92% decrease in intake per additional pig, in the range 3–15 pigs per pen for weaners, 0.25% for growing pigs and 0.32% for finishers.

NRC (1987) give examples of the use of these prediction equations for pigs (pp. 36–37), but acknowledge that the agreement with published results was not always good.

# Ruminants

Prediction of intake by ruminants is often difficult because of the interactions between animal and diet and is particularly so under conditions where few reliable data are available on which to base equations, e.g. grazing. Despite these difficulties there have been numerous attempts at prediction of the voluntary intake of sheep and cattle. Because it is clear that intake is influenced by live weight, energy demand and food quality, it is natural that multiple regression analysis should be applied to data from sheep and cattle, particularly dairy cows.

The major interest has been for the lactating dairy cow; Conrad (1987) has summarized the prediction of food intake by dairy cows under North American conditions whereas the review by Forbes (1988a) covers the British situation.

## Food characteristics

Voluntary food intake is dependent to a considerable extent on the chemical and physical characteristics of the food(s) being eaten. It is likely, therefore, that incorporation of some measure(s) of food quality will improve the predictive ability of multiple regression equations. Parameters such as digestibility and rate of passage of food are functions of the animal and the food and should, in theory at least, be capable of being predicted from primary measurements made separately on the animal and the food. However, digestibility and rate of passage are to some extent dependent on the level of food intake so direct measurement is preferable to prediction until we have better understanding of the causal relationships between all of these factors.

## Cell wall constituents

As observed in Chapter 10, forage intake is inversely related to the cell wall constituents (CWC) content of the food. The observation that sheep ate a fairly constant quantity of CWC ($35 \, g \, kg^{-0.75} \, day^{-1}$) over a range of CWC contents from 350 to $750 \, g \, kg^{-1}$ (Mertens, 1973) further confirms the generality that forage intake is limited by the bulk of indigestible, or slowly digested, dietary constituents.

Van Soest (1982) has championed the cause of using the neutral detergent fibre method to measure CWC, as it gives a better estimate of extent of occupancy of food particles in the rumen than other measures such as crude fibre.

## Indigestible organic matter

Before the 1960s, several prediction equations had been derived, all based on the idea that ruminants ate until they were 'full'. Lehmann (1941; quoted in Balch and Campling, 1962) proposed a 'ballast' theory based on the observation that, on average, cows weighing $500 \, kg$ ate $4.3 \, kg \, day^{-1}$ of indigestible organic matter (IOM). Faecal output, included in the first equation of Conrad *et al.* (1964) is essentially IOM, and Hopkins (1985) used this to develop a practical system for predicting intake by dairy cows under British conditions. He accepted that with high energy diets the metabolic controls of intake are of prime importance, but argued that this is of academic interest in view of the need to feed as much forage as possible in order to reduce concentrate requirements. From a review of the literature Hopkins calculated that a mature cow can eat $6 \, g \, kg^{-1}$ body weight $day^{-1}$ of forage IOM whereas growing heifers and beef cattle only eat $4.5 \, g \, kg^{-1}$ of their body weight. When compound foods are offered the substitution rate which results is appropriate to an IOM concentration of $110 \, g \, kg^{-1}$ of concentrate dry matter (DM). Comparison of observed and predicted substitution rates showed that agreement is moderately good.

*Artificial mastication*

Smaller food particles disappear from the rumen faster than larger ones so that the ease with which a food can be masticated will affect rate of passage and thus food intake. Troelson and Bigsby (1964) developed a method of artificial mastication which involved gentle passage of the wetted food between gears followed by drying and estimation of particle size index ($P$). The close relationship ($r=0.94$) with intake by sheep ($DMI$ intake, g day$^{-1}$) was:

$$DMI = 353P - 14 \qquad\qquad (17.16)$$

which predicted forage intake by a 45 kg sheep to within 127 g day$^{-1}$.

*Density*

Baile and Pfander (1967) found a remarkably close correlation ($r=0.99$) between intake of a range of forage foods by sheep ($DMI$, ml weight$^{-0.66}$ day$^{-1}$) and food density ($p$, g ml$^{-1}$):

$$DMI = 73p - 1.20 \qquad\qquad (17.17)$$

Despite the likelihood that this would be a widely applicable equation, very few studies on density have been published. However, given that more fibrous material has a lower bulk density, other measures such as crude fibre and neutral detergent fibre are probably just as useful.

*Near infra red spectroscopy*

There is a need for better methods of food analysis, both to give results more quickly, preferably on the farm, and to give results which are better predictors of nutritive value and voluntary food intake than the laboratory methods currently in use. Near infra red spectroscopy (NIRS) is a promising tool for this purpose as it quickly and cheaply provides information on the whole chemistry of a food rather than the few specific moieties normally monitored. However, a large data bank of NIRS spectra for foods with known intake characteristics must be built up as this it not yet available.

**Animal/food interactions**

It could not be expected that only animal factors or only food factors could give reliable predictions of voluntary intake, when the control of intake is itself so dependent on both animal and food characteristics. However, methods which require measurements with animals, such as digestibility or rate of passage, will never be as useful as those which can be carried out more simply in the laboratory.

## Digestibility

Curren *et al.* (1970) used data from several experiments with dairy cows and found that forage digestibility and the weight of concentrates fed were the most effective predictors of forage intake, live weight and live weight change being of little value. During the last 4 weeks of pregnancy the best equation was

$$DOMI = 25D - 0.19D^2 - 847 \tag{17.18}$$

where *D* is digestibility (g per 100 g), which predicted intake of a single cow with an accuracy of 17%.

The analysis by Conrad *et al.* (1964) (see Chapter 10 for interpretation) showed two relationships dependent on the digestibility of the food:

$$\log I = 1.53\log D + 1.01\log F + 0.99\log LW - 5.3 \tag{17.19}$$

where *I* is intake (lb day$^{-1}$), *D* is DM digestibility (g per 100 g), *F* is a faecal DM output (lb day$^{-1}$) and *LW* is live weight (lb). This equation was appropriate for DM digestibilities below 67% for cows with moderate milk yields (17 kg day$^{-1}$), whereas for digestibilities above 67% the following was the best fit to the data:

$$\log I = 1.48 - 1.19\log D + 0.62\log LW + 0.27\log E \tag{17.20}$$

where *E* is estimated energy requirement (Mcal day$^{-1}$). The first of these shows that with poor and medium quality forages, intake is predicted very well by factors which described physical limits to intake, i.e. diet digestibility, faecal output (an index of physical capacity) and live weight. The form of this equation is multiplicative and this makes it difficult to reconcile with the concept of additivity of factors involved in feed intake control (Chapter 7).

The second equation shows intake to be well predicted by factors which describe metabolic factors, i.e. live weight$^{0.62}$ and energy required for lactation, although the latter is raised to a power of only 0.27; again the form of the equation is multiplicative and interpretation of its biological meaning is difficult.

Even highly digestible diets, for which physical factors should have little relevance, are eaten in smaller quantities by fatter animals and there is considerable evidence for a negative feedback from adipose tissue on food intake, although the mechanisms have not been fully elucidated (Chapter 8). One difficulty is that animals are often studied as they fatten so that they are younger when thin than when fat and may be in a different season of the year and on a different quality of food. Bines *et al.* (1969) overcame this by purposely underfeeding cows to make them thin or feeding a highly digestible food *ad libitum* to allow them to fatten; the treatments were then reversed so that each animal was studied in both fat and thin conditions. For cows in both conditions, intakes of a poor quality food were similar, but increased at different rates with increasing digestibility of the diet:

$$\text{Thin cows: } DMI = 0.026D - 7.14 \tag{17.21}$$
$$\text{Fat cows: } DMI = 0.019D - 4.55 \tag{17.22}$$

where *DMI* is intake (kg DM day$^{-1}$) and *D* is digestibility (g kg). This suggests that the metabolic feedback from fat, which can exert an effect on the intake of highly digestible foods, is more important than any physical effect. However, the poorly digestible food in this work was low in protein and it is likely that this limited the amount eaten rather than the animals' degree of fatness.

*Digestible energy*

With the increasing agricultural use of cereal-based rations for ruminants in the early 1960s, experiments were carried out which included foods with a wider range of digestibilities than had previously been used. Donefer *et al.* (1963) found a relatively constant digestible energy (DE) intake by sheep on foods containing 0–60% barley and having DM digestibilities of between 54 and 69%.

Figure 17.1 summarizes the results obtained by Dinius and Baumgardt (1970), who fed sheep on pellets containing various proportions of cereals and inert fillers. These results agreed with those of Conrad *et al.* (1964) in that intake (g day$^{-1}$) was positively related to DE concentration (proportional to DM digestibility) for diets with less than 10.5 kJ DE g$^{-1}$ DM:

$$\text{Intake} = 619DEC - 660 \tag{17.23}$$

where intake is kJ DE kg BW$^{0.66}$ and *DEC* is DE concentration in kJ g$^{-1}$. Above 10.5 kJ DE g$^{-1}$ intake of DE was almost constant:

$$\text{Intake} = 1007 - 50DEC \tag{17.24}$$

showing that intake was controlled to match energy requirements when physical constraints were not important.

Grovum (1987) suggests that the tendency for a negative slope on the latter relationship and in other published work indicates that intake is not perfectly controlled by metabolic mechanisms. The curvilinear nature of the data points around 10 KJ g$^{-1}$ must also be

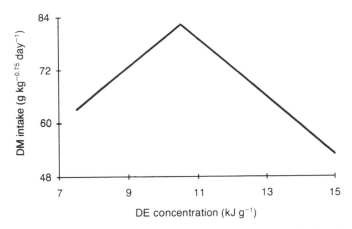

**Fig. 17.1.** Relationship between the digestible energy content of the food and its intake by sheep (Dinius and Baumgardt, 1970).

noted as an indication that the transition from physical to metabolic control of intake is not as clear-cut as was at one time imagined.

*Rates of degradation and passage*

Digestibility is relatively easy to measure but is probably not the most useful animal/food measurement for predicting intake. This is because some foods may be poorly digested but pass through the digestive tract relatively quickly, thereby occupying space for less time than a more digestible food with a slower rate of passage. For example, grinding a poor quality forage increases its rate of passage and intake but, because particles spend less time in the tract, they are less well digested. Rate of passage through the whole tract is not a good predictor of intake, however, but a more useful measurement is the rate of degradation of food in the rumen, carried out by suspension of nylon bags containing food samples in the rumen of fistulated animals. Carro *et al.* (1991) monitored the intakes of hays by sheep and the degradation characteristics, both for DM and for neutral detergent fibre (NDF). Disappearance from the bag was fitted to the equation of Ørskov and McDonald (1979):

$$y = a + b(1 - e^{-ct}) \qquad (17.25)$$

where $y$ is the DM or NDF disappearance (g kg$^{-1}$) from the bag after time $t$, $a$ represents the immediately soluble material, $b$ is the insoluble but potentially degradable material and $c$ is the rate of degradation. Carro *et al.* (1991) found significant relationships between voluntary intake and the soluble fraction of the DM, the rate of degradation of DM and the rate of degradation of NDF. The best fit, however, was

$$DMI = 21.3 + 0.073PSOL + 138DINSOL \qquad (17.26)$$

where *DMI* is voluntary DM intake (g kg$^{-0.75}$ day$^{-1}$), *PSOL* is the proportion of solubles in the DM and *DINSOL* is the rate of degradation of the insoluble potentially degradable fraction of the DM. Although NDF degradation characteristics were not as closely related to intake as those for DM in this set of forages, the simple correlation between intake and NDF content was highly significant ($r = -0.84$) which reinforces the importance of routinely measuring NDF in forage evaluation programmes.

Rate of digestion seems to be a better predictor of intake than digestibility but requires rumen-fistulated animals; what use is this when such variables cannot be measured on the farm which requires prediction? An *in vitro* method which can be automated and gives results which are almost as closely correlated with digestibility and intake as is degradation rate is the kinetics of gas production from samples of food incubated with rumen contents (Khazaal *et al.,* 1993). Gas pressure can either be read at various time intervals or monitored continuously by computer. The best prediction of voluntary intake of 10 hays by sheep ($R^2 = 0.63$) was provided by:

$$DMI = -47.7 + 4.25a + 2.12b + 444.5c \qquad (17.27)$$

where *DMI* is DM intake (g kg$^{-0.75}$), *a, b* and *c* are constants in equation 17.25. Direct measurement of degradation kinetics using nylon bags gave better results ($R^2 = 0.78$) but for considerably more labour and using more rumen-fistulated animals:

$$DMI = 10.3 + 0.53A + 0.70B + 199.4c \qquad (17.28)$$

where *A* is the water-soluble fraction lost in washing and *B* is the insoluble but fermentable fraction, $(a + b) - A$.

Mean retention time of organic matter in the rumen (*RTOM*, h) was closely ($r = -0.96$) related with intake of digestible organic matter (*DOMI*, g day$^{-1}$) for eight grasses and six legumes (Thornton and Minson, 1973):

$$DOMI = 1276 - 50.7RTOM \qquad (17.29)$$

## Growing cattle

Between-species comparison of the voluntary food intake of adult animals shows that intake is related to live weight$^{0.73}$ (metabolic live weight, Kleiber, 1961). Within a species the level of intake may also be

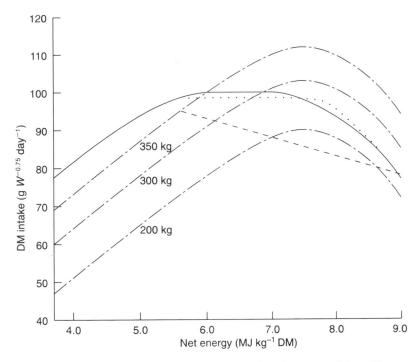

**Fig. 17.2.** Dry matter intake by growing cattle of foods with a range of digestible energy concentrations (four different studies, reported in NRC, 1987).

related to metabolic live weight, as observed for sheep by Blaxter *et al.* (1961) but the exponent is greater, the less digestible the food. This generally accepted relationship between intake and live weight does not hold good as a group of animals grow or fatten, however, as discussed in Chapter 8. For example:

$$DMI\,(\text{g day}^{-1}) = 172LW^{0.61} \tag{17.30}$$

calculated from the cattle data used by ARC (1980).

NRC (1986) show predictions of intake against net energy content of diet (Fig. 17.2). Intake per unit of metabolic body weight is stable or rising up to about 350 kg body weight, but falls above this weight.

Neal *et al.* (1988) used the ARC equation for prediction of intake in a computer program to ration beef cattle as this equation had been found to have lower prediction errors than several others tested:

$$DMI = 106.5q + 37C + 24.1 \tag{17.31}$$

where *DMI* is DM intake (g kg body weight$^{-0.75}$ day$^{-1}$), *q* is the metabolizability of the ration (MJ kg$^{-1}$ DM) and *C* is the proportion of concentrate in the ration (kg kg$^{-1}$). As they observed that this over-predicted by an average of 26% when compared with experimental data they used this equation but reduced by a factor of 0.26. Predicted silage intakes were still higher than those observed in several experiments, especially for short-chopped silage, and substitution rates were in a narrower range than actually observed. The authors suggested that the model would be much improved by inclusion of indices of silage quality and degradability.

Probably the most comprehensive study of intake prediction for beef cattle, which includes many chemical measures on silage (but not degradability), has been carried out by A.J. Rook and colleagues (Rook and Gill, 1990; Rook *et al.*, 1990a, b). They obtained data from almost 700 animals on over 60 silages and used live weight, intake and 16 silage characteristics in their predictions. In order to validate the predictions, data from another 57 silages, some fed to individuals, others to groups, were used. Ordinary least squares multiple linear regression had the major disadvantage of collinearity between variates leading to unstable estimates of regression coefficients and poor prediction in independent data sets. In order to produce better estimates, ridge regression methods were used which gave smaller errors than ordinary regression. The best equation using parameters which could be relatively easily measured was:

$$I = -5.84 - 0.615CDMI + 0.098TDM + 8.65\text{pH} - 0.049\text{NH}_3\text{-N}$$
$$+ 0.429\text{N} + 0.32DOMD \tag{17.32}$$

where $I$ is intake (g kg LW$^{-0.75}$), $CDMI$ is concentrate DM intake (g kg$^{-0.75}$ day$^{-1}$), $TDM$ is toluene DM (g kg$^{-1}$ fresh), NH$_3$-N is ammonia nitrogen (g kg$^{-1}$ N), N is total nitrogen (g kg$^{-1}$ TDM$^{-1}$) and $DOMD$ is the digestible OM in the DM (g kg$^{-1}$ TDM).

When the ridge regression equations were compared for their predictive ability with the ordinary regressions and with ordinary regressions with fewer variables, the mean square prediction errors (MSPE) were smaller for the ridge models and the reduced ordinary models (11% of the actual intakes) whereas the performance of the equations of ARC (1980) and Lewis (1981) was not so good (MSPEs of 18 and 16%, respectively); the multiple regression including all variables gave an intermediate error of 14%. Thus, it is not automatically better to include as many variables as possible in prediction equations; however, Rook's work did not clearly indicate which is the best subset of silage characteristics to measure and so does not lead immediately to reduced analytical costs.

## Dairy cows

Lactation generates a large increase in nutrient demands, especially in dairy cows which have been bred for high milk yields. Correlation coefficients for relationships between voluntary intake and milk yield have varied from less than 0.2 to 0.8 and intake is often more closely related to live weight than it is to milk yield. Simple relationships are unlikely to account for all the variations in intake which occur.

An approximate prediction of intake by dairy cows, taking live weight and milk yield into consideration, is provided by:

$$DMI = 0.025LW + 0.1MY \qquad (17.33)$$

or, for high-yielding cows

$$DMI = 0.022LW + 0.2MY \qquad (17.34)$$

(MAFF, 1975), where $DMI$ is total DM intake (kg day$^{-1}$), $LW$ is live weight (kg) and $MY$ is milk yield (kg day$^{-1}$).

A large set of data was assembled by Vadiveloo and Holmes (1979) from 385 cows in 26 experiments at five sites. Of the many regression models fitted, the one which explained most variation was their equation 2:

$$FDMI = 0.015LW + 0.21MY - 0.57C - 0.095WL$$
$$+ 4.04\log WL - 4.14 \qquad (17.35)$$

where $FDMI$ is forage DM intake (kg day$^{-1}$), $C$ is the amount of concentrate supplement (kg day$^{-1}$) and $WL$ is the week of lactation. The constant for milk yield is similar for the equations from MAFF (1975) and to the ME requirement for milk secretion and suggests that cows can adjust intake quite well to compensate for increased energy requirements when fed supplements according to recommendations.

In a comprehensive study (Rook *et al.*, 1991), data from 251 lactations of cows fed 14 different silages were used for prediction. Concentrates were given at flat rates not closely related to milk yield. Data from 192 lactations on 15 silages were used for validation. Five food variables were available (cf. 15 for the beef cattle study) and with this reduced number of variables no problems of collinearity among them were found. The negative relationship between level of concentrate supplementation and silage intake was linear over the range of conditions studied, with a coefficient (i.e. substitution rate) of −0.39 kg kg$^{-1}$. Live weight was best handled by using postcalving weight as an index of frame size and deviations from this as an index of body condition change. Better prediction was obtained using yield of milk fat plus protein than simply milk yield, milk fat or milk energy. There were no important effects of silage composition variables. The best model

(model 6 of Rook *et al.*, 1991), overall, was:

$$I = -3.74 - 0.39CDMI + 1.49(MF + MP) + 0.007LW \qquad (17.36)$$

where $I$ is silage intake (g DM day$^{-1}$), $CDMI$ is concentrate allowance (kg DM day$^{-1}$), $MF$ is milk fat (g kg$^{-1}$), $MP$ is milk protein (g kg$^{-1}$) and $LW$ is live weight (kg). This equation gave a mean square prediction error (MSPE) for weeks 3–9 of 1.88 (kg day$^{-1}$)$^2$ and for weeks 10–20, 1.52 (kg day$^{-1}$)$^2$. At 17 and 15% of mean intake, these MSPE values were better than those of Vadiveloo and Holmes (1979) (19 and 16% for early and mid-lactation, respectively).

There was greater variation in intakes in early lactation and improvement was obtained by considering weeks 3–9 separately and fitting time effects explicitly. The comprehensive equation for weeks 3–9 (equation 7 of Rook *et al.*, 1991) was:

$$I = -4.28 - 0.46CDMI + 1.44 (MF + MP) + 0.006PCLW + 0.01LWD$$
$$-0.0002LWD^2 - 0.0005NH_3\text{-}N + 0.012DOMD + 0.77WL$$
$$-0.04WL^2 \qquad (17.37)$$
$$(\text{MSPE } 2.12 \text{ (kg day}^{-1}\text{)}^2)$$

where $PCLW$ is postcalving live weight (kg). $LWD$ is live weight deviation from postcalving weight (kg), $NH_3\text{-}N$ is ammonia nitrogen (g kg$^{-1}$N), $DOMD$ is digestible organic matter in the DM (g kg$^{-1}$) and $WL$ is week of lactation.

For weeks 10–20 (equation 8 of Rook *et al.*, 1991) it was:

$$I = -57.7 - 0.48C + 3.09(MF + MP) + 0.006PCLW + 0.011LWD$$
$$-0.00003LWD^2 + 0.184 DOMD - 0.0001DOMD^2 \qquad (17.38)$$
$$(\text{MSPE } 1.74 \text{ (kg day}^{-1}\text{)}^2)$$

However, there was discontinuity between these models of the two stages of lactation and discrepancy in prediction of intake at the intersection (9–10 weeks of lactation). The remaining error was mainly due to random variation rather than consistent bias and suggests that emphasis should be given to obtaining more and better data rather than developing more sophisticated models. Rook *et al.* (1991) speculated that great improvements in prediction should not be expected as for groups of animals it was probably much better than for individuals; however, they did not test this proposition.

Investigation of lag between change in milk yield and change in intake, and possibility of autocorrelation between successive weeks did not yield any improvements in the models. The authors suggest that specific models for different situations be developed rather than a global equation.

*Stage of lactation*

Odwongo and Conrad (1983) found that intakes (*DMI*, kg DM day$^{-1}$) of groups of cows averaged over 2-week periods fit a quadratic equation with stage of lactation (*Days*) well, but individual cows show wide variation from this curve:

$$DMI = 11.21 + 0.11Days - 0.0003Days^2 \qquad (17.39)$$

From such intake prediction equations it is possible to derive predictions of the digestible energy concentration of food (*DEC*, Mcal kg$^{-1}$) necessary to allow maximum intake (Odwongo and Conrad, 1983):

$$DEC = 0.453LW^{0.59}M^{0.33}e^{0.16LWC}$$

where *M* is milk yield (kg day$^{-1}$), from which food intake can be calculated.

Although the curves of milk yield and voluntary food intake of cows during early lactation are approximately parallel there is usually a lag in voluntary intake and simple regression is not adequate to describe the relationship (Bines, 1979). The goodness of fit has often been found to be improved by inclusion of a term for the stage of lactation. Cows are usually given supplementary feeding during lactation and this invariably depresses forage intake; concentrate allowance is therefore a useful additional term to include in prediction equations.

The equation of Brown *et al.* (1977), in addition to animal factors (live weight, milk yield, milk fat, stage of lactation) included a quadratic relationship with the crude fibre content of the food:

$$\ln DMI = 0.52 - 0.00083DL + 0.148\ln DL + 0.339\ln MY + 0.099MF$$
$$+ 0.00068LW + 0.018CF - 0.00056CF^2 \qquad (17.40)$$

These authors state that milk yield is the most important factor in the prediction of voluntary intake.

*Live weight change*

In early lactation it is common for cows to mobilize body reserves which substitute for ingested food, and later in lactation to replenish these reserves by eating more than required for maintenance and lactation. The importance of live weight change as one of the predictors of intake was realized by Bines *et al.* (1977) whose equation for heifers was:

$$DMI = 0.16MY + 2.45LWC + 0.011LW + 4.25 \qquad (17.41)$$

where *LWC* is live weight change (kg day$^{-1}$).

However, live weight change is difficult to measure over short periods in ruminants and its interpretation is uncertain due to short-term effects of gut fill. Also, there is considerable uncertainty in most situations as to whether mobilization is the cause or the effect of a change in food intake.

Curran *et al.* (1970) found that for cows in the first 4 weeks of lactation live weight did not contribute usefully and the best equation was:

$$DOMI = 0.22LWC + 0.64CDM + 4.6D - 0.17MY$$
$$+ 0.003MY^2 - 6.8 \tag{17.42}$$

where *DOMI* is digestible organic matter intake (kg day$^{-1}$), *LWC* is live weight change (kg day$^{-1}$), *D* is digestibility (g kg$^{-1}$) and *MY* is milk yield (kg day$^{-1}$) with a limit of prediction for a single cow of 13%. The list of independent variables to be included to obtain the best correlation varied at different stages of the investigation, demonstrating the inadequacy of this approach to the general prediction of intake. The predominance of digestibility as a predictor in these equations demands that this parameter be known (or predicted with accuracy) and this is not feasible in practice; in the work of Curran *et al.* (1970) digestibility was estimated from regression equations based on dry cows and wether sheep data. These authors concluded that '... attempts to predict the intake of single cows are unlikely to be worthwhile in practice ... but the mean intakes of groups of 30 similar cows could be predicted with an acceptable level of accuracy for practical applications'. A similar conclusion was drawn from analysis of data from 72 grazing cows in which individual intakes could be predicted with tolerance limits of about 25% (Curran and Holmes, 1970).

*Comparisons of prediction equations*

There have been a few published comparisons of predictions by the equations described and observed intakes by cows. Brigstocke *et al.* (1982) found that Jersey cows in the seventh week of lactation ate 19.2 kg DM day$^{-1}$, much more than predicted by the equations of MAFF (1975) (13.3 kg), Vadiveloo and Holmes (1979) (17.6 kg; 18.5 for fat-corrected milk, FCM) or Bines *et al.* (1977) (12.5 kg). In late lactation, when intake was 12.8 kg DM day$^{-1}$, the equations predicted intakes of 11.7, 9.9 (10.3 for FCM) and 11.7, respectively. The Jersey is a lean breed with a high propensity to produce milk, both factors that tend to increase food intake. The great majority of dairy cows in Europe, however, are Friesians, which have a greater tendency to fatten, although much Holstein blood has been introduced from North

America which increases milking potential.

For North American conditions NRC (1987) compared predictions of six equations with a range of milk yields but offer no validation by comparison with independent data.

The most comprehensive comparison of prediction equations for dairy cows has been that of Neal *et al.* (1984). These authors used data collected over a period of nine years from British Friesian cows fed silage *ad libitum* plus various supplements, to compare with the predictions of seven equations. In addition to those mentioned above (MAFF, 1975, for average and high-yielding cows; Vadiveloo and Holmes, 1979, equation 2; Bines *et al.*, 1977), the others were:

$$TDMI = \{0.135LW^{0.75} + 0.2[MY - Y5000\,(n)]\}\,M \qquad (17.43)$$

(ARC, 1980, where Y5000 is the average milk yield for week $n$ with a total lactation yield of 5000 kg and $M$ is the adjustment for the month of lactation).

$$TDMI = 0.076 + 0.404C + 0.013LW - 0.129WL$$
$$+ 4.129\log WL + 0.140MY \qquad (17.44)$$

(Vadiveloo and Holmes, 1979, equation 1)

$$TDMI = SDMI.LW^{**}0.75)/1000 + C + 0.00175MY^{**}2 \qquad (17.45)$$

(Lewis, 1981) where

$$SDMI = 1.086I - 0.00247C'I - 0.00337(C')^{**}2 - 10.9 \qquad (17.46)$$

where

$$SI = 0.103SDM + 0.0516D - 0.05AN + 45.0 \qquad (17.47)$$

Actual and predicted weekly intakes were compared by calculating the MSPE:

$$MSPE = 1/t\,\text{sigma}\,(A - P)^{**}2 \qquad (17.48)$$

where $A$ is the actual intake and P the predicted intake.

When the observed weekly live weights were used both equations 1 and 2 of Vadiveloo and Holmes and that of Lewis gave the fewest MSPEs. Table 17.1 includes the MSPEs for four most widely-quoted equations, from the work of Neal *et al.* (1984) and also from that of Rook *et al.* (1991) who used different data for validation.

Many farms have no facilities for weighing cows; when the estimated weight after calving was used, together with notional live weight changes, equation 1 of Vadiveloo and Holmes was the best. Equations which gave the best predictions were all those which were derived from cows in similar conditions to those used for this comparison; they all also included some aspect of food quality, though

**Table 17.1.** Mean square prediction errors (MSPEs) for equations predicting the voluntary intake of cows, compared with independent data (Neal *et al.*, 1984; Rook *et al.*, 1991).

| Source | Equation | MSPE (kg DM day$^{-1}$)$^2$ | | | |
|---|---|---|---|---|---|
| | | All cows | Heifers | Adult cows | Weeks 10–26 |
| Vadiveloo and Holmes (1979) (equation 1) | 17.44 | 2.1 | 2.1 | 2.2 | 1.74 |
| Lewis (1981) | 17.45 | 2.5 | 2.0 | 2.8 | 2.11 |
| MAFF (1975) (mean yield) | 17.34 | 3.3 | 2.7 | 3.7 | 3.05 |
| ARC (1980) | 17.43 | 3.5 | 3.5 | 4.3 | 5.75 |
| Rook *et al.* (1991) (equation 8) | 17.38 | | | | 1.74 |

only that of Lewis specifically incorporated indices of silage quality and Rook *et al.* (1991) found little advantage in including silage characteristics in prediction equations for dairy cows.

Those equations which have no term for stage of lactation have high MSPEs in early lactation when intake is lower than expected. Least MSPE in the comparisons of Neal *et al.* (1984) was 1.8 kg DM$^2$ for heifers and 2.2 kg DM$^2$ for cows when weekly live weights were used; this lack of accuracy is a cause for concern but, in view of the complex factors affecting and controlling intake, it is doubtful whether further empirical investigations will be of benefit. Neilson *et al.* (1983) compared data collected from Friesian cows fed on a complete diet with five of the prediction equations outlined above. Although the observed DM intakes were not significantly different from any of the predictions, the errors were relatively large in some cases; the most suitable equation will depend on the variates available to be included.

Satter (quoted by NRC, 1987, p. 52) compared the predictions of the equation of Odwongo and Conrad (1983) with 10 sets of independent data and found a mean prediction error of 0.32 kg DM day$^{-1}$ (range −0.58 to +1.93). This is good agreement but it should be borne in mind that the validation data and the equations were for the same North American conditions, i.e. corn silage with high levels of concentrate supplementation.

AFRC (1991) reviewed prediction of silage intake by beef cattle and dairy cows. Prediction can be improved by (i) using a more comprehensive data set; (ii) using more variables; and (iii) using better models. For beef cattle, the ARC (1980) equation gave quite large mean prediction errors of 18% whereas that of Lewis (1981) gave 16%. The INRA fill system gave poorer predictions but the data were not designed to be used with this system and a number of assumptions were made concerning fill capacities of animals; to adopt this system in the UK would mean that more data would have to be collected.

### Prediction from early lactation measurements

Prediction will be much better if previous records are available from individual or groups of animals. Although typically this would be milk production and live weights in previous lactations, Persaud and Simm (1991) found that intake and efficiency recorded for a few weeks in early or mid-lactation are well correlated with these measures over the whole of the same lactation. Specifically with regard to voluntary intake, Simm *et al.* (1991) regressed food intake over the first 38 weeks of lactation on intake measured over shorter periods within that time and found intake in weeks 5–10 of lactation to be highly correlated ($r^2$ = 0.76) with intake over the whole 38 weeks. Thus, it is possible to monitor intakes for a short period (e.g. using the LUCIFIR system, Chapter 2) and to use these in the index for selecting heifers for a breeding programme.

### Sheep

A model was developed by Neal *et al.* (1985) to predict hay intake of pregnant ewes from the results of Orr and Treacher (1984) but linearized to enable the use of linear programming techniques:

$$HOMI = COMI(1.90 - 0.076WEEK - 1.87HOMD)$$
$$+ 2069HOMD - 88LS + 17.4LW - 1325 \qquad (17.49)$$

where *HOMI* is hay organic matter (OM) intake (g day$^{-1}$), *HOMD* is hay OM digestibility (g DOM g OM$^{-1}$). Rations were formulated to include the maximum proportion of hay while remaining within the intake limits provided by the equation; requirements are calculated from ARC (1980). The model was validated by comparison with other experimental results and found to perform reasonably well, but in general to predict lower voluntary intakes of hay than often observed which the authors ascribe to the high level of wastage in many large-scale experiments.

From a series of eight experiments, each with 48 ewes, Bocquier *et al.* (1987) derived the equation:

$$HDMI = 346 \pm 58A \pm 45B + 672W - 28.9WEEK \times WEEK - 1.53EC$$
$$+ 12.8EBW + 39.9EBWC + 1.72LGR - 1.28NDF - 0.55W \times NDF$$
$$+ 0.002EC \times NDF - 0.07W \times EC \qquad (17.50)$$

where *HDMI* is hay DM intake (g day$^{-1}$), $A = +$ for mature, $-$ for old ewes, $B = +$ for Romanov cross ewes, $-$ for Limousines, $EC =$ concentrate allowance (g day$^{-1}$), $EBW$ = ewe body weight at lambing (kg), $EBWC$ = ewe body weight change during lactation (kg per 6 weeks), $NDF$ = neutral detergent fibre content of hay (g kg$^{-1}$ DM), and $LGR$ = litter daily gain from 7 to 28 days (g day$^{-1}$). Despite the complexity of this equation it only accounted for 53% of the variation in hay intake.

Similarly, Orr and Treacher (1989) compiled results from several of their experiments with pregnant ewes fed silage and produced the equation:

$$SOMI = 1063COMI + 2882\ SOMD - 3.20SOMD \times COMI$$
$$+ 462\ WEEK - 14.71WEEK \times WEEK + 0.034\ WEEK \times COMI$$
$$+ 1.92SDM - 71.7\ LS + 9.08\ W - 5516$$

where $SOMI$ is silage OM intake (g day$^{-1}$), $COMI$ is intake of concentrates (g day$^{-1}$), $SOMD$ is OM digestibility of silage (g g$^{-1}$), $WEEK$ is week of pregnancy, $SDM$ is silage DM (g g$^{-1}$), $LS$ is litter size, and $W$ is body weight of the ewe 8 weeks before lambing.

## Combinations of relationships into predictive models

Even the most complex equation cannot adequately represent what we know to be the range of factors which affect intake and can therefore be used in its prediction. Some of these factors are discontinuous whereas others are conditional. Several prediction systems have been developed with the aim of making them more flexible and general than any one single equation. Some approaches involve iterative calculations and are as much to explore the limits of our understanding as they are to be used for predictions under practical conditions.

### Institut National de la Recherche Agronomique, France

A comprehensive documented system of prediction of food intake by ruminants has been developed by Jarrige and his colleagues of the National Institute for Agricultural Research of France (INRA, 1979; Jarrige *et al.*, 1986). This system depends on knowledge or prediction of the animal's ingestion capacity for a standard food, the ingestibility of a food relative to that of a standard food by a standard animal and substitution rates for concentrates in place of forages.

### The animal's ingestion capacity for a standard food
Observations of food intake of cows on 59 different dietary regimes, corrected to 600 kg live weight, showed that the ingestion capacity (bulk units for cattle, $BUC$) was closely related ($r = 0.88$) to milk yield

(kg of fat-corrected milk day$^{-1}$, $MY$):

$$BUC = 10.43 + 0.26MY \qquad (17.51)$$

The data were for cows having a mean yield of 17 kg day$^{-1}$ (range 10–28) at which level the capacity is 14.9 BUC. During the first month of lactation, and for the whole of the first lactation, ingestion capacity is reduced by 0.15 because heifers and recently calved cows have low voluntary intakes.

Coulon *et al.* (1989) found, for lactating dairy cows:

$$IC = 22 - 8.25 \exp(-0.02MP) + 0.01(LW - 600) \qquad (17.52)$$

where $IC$ is intake capacity (kg day$^{-1}$), $MP$ is milk production (kg FCM day$^{-1}$) and $LW$ is live weight (kg). Ingestion capacities for suckler beef cows are also tabulated by INRA (1979).

*The ingestibility of a food relative to that of a standard food by a standard animal*

The ingestibilities of some 2500 forages by 'standard' sheep (castrated males aged 1 to 3 years and weighing 40–75 kg) have been determined. A pasture grass which was used as the standard food had a mean intake by such sheep of 75 g kg$^{-0.75}$; on average this grass contained 150 g kg$^{-1}$ of crude protein and 250 g kg$^{-1}$ of crude fibre with an organic matter digestibility of 770 g kg$^{-1}$. By definition, 1 kg DM of this standard food has a bulk value of 1 bulk unit for sheep (BUS). Thus the BUS value for other forages is 75 divided by the amount of that forage consumed by the standard sheep per unit of metabolic live weight. Typically green leguminous plants have a BUS of around 0.8 whereas straws are 2–2.5 BUS.

The ingestibility of forages by cattle is higher than by sheep, for any given food. Data from a large number of feeding trials in which the same forage was offered *ad libitum* to both sheep and cattle were used to allow BUC to be predicted from BUS:

$$BUC = 57 + 0.87BUS \qquad (17.53)$$

Thus the standard grass has an ingestibility for cows of 122.6 g DM kg$^{-0.75}$ which for a 600 kg cow is 14.9 kg DM. The bulk value for a forage for cattle is therefore 122.6 divided by its ingestibility in cattle.

*Substitution rates for concentrates in place of forages*

The extent to which a unit of concentrate food will replace forage depends on the ingestibilities of both foods. A summary of 30 sets of data showed that substitution rates in dairy cows (kg change in forage

intake per kg concentrate increment, S) was related ($r = 0.87$) to the bulk
value of the forage as follows:

$$S = 1 - (BUC - 0.975)^{0.33} \qquad (17.54)$$

Substitution rates are low (0.2–0.4) for forages of poor to medium
ingestibility, but approach unity with high quality forages; this is
similar to the range of substitution rates normally encountered (Chapter 10).

Substitution is negatively related to the difference between the
energy of the forage fed alone and the animals' energy requirements –
the wider this gap, the lower the substitution rate. It is lower for high-
than low-producing animals.

$$S = 0.673 + 1.134OMD - 0.665FFV + 126.2PC - 118.2PC^2 \qquad (17.55)$$

where $S$ is substitution rate, $OMD$ is digestibility of OM ($g\,g^{-1}\,DM$),
$FFV$ is fill value of forage ($g\,g^{-1}\,DM$) and $PC$ is proportion of concentrates in ration ($g\,g^{-1}$).

As with the system of Hopkins (1985), that devised by INRA (1979)
is designed to be used in situations where physical factors are
predominant in the control of intake. That is, forages are to be used as
much as possible, concentrate supplements being given only to the
extent demanded by the desired level of production. However, there is
now a recognition that nutrient demand can exert some influence on
voluntary intake so it will be interesting to see how well the principles
and procedures adopted in the INRA system cope with the needs of the
farmer and his advisers.

### National Research Council, USA

NRC (1987) outline seven equations for predicting the food intakes of
beef cattle and give the limitations of each. Having concluded that none
of them includes all the important variables, NRC adopts a factorial
approach and presents equations and tables for adjusting predicted
intake for diet energy concentration, body fat, initial body weight,
breed, genetic variance, anabolic agents, food additives, particle size of
diet, environmental temperature, muddiness of ground, forage availability, grazing system, milk production, milk intake, pregnancy and
water intake. Space precludes a detailed synopsis of this work, but the
interested reader is strongly recommended to study it.

### Integration of physical and metabolic factors

Although physical limitation is undoubtedly predominant during the
first half of lactation with all but highly concentrated foods, a

comprehensive model should incorporate considerations of metabolic control. From a sheep model which predicts daily intake (Forbes, 1977a), a dairy cow model has been developed which includes both aspects (Forbes, 1977b). (Fig. 7.7). The primary purpose of the model was to explore the feasibility of integrating physical and metabolic controls of intake, but the predictions are at least as close to reality as those of several multiple regression equations.

ME requirements were calculated from estimates of requirements (MAFF, 1975) and ME intake matches these ME requirements when physical limits to intake are not operating. The physical limit was calculated from the equation (17.23) of Conrad *et al.* (1964, see above) and the capacity to handle bulk was varied inversely with the cow's fatness. The parameters of these equations will be improved as more data become available. Pregnancy, included in the sheep model (Forbes, 1977a), was not incorporated in the original cow model (Forbes, 1977b) but can be simulated by increases in ME requirements and by competition for abdominal space. The model was programmed to run iteratively so that the predictions for 1 day are used as the starting values for the next. A lactation curve of average shape (Wood, 1969) was

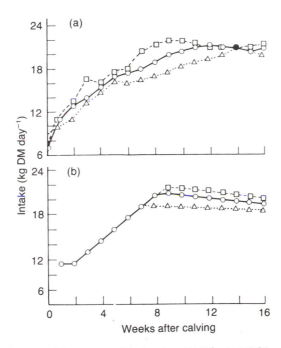

**Fig. 17.3.** Predictions of the cow model of Forbes (1977b, 1983) (b) and observed intakes of cows that were in fat (△), medium (○) and thin (□) condition at calving (Garnsworthy and Topps, 1982) (a).

taken, accepting that this was derived from cows which were fed mainly according to yield and may not be the optimum shape. Figure 17.3 shows (b) the predictions of voluntary intake for cows of different fatness at calving from this model compared with (a) the observations of Garnsworthy and Topps (1982). It can be seen that there is quite good agreement although it must now be accepted that it is not likely that all of the effect of body fat on food intake is via physical limitation, as supposed in this model.

The model of Illius and Gordon (1991) is discussed in Chapter 7. Although it includes 'Prediction of intake' in the title and deals with interactions between the ruminant animal and its food, it is more of a research tool than a practical method of prediction. The same could be said about the approaches of Fisher *et al.* (1987) and Poppi *et al.* (1994), which are also discussed in Chapter 7.

## Prediction of intake in grazing simulation models

### Cattle

When cattle are grazing herbage there are factors, such as the height or mass of the sward (Chapter 16) and the energy costs of grazing and walking (Chapter 15), which are additional to those which affect the intake of prepared foods indoors. Models of grazing behaviour are discussed in Chapter 16.

Caird and Holmes (1986) analysed data from several grazing experiments and found the equations with smallest prediction errors to be:

for rotationally-grazed dairy cows

$$TOMI = 0.323 + 0.177MY + 0.010LW + 1.636C - 1.008HM$$
$$+ 0.540HAL - 0.006HAL^2 - 0.048HAL \times C \qquad (17.56)$$

and for continuously grazed cows

$$TOMI = 8.228 + 0.208MY + 0.004LW + 0.609WL - 0.118C$$
$$- 0.289SHT + 0.133C \times SHT - 0.011WEEK \qquad (17.57)$$

where *HM* is herbage mass (tonnes OM ha$^{-1}$), *HAL* is herbage allowance (kg OM head$^{-1}$ day$^{-1}$), *SHT* is sward height (cm) and *WEEK* is week of calendar year.

When it is considered that these two equations were derived from cows of similar type and all under UK conditions, there are some remarkable differences. Concentrate supplementation gives a large increase in total DM intake under rotational grazing but has almost no effect (substitution rate close to 1) with continuous grazing; these are below and above, respectively, the normal range of substitution rates consistently encountered when feeding cows indoors. Also, the sets of variables found to explain most of the variation in intake are very different for the two grazing conditions, making it very difficult to see how they could be used except under conditions very close to those from which the equations were derived.

*Sheep*

The types of model described for indoor conditions must be developed to incorporate the seasonal changes in quality and availability of grass. There have been several modelling approaches to predicting intake and performance of sheep at grass, rather than the multiple regression approach predominantly used for cows.

Rice *et al.* (1974) estimated intake from the digestibility of the available herbage and used known relationships between dietary quantity and quality and rumen fermentation to predict yields of nutrients and rumen capacity available to receive food the next day. Incorporated into a comprehensive model of range management, this system of predicting intake gave a high correlation ($r=0.93$) between predicted and observed weight gains of sheep.

Neither of these approaches to the simulation of grazing intake included any acknowledgement that intake is affected by the nutrient requirements of the grazing animal. This was taken into account in the comprehensive simulation of forage intake by sheep which was undertaken by Vera *et al.* (1977). The relationship used between voluntary intake ($I$) and green herbage on offer ($x$) was:

$$I = A[1 - B\exp(kx)] \tag{17.58}$$

where $A$ is the mature weight of the animal and with $B$ set to 1 and $k$ to 0.025. Intake of dead forage increased asymptotically with the amount of dead material and decreased with the amount of green material on offer. Maximum intake was taken to be $81\,\text{g DM kg}^{-0.75}$ day$^{-1}$. Pregnancy was not considered to affect intake whereas for lactation the relationships found by Hadjipieris and Holmes (1966) were used to calculate a modulator for intake, adjusted for the mean differences in milk yield between breeds. The effects of body weight on intake were included by calculating the expected weight-for-age from a Gompertz growth curve and adjusting intake upwards for animals which were lighter than expected and downwards for overweight animals. This neatly simulates the high intake during compensatory growth and the low intake of fat ewes. The digestibility of herbage was estimated and the digestible organic matter intake was derived from estimates of ash content. An attempt was then made to partition nutrients between growth and lactation and this, together with any changes in availability and digestibility of the grass were used in the calculation of intake for the next iteration. Within the limits of Merino ewes and swards of perennial ryegrass, the simulations agree closely with observed performance.

In the model of Arnold *et al.* (1977) potential DM intake per kg of live weight of ewes was inversely related to live weight by an equation derived from field data with a reduction for young ewes:

$$\text{Potential OMI(g day}^{-1}) = \text{lwt}\{47.8 + 0.98[1.0 - \exp(-0.052\text{lwt})]\} \quad (17.59)$$

This was then adjusted for ratios of green:dead material and clover:grass, for digestibility and for nitrogen content.

Although a negative effect of live weight on intake is appropriate for wether sheep, potential intake should be predicted according to physiological state in the breeding ewe. Such a relationship is a feature of the comprehensive model of lamb production developed by Edelsten and Newton (1977); the depressing effect of concentrate supplementation on grass intake is also incorporated.

Sibbald *et al.* (1979) used a positive linear relationship between intake and digestibility and based digestibility of the whole diet on the proportions of green and dead material in the sward. The level of intake predicted by this equation was then reduced according to the fatness of the grazing mature sheep and was also reduced if there was less than 1000 kg DM available herbage per hectare. In addition, the proportion of green:dead material was calculated from the time of year and the grazing pressure and this ratio was used in the determination of digestibility for the next iteration. This model adequately simulated the real situation for two stocking rates.

*Australian system for predicting herbage intake*

In a comprehensive consideration of factors affecting voluntary intake by ruminants, the Australian Standing Committee on Agriculture; Ruminant Subcommittee (1990) have incorporated a series of equations into a model for prediction of intake by grazing ruminants with or without supplements. This information will also be useful for housed animals on forage diets, but not for concentrates. Two factors are considered to affect intake: the potential intake by the animals and the relative intake offered by the pasture.

*Potential intake of the animal*
Potential is clearly proportional to the size of the animal, to which nutrient demand and physical capacity are both related. Within a species they consider there is little justification for using an exponent

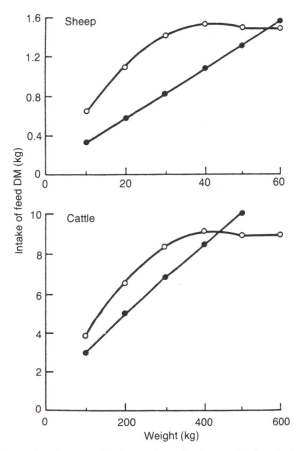

**Fig. 17.4.** Relationships between body weight and voluntary food intake by sheep and cattle; ○, Australian Standing Committee on Agriculture; Ruminant Subcommittee (1990); ●, ARC (1980).

of live weight other than 1.0. To allow for the fact that a fat animal has a lower potential intake than a thin animal of the same body weight, potential intake is predicted from the standard reference weight (SRW) of the animal (i.e. mature and in the middle of the condition score range) and the current size relative to the mature size. Figure 17.4 presents predicted intakes from this equation and those from ARC (1980) compared to which predictions are higher for young animals, but similar for animals at maturity. The INRA system appears also to underpredict intake by immature animals. No effect of pregnancy is incorporated as it was felt that any influence of increased nutrient requirements would be balanced by inhibition due to space restriction and/or hormones.

For predicting intake during lactation a multiplier is calculated and applied to potential intake based on ewe size and fatness and on herbage characteristics:

$$\text{ewes: multiplier}=1.0+0.025n(T^{1.4})\exp(-0.05T) \qquad (17.60)$$
$$\text{cows: multiplier}=1.0+aT^{1.7}\exp(-0.021T) \qquad (17.61)$$

where $n$ is 1.0 for a single lamb and 1.35 for twins; $a$ is 0.0013 for beef cows and 0.0024 for dairy cows; and $T$ is time from parturition in days. For dairy cows, the multiplier is appropriate for a yield of $SRW/20$ kg FCM per day, and for a different potential yield, $Y$, the value of the multiplier is increased by 0.013 ($Y-SRW/20$).

In young animals, intake depends on the degree of rumen development rather than on body weight and a multiplier for potential intake, $s$, is used:

$$s=1.0/(1.0+\exp(0.2(X-T))) \qquad (17.62)$$

where $T$ is days from birth and $X$ is 25 days for lambs and 60 for calves.

It was acknowledged that it is difficult to predict the effects of high temperatures, but for cattle of temperate breeds intake is reduced by 2% for each degree increase in temperature over 25°C whereas for Brahman cattle and sheep the reduction is 1% per degree. In cold conditions it was assumed that the increase in energy requirements is offset by effects of rain and mud, and no attempt at modifying predictions for cold weather were made.

*Relative intake offered by the pasture*
This is influenced by the chemical composition of sward and physical features which limit eating.

The weight of herbage eaten is a function of rate of eating and time spent eating which in turn is a function of herbage availability:

$$F = ET = [1.0-\exp(-aH)][1.0+b.\exp(-kH^2)] \qquad (17.63)$$

where $F$ is relative availability (g day$^{-1}$), $E$ is rate of eating (g min$^{-1}$), $T$ is time spent grazing (min day$^{-1}$), $H$ is the weight of herbage available (tonnes h$^{-1}$) and $a$, $b$ and $k$ are constants which for sheep are 1.5, 0.6 and 1.4, respectively. Over 2 tonnes of herbage per hectare feeding is considered not to be limited by availability. Figure 17.5 shows the relative values of $F$, $E$ and $T$ for different amounts of available herbage for sheep of a standard type.

It is not sufficient to assume that all herbage material is the same; material must be classified into several compartments and then 'rules' determined concerning animals' responses to the presence of different amounts of various types of material. New growth enters the first class and then, after a given number of days, if it has not been eaten, enters

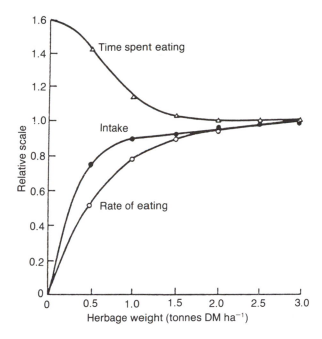

**Fig. 17.5.** Effect of herbage availability on herbage intake rate of eating and time spent eating by sheep. (Australian Standing Committee on Agriculture; Ruminant Subcommittee, 1990).

the second, and so on, each class having a lower digestibility and desirability than the one before. An animal attempts to satisfy its requirements from each class in turn, starting with the youngest.

Take the case where the digestibilities of the five classes are 0.8, 0.7, 0.6, 0.5 and 0.4 and the weights of the five classes are 0.20, 0.44, 0.12, 0.04 and 0.0. The relative capacity for class 1 is 1.0 and relative availability, as defined in equation 17.65, is 0.41 so that the relative intake is $1.0 \times 0.41 = 0.41$. Thus, the relative capacity for class 2 is $1 - 0.41 = 0.59$, and so on. To predict daily intake the total intake of all classes is multiplied by the potential intake as calculated from the animal factors. The overall digestibility of the diet is calculated from the weight of each class eaten multiplied by its digestibility, adding all these and then dividing by total intake.

$$\text{Relative intake} = FC[1.0 - H(0.8 - D) + 0.17G] \qquad (17.64)$$

where $H = 1.7$ for introduced grasses (ryegrass, etc.) or 1.0 for native Australian grasses and $G$ is the proportion of legume in the sward.

Where the sward is relatively stable, daily iteration is satisfactory but where the situation is changing rapidly, e.g. short rotational systems, it may be necessary to do calculations every hour or two where herbage availability is falling measurably during the day. Estimation of the amount of herbage available is by eye or by meter (e.g. rising plane meter). Digestibility should be measured but this is normally impractical, so educated guesses have to suffice.

The requirement for rumen degradable protein (RDP) is $8.4$ g $MJ^{-1}$ of ME and predicted intake falls in proportion to the deficit in RDP. Deficiencies of sulphur and other minerals are also important but quantitative relationships are not reliable and have therefore not been incorporated in the model.

As for substitution rate, it is simply assumed that the animal will select the supplement before it starts to select herbage, i.e. the supplement is class zero in the above-mentioned classification of herbage. Table 17.2 shows the effect of offering 200 g of high quality supplement per day to sheep. The predictions are for substitution rate to rise from 0 when no herbage is available, rising quite steeply to a value of about 0.8 at 1 tonne of herbage per acre, then slowly approach 1.0 at an infinite amount of herbage for a pasture digestibility of 700 g $kg^{-1}$. For a pasture of 500 g $kg^{-1}$ digestibility, substitution rate never goes above about 0.5 for a supplement with a high digestibility (800 g $kg^{-1}$). For a supplement of low digestibility (600 g $kg^{-1}$) there is predicted to be a much higher substitution rate for poor pastures and refusals of good pasture. In protein-limiting swards, high protein supplements increase intake up to the

**Table 17.2.** Calculation of substitution rate in the Australian system for predicting the intake of grazing ruminants (Australian Standing Committee on Agriculture; Ruminant Subcommittee, 1990). See text for details.

|  | Supplement | | | | | |
|---|---|---|---|---|---|---|
| Herbage class | 0 | 1 | 2 | 3 | 4 | 5 |
| Digestibility (g $kg^{-1}$) | 800 | 800 | 700 | 600 | 500 | 400 |
| Weight of herbage |  | 0.2 | 0.44 | 0.12 | 0.04 | 0.0 |
| Weight of supplement | 0.2 |  |  |  |  |  |
| Relative capacity |  | 1.0 | 0.89 | 0.52 | 0.15 | 0.11 |
| Relative availability |  | (0.11) | 0.37 | 0.36 | 0.04 | 0.01 |
| Relative intake |  | 0.37 | 0.30 | 0.03 | <0.01 |  |
| Cumulative intake |  | 0.37 | 0.67 | 0.70 |  |  |
| Actual intake (kg) | 1.05 |  |  |  |  |  |
| Reduction in herbage intake | 0.12 |  |  |  |  |  |
| Substitution rate | 0.60 |  |  |  |  |  |

FC for supplement is proportion of relative capacity which is satisfied by the supplement.

point where RDP is sufficient. The committee's opinion is that more critical work is needed, particularly in the area of substitution rate.

## Conclusions

For the prediction of intake in a situation where a large body of data is already available the use of regression equations is valid. The important independent variables for dairy cows usually include live weight, milk yield, live weight change and some index of forage quality.

A more complex system of prediction has been developed in France, based on forage fill units, whereas in the USA the quantitative effects of numerous factors affecting intake have been compiled but not developed into an integrated production system.

A more fundamental approach involves combining relationships between metabolic and physiological parameters at a lower level of organization than the whole animal and constructing a model. Such an approach is potentially applicable to any situation but so far has not yielded simulations which are sufficiently accurate for general use, although the grazing model developed in Australia seems promising.

# 18 EPILOGUE

- Sensing the environment
- Gastrointestinal receptors
- Metabolic receptors
- Central nervous involvement
- Future experimentation
- Practical considerations for farm animals

This chapter brings together various threads which have been running through the rest of the book and provides a personal view of how voluntary food intake and diet selection might be controlled. We can no longer look upon the various theories of intake control as alternatives but rather as complementary and contributing to a multifactorial control system. No single factor is essential for normal feed intake and many manipulations which stay within the physiological range have effects which can only be picked up by close attention to details of feeding behaviour. As Novin (1983) says, there are no necessities to satiety, only sufficiencies.

## Sensing the Environment

### General senses

The first primitive organisms to evolve the capacity to move must also have developed receptors to inform them of the environment in which they found themselves, otherwise they would have no reason to use the new-found ability of locomotion. Initially the receptors would be likely

416

to sense chemicals to which the proto-animal would respond by moving towards (food) or away from (toxins). Multicellular organisms developed a coelom and eventually a digestive system in which to store and digest food. The contents of the digestive system are outside the body proper and their composition is still sensed, but now a mechanism is required to encourage the ingestion of some substances (food) and to avoid ingesting others (toxins). Special senses developed to allow the animal to sense the outside world separately from the world within the digestive tract and to allow it to make decisions about what (and how much?) to eat, based either on innate preferences or on previous experience.

*Special senses*

In mammals, the taste of potential food is used as a powerful cue to its nutritive value. In some cases (e.g. sugar) the connection between the taste and the nutritive value is close and an innate link can be established. In other cases the nutrient cannot itself be sensed and the animal must learn to rely on some other, proximate, feature of a food source to determine whether it is likely to provide the nutrient in question. Thus, learned associations between the sensory properties of foods and their nutritive value are likely to be very primitive ones which can function at the subconscious level. For example, the ability of the effects of a painful stimulus administered to an anaesthetized animal to become associated with the food available just before anaesthetization (Provenza *et al.*, 1994a).

What are the most appropriate means of differentiating foods for different types of animal? We know that mammals are more sensitive to taste whereas vision is more important in birds, but are there particular characteristics which make it easier for animals to learn to associate a food with the metabolic consequences of eating that food? Is a combination of cues, e.g. colour and taste, more effective than one single cue?

# Gastrointestinal Receptors

As the receptors in the wall of the digestive tract are no longer in direct contact with the external environment the information they provide cannot be used directly to seek or reject food (except in the case of vomiting). However, their responses can be used as the conditioning stimulus for learned preference or aversion to food with a particular taste, or other characteristic sensory property such as colour. Nausea or other feelings of illness, especially when of abdominal origin, are powerful conditioning stimuli presumably because they presage more serious illness and/or vomiting. Vomiting is so aversive because when repeated it causes severe damage to mouth and teeth due the acid and enzymes from the stomach; also to expend resources seeking and eating food and then not to obtain any nutritive value from that food is wasteful in the extreme and waste is minimized by evolution.

The visceral organs of the ruminant are well supplied with receptors for mechanical, chemical and (probably) osmotic stimuli, with afferent information passing to the central nervous system (CNS) by the vagal and splanchnic routes. Although numerous experiments have been performed in which the natural stimulation of these receptors by digesta has been augmented by balloon distension or introduction of chemicals into the rumen, these have often generated conflicting results. Specifically, how does osmolality exert its effect on food intake via the rumen when it has proved to be so difficult to identify osmoreceptors? Of the three major volatile fatty acids, why does butyrate exert least effect on feeding when infused into the rumen but have the greatest effect on chemoreceptors?

## Metabolic Receptors

The gastrointestinal receptors cannot be expected to guide the animal to eat amounts and mixtures of foods which meet the animals' requirements. Such control must come from within the animal and receptors must exist which monitor the supply in relation to the demand. It is unlikely that there is a specific receptor for each of the 50 or so essential nutrients and even if there were such prolificacy of receptor types, how would each one know whether the level of the nutrient it sensed was sufficient or not? Nutrients are essential when they act either as substrates for, or enzymes and cofactors in, essential metabolic pathways, so it would seem sensible to look for ways in which the CNS could be informed about the state of a few critical metabolic pathways. One such appears to be the pathway whereby energy is made available in the liver (Chapter 3).

The concept of a requirement for a nutrient is difficult to sustain when an animal functions quite well over a range of levels of supply of each nutrient, adapting to an excess by eliminating or storing the unwanted material and to a deficiency by reducing the rate of the pathway in question. The concept of 'responses to nutrients' and hypotheses that animals endeavour to eat quantities of nutrients which support maximum growth or milk production or that they eat to optimum efficiency do not seem realistic. Rather, animals eat to achieve the most comfortable situation metabolically which does, in practice, often mean that they eat that amount and proportion of foods which allows them to be most efficient.

Whatever their nature, the signals generated by the animals' metabolism can be used as conditioning stimuli for learned preferences for food, both in terms of quality and quantity. An animal whose metabolism is provided with too much glucose in relation to lysine may attempt to redress the balance by eating more food (to increase the lysine supply), eating less food (to reduce the glucose supply), or eating a different mixture of foods, if it has the choice (to correct the glucose:lysine imbalance). Which of these actions it takes will depend not only on its immediate circumstances (is there a choice of foods available?) but on its nutritional and metabolic history (what has it learned previously about how to cope with the imbalanced situation?).

Despite our appreciation of the importance of learning and our knowledge of receptors in the visceral organs, we are still left with the problem of knowing how animals are able to regulate food intake with such apparent accuracy in relation to their requirements for normal growth, reproduction and fattening. We know, for example, that pigs in the UK used to become very fat if fed *ad libitum*, so they clearly had the capacity to eat, digest and metabolize great quantities of nutrients. Genetic selection for leanness over the last few decades has produced pigs which have a low level of food intake so presumably the lower propensity to fatten has caused the lower food intake – intake is responding to demand. Reduced fat synthesis results in reduced uptake of precursors into adipose tissue and this must lead to metabolic discomfort which, in turn, reduces voluntary intake. Is the metabolic discomfort in this case simply an excess of fatty acids for oxidation in the liver?

A related issue is the ability of animals to select between two foods, a mixture of which provides the most appropriate intake of energy and another nutrient, e.g. protein. Pigs with greater potential rates of lean tissue deposition choose to eat food with a higher protein:energy ration than pigs with a greater propensity to fatten. Again, this must be related to the ability of the foods to provide metabolic comfort.

How are we to proceed experimentally to unravel the concept of metabolic comfort?

## Central Nervous Involvement

In higher animals all the capabilities of learning are concentrated in the brain and closely related structures (CNS). The CNS is provided with information by the special senses, gastrointestinal receptors and metabolic sensations and it can use any or all of these as conditioning agents.

It may learn, for example, that food with certain sensory characteristics leads to certain unpleasant gastrointestinal consequences and avoid eating it on that basis. Another food may be recognized as one which alleviates a metabolic imbalance and become preferred for that reason.

It is also likely that the CNS is directly sensitive to its own nutrient supply, particularly to energy deficit. However, it is the duty of much of the rest of the body, particularly the liver, to prevent shortages of nutrient supply to the brain (excesses are not so damaging) so the CNS should not normally have to take action to eat food, or avoid eating food, based on its own metabolic status.

# Future Experimentation

## Experimental design

Attempts to understand what causes animals to stop eating have often involved injection of putative satiety factors into parts of the digestive or vascular systems with observation of food intakes during and after the injection period. In a 'well-designed' experiment each animal is given each treatment only once before it is given control and other treatments in a Latin square design. Thus, the animals are not given the opportunity to learn to associate the effects of the injection with any characteristic of the food and are denied an important route of control which is normally open to them, namely learned associations between the sensory properties of the food, its eventual visceral effects and yields of metabolites. It is postulated that many such experiments have either under- or overestimated the satiating effects of metabolites; some may even have shown no effects of a factor which is, under 'natural' circumstances, actually quite important and vice versa. Consider the dilemma of an experimental animal who, despite continuing to eat the same safe food as usual, suddenly feels ill (or metabolically uncomfortable) due to an infusion of an imbalancing nutrient. The immediate effect of the feeling of illness is to depress food intake but a longer-term effect might be to render that food aversive, especially if the treatment is repeated on other days. However, on non-experimental days, or during control infusions, the same food is once again safe. Does the animal learn to associate the presence of the white-coated experimenter with illness and the blue-overalled technician with well-being? Whatever the outcome, it would hardly be surprising if it became very confused and gave results which were difficult to interpret.

If we are to discover the real significance of putative factors involved in the control of food intake we must give animals the chance to learn about their effects in a much more natural way than the change-over experiments outlined above. During the periods when the animals are exposed to the experimental treatment they should be given a food with distinctive sensory properties, different from the one they normally eat. The treatment–food pairing should be repeated on several occasions to allow the association to be established and, in addition to recording intake during these treatment periods, the animal should be allowed to demonstrate its feelings for the experimental food, either by recording intake of the stimulus paired food in the absence of the treatment stimulus or by assessing the animal's preference for this food against another distinctive food which has been paired with a control treatment. For example, not only does cholecystokinin (CCK) depress food intake in broiler chickens but it also leads to a conditioned aversion for the colour of food on offer after the injection of CCK, relative to a food of a different colour which was available after saline injections (Covasa and Forbes, 1994a). Although learned aversions to novel foods by farm animals have been demonstrated many times, particularly by Provenza and colleagues, learned preferences are just starting to be studied (F.D. Provenza, personal communication). However, the development of specific appetites for nutrients, where animals not only avoid eating too much of a substance but also avoid eating too little, are clear evidence that learning to balance the diet is possible; indeed it is much more important than unrefined learned aversion or learned preference.

### Experimental complexity and the role of modelling

The complexity of the control of food intake suggests that complex experiments must be performed to advance our understanding of the system. However, the more elaborate the experiment the more likelihood there is of problems occurring where the main parameter to be measured is voluntary food intake, subject as it is to large between- and within-animal variation and to the well-being of the experimental animals. Although some complicated experiments may still be necessary, progress can be made by an alternative strategy involving testing of simple hypotheses and linking of ideas and data by simulation models. Toates and Booth (1974) were the first to adopt this approach for the rat, and assumed additivity of effects of the energy yielded by a meal and its distending effects in the viscera. Their model generated realistic predictions concerning meal size and interval. A similar approach was adopted for ruminants by Forbes (1980) but assuming that feeding was inhibited either by energy-yielding products of digestion or by rumen fill. Again the predictions were reasonably realistic but clearly this model needs to be updated to take account of the likely additivity of negative feedback effects, rather than their exclusivity.

We need to perform well-controlled, critical experiments to clarify individual parts of the jigsaw, and to integrate this with models and to validate the models with other, independent results. Given the key role of learning in the control of food intake and diet selection, it will be necessary to use artificial intelligence techniques in future models, but such applications are only just beginning. It may well be that intake control is so complex that it will not be fully understood until we have models as complex as animals themselves.

## Practical Considerations for Farm Animals

### A balanced diet

Voluntary intake of a single food will be likely to be at an adequate level to meet most closely the animal's 'requirements' when it provides nutrients in a ratio which is close to that with which the animal uses those nutrients, i.e. a well-balanced food. Where the food is imbalanced then intake might increase and the animals thereby take in too much energy and become fat, or intake might decrease if the imbalance causes severe metabolic discomfort. The problem of deciding when a food is balanced is particularly difficult in the case of ruminants, in which considerable modification of some food constituents takes place before absorption. The relative amounts of acetate, propionate and butyrate produced by rumen fermentation are unlikely to match exactly the amounts required for the animal's metabolic processes, resulting in a situation of imbalance. Although the amount of acetate absorbed from the rumen of a lactating cow offered forage might be adequate to support the synthesis of milk fat, the amount of propionate might be insufficient for gluconeogenesis to support milk lactose synthesis. An increase in voluntary intake to supply the propionate would result in overproduction of acetate and either a return to undereating or an increase in body fat deposition. The practical solution is to supplement the forage with concentrates which provide a higher propionate:acetate ratio thus balancing the forage and overcoming the imbalance.

It is possible that a rumen fermentation modifier, by increasing the propionate:acetate ratio, might increase the intake of a forage. However, the forage may well have other imbalances, such as a gross deficiency of protein or an imbalance in the ratio of amino acids, which prevent a higher level of voluntary intake even when the VFA balance is corrected. The problem of amino acid supply is of particular importance in ruminants in which dietary nitrogen sources are considerably metabolized by the rumen microflora to produce an imbalanced mixture of absorbed amino acids even when the dietary amino acid mixture was balanced. Hence the importance of providing sources of some essential amino acids which escape rumen degradation (UDP) as well as sufficient sources of degradable nitrogen so as not to limit microbial activity in the rumen (RDP).

Adequate ways of predicting the yields of absorbed nutrients from the composition of the diet and the characteristics of the animal are therefore of the utmost importance and dynamic modelling, supported by appropriate experimentation, provides the best chance of achieving this.

## Choice feeding

Chapters 13 and 14 have provided many examples of the ability of animals to correct nutritional imbalances by making appropriate choices from two or more foods. Although there is some commercial interest in choice-feeding using whole cereal grains for poultry, it is with ruminants that the greatest potential lies, given our relative ignorance of the ability of forage foods to provide a balanced diet in most situations. We have ample evidence that ruminants are capable of making nutritionally wise choices between foods but, as yet, no attempts have been made to develop choice-feeding to answer the problems outlined above. There is a rational fear that, given free access to concentrates, animals would gorge themselves in the short term and eat wastefully large amounts in the long term. However, it may be that offering choices between two forages or a forage and a by-product such as brewer's grains would actually reduce the need for concentrate supplementation.

It would be a mistake to expect choice feeding to solve all the problems of nutrition of farm animals. We do not yet know the limits to animals' ability to select appropriately in situations where one food is scarce or where one food contains innately-aversive compounds, even where these are not toxic. As shown in Fig. 13.2 apparently similar animals can show quite different levels of intake and dietary preference and it is not known to what extent this is due to differences in their nutritional history and nutrient requirements and to what extent it is inexplicable, random, variation.

## Welfare

In the wild most animals have access to, and eat from, a variety of food materials. Two of the 'five freedoms' to which farm animals are entitled are 'freedom from hunger and thirst' and 'freedom to indulge in most natural forms of behaviour'. Where a dietary imbalance exists, which according to the discussion above causes metabolic discomfort, choice feeding is clearly good for the welfare of animals. What is less certain is whether the welfare of animals given a completely balanced diet *ad libitum* can be improved by access to a choice in order to allow them to indulge in the natural behaviour of diet selection and to be given a feeling of some control over their own lives.

# Appendix 1
# Particular Features of
# Poultry and Ruminant
# Animals

The structure and function of the digestive tract and its associated organs and the metabolism of nutrients in omnivorous species such as the pig, rat and man are described in standard texts (e.g. Davenport, 1966). A brief description of the ways in which digestion differs in poultry and ruminants is given in the following pages.

## Poultry

The avian species commonly used as farm animals are omnivorous and include the domestic fowl (chicken), turkey, duck, goose and quail. Sturkie (1976) gives a comprehensive account of avian physiology.

Birds secrete saliva but do not chew their food. There is a pouch in the wall of the lower oesophagus, the crop, which can store food and where a small degree of fermentation can occur. In chickens the crop is often filled before dusk and empties slowly during the night-time fast (Savory, 1979). The true stomach is the proventriculus which is followed by the gizzard, a thick-walled, muscular organ in which particles of food, particularly seeds, can be ground with pieces of grit which the bird eats. The small intestine is short (1200 mm) in relation to the size of the bird. There are two long narrow caecae and the rectum opens into a cloaca so the faeces and urine are mixed before being voided (Hill, 1976).

The modern hybrid laying hen, weighting about 2.2 kg lays about 280 eggs per year which involves the secretion of some eight times its body protein, six times its body fat and 32 times its body calcium (Fisher, 1983).

*Appendix 1*

A major difference from mammalian metabolism is the fact that lipids are synthesized in the liver as well as in adipose tissue to be transported in the blood to adipose tissue or to the ovary (for yolk formation); plasma lipid levels are, therefore, very high especially in the laying hen. Further differences lie in the very high plasma glucose concentrations (220–250 mg 100 ml$^{-1}$), the small change in blood glucose during fasting and the relative lack of effect of insulin on blood glucose levels. Glucagon appears to play an important part in the control of energy metabolism in birds.

# Ruminant Animals

Ruminants, like pigs, are even-toed ungulates but with jaws and teeth modified for harvesting grass in addition to the adaptations of the digestive tract. The lower front teeth are sharp and press grass against the hard pad of the upper jaw. The molar teeth grind, both during eating and rumination. Grazing accounts for 20,000–40,000 bites per day and rumination for a further 15,000–20,000 jaw movements. Grazing takes 6–12 h, ruminating 4–6 h and a cow walks 3–4 km in order to harvest the 12–16 kg DM she needs.

Ruminants have also evolved a complex set of four stomachs to enable them to take advantage of symbiotic microorganisms to ferment fibrous materials such as grass. (Church, 1975, gives a comprehensive coverage of ruminant digestive anatomy and physiology.) The first and largest of these stomachs is the rumen; it has a capacity of up to 12 l in sheep and 140 l in cattle (i.e. up to 250 g kg$^{-1}$ live weight) and is normally almost full of digesta, with a low dry matter content (around 120 g kg$^{-1}$) and a pH of about 5.5.

The acid nature of rumen contents is due largely to the products of fermentation of food by the huge population of bacteria (5000–20,000 million ml$^{-1}$) and protozoa (0.1–2 million ml$^{-1}$) inhabit the rumen. Hungate (1966) gives a comprehensive treatise on rumen microbiology. Major products of fermentation are short-chain fatty acids (acetate, propionate, butyrate, valerate; Rook and Thomas, 1983), which are absorbed and used as energy sources in several metabolic processes; ammonia, which is converted into urea in the liver (to be secreted in saliva and thus recycled, as well as being excreted by the kidneys); methane and carbon dioxide which are eructated (belched) via the mouth. The microbes secrete cellulases which digest plant fibre and give their ruminant hosts access to a greater proportion of plant material than would be possible with mammalian digestive enzymes alone. Microbial action is inefficient, however, and yields large amounts of metabolites, such as the short-chain fatty acids, to which mammalian metabolism is not fully adapted. This mode of digestion can also lead to deficiencies or less-efficient production where the microbes degrade essential nutrients such as glucose. Fibrous materials reside in the rumen for long periods (half-life can exceed 100 h) and their breakdown is assisted by rumination – remastication of a bolus of digesta which has been regurgitated in response to physical stimulation of the anterior rumen and reticulum by coarse particles of food (Wyburn, 1980, gives a description of rumen contractions).

The reticulum is the second stomach, with a capacity of around 1 l in the sheep and 15 l in cattle, which is a forward continuation of the rumen separated from it by a fold of tissue which acts like a dam. The stream of fluid which flows over this dam carries with it small particles of food which can then pass through the reticulo-omasal orifice to the omasum, the third stomach, whose lumen is filled with 100 or so leaves of tissue with the main function of water absorption. The fourth stomach, the abomasum, is the true stomach and is directly analogous to the simple stomach in its acid and enzyme secretion. The first three stomachs do not secrete gastric juice (Church, 1975).

There is copious production of saliva which serves to prevent excessive changes in the pH of rumen fluid and to replace water lost by absorption and onward flow.

Some digestible nutrients, including the microbes which have flowed into the abomasum and been killed by its acid secretions, reach the intestines to yield glucose and amino acids. However, the rate of glucose absorption is often insufficient for the needs of the animal, especially if she is lactating. The shortfall is normally made up by hepatic gluconeogenesis from propionate and amino acids taken up from the hepatic portal blood; with normal diets little propionate escapes into the general circulation. Of the butyrate absorbed from the rumen, most is converted into 3-hydroxybutyrate as it passes through the rumen wall. Acetate, normally produced in the greatest quantities of the short-chain fatty acids, passes into the general circulation largely unchanged and is used in fat synthesis and generally as an energy source.

The rumen microbes can synthesize proteins from non-protein nitrogen, usually urea of salivary origin, and low protein feeds can be supplemented with non-protein nitrogen, usually in the form of urea. Quantitative aspects of digestion and metabolism in ruminants are detailed in Forbes and France (1993).

# Appendix 2
# Outline Program to Identify and Store Meals from the Identities of Animals and Weights of Food Containers (Forbes *et al.*, 1987)

```
begin { main program }
  initialize;   { procedure to initialize variables }
  openfile;   { procedure to open data files }
  repeat { for ever! }
    repeat { until a key is pressed }
      updatetime; { get current time from system clock }
      if startofnewday then
        begin
          closefile; { close old data file }
          openfile; { open new data file }
        end;
      for thischan := 1 to MAXWEIGHER do
        if outofuse = false then
          begin
            thisweight[thischan] := inputweight(thischan); { get current weight on thischan }
            if (lastweight[thischan]<>thisweight[thischan]) then { eating in progress }
              begin
                if (endpending = false) then { meal starts }
                  mealstarts(thischan)
                else { meal continues }
                  mealcontinues(thischan);
              end
            else  { not eating }
              begin
                if (mealinprogress = true) then { end of meal? }
                  mealends(thischan)
                else
```

```
begin { not eating but check to see if within minimum intermeal interval }
  if (endpending = true) and ((thistime − imi) > endtime) then
                                        { less than interval specified for minimum
                                        { intermeal interval since end of meal }
      savemeal(thischan)
  else
      { do nothing } ;
    end;
  end; { of not eating }
  lastweight[thischan] := thisweight[thischan];
  end; {of thischan}
until keypressed;
dealwithkey; { procedure to interpret and act on whichever key was pressed }
until true = false;
end.
```

# REFERENCES

Abasiekong, S.F. (1989) Seasonal effect of wet rations on performance of broiler poultry in the tropics. *Archives of Animal Nutrition, Berlin* 39, 507–514.

Abrams, S.M., Harpster, H.W., Wangsness, P.J., Shenk, J.S., Keck, E. and Rosemberger, J.L. (1987) Use of a standard forage to reduce effects of animal variation on estimates of mean voluntary intake. *Journal of Dairy Science* 70, 1235–1240.

Ackroff, K. (1992) Foraging for macronutrients, effects of protein availability and abundance. *Physiology and Behavior* 51, 533–542.

Adam, I., Young, B.A., Nicol, A.M. and Degen, A.A. (1984) Energy cost of eating in cattle given diets in different form. *Animal Production* 38, 53–56.

Adams, D.C., Nelson, T.C., Reynolds, W.L. and Knapp, B.W. (1986) Winter grazing activity and forage intake of range cows in the northern Great Plains. *Journal of Animal Science* 62, 1240.

Adams, G.B. and Forbes, J.M. (1981) Additivity of effects of ruminal acetate and either portal propionate or rumen distension on food intake in sheep. *Proceedings of the Nutrition Society* 40, 44A.

Adams, G.B. and Forbes, J.M. (1982) Metabolite levels in hepatic portal blood of sheep during ad libitum feeding. *Journal of Physiology* 330, 47–48P.

Adams, G.B., Jones, R. and Forbes, J.M. (1983) Voluntary intake and growth of lambs offered fresh food one or four times per day. *Animal Production* 36, 508.

Adams, R.L., Andrews, F.N., Rogler, J.C. and Carrick, C.W. (1962) The protein requirement of 4-week-old chicks as affected by temperature. *Journal of Nutrition* 77, 121–126.

Adolph, E.F. (1947) Urges to eat and drink in rats. *American Journal of Physiology* 151, 110–125.

AFRC (Agriculture and Food Research Council) (1991) Voluntary intake of cattle. *Nutrition Abstracts and Reviews* 61, 815–823.

Aherne, F.X., Danielsen, V. and Nielsen, H.E. (1982) The effects of creep feeding on pre- and post-weaning pig performance. *Acta Agriculturae Scandinavica* 32, 155–160.

Aitken, J.N. and Preston, T.R. (1964) The self-feeding of complete milled rations to dairy cattle. *Animal Production* 6, 260.

Alawa, J.P., Fishwick, G., Parkins, J.J. and Hemingway, R.G. (1986) Influence of energy source and dietary protein degradability on the voluntary intake and digestibility of barley straw by pregnant beef cows. *Animal Production* 43, 201–209.

Alawa, J.P., Fishwick, G., Parkins, J.J. and Hemingway, R.G. (1987) A note on the effects of dietary protein degradability in the rumen on the voluntary intake and digestibility of barley straw by lactating beef cows. *Animal Production* 44, 446–449.

Al Bustany, Z. and Elwinger, K. (1988) Whole grains, unprocessed rapeseed and β-gluconase in diets for laying hens. *Swedish Journal of Agricultural Research* 18, 31–40.

Aldrich, C.G., Rhodes, M.T., Miner, J.L., Kerley, M.S. and Paterson, J.A. (1993) The effects of endophyte-infected tall fescue consumption and use of a dopamine antagonist on intake, digestibility, body temperature and blood constituents in sheep. *Journal of Animal Science* 71, 158–163.

Aldringer, S.M., Sper, V.C., Hays, V.W. and Catron, D.V. (1959) Effect of saccharin on consumption of starter rations by baby pigs. *Journal of Animal Science* 18, 1350–1355.

Allden, W.G. (1968) Undernutrition of the Merino sheep and its sequelae. 1. Growth and development of lambs following prolonged periods of nutritional stress. *Australian Journal of Agricultural Research* 19, 621–638.

Allden, W.G. and Whittaker, I.A.M. (1970) The determinants of herbage intake by grazing sheep: the interrelationships of factors influencing herbage intake and availability. *Australian Journal of Agricultural Research* 21, 755–766.

Amar-Sahbi, R. (1987) The diet selection of female broilers. PhD thesis, University of Aberdeen.

Ammerman, C.B., Chicco, C.F., Moore, J.E., Van Wallegheim, P.A. and Arrington, L.R. (1971) Effect of dietary magnesium on voluntary feed intake and rumen fermentation. *Journal of Animal Science* 54, 1288–1293.

Anderson, D.M. (1990) Diet selection of bonded and non-bonded free-ranging sheep and cattle. *Applied Animal Behaviour Science* 26, 231–242.

Anderson, G.H. (1979) Control of protein and energy intake; role of plasma amino acids and brain neurotransmiters. *Canadian Journal of Physiology and Pharmacology* 57, 1043–1057.

Andersson, B. (1978) Regulation of water intake. *Physiological Reviews* 58, 582–603.

Andersson, B. and Larsson, B. (1961) Influence of local temperature changes in the preoptic area and rostral hypothalamus on the regulation of food and water intake. *Acta Physiologica Scandinavica* 52, 75–89.

Andrews, F.N. and Beeson, W.M. (1953) The effect of various methods of estrogen administration on the growth and fattening of wether lambs. *Journal of Animal Science* 12, 182–187.

Andrews, R.P. and Kay, M. (1967) The effect of the energy concentration of the diet on voluntary intakes and performance of intensively fed lambs. *Animal Production* 9, 275–276.

Anil, M.H. and Forbes, J.M. (1980a) Feeding in sheep during intraportal infusions of short-chain fatty acids and the effect of liver denervation. *Journal of Physiology* 298, 407–414.

Anil, M.H. and Forbes, J.M. (1980b) Effects of insulin and gastro-intestinal hormones on feeding and plasma insulin levels in sheep. *Hormone and Metabolic Research* 12, 234–236.

Anil, M.H. and Forbes, J.M. (1987) Neural control and sensory functions of the liver. *Proceedings of the Nutrition Society* 46, 125–133.

Anil, M.H. and Forbes, J.M. (1988) The roles of hepatic nerves in the reduction of food intake as a consequence of intraportal sodium propionate administration in sheep. *Quarterly Journal of Experimental Physiology* 73, 539–546.

Anil, M.H., Jessop, N. and Forbes, J.M. (1987) Control of liver enzyme activity by the autonomic nerves in sheep. *Proceedings of the Nutrition Society* 45, 77A.

Anil, M.H., Mbanya, J.N., Symonds, H.W. and Forbes, J.M. (1993) Responses in the voluntary intake of hay or silage by lactating cows to intraruminal infusions of sodium acetate, sodium propionate or rumen distension. *British Journal of Nutrition* 69, 699–712.

Antin, J., Gibbs, J., Holt, J., Young, R. and Smith, G.P. (1975) Cholecystokinin elicits the complete behavioural sequence of satiety in rats. *Journal of Comparative and Physiological Psychology* 89, 784–790.

Appleby, M.C., Pajor, E.A. and Fraser, D. (1991) Effects of management options on creep feeding by piglets. *Animal Production* 53, 361–366.

Appleby, M.C., Hughes, B.O. and Elson, H.A. (1992a) *Poultry Production Systems, Behaviour, Management and Welfare.* CAB International, Wallingford.

Appleby, M.C., Pajor, E.A. and Fraser, D. (1992b) Individual variation in feeding and growth of piglets, effects of increased access to creep feed. *Animal Production* 55, 147–152.

Arave, C.W., Purcell, D. and Engstrom, M. (1989) Effect of feed flavours on improving choice for a ten per cent meat and bonemeal dairy concentrate. *Journal of Dairy Science* 72 (Suppl 1), 563.

ARC (Agricultural Research Council) (1980) *The Nutrient Requirements of Ruminant Livestock.* Commonwealth Agricultural Bureaux, Slough, 351pp.

ARC (Agricultural Research Council) (1981) *The Nutrient Requirements of Pigs.* Commonwealth Agricultural Bureaux, Farnham Royal, 307pp.

Argo, C.M. and Smith, J.S. (1983) Relationship of energy requirements and seasonal cycles of food intake in Soay rams. *Journal of Physiology* 343, 23–23P.

Armitage, G., Hervey, G.R., Rolls, B.J., Rowe, E.A. and Tobin, G. (1983) The effects of supplementation of the diet with highly palatable foods upon energy balance in the rat. *Journal of Physiology* 342, 229–251.

Armstrong, S. (1980) A chronometric approach to the study of feeding behaviour. *Neuroscience and Biobehavioral Reviews* 4, 27–53.

Arnold, G.W. (1966a) The special senses in grazing animals. 1. Sight and dietary habits in sheep. *Australian Journal of Agricultural Research* 17, 521–529.

Arnold, G.W. (1966b) The special senses in grazing animals. 2. Smell, taste, and touch and dietary habits in sheep. *Australian Journal of Agricultural Research* 17, 531–542.

Arnold, G.W. (1970) Regulation of food intake in grazing ruminants. In: Phillipson, A.T. (ed.) *Physiology of Digestion and Metabolism in the Ruminant,* Oriel Press, Newcastle, pp. 264–276.

Arnold, G.W. and Dudzinski, M.C. (1967) Studies on the diet of the grazing animal. 2. The effect of physiological status in ewes and pasture availability on herbage intake. *Australian Journal of Agricultural Research* 18, 349–359.

Arnold, G.W. and Dudzinski, M.L. (1978) *Ethology of Free Ranging Domestic Animals.* Elsevier, Amsterdam.

Arnold, G.W. and Maller, R.A. (1977) Effects of nutritional experience in early and adult life on the performance and dietary habits of sheep. *Applied Animal Ethology* 3, 5–26.

Arnold, G.W., McManus, W.R. and Bush, I.G. (1964) Studies in the wool production of grazing sheep. 1. Seasonal variation in feed intake, liveweight and wool production. *Australian Journal of Experimental Agriculture and Animal Husbandry* 4, 392–403.

Arnold, G.W., Campbell, N.A. and Galbraith, K.A. (1977) Mathematical relationships and computer routines for a model of food intake, liveweight change and wool production in grazing sheep. *Agricultural Systems* 2, 209–226.

Arnold, G.W., de Boer, E.S. and Boundy, C A.P. (1980) The influence of odour and taste on the food preferences and food intake of sheep. *Australian Journal of Agricultural Research* 31, 489–509.

Aronen, J. and Vanhatalo, A. (1992) Heat–moisture treatment of rapeseed meal, effect on digestibility of the diet, voluntary grass silage intake and growth rate of Ayrshire bulls. *Acta Agriculturae Scandinavica, Section A, Animal Science* 42, 157–166.

Ash, R.W. (1959) Inhibition and excitation of reticulo-ruminal contractions following the introduction of acids into the rumen and abomasum. *Journal of Physiology* 147, 58–73.

Ash, R.W. and Kay, R.N.B. (1957) Stimulation and inhibition of reticulum contractions, rumination and parotid secretion from the forestomach of conscious sheep. *Journal of Physiology* 149, 43–57.

Ashcraft, D.W. (1930) Correlative activities of the alimentary canal in fowls. *American Journal of Physiology* 93, 105–110.

Auffray, P. (1969) Effect of ventromedial hypothalamic lesions on food intake in the pig. *Annales de Biologie Animale, Biochimie et Biophysique* 9, 513–526.

Auffray, P. and Blum, J.C. (1970) [Hyperphagia and fatty liver in the goose after ventromedial hypothalamic lesions.] *Compte Rendues Hebdomadaire des Seances de l'Academie des Sciences, Paris, serie D* 270, 2362–2365.

Auffray, P. and Gallouin, F. (1971) [Obesity and fatty liver caused by injection of 6-hydroxydopamine into the brain of the goose.] 10th Congress Mondiale Zootechnique, Versailles, theme VII.

Auffray, P. and Marcilloux, J.C. (1980) [Analysis of feeding patterns of pigs from weaning to maturity.] *Reproduction, Nutrition, Developpement* 20, 1625–1652.

Auffray, P. and Marcilloux, J.C. (1983) [Studies of feeding behaviour in the adult pig.] *Reproduction, Nutrition, Developpement* 23, 517–524.

Aumaitre, A. (1980) Palatability of piglet feeds, trial methods and practical results. In: *Palatability and Flavour Use in Animal Feeds.* First International Symposium on Palatability and Flavour use in Animal Feeds, Zurich; pp. 86–95.

Austic, R.E. and Scott, R.L. (1975) Involvement of food intake in the lysine–

arginine antagonism in chicks. *Journal of Nutrition* 105, 1122–1131.

Aydintug, S. and Forbes, J.M. (1985) Additive effects of intraventricular injection of noradrenaline and intraruminal infusion of sodium acetate on food intake of sheep. *Proceedings of the Nutrition Society* 44, 48A.

Azahan, E.A.E. (1988) Voluntary food intake of chickens and sheep in relation to energy metabolism, metabolite solutions and choice feeding. PhD thesis, University of Leeds, 212pp.

Azahan, E.A.E. and Forbes, J.M. (1989) Growth, food intake and energy balance of layer and broiler chickens offered glucose in the drinking water and the effect of dietary protein content. *British Poultry Science* 30, 907–917.

Azahan, E.A.E. and Forbes, J.M. (1992) The effects of intraruminal infusions of sodium salts on the selection of hay and concentrate foods by sheep. *Appetite* 18, 143–154.

Babapour, V. and Bost, J. (1973) [Effect of gold thioglucose on glycaemia in sheep.] *Annales de Biologie Animale, Biochimie et Biophysique* 13, 753–754.

Badamana, M.S. and Sutton, J.D. (1992) Hay intake, milk production and rumen fermentation in British Saanen goats given concentrates varying widely in protein concentration. *Animal Production* 54, 395–403.

Badamana, M.S., Sutton, J.D., Oldham, J.D. and Mowlem, A. (1990) The effect of amount of protein in the concentrates on hay intake and rate of passage, diet digestibility and milk production in British Saanen goats. *Animal Production* 51, 333–342.

Baidoo, S.K., McIntosh, M.K. and Aherne, F.X. (1986) Selection preference of starter pigs fed canola meal and soyabean meal supplemented diets. *Canadian Journal of Animal Science* 66, 1039–1049.

Baile, C.A. (1971) Metabolites as feedbacks for control of feed intake and receptor sites in goats and sheep. *Physiology and Behavior* 7, 819–826.

Baile, C.A. (1975) Control of feed intake in ruminants. In: McDonald, I.W. and Warner, A.C.I. (eds), *Digestion and Metabolism in the Ruminant*, University of New England, Armidale, N.S.W., pp. 332–350.

Baile, C.A. and Forbes, J.M. (1974) Control of feed intake and regulation of energy balance in ruminants. *Physiological Reviews* 54, 160–214.

Baile, C.A. and Mahoney, A.W. (1967) Hypothalamic function in ruminant food intake regulation. *Proceedings of the 17th International Congress of Nutrition* 2, 67–72.

Baile, C.A. and Martin, F.H. (1971) Hormones and amino acids as possible factors in the control of hunger and satiety in sheep. *Journal of Dairy Science* 54, 897–905.

Baile, C.A. and Martin, F.H. (1972) Effect of local anesthetic on taste and feed intake. *Journal of Dairy Science* 55, 1461–1463.

Baile, C.A. and Martin, F.H. (1973) Relationship between prostaglandin $E_1$, polyphloretin phosphate and α- and β- adrenoceptor-bound feeding loci in the hypothalamus of sheep. *Pharmacology, Biochemistry and Behavior* 1, 539–545.

Baile, C.A. and Martin, F.H. (1974) Parotid secretion and feeding in sheep following intraventricular injections of l-norepinephrine, dl-isoproterenol, pentobarbital and carbachol. *Journal of Dairy Science* 57, 308–313.

Baile, C.A. and Mayer, J. (1966) Hyperphagia in ruminants induced by a depressant. *Science* 151, 458–459.

Baile, C.A. and Mayer, J. (1968a) Effects of intravenous versus intraruminal injections of acetate on feed intake of goats. *Journal of Dairy Science* 51, 1490–1494.

Baile, C.A. and Mayer, J. (1968b) Hypothalamic temperature and the regulation of feed intake in goats. *American Journal of Physiology* 214, 677–684.

Baile, C.A. and Mayer, J. (1968c) Effects of insulin-induced hypoglycaemia and hypoacetonemia on eating behavior in goats. *Journal of Dairy Science* 51, 1495–1499.

Baile, C.A. and Mayer, J. (1969) Depression of feed intake of goats by metabolites injected during meals. *American Journal of Physiology* 217, 1830–1836.

Baile, C.A. and McLaughlin, C.L. (1970) Feed intake during volatile fatty acid injections into four gastric areas. *Journal of Dairy Science* 53, 1058–1063.

Baile, C.A. and McLaughlin, C.L. (1987) Mechanisms controlling feed intake in ruminants: a review. *Journal of Animal Science* 63, 915–922.

Baile, C.A. and Pfander, W.H. (1967) Ration density as a factor controlling food intake in ruminants. *Journal of Dairy Science* 50, 77–80.

Baile, C.A., Mahoney, A.W. and Mayer, J. (1967) Placement of electrodes in the hypothalamus of goats. *Journal of Dairy Science* 50, 576–578.

Baile, C.A., Mahoney, A.W. and Mayer, J. (1968) Induction of hypothalamic aphagia and adipsia in goats. *Journal of Dairy Science* 51, 1474–1480.

Baile, C.A., Mayer, J., Mahohey, A.W. and McLaughlin, C. (1969) Hypothalamic hyperphagia in goats and some observations of its effect on glucose utilisation rate. *Journal of Dairy Science* 52, 101–109.

Baile, C.A., Mayer, J., Baumgardt, B.R. and Peterson, A. (1970) Comparative goldthioglucose effects on goats, sheep, dogs, rats and mice. *Journal of Dairy Science* 53, 801–807.

Baile, C.A., Simpson, C.W., Krabill, L.F. and Martin, F.H. (1972) Adrenergic agonists and antagonists and feeding in sheep and cattle. *Life Science* 11, 661–668.

Baile, C.A., McLaughlin, C.L., Krabill, L.F. and Beyea, J.S. (1974a) Phenobarbital – a feed intake stimulant in sheep. *Proceedings of the International Union of Physiological Sciences* 11, 403.

Baile, C.A., Martin, F.H., Simpson, C.A., Forbes, J.M. and Beyea, J.S. (1974b) Feeding elicited by α- and β-andrenoceptor agonists injected intrahypothalamically in sheep. *Journal of Dairy Science* 57, 68–80.

Baile, C.A., Martin, F.H., Forbes, J.M., Webb, R.L. and Kingsbury, M. (1974c) Intrahypothalamic injections of prostaglandins and prostaglandin antagonists and feeding in sheep. *Journal of Dairy Science* 57, 81–88.

Baile, C.A., Beyea, J.S., Krabill, L.F. and Della-Fera, M.A. (1979a) Intracranial injections of 5-HT and db cAMP and feeding in sheep and cattle. *Journal of Animal Science* 49, 1076–1084.

Baile, C.A., McLaughlin, C.L., Potter, E.L. and Chalupa, W. (1979b) Feeding behavior changes of cattle during introduction of monensin with roughage or concentrate diets. *Journal of Animal Science* 48, 1501–1508.

Baile, C.A., Keim, D.A., Della-Fera, M.A. and McLaughlin, C.L. (1981) Opiate antagonists and agonists and feeding in sheep. *Physiology and Behavior* 26, 1019–1023.

Baile, C.A., Della-Fera, M.A. and McLaughlin, C.L. (1983) Hormones and feed intake. *Proceedings of the Nutrition Society* 42, 113–127.

Baile, C.A., McLaughlin, C.L. and Della-Fera, M.A. (1986) Role of cholecystokinin and opioid peptides in control of food intake. *Physiological Reviews* 66, 172–234.

Baile, C.A., McLaughlin, C.A., Buonomo, F.C., Lauterio, T.J., Marson, L. and Della-Fera, M.A. (1987) Opioid peptides and the control of feeding in sheep. *Federation Proceedings* 46, 173–177.

Bailey, M. (1990) The water requirements of poultry. In: *Recent Advances in Animal Nutrition*, Butterworths, London, pp. 137–176.

Baker, B., Booth, D.A., Duggan, J.P. and Gibson, E.L. (1987) Protein appetite demonstrated. Learned specificity of protein-cue preference to protein need in adult rats. *Nutrition Research* 7, 481–487.

Baker, D.H., Katy, R.S. and Easter, R.A. (1975) Lysine requirement of growing pigs at two levels of dietary protein. *Journal of Animal Science* 40, 851–856.

Balch, C.C. and Campling, R.C. (1962) Regulation of voluntary food intake in ruminants. *Nutrition Abstracts and Reviews* 32, 669–686.

Baldwin, B.A. (1976) Quantitative studies on taste preference in pigs. *Proceedings of the Nutrition Society* 35, 69–73.

Baldwin, B.A. (1979) Operant studies on the behavior of pigs and sheep in relation to the physical environment. *Journal of Animal Science* 49, 1125–1134.

Baldwin, B.A. (1985) Neural and hormonal mechanisms regulating food intake. *Proceedings of the Nutrition Society* 44, 303–311.

Baldwin, B.A. and Cooper, T.R. (1979) The effects of olfactory bulbectomy on feeding behavior in pigs. *Applied Animal Ethology* 5, 153–159.

Baldwin, B.A. and Parrott, R.F. (1979) Studies on intracranial electrical self-stimulation in pigs in relation to ingestive and exploratory behaviour. *Physiology and Behavior* 22, 723–730.

Baldwin, B.A. and Parrott, R.F. (1982) Self-stimulation in the sheep, interactions with ingestive behaviour and light cycle. *Physiology and Behavior* 28, 77–81.

Baldwin, B.A. and Parrott, R.F. (1985) Effects of intracerebroventricular injection of naloxone on operant feeding and drinking in pigs. *Pharmacology, Biochemistry and Behavior* 22, 37–40.

Baldwin, B.A., Grovum, W.L., Baile, C.A. and Brobeck, J.R. (1975) Feeding following intraventricular injection of $Ca^{++}$, $Mg^{++}$ or pentobarbital in pigs. *Pharmacology, Biochemistry and Behavior* 3, 915–918.

Baldwin, B.A., Cooper, T.R. and Parrott, R.F. (1983a) Intravenous cholecystokinin octapeptide in pigs reduces operant responding for food, water, sucrose solution or radiant heat. *Physiology and Behavior* 30, 399–403.

Baldwin, B.A., Ingrey, C.C., Parrott, R.F. and Toner, J.N. (1983b) A method for the quantitative recording of ingestive behaviour in sheep, using closed circuit television. *Journal of Physiology* 343, 5P.

Baldwin, B.A., De La Riva, C. and Ebenezer, I.S. (1990a) Effects of intracerebroventricular injection of dynorphin, leumorphin and α neo-endorphin on operant feeding in pigs. *Physiology and Behavior* 48, 821–824.

Baldwin, B.A., Ebenezeer, I.S. and De La Riva, C. (1990a) Effects of intracerebroventricular injection of muscimol or GABA on operant feeding in pigs. *Physiology and Behavior* 48, 417–421.

Balnave, D. and Abdoellah, T.M. (1990) Self-select feeding of commercial pullets using a complete layer diet and a separate protein concentrate at cool and hot temperatures. *Australian Journal of Agricultural Research* 41, 549–555.

Balog, J.M. and Millar, R.I. (1989) Influence of the sense of taste on broiler chick feed consumption. *Poultry Science* 68, 1519–1526.

Bampton, P.R. (1991) Relationships between growth performance and feeding pattern of pigs using electronic feeding stations. *Animal Production* 52, 562.

Barach, I., Nitsan, Z. and Nir, I. (1992) Metabolic and behavioural adaptation of light-bodied chicks to meal feeding. *British Poultry Science* 33, 271–278.

Barbato, G.F., Siegel, B. and Cherry, J. (1982) Genetic analysis of gustation in the fowl. *Physiology and Behavior* 27, 29–33.

Barbato, G.F., Cherry, J.A., Siegel, P.B. and Van Krey, H.P. (1984) Selection for body weight at eight weeks of age. 17. Overfeeding. *Poultry Science* 63, 11–18.

Barber, J., Brooks, P.H. and Carpenter, J.L. (1989) The effects of water delivery on the voluntary food intake, water use and performance of early weaned pigs from 3 to 6 weeks of age. In: Forbes, J.M., Varley, M.A. and Lawrence, T.L.J. (eds), *The Voluntary Food Intake of Pigs*, Occasional Publication of the British Society of Animal Production, pp. 103–104.

Barber, J., Brooks, P.H. and Carpenter, J.L. (1991) The effect of four levels of food on the water intake and water to food ratio of growing pigs. *Animal Production* 52, 602.

Barber, R.S., Braude, R., Mitchell, K.G. and Pittman, R.J. (1978) The value of virginiamycin (Eskalin) as a feed additive for growing pigs in diets with or without a high copper supplementation. *Animal Production* 26, 151–155.

Bargeloh, J.F., Hibbs, J.W. and Conrad, H.R. (1975) Effect of prepartal hormone administration on feed intake and mineral metabolism of cows. *Journal of Dairy Science* 58, 1701–1707.

Bark, L.J., Crenshaw, T.D. and Leibbrandt, V.D. (1986) The effect of meal intervals and weaning on feed intake of early weaned pigs. *Journal of Animal Science* 62, 1233–1239.

Barrio, J.P., Bapat, S.T. and Forbes, J.M. (1991) The effect of drinking water on food-intake responses to manipulations of rumen osmolality in sheep. *Proceedings of the Nutrition Society* 50, 98A.

Barry, T.N. (1975) Effect of treatment with formaldehyde, formic acid and formaldehyde–acid mixtures on the chemical composition and nutritive value of silage. *New Zealand Journal of Agricultural Research* 18, 285–294.

Barry, T.N. (1976) Effects of intraperitoneal injections of DL-methionine on the voluntary intake and wool growth of sheep fed sole diets of hay, silage and pasture differing in digestibility. *Journal of Agricultural Science* 86, 141–149.

Barry, T.N. and Manley, T.R. (1984) The role of condensed tannins in the nutritional value of *Lotus pedunculatus* for sheep. 1. Voluntary intake. *British Journal of Nutrition* 51, 485–492.

Barry, T.N. and Manley, T.R. (1986) Glucose and protein metabolism during late pregnancy in triplet-bearing ewes given fresh forages. 1. Voluntary intake and birth weight. *British Journal of Nutrition* 54, 521–534.

Barton, M.A. and Broom, D.M. (1985) Social factors affecting the performance of teat-fed calves. *Animal Production* 40, 525A.

Bass, J.M. (1982) A note on the effects of various diets on the drinking behaviour of wether sheep. *Animal Production* 35, 293–294.

Bassett, J.M. (1960) The influence of maintenance feeding and subsequent compensatory effects on the pattern of growth and development in lambs. PhD thesis, University of Reading.

Bassett, J.M. (1963) The influence of cortisol on food intake and glucose metabolism in the sheep. *Journal of Endocrinology* 26, 539–553.

Bassett, J.M. (1975) Dietary and gastro-intestinal control of hormones regulating carbohydrate metabolism in ruminants. In: McDonald, I.W. and Warner, A.C.I. (eds), *Digestion and Metabolism in the Ruminant*, University of New England Press, Armidale, pp. 383–398.

Bate, L.A. (1992) Sound stimuli to enhance ingestive behaviour of young turkeys. *Applied Animal Behaviour Science* 34, 189–194.

Bath, D.L., Gall, G.A.E. and Ronning, M. (1974) Voluntary alfalfa hay wafer intake by lactating dairy cows fed varying concentrate amounts. *Journal of Dairy Science* 57, 19–204.

Bauman, D.E. (1984) Regulation of nutrient partitioning. In: Gilchrist, F.M.C. and Mackie, R.I. (eds) *Herbivore Nutrition in the Subtropics and Tropics*, The Science Press, Craighill, South Africa, pp. 505–524.

Bauman, D.E., Eppard, P.J., DeGeeter, M.J. and Lanza, G.M. (1984) Responses of high producing dairy cows to long term treatment with pituitary- and recombinant-growth hormone. *Journal of Dairy Science* 68, 1352–1362.

Baumgardt, B.R. and Peterson, A.D. (1971) Regulation of food intake in ruminants. 1. Caloric density of diets for young growing lambs. *Journal of Dairy Science* 54, 1191–1194.

Baumont, R., Malbert, C.H. and Ruckebusch, Y. (1990a) Mechanical stimulation of rumen fill and alimentary behaviour in sheep. *Animal Production* 50, 123–128.

Baumont, N., Seguier, N. and Dulphy, J.P. (1990b) Rumen fill, forage palatability and alimentary behaviour in sheep. *Journal of Agricultural Science* 115, 277–284.

Bazely, D.R. (1988) Foraging behaviour of sheep (*Ovis aries* L.) grazing on swards of perennial ryegrass (*Lolium perenne* L.). PhD thesis, University of Oxford, 180pp.

Bazely, D.R. and Ensor, C.V. (1989) Discrimination learning in sheep with cues varying in brightness and hue. *Applied Animal Behaviour Science* 23, 293–299.

Bechdel, S.I., Landsberg, K.G. and Hill, O.J. (1933) Rickets in calves. *Pennsylvania State College School of Agriculture and Experiment Station Technical Bulletin* no. 29.

Bechet, G. (1978) Enregistrement des activities alimentaires et meryciques des ovins au paturage. *Annales de Zootechnie* 27, 107–113.

Beh, B.L. (1981) PhD thesis, University of London.

Bekverlin, S.K., Havstad, K.M., Ayers, E,L. and Petersen, M.K. (1989) Forage intake responses to winter cold exposure of free-ranging beef cows. *Applied Animal Behaviour Science* 23, 75–85.

Bell, F.R. (1959) The sense of taste in domestic animals. *Veterinary Record* 71, 1071–1081.

Bell, F.R. and Sly, J. (1979) The metabolic effects of sodium depletion in calves on salt appetite assessed by operant methods. *Journal of Physiology* 295, 431–443.

Bell, F.R. and Sly, J. (1983) The olfactory detection of sodium and lithium salts by sodium deficient cattle. *Physiology and Behavior* 31, 307–313.

Bellin, S.I. and Ritter, S. (1981a) Disparate effects of infused nutrients on delayed glucoprivic feeding and hypothalamic norepinephrine turnover. *Journal of Neuroscience* 1, 1347–1353.

Bellin, S.I. and Ritter, S. (1981b) Insulin-induced elevation of hypothalamic norepinephrine turnover persists after glucorestoration unless feeding occurs. *Brain Research* 217, 327–337.

Bellinger, L.L. and Mendel, V.E. (1988) Ingestion, body weight and activity of rats receiving repeated intracerebroventricular infusions of rat satietin. *Physiology and Behavior* 44, 445–452.

Bellinger, L.L., Mendel, V.E., Williams, F.E. and Castonguay, T.W. (1984) The effect of liver denervation on meal patterns, body weight and body composition of rats. *Physiology and Behavior* 33, 661–667.

Beranger, C. and Micol, D. (1980) Intake in relation to the animal. *Annales de Zootechnie* 29, 209–226.

Bergen, W.G. (1972) Rumen osmolality as a factor in feed intake control in sheep. *Journal of Animal Science* 34, 1054–1060.

Bermudez, F.F., Forbes, J.M. and Injidi, M.H. (1983) Involvement of melatonin and thyroid hormones in the control of sleep, food intake and energy metabolism in the domestic fowl. *Journal of Physiology* 337, 19–27.

Bermudez, F.F., Sans Arias, R. and Forbes, J.M. (1984) Effect of feed quality on the growth check at weaning in artificially reared lambs. *Research and Development in Agriculture* 1, 113–117.

Bernstein, I.L. (1994) Development of food aversion during illness. *Proceedings of the Nutrition Society* 53, 131–137.

Berthoud, H.R., Kressel, M. and Neuhuber, W.L. (1992) An anterograde tracing study of the vagal innervation of rat liver, portal vein and biliary system. *Anatomy and Embryology* 186, 431–442.

Beyea, J.S., Krabill, L.F. and Baile, C.A. (1975) Pentobarbital elicited feeding of concentrates, roughage and protein deficient rations in sheep at 22 and 32°C room temperatures. *Federation Proceedings* 34, 902.

Bhargava, P.K., Orskov, E.R. and Walli, T.K. (1988) Rumen degradation of straw. 4. Selection and degradation of morphological components of barley straw by sheep. *Animal Production* 47, 105–110.

Bhattacharya, A.N. and Warner, R.G. (1967) Rumen pH as a factor for controlling feed intake in ruminants. *Journal of Dairy Science* 50, 1116–1119.

Bhattacharya, A.N. and Warner, R.G. (1968a) Influence of varying rumen temperature on central cooling or warming and on regulation of voluntary feed intake in dairy cattle. *Journal of Dairy Science* 51, 1481–1489.

Bhattacharya, A.N. and Warner, R.G. (1968b) Voluntary feed intake of pelletted diets for cattle, sheep and rabbits as affected by different alkali supplements. *Journal of Animal Science* 27, 1418–1425.

Bhatti, B.M. and Morris, T.R. (1978) The effect of ahemeral light and dark cycles on patterns of food intake by the laying hen. *British Poultry Science* 19, 125–128.

Bianca, W. (1966) Heat tolerance in dehydrated steers. *Journal of Agricultural Science* 66, 57–60.

Bierer, B.W., Eleazer, T.H. and Barnett, B.D. (1966) The effect of feed and water deprivation on water and feed consumption, body weight and mortality in broiler chickens of various ages. *Poultry Science* 45, 1045–1051.

Bines, J.A. (1979) Voluntary food intake. In: Broster, W.H. and Swan, H. (eds) *Feeding Strategy for the High Yielding Dairy Cow,* Granada, London, pp. 23–48.

Bines, J.A. (1985) Feeding systems and food intake by housed dairy cows. *Proceedings of the Nutrition Society* 44, 355–362.

Bines, J.A., Suzuki, S. and Balch, C.C. (1969) The quantitative significance of long-term regulation of food intake in the cow. *British Journal of Nutrition* 23, 695–704.

Bines, J.A., Jones, P.A. and Napper, D.J. (1973) The effect of a long-term reduction in rumen capacity on the intake of hay by a cow. *Proceedings of the Nutrition Society* 32, 75–76A.

Bines, J.A., Napper, D.J. and Johnson, V.W. (1977) Long-term effects of level of intake and diet composition on the performance of lactating dairy cows. 2. Voluntary intake and ration digestibility in heifers. *Proceedings of the Nutrition Society* 36, 146A.

Biquard, S. and Biquard-Guyot, V. (1992) The influence of peers, lineage and environment on food selection of the Criollo goat (*Capra hircus*). *Applied Animal Behaviour Science* 34, 231–245.

Birrell, H.A. (1984) Effects of pasture availability and liveweight on the feeding of grass hay to grazing sheep. *Australian Journal of Experimental Agriculture and Animal Husbandry* 24, 26–33.

Black, J.L. and Kenney, P.A. (1984) Factors affecting diet selection by sheep. II Height and density of pasture. *Australian Journal of Agricultural Research* 35, 565–578.

Blair-West, J.R. and Brook, A.H. (1969) Circulatory changes and renin secretion in sheep in response to feeding. *Journal of Physiology* 204, 15–30.

Blair-West, J.R., Denton, D.A., Gellatly, D.R., McKinley, M.J., Nelson, J.F. and Weisinger, R.S. (1987) Changes in sodium appetite in cattle induced by changes in CSF sodium concentration and osmolality. *Physiology and Behavior* 39, 465–469.

Blake, A.G., Mather, F.B. and Gleaves, E.W. (1984) Dietary self-selection of laying hens inadequate to overcome the effects of high environmental temperature. *Poultry Science,* 63, 1346–1349.

Blaxter, K.L. (1962) *The Energy Metabolism of Ruminants,* Hutchinson, London, 329pp.

Blaxter, K.L. and Boyne, A.W. (1982) Fasting and maintenance metabolism of sheep. *Journal of Agricultural Science* 99, 611–620.

Blaxter, K.L. and Gill, J.C. (1979) Voluntary intake of feed and equilibrium body-weight in sheep. *Proceedings of the Nutrition Society* 38, 150A.

Blaxter, K.L. and Wilson, R.S. (1963) The assessment of a crop husbandry technique in terms of animal production. *Animal Production* 5, 27–42.

Blaxter, K.L., Wainman, F.W. and Wilson, R.S. (1961) The regulation of food intake by sheep. *Animal Production* 3, 51–61.

Blaxter, K.L., Fowler, V.R. and Gill, J.C. (1982) A study of the growth of sheep to maturity. *Journal of Agricultural Science* 98, 405–420.

Blummel, M. and Orskov, E.R. (1993) Comparison of in vitro gas production and nylon bag degradability of roughages in predicting food intake in cattle. *Animal Feed Science and Technology* 40, 109–119.

Blundell, J.E. (1988) Role of monoamine systems in the control of food intake and nutrient selection. In: Morley, J.E., Sterman, M.B. and Walsh, J.H. (eds) *Nutritional Modulation of Neural Function*, Academic Press, New York, pp. 95–123.

Bocquier, F., Theriez, M. and Brelurut, A. (1987) The voluntary intake by ewes during the first weeks of lactation. *Animal Production* 44, 387–394.

Boda, J.M. and Riley, R.W. (1961) Observations of some effects of glucose infusion in sheep. *Proceedings of the New Zealand Society of Animal Production* 21, 176–177.

Boling, J.A., Kowalczyck, T. and Hauser, E.R. (1969) Short-term voluntary feed intake and rumen volatile fatty acids of steers fed diets diluted with polyethylene particles. *Journal of Animal Science* 28, 84–89.

Bolton, J.R., Merrit, A.M., Carlson, G.M. and Donawick, W.J. (1976) Normal abomasal electromyography and emptying in sheep and the effects of intra-abomasal volatile fatty acid infusion. *American Journal of Veterinary Research* 37, 1387–1392.

Boorman, K.N. (1979) Regulation of protein and amino acid intake. In: Boorman, K.N. and Freeman, B.M. (eds) *Food Intake Regulation in Poultry*, Longman, Edinburgh, pp. 87–126.

Booth, D.A. (1972a) Satiety and behavioral caloric compensation following intragastric glucose loads in the rat. *Journal of Comparative and Physiological Psychology* 78, 412–432.

Booth, D.A. (1972b) Postabsorptively induced suppression of appetite and the energostatic control of feeding. *Physiology and Behavior* 9, 199–202.

Booth, D.A. (1978) Prediction of feeding behaviour from energy flows in the rat. In: Booth, D.A. (ed.) *Hunger Models. Computable Theory of Feeding Control*, Academic Press, London, pp. 227–278.

Booth, D.A. (1979) Feeding control systems within animals. In: Boorman, K.N. and Freeman, B.M. (eds) *Food Intake Regulation in Poultry*, Longman, Edinburgh, pp. 13–62.

Booth, D.A. (1987) Central dietary 'Feedback onto nutrient selection', not even a scientific hypothesis. *Appetite* 8, 195–201.

Booth, D.A. and Mather, P. (1978) Prototype model of human feeding, growth and obesity. In: Booth, D.A. (ed.) *Hunger Models. Computable Theory of Feeding Control*, Academic Press, London, pp. 279–322.

Bordas, A. and Merat, P. (1976) Effect of laying on food and water intake in dwarf and normal hens. *British Poultry Science* 17, 415–426.

Bosticco, A., Amich-Gali, J. and Tartari, E. (1975) The effect of feed grade fat (F.G.A.F.) in liquid feeding for swine. *Nutrition Abstracts and Reviews* 45, 163.

Boucquier, F., Theriez, M. and Brelurut, A. (1987) The voluntary intake by ewes during the first weeks of lactation. *Animal Production* 44, 387–394.

Bouissou, M.F. (1970) [The role of physical contact in the manifestation of dominance in cattle, practical consequences.] *Annales de Zootechnie* 19, 279.

Bown, M.D., Poppi, D.P. and Sykes, A.R. (1989) The effect of post-ruminal infusion of protein or energy on the pathology of *Trichostrongylus colubriformis* infection and body composition in lambs. *Proceedings of the New Zealand Society of Animal Production* 46, 27–30.

Bradford, M.M.V. and Gous, R.M. (1991) The response of growing pigs to a choice of diets differing in protein content. *Animal Production* 52, 185–192.

Bradford, M.M.V. and Gous, R.M. (1992) The response of weaner pigs to a choice of foods differing in protein content. *Animal Production* 55, 227–232.

Braude, R. and Rowell, J.G. (1967) Comparison of dry and wet feeding of growing pigs. *Journal of Agricultural Science* 68, 325–330.

Brigstocke, T.D.A., Lindeman, M.A., Cuthbert, N.H., Wilson, P.N. and Cole, J.P.L. (1982) A note on the dry-matter intake of Jersey cows. *Animal Production* 35, 285–287.

Brink, D.R. (1975) Effect of ambient temperature on lamb performance. MS thesis, Kansas State University, Manhattan.

Brobeck, J.R. (1948) Food intake as a mechanism of temperature regulation. *Yale Journal of Biology and Medicine* 20, 545–552.

Brody, S. (1945) *Bioenergetics and Growth*, Reinhold, New York, 1023pp.

Brody, T.B., Chery, J.A. and Siegal, P.B. (1984) Responses to dietary self selection and calories in liquid form by weight selected lines of chickens. *Poultry Science* 63, 1626–1633.

Brooks, P.H. and Carpenter, J.L. (1990) The water requirement of growing-finishing pigs – theoretical and practical considerations. In: Haresign, W. and Cole, D.J.A. (eds) *Recent Advances in Animal Nutrition*, Butterworths, London, pp. 115–136.

Broom, D.M. (1982) Husbandry methods leading to inadequate social and maternal behaviour in cattle. In: Bessei, W. (ed.) *Disturbed Behaviour in Farm Animals, Hohenheimer Arbeiten* 121, 42–50.

Broom, D.M. and Arnold, G.W. (1986) Selection by grazing sheep of pasture plants at low herbage availability and responses of the plants to grazing. *Australian Journal of Agricultural Research* 37, 527–538.

Broom, D.M., Pain, B.F. and Leaver, J.D. (1975) The effects of slurry on the acceptability of swards to grazing cattle. *Journal of Agricultural Science* 85, 331–336.

Broster, W.H., Clough, P.A., Clements, A.J. and Siviter, J.W. (1982) Electronically controlled feeding troughs for dairy cows: some nutritional implications. *Journal of Dairy Research* 49, 545–557.

Brouns, F., Edwards, S.A. and English, P.R. (1991) Fibrous raw materials in sow diets, effects on voluntary food intake, digestibility and diurnal activity patterns. *Animal Production* 52, 598.

Brouns, F., Edwards, S.A. and English, P.R. (1992a) Feeding motivation of sows fed a sugarbeet pulp diet. *Animal Production* 54, 486–487.

Brouns, F., MacMenemy, F. and Edwards, S.A. (1992b) Dominance hierarchies in sows and the consequences for liveweight gain in competitive and non-competitive feeding systems. *Animal Production* 54, 486.

Brown, A.N.R. and Henderson, M. (1989) Development of an ad libitum food-intake recording system for pigs, pigs from 3 to 6 weeks of age. In: Forbes, J.M., Varley, M.A. and Lawrence, T.L.J. (eds) *The Voluntary Food Intake of*

*Pigs*, Occasional Publication of the British Society of Animal Production, p. 111.

Brown, C.A., Chandler, P.T. and Holter, J.B. (1977) Development of predictive equations for milk yield and dry matter intake in lactating cows. *Journal of Dairy Science* 60, 1739–1754.

Brown, D., Salim, M., Chavalimu, E. and Fitzhugh, H. (1988) Intake, selection, apparent digestibility and chemical composition of *Pennisetum purpureum* and *Cajanus cajan* foliage as utilized by lactating goats. *Small Ruminant Research* 1, 59–65.

Bryant, J.J. and Ewbank, R. (1974) Effect of stocking rate upon performance, general activity and ingestive behaviour of growing pigs. *British Veterinary Journal* 130, 139–149.

Buchanan-Smith, J.G. (1990) An investigation into palatability as a factor responsible for reduced intake of silage by sheep. *Animal Production* 50, 253–260.

Buchanan-Smith, J.G. and Phillip, L.E. (1986) Food intake in sheep following intraruminal infusion of extracts from lucerne silage with particular reference to organic acids and products of protein degradation. *Journal of Agricultural Science* 106, 611–617.

Bueno, L. (1975) [Role of dl-lactic acid in the control of food intake in the sheep.] *Annales de Recherches Veterinaires* 6, 325–336.

Bueno, L., Duranton, A. and Ruckebusch, Y. (1983) Antagonistic effects of naloxone on CCK-octapeptide induced satiety and rumino-reticular hypo-motility in sheep. *Life Sciences* 32, 855–863.

Bunk, M.J. and Coombs, C.F. (1980) Effect of selenium on appetite in the selenium-deficient chick. *Journal of Nutrition* 110, 743–749.

Burghardi, S.R., Goodrich, R.D., Meiske, J.C., Thonney, M.L., Theuninck, D.H., Kahlon, T.S., Pamp, D.E. and Kraiem, K. (1982) Free choice consumption of minerals by lambs fed calcium-adequate or calcium-deficient diets. *Journal of Animal Science* 54, 410–418.

Burkhart, C.A., Cherry, J.A., Van Krey, H.P. and Siegel, P.B. (1983) Genetic selection for growth rate alters hypothalamic satiety mechanisms in chickens. *Behaviour and Genetics* 13, 295–300.

Burritt, E.A. and Provenza, F.D. (1990) Food aversion learning in sheep, persistence of conditioned taste aversions to palatable shrubs (*Cercocarpus montagnus* and *Amelanchier alnifolia*). *Journal of Animal Science* 68, 1003–1007.

Byerly, T.C. (1979) Prediction of the food intake of laying hens. In: Boorman, K.N. and Freeman, B.M. (eds) *Food Intake Regulation in Poultry*, Longman, Edinburgh, pp. 327–363.

Bywater, A.C. (1984) A generalised model of feed intake and digestion in lactating cows. *Agricultural Systems* 13, 167–186.

Caird, L. and Holmes, W. (1986) The prediction of voluntary intake of grazing dairy cows. *Journal of Agricultural Science* 107, 43–54.

Calder, F.W., Nicholson, J.W.G. and Cunningham, H.M. (1964) Water restriction for sheep on pasture and rate of consumption with other feeds. *Canadian Journal of Animal Science* 44, 266–271.

Caldwell, J.M., Lyons, J.J. and Vandepopulier, J.M. (1986) Methane digester effluent as feedstuff for layers. *Poultry Science* 65, 147–152.

Campbell, R.G. (1976) A note on the use of a feed flavour to stimulate the feed intake of weaner pigs. *Animal Production* 23, 417–419.

Campfield, L.A. and Smith, F.J. (1986) Functional coupling between transient declines in blood glucose and feeding behavior:temporal relationships. *Brain Research Bulletin* 174, 427–433.

Campling, R.C. (1966a) The intake of hay and silage by cows. *Journal of the British Grassland Society* 21, 41–48.

Campling, R.C. (1966b) A preliminary study of the effect of pregnancy and of lactation on the voluntary intake of food by cows. *British Journal of Nutrition* 20, 25–39.

Campling, R.C. and Balch, C.C. (1961) Factors affecting the voluntary feed intake of the cow. 1. Preliminary observations on the effect, on the voluntary intake of hay, of changes in the amount of the reticulo-ruminal contents. *British Journal of Nutrition* 15, 523–530.

Campling, R.C. and Freer, M. (1966) Factors affecting the voluntary intake of food by cows. 8. Experiments with ground, pelletted roughages. *British Journal of Nutrition* 20, 229–244.

Campling, R.C. and Murdoch, J.C. (1966) The effect of concentrates on the voluntary intake of roughages by cows. *Journal of Dairy Research* 33, 1–11.

Canbeyli, R.S. and Koopmans, H.S. (1984) Comparison of gastric, duodenal and jejunal contributions to the inhibition of food intake in the rat. *Physiology and Behavior* 33, 951–958.

Cannon, W.B. and Washburn, A.L. (1912) An explanation of hunger. *American Journal of Physiology* 29, 441–443.

Carlisle, H.J. and Ingram, D.L. (1973) The effects of heating and cooling the spinal cord and hypothalamus on thermoregulatory behaviour in the pig. *Journal of Physiology* 231, 353–364.

Carr, S.B. and Jacobson, D.K. (1967) Intraruminal addition of mass or removal of rumen contents on voluntary intake of the bovine. *Journal of Dairy Science* 50, 1814–1818.

Carro, M.D., Lopez, S., Gonzalez, J.S. and Ovejero, F.J. (1991) The use of the rumen degradation characteristics of hay as predictors of voluntary intake by sheep. *Animal Production* 52, 133–139.

Carroll, F.D., Powers, S.B. and Clegg, M.T. (1963) Effect of cortisone acetate on steers. *Journal of Animal Science* 22, 1009–1011.

Carter, R.R. and Grovum, W.L. (1990) Factors affecting the voluntary intake of food by sheep. 5. The inhibitory effect of hypertonicity in the rumen. *British Journal of Nutrition* 64, 285–299.

Castle, M.E. (1976) A simple disc instrument for estimating herbage yield. *Journal of the British Grassland Society* 31, 37–40.

Castle, M.E. (1983) Feeding high-quality silage. In: *Silage for Milk Production*, Technical Bulletin No. 2, NIRD, HRI, pp. 127–150.

Castle, M.E. and Watson, J.N. (1975) Silage and milk production. A comparison between barley and dried grass as supplements to silage of high digestibility. *Journal of the British Grassland Society* 30, 217–222.

Castle, M.E. and Watson, J.N. (1976) Silage and milk production. A comparison between barley and groundnut cake as supplements to silage of high digestibility. *Journal of the British Grassland Society* 31, 191–195.

Castle, M.E. and Watson, J.N. (1979) Silage and milk production: a comparison between soya, groundnut and single-cell protein as silage supplements. *Grass and Forage Science* 34, 101–106.

Castle, M.E., Retter, W.C. and Watson, J.N. (1979) Silage and milk production: comparisons between three silages of different chop lengths. *Grass and Forage Science* 34, 293–301.

Castle, M.E., Reid, D. and Watson, J.N. (1983) Silage and milk production: studies with diets containing white clover silage. *Grass and Forage Science* 38, 193–200.

Castonguay, C.J., Kaiser, L.L. and Stern, J.S. (1986) Meal pattern analysis; artifacts, assumptions and implications. *Brain Research Bulletin* 17, 439–444.

Cave, N.A.G. (1978) The influence of non-esterified fatty acids on feeding activity of chicks. *Poultry Science* 57, 1124.

Cave, N.A.G. (1982) Effect of dietary short- and medium-chain fatty acids on feed intake by chicks. *Poultry Science* 61, 1147–1153.

Chacon, E. and Stobbs, T.H. (1976) Influence of progressive defoliation of a grass sward on the eating behaviour of cattle. *Australian Journal of Agricultural Research* 27, 709–725.

Chah, C.C. and Moran, E.T. (1985) Egg characteristics of high performance hens at the end of lay when given cafeteria access to energy, protein and calcium. *Poultry Science* 64, 1696–1712.

Chalmers, J.S., Moisey, F.R. and Leaver, J.D. (1984) The performance of dairy cows with access to self-feed silage offered concentrates from a free-access dispenser. *Animal Production* 39, 17–23.

Chalupa, W., Baile, C.A., McLaughlin, C.L. and Brand, J.G. (1979) Effect of introduction of urea on feeding behavior of Holstein heifers. *Journal of Dairy Science* 62, 1278–1284.

Chambers, A.R.M., Hodgson, J. and Milne, J.A. (1981) The development and use of equipment for the automatic recording of ingestive behaviour in sheep and cattle. *Grass and Forage Science* 36, 97–105.

Chapman, H.W. and Grovum, W.L. (1982) Studies on the palatability of salt and urea in sheep. *Proceedings of the Nutrition Society* 41, 73A.

Chapple, R.S. and Lynch, J.J. (1986) Behavioural factors modifying acceptance of supplementary foods by sheep. *Research and Development in Agriculture* 3, 113–120.

Chapple, R.S., Wodzika-Tomaszewska, M. and Lynch, J.J. (1987a) The learning behaviour of sheep when introduced to wheat. I. Wheat acceptance by sheep and the effect of trough familiarity. *Applied Animal Behaviour Science* 18, 157–162.

Chapple, R.S., Wodzika-Tomaszewska, M. and Lynch, J.J. (1987b) The learning behaviour of sheep introduced to wheat. II. Social transmission of wheat feeding and the role of the senses. *Applied Animal Behaviour Science* 18, 163–172.

Charnov, E.L., Orians, G.H. and Hyatt, K. (1976) The ecological implications of resources depression. *American Naturalist* 110, 247–259.

Chase, L.E., Wangsness, P.J. and Baumgardt, B.R. (1976) Feeding behavior of steers fed a complete mixed ration. *Journal of Dairy Science* 59, 1923–1928.

Chase, L.E., Wangsness, P.J. and Martin, R.J. (1977) Portal blood insulin and metabolite changes with spontaneous feeding in steers. *Journal of Dairy Science* 60, 410–415.

Chenost, M. and Demarquilly, C. (1982) Measurement of herbage intake by housed animals. In: Leaver, J.D. (ed.) *Herbage Intake Handbook*, British Grassland Society, Maidenhead, Berks, pp. 95–112.

Cherry, J.A. (1979) Adaptation in food intake after changes in dietary energy. In: Boorman, K.N. and Freeman, B.M. (eds) *Food Intake Regulation in Poultry*, Longman, Edinburgh, pp. 77–86.

Cherry, P. and Barwick, M.W. (1962) The effect of light on broiler growth: II. Light patterns. *British Poultry Science* 3, 41–50.

Chestnutt, D.M.B. (1989) The effect of contrasting silages offered in mid and late pregnancy on the performance of breeding ewes. *Animal Production* 49, 435–441.

Choung, J.J. and Chamberlain, D.G. (1992) The effects of postruminal supplements of casein and of soya-protein isolate with or without additional amino acids on silage intake and milk production in dairy cows. *Animal Production* 54, 502.

Christopherson, R.J. and Kennedy, P.M. (1983) Effects of the thermal environment on digestion in ruminants. *Canadian Journal of Animal Science* 63, 477–496.

Christopherson, R.J. and Webster, A.J.F. (1972) Changes during eating in oxygen consumption, cardiac function and body fluids in sheep. *Journal of Physiology* 221, 441–507.

Church, D.C. (1975) *Digestive Physiology and Nutrition of Ruminants*. Vol 1 – *Digestive Physiology*. D.C. Church, Corvallis, Oregon, 350pp.

Clancy, M., Bull, L.S., Wangsness, P.J. and Baumgardt, B.R. (1976) Digestible energy intake of complete diets by wethers and lactating ewes. *Journal of Animal Science* 42, 960–969.

Clancy, M., Wangsness, P.J. and Baumgardt, B.R. (1977) Effect of silage extract on voluntary intake, rumen fluid constituents, and rumen motility. *Journal of Dairy Science* 60, 580–590.

Clarke, R.T.J. and Reid, C.S.W. (1970) Legume bloat. In: Phillipson, A.T. (ed.)*Physiology of Digestion and Metabolism in the Ruminant*, Oriel Press, Newcastle upon Tyne, pp. 599–606.

Classen, H.L. and Scott, T.A. (1982) Self-selection of calcium during the rearing and early laying periods of White leghorn pullets. *Poultry Science* 61, 2065–2074.

Clifton, P.G. (1979) Patterns of feeding in the domestic chick. 2. An operant feeding situation. *Animal Behaviour* 27, 821–828.

Close, W.H. (1989) The influence of the thermal environment on the voluntary food intake of pigs. In: Forbes, J.M., Varley, M.A. and Lawrence, T.L.J. (eds) *The Voluntary Food Intake of Pigs*, Occasional Publication of the British Society of Animal Production, pp. 87–96.

Close, W.H., Mount, L.E. and Start, I.B. (1971) The influence of environmental temperature and plane of nutrition on heat loss from groups of growing pigs. *Animal Production* 13, 285–294.

Clough, P.A. (1972) Feeding 'porridge' in the parlour. *Dairy Farmer* 19, 18–21.

Colburn, M.W., Evans, J.L. and Ramage, C.H. (1968) Ingestion control in growing ruminant animals by the components of cell-wall constituents. *Journal of Dairy Science* 51, 1458–1464.

Colditz, P.J. and Kellaway, R.C. (1972) The effect of diet and heat stress on feed intake, growth and nitrogen metabolism in Friesian, F1 Brahman × Friesian, and Brahman heifers. *Australian Journal of Agricultural Research* 23, 717–725.

Cole, D.J.A. (1984) The nutrient density of pig diets – allowances and appetites. In: Wiseman, J. (ed.) *Fats in Animal Nutrition*, Butterworths, London, pp. 301–311.

Cole, D.J.A. and Chadd, S.A. (1989) Voluntary food intake of growing pigs. In: Forbes,J.M., Varley, M.A. and Lawrence, T.L.J. (eds) *The Voluntary Food Intake of Pigs*, Occasional Publication of the British Society of Animal Production, pp. 61–70.

Cole, D.J.A., Duckworth, J.E. and Holmes, W. (1967) Factors affecting voluntary feed intake in pigs. 1. The effect of digestible energy content of the diet on the intake of castrated male pigs housed in holding pens and in metabolism crates. *Animal Production* 9, 141–148.

Cole, D.J.A., Duckworth, J.E., Holmes, W. and Cuthbertson, A. (1968) Factors affecting voluntary feed intake in pigs. 3. The effect of a period of feed restriction, nutrient density in the diet and sex on intake, performance and carcass characteristics. *Animal Production* 10, 345–357.

Cole, D.J.A., Clent, E.G. and Luscombe, J.R. (1969) Single cereal diets for bacon pigs. 1. The effects of diets based on barley, wheat, maize meal, flaked maize or sorghum on performance and carcass characteristics. *Animal Production* 11, 325–335.

Cole, D.J.A., Hardy, B. and Lewis, D. (1972) Nutrient density in pig diets. In: Cole, D.J.A. (ed.) *Pig Production*, Butterworths, London, pp. 243–257.

Collier, G.H. (1985) Satiety, an ecological perspective. *Brain Research Bulletin* 14, 693–700.

Colvin, H.W., Digesti, R.D. and Louvier, J.A. (1978) Effect of succulent and nonsucculent diets on rumen motility and pressure before, during and after eating. *Journal of Dairy Science* 61, 1414–1421.

Conrad, H.R. (1987) Dairy cattle. In: *Predicting Feed Intake of Food-Producing Animals*, NRC Committee on Animal Nutrition, Washington, National Academy Press, pp. 48–55.

Conrad, H.R., Pratt, A.D. and Hibbs, J.W. (1964) Regulation of feed intake in dairy cows. 1. Change in importance of physical and physiological factors with increasing digestibility. *Journal of Dairy Science* 47, 54–62.

Conrad, H.R., Baile, C.A. and Mayer, J. (1977) Changing meal patterns and suppression of feed intake with increasing amounts of dietary nitrogen in ruminants. *Journal of Dairy Science* 60, 1725–1733.

Cooper, S.J. (1985) Neuropeptides and food and water intake. In: Sandler, M. and Silverstone, T. (eds) *Psychopharmacology of Food*, Oxford University Press, Oxford, pp. 17–58.

Cooper, R.A., Evans, S. and Kirk, J.A. (1991) Effects of water additives on water consumption, urine output and urine mineral levels in Angora goats. *Animal Production* 52, 609.

Cooper, S.D.B. and Kyriazakis, I. (1993) The diet selection of lambs offered food choices of different nutrient density. *Animal Production* 56, 469A.

Cooper, S.D.B., Kyriazakis, I., Anderson, D.H. and Oldham, J.D. (1993) The effect of physiological state (late pregnancy) on the diet selection of ewes. *Animal Production* 56, 469A.

Coppock, C.E., Noller, C.H., Wolfe, S.A., Callaghan, C.J. and Baker, J.S. (1972) Effect of forage–concentrate ratio in complete feeds fed ad libitum on feed intake prepartum and the occurrence of abomasal displacement in dairy cows. *Journal of Dairy Science* 55, 783–789.

Costain, R.A. and Lloyd, L.E. (1962) Consequences of the addition of zinc bacitracin to early weaned pig rations. *Journal of Animal Science* 21, 963–965.

Cottrell, D. (1993) *Nutrient Requirements of Ruminant Animals: Protein*, Commonwealth Agricultural Bureaux International, Wallingford, Oxford, 71pp.

Cottrell, D.D. and Iggo, A. (1984a) Mucosal enteroceptors with vagal afferent fibers in the proximal jejunum of sheep. *Journal of Physiology* 354, 497–522.

Cottrell, D.F. and Iggo, A. (1984b) Tension receptors with vagal afferent fibres in the proximal duodenum and pyloric sphincter of sheep. *Journal of Physiology* 354, 457–475.

Coulon, J.B., Hoden, A., Faverdin, P. and Journet, M. (1989) Dairy cows. In: Jarrige, R. (ed.) *Ruminant Nutrition, Recommended Allowances and Feed Tables*, INRA, Paris, pp. 73–91.

Covasa, M. and Forbes, J.M. (1993) The effect of food deprivation, time of exposure and type of food on diet selection of broiler chickens. *Proceedings of the Nutrition Society* 52, 380A.

Covasa, M. and Forbes, J.M. (1994a) Exogenous cholecystokinin octapeptide in broiler chickens: satiety, conditioned colour aversion and vagal mediation. *Physiology and Behavior* 56, 39–49.

Covasa, M. and Forbes, J.M. (1994b) Effects of the CCK receptor antagonist MK-329 on food intake in broiler chickens. *Pharmacology, Biochemistry and Behavior* 48, 476–486.

Covasa, M. and Forbes, J.M. (1995) The effects of social interaction on selection of feeds by broiler chickens. *British Poultry Science* (in press).

Cowan, P.J. and Michie, W. (1977a) Choice feeding of the turkey: use of a high-protein concentrate fed with either whole wheat, barley, oats or maize. *Zeitschrift fur Tierphysiologie, Tierernahrung und Futtermittelkunde* 39, 124–130.

Cowan, P.J. and Michie, W. (1977b) Environmental temperature and choice feeding of broilers. *British Journal of Nutrition* 40, 311–314.

Cowan, P.J. and Michie, W. (1978) Environmental temperature and broiler performance, the use of diets containing increasing amount of protein. *British Poultry Science* 19, 601–605.

Cowan, P.J., Michie, W. and Roele, D.J. (1978) Choice feeding of the egg-type pullet. *British Poultry Science* 19, 153–157.

Cowan, R.T., Robinson, J.J., McDonald, I. and Smart, R. (1980) Effects of body fatness at lambing and diet in lactation on body tissue loss, feed intake and milk yield of ewes in early lactation. *Journal of Agricultural Science* 95, 497–514.

Cowan, R.T., Reid, G.W., Greenhalgh, J.F.D. and Tait, C.A.G. (1981) Effects of feeding level in late pregnancy and dietary protein concentration during early lactation on food intake, milk yield, liveweight change and nitrogen balance of cows. *Journal of Dairy Research* 48, 201–212.

Crampton, E.W., Donefer, E. and Lloyd, L.E. (1960) A nutritive value index for forages. *Journal of Animal Science* 19, 538–544.

Crichlow, E.C. (1988) Ruminal lactic acidosis, forestomach epithelial receptor activation by undissociated volatile fatty acids and rumen fluids collected during loss of reticuloruminal motility. *Research in Veterinary Science* 45, 364–368.

Crichlow, E.C. and Leek, B.R. (1981) The importance of pH in relation to the acid-excitation of epithelial receptors in the reticulo-rumen of sheep. *Journal of Physiology* 310, 60P–61P.

Cropper, M.R. (1987) Growth and development of sheep in relation to feeding strategy. PhD thesis, University of Edinburgh.

Cropper, M.R. and Poppi, D.P. (1992) The effect of ambient temperature on feed intake and diet selection in growing lambs. *Animal Production* 54, 492.

Cropper, M., Lloyd, M.D. and Emmans, G.C. (1985) An investigation into the relationship between nutrient requirements and diet selection in growing lambs. *Animal Production* 40, 562.

Cropper, M., Lloyd, M., Emmans, G.C. and Hinks, C.E. (1986) Choice feeding as a method of determining lamb nutrient requirements and growth potential. *Animal Production* 42, 453–454.

Cumming, R.B. (1983) Further experiments on choice feeding in poultry. *Recent Advances in Animal Nutrition in Australia 1983*, pp. 313–316.

Cumming, R.B. (1984) Choice feeding of laying birds. *Proceedings of the 1984 Symposium of the Poultry Husbandry Research Foundation Within the University of Sydney.*

Cumming, R. (1987) The effect of dietary fibre and choice feeding on coccidiosis in chickens. *Proceedings of the 4th AAAP Animal Science Congress*, p. 216.

Cumming, R.B. (1992) Mechanisms of biological control of coccidiosis in chickens. *Australian Poultry Science Symposium*, University of Sydney, pp. 46–51.

Cumming, R.B., Mastika, I.M. and Wodzika-Tomaszewska, M. (1987) Practical aspects of choice feeding in poultry and its future role. *Recent Advances in Animal Nutrition in Australia 1987.*

Curll, M.L., Wilkins, R.J., Snaydon, R.W. and Shanmugalingham, V.S. (1985) The effects of stocking rate and nitrogen fertilizer on a perennial ryegrass–clover sward. 1. Sward and sheep performance. *Grass and Forage Science* 40, 129–140.

Curran, M.K. and Holmes, W. (1970) Prediction of the voluntary intake of food by dairy cows. 2. Lactating grazing cows. *Animal Production* 12, 213–224.

Curran, M.K., Campling, R.C. and Holmes, W. (1967) The feed intake of milk cows during pregnancy and early lactation. *Animal Production* 9, 266.

Curran, M.K., Wimble, R.H. and Holmes, W. (1970) Prediction of the voluntary intake of food by dairy cows. 1. Stall-fed cows in late pregnancy and early lactation. *Animal Production* 12, 195–212.

D'Mello, J.P. and Lewis, D. (170) Amino acid interactions in chick nutrition:

growth, food intake and plasma amino acid patterns. *British Poultry Science* 12, 345–358.

Dalby, J.A., Forbes, J.M., Varley, M.A. and Jagger, S. (1994a) Diet selection of weaned piglets – is a training period necessary? *Animal Production* 58, 435–436 (abstract).

Dalby, J.A., Forbes, J.M., Varley, M.A. and Jagger, S. (1994b) Diet selection of weaned piglets for lysine using flavour as a cue. *Proceedings of the 45th Annual Meeting of the European Association of Animal Production.*

Dalton, D.C. (1964) Dilution of the diet and feed intake in the mouse. *Nature* 205, 807.

Dargie, J.D. (1980) The pathophysiological effects of gastrointestinal and liver parasites in sheep. In: Ruckebusch, Y. and Thivend, P. (eds) *Digestive Physiology and Metabolism in Ruminant,* MTP Press, Lancaster, pp. 349–371.

Darre, M.J., Hanson, H.C. and Cogburn, L.A. (1978) The effect of pinealectomy on feed and oxygen consumption in immature cockerels. *Poultry Science* 57, 1132.

Davenport, H.W. (1966) *Physiology of the Digestive Tract.* Year Book Medical Publishers, Chicago, 230pp.

Davey, A.W.F. and Holmes, C.W. (1977) The effects of shearing on the heat production and activity of sheep receiving dried grass or ground hay. *Animal Production* 24, 355–361.

Davies H.L. (1962) Intake studies in sheep involving high fluid intake. *Proceedings of the Australian Society of Animal Production* 4, 167–171.

Davies, M.H. and Wade, A.P. (1993) Effect of extended daylength on appetite, liveweight performance and attainment of slaughter weight in weaned deer stag calves. *Animal Production* 56, 473.

Davis, J.D. and Smith, G.P. (1988) Analysis of lick rate measures the positive and negative feedback effects of carbohydrate on eating. *Appetite* 11, 229–238.

Davis, R.H., Hassann, O.E.M. and Sykes, A.H. (1973) Energy utilisation in the laying hen in relation to ambient temperature. *Journal of Agricultural Science* 81, 173–177.

Davis, S.L., Hossner, K.L. and Ohlson, D.L. (1984) Endocrine regulation of growth in ruminants. In: Roche, J.F. and O'Callaghan, D. (eds) *Manipulation of Growth in Farm Animals,* Martinus Nijhoff, Boston, pp. 151–178.

Dawkins, M.S. and Beardsley, T.M. (1986) Reinforcing properties of access to litter in hens. *Applied Animal Behaviour Science* 15, 351–364.

Deaton, J.W., Reece, F.N. and Naughton, J.L. (1978) The effect of temperature during the growing period on broiler performance. *Poultry Science* 57, 1070–1074.

Deetz, L.E. and Wangsness, P.J. (1980) Effect of intrajugular administration of insulin on feed intake, plasma glucose and plasma insulin of sheep. *Journal of Nutrition* 110, 1976–1982.

Deetz, L.E., Wangsness, P.J., Kavanaugh, J.F. and Griel, L.C. (1980) Effect of intraportal and continuous intrajugular administration of insulin on feeding in sheep. *Journal of Nutrition* 110, 1983–1991.

Degen, A.A., Kam, M., Rosenstrauch, A. and Plavnik, I. (1991) Growth rate, total body water volume, dry-matter intake and water consumption of domesticated ostriches (*Struthio camelus*). *Animal Production* 52, 225–232.

de Groot, G. (1972) A marginal income and cost analysis of the effect of nutrient density on the performance of White Leghorn hens in battery cages. *British Poultry Science* 13, 503–520.

de Haer, L.C.M. and Merks, J.W.M. (1992) Patterns of daily food intake in growing pigs. *Animal Production* 54, 95–104.

de Jong, A. (1981a) Regulation of food intake in the goat. PhD thesis, University of Groningen, 151pp.

de Jong, A. (1981b) Short- and long-term effects of eating on blood composition in free-feeding goats. *Journal of Agricultural Science* 96, 659–668.

de Jong, A. (1986) The role of metabolites and hormones as feedbacks in the control of food intake in ruminants. In: Milligan, L.P., Grovum, W.L. and Dobson, A. (eds) *Control of Digestion and Metabolism in Ruminants*, Prentice-Hall, Englewood Cliffs, NJ, pp. 459–478.

de Jong, A., Steffens, A.B. and de Ruiter, L. (1981) Effects of portal volatile fatty acid infusions on meal patterns and blood composition in goats. *Physiology and Behavior* 27, 683–689.

Della-Fera, M.A. and Baile, C.A. (1980) Cerebral ventricular injections of CCK-octapeptide and feed intake: the importance of continuous injection. *Physiology and Behavior* 24, 1133–1138.

Della-Fera, M.A., McLaughlin, C.A., Weston, R.H., Bender, P.E., Baile, C.A. and Chalupa, W.V. (1977) Rumen function during Elfazepam and 9-AZA-Cannabinol elicited feeding in sheep. *Federation Proceedings* 36, 1141.

Della-Fera, M.A., Baile, C.A. and Peikin, S.R. (1981) Feeding elicited by injection of the cholecyctokinin antagonist dibutyryl cyclic GMP into the cerebral ventricles of sheep. *Physiology and Behavior* 26, 799–801.

Della-Fera, M.A., Baile, C.A., Miner, J.L , Coleman, B. and Patterson, J.A. (1990) Feeding after bolus or continuous intracerebroventricular (icv) injection of Neuropeptide Y (NPY). *Journal of Animal Science* 68 Suppl 1, 257–258.

Demarquilly, C. (1973) [Chemical composition, fermentative characteristics, digestibility and amounts eaten of silage, modification by the proportion of the original green herbage.] *Annales de Zootechnie* 22, 1–35.

Demment, M.W. and Greenwood, G.B. (1988) Forage ingestion, effects of sward characteristics and body size. *Journal of Animal Science* 66, 2380–2392.

Denbow, D.M. (1985) Food intake control in birds. *Neuroscience and Biobehavioral Reviews* 9, 23–232.

Denbow, D.M. (1989) Peripheral and central control of food intake. *Poultry Science* 68, 938–947.

Denbow, D.M.and Myers, R.D. (1982) Eating, drinking and temperature responses to intracerebroventricular cholecystokinin in chicks. *Peptides* 3, 739–743.

Denbow, D.M., Van Krey, H.P. and Cherry, J.A. (1982) Feeding and drinking response of young chicks to injections of serotonin into the lateral ventricle of the brain. *Poultry Science* 61, 150–155.

Denbow, D.M., Van Krey, H.P., Lacy, M.P. and Dietrick, T.J. (1983) Feeding, drinking and body temperature of Leghorn chicks: effects of ICV injections of biogenic amines. *Physiology and Behavior* 31, 85–90.

Denbow, D.M., Van Krey, H.P. and Siegel, P.B. (1986) Selection for growth alters the feeding response to injections of biogenic amines. *Pharmacology, Biochemistry and Behavior* 24, 39–42.

Denton, D.A. (1982) *The Hunger for Salt.* Springer Verlag, Berlin, 650pp.

Deswysen, A.G. and Ellis, W.C. (1990) Fragmentation and ruminal escape of particles as related to variations in voluntary intake, chewing behaviour and extent of digestion of potentially digestible NDF in heifers. *Journal of Animal Science* 68, 3871–3879.

Deswyssen, A., Vanbelle, M. and Focant, M. (1978) The effect of silage chop length on the voluntary intake and rumination behaviour of sheep. *Journal of the British Grassland Society* 33, 107–115.

Deswysen, A.G., Dutilleul, P.A. and Ellis, W.C. (1989) Quantitative analysis of nycterohemeral eating and ruminating patterns in heifers with different voluntary intakes and effects of monensin. *Journal of Animal Science* 67, 2751–2761.

Devilat, J., Pond, W.G. and Miller, P.D. (1970) Dietary amino acid balance in growing-finishing pigs – effect on diet preference and performance. *Journal of Animal Science* 30, 536–543.

de Vries, A.G. and Kanis, E. (1992) A growth model to estimate economic values for food intake capacity in pigs. *Animal Production* 55, 241–246.

Dinius, D.A. and Baile, C.A. (1977) Beef cattle response to a feed intake stimulant given alone and in combination with a propionate enhancer and an anabolic agent. *Journal of Animal Science* 45, 147–153.

Dinius, D.A. and Baumgardt, B.R. (1970) Regulation of food intake in ruminants. 6. Influence of caloric density of pelletted rations. *Journal of Dairy Science* 53, 311–316.

Dinius, D.A., Kavanaugh, J.F. and Baumgardt, B.R. (1970) Regulation of food intake in ruminants. 7. Interrelations between food intake and body temperature. *Journal of Dairy Science* 53, 438–445.

Dirven, J.G.P. and Deinum, B. (1977) The effect of temperature on the digestibility of grasses: an analysis. *Forage Research* 3, 1–17.

Dodsworth, T.L. and Campbell, W.H.M. (1953) Report on a further experiment to compare the fattening values, for beef cattle, of silage made from grass cut at different stages of growth, together with the results of some supplementary experiments. *Journal of Agricultural Science* 43, 166–177.

Dominigue, B.M.F., Wilson, P.R., Dellow, D.W. and Barry, T.N. (1992) Effects of subcutaneous melatonin implants during long daylengths on voluntary feed intake, rumen capacity and heart rate of red deer (*Cervus elephas*) fed on a forage diet. *British Journal of Nutrition* 68, 77–88.

Donefer, E., Lloyd, L.E. and Crampton, E.W. (1963) Effect of varying alfalfa:barley ratios on energy intake and volatile fatty acid production by sheep. *Journal of Animal Science* 22, 425–428.

Donnelly, J.R., Davison, J.L. and Freer, M. (1974) Effect of body condition on the intake of food by mature sheep. *Australian Journal of Agricultural Research* 25, 813–823.

Dourmand, J.Y. (1991) Effect of feeding level in the gilt during pregnancy on voluntary feed intake during lactation and changes in body composition during gestation and lactation. *Livestock Production Science* 27, 309–319.

Dourmand, J.Y. (1993) Standing and feeding behaviour of the lactating sow: effect of feeding level during pregnancy. *Applied Animal Behaviour Science* 37, 311–319.

Dove, W.F. (1935) A study of individuality in the nutritive instincts and of the effects of variations in the selection of food. *American Naturalist* 69, 469–544.

Dove, H. and Mayes, R.W. (1991) The use of plant wax alkanes as marker substances in studies of the nutrition of herbivores: a review. *Australian Journal of Agricultural Research* 42, 913–952.

Dove, H. and Milne, J.A. (1991) An evaluation of the effects of incisor dentition and of age on the performance of lactating ewes and their lambs. *Animal Production* 53, 183–190.

Dowden, D.R. and Jacobson, D.R. (1960) Inhibition of appetite in dairy cattle by certain intermediate metabolites. *Nature, London* 188, 148–149.

Driver, P.M. and Forbes, J.M. (1981) Episodic growth hormone secretion in sheep in relation to time of feeding, spontaneous meals and short term fasting. *Journal of Physiology* 317, 413–424.

Driver, P.M. and Forbes, J.M. (1982) Feeding and GH after ventricular carbachol in sheep. *Annales de Recherches Veterinaire* 12, 99–101.

Driver, P.M., Forbes, J.M. and Scanes, C.G. (1979) Hormones, feeding and temperature in sheep following cerebroventricular injections of neuro-transmitters and carbachol. *Journal of Physiology* 290, 399–411.

Ducker, M.J., Kendall, P.T., Hemingway, R.G. and McClelland, T.H. (1981) An evaluation of feedblocks as a means of providing supplementary nutrients to ewes grazing upland/hill pastures. *Animal Production* 33, 51–57.

Duckworth, J.E. and Shirlaw, D.W. (1958) A study of factors affecting feed intake and the eating behaviour of cattle. *Animal Behaviour* 6, 147–154.

Dulphy, J.P. and Demarquilly, C. (1973) [Effect of type of forage harvester and chopping fineness on the feeding value of silages.] *Annales de Zootechnie* 22, 199–217.

Dulphy, J.P. and Faverdin, P. (1987) [Voluntary feed intake in ruminants, feeding patterns and associated phenomena.] *Reproduction, Nutrition, Developpement* 27, 129–155.

Dulphy, J.P., Remond, B. and Theriez, M. (1980) Ingestive behaviour and related activities in ruminants. In: Ruckebusch, Y. and Thivend, P. (eds) *Digestive Physiology and Metabolism in Ruminants*, MTP Press, Lancaster, pp. 103–122.

Duncan, I.J.H. and Hughes, B.O. (1975) Feeding activity and egg formation in hens lit continuously. *British Poultry Science* 16, 145–155.

Duncan, I.J.H., Horne, A.R., Hughes, B.O. and Wood-Gush, D.G.M. (1970) The pattern of food intake in female Brown Leghorn fowls as recorded in a Skinner box. *Animal Behaviour* 18, 245–255.

Dunlop, R.H. and Hammond, P.B. (1965) D-Lactic acidosis of ruminants. *Annales of the New York Academy of Science* 119, 1109–1132.

Duquette, P.F. and Muir, L A. (1979) Monitoring the effects of selected compounds on feeding behavior of sheep. *Journal of Animal Science* 49, 1120–1124.

Duranton, A. and Bueno, L. (1985) Influence of regimen (roughage vs. concentrate) on satiety and forestomach motility in sheep. *Physiology and Behavior* 35, 105–108.

du Toit, J.T., Provenza, F.D. and Nastis, A. (1991) Conditioned taste aversions:

how sick must a ruminant get before it learns about toxicity in foods? *Applied Animal Behaviour Science* 30, 35–46.

Dynes, R.A. (1993) Factors causing feed intake depression in lambs infected by gastrointestinal parasites. PhD Thesis, Lincoln University, 194pp.

Dynes, R.A., Ankersmit, A.E.L., Poppi, D.P., Barrell, G.K. and Sykes, A.R. (1990) Studies on the physiological basis of appetite depression in nematode infection in sheep. *Proceedings of the New Zealand Society of Animal Production* 50, 249–253.

Ebenezer, I.S., de la Riva, C. and Baldwin, B.A. (1990) Effects of the CCK receptor antagonist MK-329 on food intake in pigs. *Physiology and Behavior* 47, 145–148.

Edelsten, P.R. and Newton, J.E. (1977) A simulation model of a lowland sheep system. *Agricultural Systems* 2, 17–32.

Edholm, O.G., Fletcher, J.G., Widdowson, E.M. and McCance, R.A. (1955) Energy expenditure and food intake of individual men. *British Journal of Nutrition* 9, 286–300.

Edmonds, M.S., Gonyou, H.W. and Baker, D.H. (1987) Effect of excess levels of methionine, tryptophan, arginine, lysine or threonine on growth and dietary choice in the pig. *Journal of Animal Science* 65, 179–185.

Edwards, S.A. and Poole, D.A. (1983) The effects of including sodium bicarbonate in the diet of dairy cows in early lactation. *Animal Production* 37, 183–188.

Edwards, S.A., Marconnet, C., Taylor, A.G. and Cadenhead, A. (1992) Voluntary intake and digestibility of distillery products for dry sows. *Animal Production* 54, 486A.

Egan, A.R. (1965a) Nutritional status and intake regulation in sheep. 2. The influence of sustained duodenal infusions of casein or urea upon voluntary intake of low-protein roughages by sheep. *Australian Journal of Agricultural Research* 16, 452–462.

Egan, A.R. (1965b) Nutritional status and intake regulation in sheep. 3. The relationship between improvement of nitrogen status and increase in voluntary intake of low-protein roughages by sheep. *Australian Journal of Agricultural Research* 16, 463–472.

Egan, A.R. (1970) Nutritional status and intake regulation in sheep. 6. Evidence for variation in setting of an intake regulatory mechanism relating to the digesta content of the reticulorumen. *Australian Journal of Agricultural Research* 21, 735–746.

Egan, A.R. (1972) Nutritional status and intake regulation in sheep. 7. Control of voluntary intake of three diets and the responses to intraruminal feeding. *Australian Journal of Agricultural Research* 23, 347–361.

Egan, A.R. and Moir, R.J. (1964) Nutritional status and intake regulation in sheep. 1. Effects of duodenally infused single doses of casein, urea and propionate upon voluntary intake of a low protein roughage. *Australian Journal of Agricultural Research* 16, 437–449.

Elkin, R.G. (1986) A review of duck nutrition and research. *World's Poultry Science Journal* 43, 84–106.

Ellington, E.F., Fox, C.W., Kennick, W.H. and Sather, L.A. (1967) Feedlot performance and carcass characteristics of lambs receiving cortisone and diethylstilbestrol. *Journal of Animal Science* 26, 462–465.

Elliot, J.M., Symonds, H.W. and Pike, B. (1985) Effect on feed intake of infusing sodium propionate or sodium acetate into a mesenteric vein of cattle. *Journal of Dairy Science* 68, 1165–1170.

Elliott, R.C. (1967) Voluntary intake of low-protein diets by ruminants. 1. Intake of food by cattle. *Journal of Agricultural Science* 69, 375–382.

Elliott, R.C. and Topps, J.H. (1963) Voluntary intake of low protein diets by sheep. *Animal Production* 5, 269–276.

Ellis, M., Smith, W.C. and Laird, R. (1979) Correlated responses in feed intake to selection for economy of production and carcass lean content in Large White pigs. *Animal Production* 28, 424.

Ellis, W.C. (1978) Determinants of grazed forage intake and digestibility. *Journal of Dairy Science* 61, 1828–1840.

Elwinger, K. and Nilsson, L. (1984) Alternative diets for laying hens. Experiments with domestic feed stuffs and on-farm feed preparation. *Report 13,8 Department of Animal Nutrition and Management, Uppsala University.*

Emmans, G.C. (1977) The nutrient intake of laying hens given a choice of diets in relation to their protein requirement. *British Poultry Science*, 18, 227–236.

Emmans, G.C. (1991) Diet selection by animals: theory and experimental design. *Proceedings of the Nutrition Society* 50, 59–64.

Emmerson, D.E., Denbow, D.M. and Hulet, R.M. (1990) Protein and energy self-selection of turkey breeder hens: reproductive performance. *British Poultry Science* 31, 283–292.

Emmerson, D.E., Denbow, D.M., Hulet, R.M., Potter, L.M. and Van Krey, P. (1991) Self-selection of dietary protein and energy by turkey breeder hens. *British Poultry Science* 32, 555–564.

Engelke, G.L., Jurgens, M.H. and Speer, V.C. (1984) Performance of growing-finishing swine fed high-moisture or artificially dried corn in complete and free-choice diets. *Journal of Animal Science* 58, 1307–1312.

English, P.B. (1966) A study of water and electrolyte metabolism in sheep. 1. External balances of water, sodium, potassium and chloride. *Research in Veterinary Science* 7, 233–257.

Etheridge, M.O., Stockdale, C.R. and Cranwell, P.D. (1993) Influence of method of conservation of lucerne on factors associated with voluntary intake in sheep. *Australian Journal of Experimental Agriculture* 33, 417–423.

Evans, A.J. (1972) The effect of protamine zinc insulin on weight gain and fat deposition in the juvenile domestic duck. *Quarterly Journal of Experimental Physiology* 57, 1–11.

Even, P. and Nicolaidis, S. (1986) Short-term control of feeding: limitation of the glucostatic theory. *Brain Research Bulletin* 17, 621–626.

Everitt, G.C. (1966) Maternal food consumption and foetal growth in Merino sheep. *Proceedings of the Australian Society of Animal Production* 6, 91–101.

Everson, R.A., Jorgensen, N.A., Crowley, J.W., Jensen, E.L. and Barrington, G.P. (1976) Input–output of dairy cows fed a complete ration of a constant or variable forage-to-grain ratio. *Journal of Dairy Science* 59, 1776–1787.

Ewan, R.C. (1983) *Voluntary Feed Intake of the Pig.* Iowa State University Cooperative Extension Service Publication NoAS-539-T, Ames, Iowa.

Faichney, G.J. (1992) Consumption of solid feed by young lambs during their transition for pre-ruminant to full ruminant function. *Applied Animal Behaviour Science* 34, 85–91.

Fairley, R.A.C., Rose, S.P. and Fuller, M.F. (1993) Selection of dietary lysine and threonine concentration of growing pigs. *Animal Production* 56, 468–469A.

Fantz, R.L. (1957) Form preference in newly hatched chicks. *Journal of Comparative and Physiological Psychology* 50, 422–430.

Farhan, S.M.A. and Thomas, P.C. (1978) The effect of partial neutralisation of formic acid silages with sodium bicarbonate on their voluntary intake by cattle and sheep. *Journal of the British Grassland Society* 33, 151–158.

Farrell, D.J., Ball, W., Thomson, E., Abdelsamie, R.E. and Pesti, G.M. (1989) How well do layers discriminate given choices of grain and protein concentrate? *Recent Advances in Animal Nutrition in Australia 1989*, 311–321.

Faust, I.M., Johnson, P.R. and Hirsch, J. (1977) Surgical removal of adipose tissue alters feeding behavior and the development of obesity in rats. *Science* 197, 393–396.

Faverdin, P. (1986a) [Variations of blood insulin at feeding in the lactating cow.] *Reproduction, Nutrition, Developpement* 26, 381–382.

Faverdin, P. (1986b) [Injections of physiological doses of insulin in the lactating cow: effects on the amount eaten and blood metabolites.] *Reproduction, Nutrition, Developpement* 26, 383–384.

Faverdin, P. (1990) [Effects of infusions of a mixture of volatile fatty acids during meals on feeding behaviour of dry and lactating cows.] *Reproduction, Nutrition, Developpement* suppl 2, 213s–214s.

Faverdin, P., Dulphy, J.P., Coulon, J.B., Verite, R., Garel, J.P., Rouel, J. and Marquis, B. (1991) Substitution of roughage by concentrates for dairy cows. *Livestock Production Science* 27, 137–156.

Felix, B., Auffray, P. and Marcilloux, J.C. (1980) [Effect of induced hypothalamic hyperphagia and forced-feeding on organ weight and tissular development in Landes geese.] *Reproduction, Nutrition, Developpement* 20, 709–717.

Ferguson, K.A. (1958) The influence of thyroxine on wool growth. *Proceedings of the New Zealand Society of Animal Production* 18, 128–140.

Fernstrom, J.D. (1987) Food-induced changes in brain serotonin synthesis: is there a relationship to appetite for specific macronutrients. *Appetite* 8, 163–182.

Filmer, D. (1991) A new system for livestock feeding. *Feeds and Feeding* July/ August, 1991.

Firman, J.D. and Keunzel, W.J. (1988) Neuroanatomical regions of the chick brain involved in monitoring amino acid deficient diets. *Brain Research Bulletin* 21, 637–642.

Fisher, C. (1983) Egg production. In: Rook, J.A.F. and Thomas, P.C. (eds) *Nutritional Physiology of Farm Animals*, Longman, London, pp. 626–638.

Fisher, D.S., Burns, J.C. and Pond, K.R. (1987) Modeling ad libitum dry matter intake by ruminants as regulated by distension and chemostatic feedbacks. *Journal of Theoretical Biology* 126, 407–418.

Flores, E.R., Provenza, F.D. and Balph, D.F. (1989a) Role of experience in the development of foraging skills of lambs browsing the shrub serviceberry. *Applied Animal Behaviour Science* 23, 271–278.

Flores, E.R., Provenza, F.D. and Balph, D.F. (1989b) Relationship between plant maturity and foraging experience of lambs grazing hycrest crested wheatgrass. *Applied Animal Behaviour Science* 23, 279–284.

Folse, L.J., Packard, J.M. and Grant, W.E. (1989) AI modelling of animal movements in a heterogeneous habitat. *Ecological Modelling* 46, 57–72.

Foot, J.Z. (1972) A note on the effect of body condition on the voluntary food intake of dried grass wafers by Scottish Blackface ewes. *Animal Production* 14, 131–134.

Foot, J.Z. and Greenhalgh, J.F.D. (1969) Effect of previous dietary restriction on the voluntary food intake of sheep in late pregnancy. *Animal Production* 11, 279–280.

Foot, J.Z. and Russel, A.J.F. (1978) Pattern of intake on three roughage diets by non-pregnant, non-lactating Scottish Blackface ewes over a long period and the effects of previous nutritional history on current intake. *Animal Production* 26, 203–215.

Foot, J.Z., Russel, A.J.F., Maxwell, T.J. and Morris, P. (1973) Variation in intake among group-fed pregnant Scottish Blackface ewes given restricted amounts of food. *Animal Production*, 17, 169–177.

Forbes, J.M. (1967) The water intake of ewes. *British Journal of Nutrition* 22, 33–43.

Forbes, J.M. (1968) The physical relationships of the abdominal organs in the pregnant ewe. *Journal of Agricultural Science* 70, 171–177.

Forbes, J.M. (1969a) The effect of pregnancy and fatness on the volume of rumen contents in the ewe. *Journal of Agricultural Science* 72, 119–121.

Forbes, J.M. (1969b) A note on the voluntary feed intake of lactating ewes, their milk yield and the growth rate of their lambs. *Animal Production* 11, 263–266.

Forbes, J.M. (1970) Voluntary food intake of pregnant ewes. *Journal of Animal Science* 31, 1222–1227.

Forbes, J.M. (1971) Physiological changes affecting voluntary food intake in ruminants. *Proceedings of the Nutrition Society* 30, 135–142.

Forbes, J.M. (1972) Effects of oestradiol-17β on voluntary food intake in sheep and goats. *Journal of Endocrinology* 52, viii–ix.

Forbes, J.M. (1974) Feeding in sheep modified by intraventricular estradiol and progesterone. *Physiology and Behavior* 12, 741–747.

Forbes, J.M. (1977a) Interrelationships between physical and metabolic control of voluntary food intake in fattening, pregnant and lactating mature sheep a model. *Animal Production* 24, 90–101.

Forbes, J.M. (1977b) Development of a model of voluntary food intake and energy balance in lactating cows. *Animal Production* 24, 203–214.

Forbes, J.M. (1980) A model of the short-term control of feeding in the ruminant: effects of changing animal or feed characteristics. *Appetite* 1, 21–41.

Forbes, J.M. (1982a) Prediction of the voluntary intake of complete foods by growing cattle. *Animal Production* 34, 372.

Forbes, J.M. (1982b) Effects of lighting pattern on growth, lactation and food intake of sheep, cattle and deer. *Livestock Production Science* 9, 361–374.

Forbes, J.M. (1983) Models for the prediction of food intake and energy balance in dairy cows. *Livestock Production Science* 10, 149–157.

Forbes, J.M. (1986a) *The Voluntary Food Intake of Farm Animals.* Butterworths, London, 207pp.

Forbes, J.M. (1986b) Effects of sex hormones and lactation on the digestive tract and food intake. in: Milligan, L.P., Grovum, W.L. and Dobson, A. (eds) *Control of Digestion and Metabolism in the Ruminant.* Prentice-Hall, New Jersey, pp. 420–435.

Forbes, J.M. (1988a) Prediction of food intake by lactating cows. In: Garnsworthy, P.C. (ed.) *Nutrition and Lactation in the Dairy Cow.* Butterworths, London, pp. 294–312.

Forbes, J.M. (1988b) Metabolic aspects of the regulation of voluntary food intake and appetite. *Nutrition Research Reviews* 1, 145–168.

Forbes, J.M. and Baile, C.A. (1974) Feeding and drinking in sheep following hypothalamic injections of carbachol. *Journal of Dairy Science* 57, 878–883.

Forbes, J.M. and Barrio, J.P. (1992) Abdominal chemo- and mechanosensitivity in ruminants and its role in the control of food intake. *Experimental Physiology* 77, 27–50.

Forbes, J.M. and Blundell, J.E. (1989) Central nervous control of voluntary food intake. In: Forbes, J.M., Varley, M.A. and Lawrence, T.L.J. (eds) *The Voluntary Food Intake of Pigs*, Occasional Publication of the British Society of Animal Production, pp. 7–26.

Forbes, J.M. and Catterall, J. (1993) Substitution of low protein for high protein food by broiler chickens. *Proceedings of the Nutrition Society* 52, 355A.

Forbes, J.M. and Covasa, M. (1995) Application of diet selection by poultry with particular respect to whole cereals. *World's Poultry Science Journal* (in press).

Forbes, J.M. and France, J. (eds) (1993) *Quantitative Aspects of Ruminant Digestion and Metabolism*, CAB International, Wallingford, 515pp.

Forbes, J.M. and Rook, J.A.F. (1970) The effect of intravenous infusion of oestrogen on lactation in the goat. *Journal of Physiology* 207, 79pp.

Forbes, J.M. and Shariatmadari, F.S. (1994) Diet selection for protein by poultry. *World's Poultry Science Journal* 50, 7–24.

Forbes, J.M., Rees, J.K. and Boaz, T.G. (1967) Silage as a feed for pregnant ewes. *Animal Production* 9, 399–408.

Forbes, J.M., Wright, J.A. and Bannister, A. (1972) A note on rate of eating in sheep. *Animal Production* 15, 211–214.

Forbes, J.M., El Shahat, A.A., Jones, R., Duncan, J.G.S. and Boaz, T.G. (1979) The effect of daylength on the growth of lambs. 1. Comparison of sex, level of feeding, shearing and breed of sire. *Animal Production* 29, 33–42.

Forbes, J.M., Brown, W.B., Al Banna, A.G.M. and Jones, R. (1981) The effect of daylength on the growth of lambs. 3. Level of feeding, age of lamb and speed of gut-fill response. *Animal Production* 32, 23–28.

Forbes, J.M., Jackson, D.A., Johnson, C.L., Stockill, P. and Hoyle, B.S. (1987) A method for the automatic monitoring of food intake and feeding behaviour of individual cows kept in a group. *Research and Development in Agriculture* 3, 175–180.

Forbes, J.M., Bermudez, F.F. and Jones, R. (1989) Feeding behaviour of sheep during pregnancy and lactation. *Appetite* 13, 211–222.

Forbes, J.M., Johnson, C.L. and Jackson, D.A. (1991) The drinking behaviour of lactating cows offered silage *ad lib. Proceedings of the Nutrition Society* 50, 97A.

Forbes, J.M., Mbanya, J.N. and Anil, M.H. (1992) Comparisons of the effects of intraruminal infusions of sodium acetate and sodium chloride on silage intake by lactating cows. *Appetite* 19, 293–301.

Forbes, T.D.A. (1988) Researching the plant–animal interface: the investigation of ingestive behavior in grazing animals. *Journal of Animal Science* 66, 2369–2379.

Forbes, T.D.A. and Beattie, M.M. (1987) Comparative studies of ingestive behaviour and diet composition in oesophageal fistulated and non-fistulated cows and sheep. *Grass and Forage Science* 42, 79–84.

Foster, L.A., Ames, N.K. and Emery, R.S. (1991) Food intake and serum insulin responses to intraventricular infusions of insulin and IGF-1. *Physiology and Behavior* 50, 745–749.

Fowler, V.R. and Gill, B.P. (1989) Voluntary food intake in the young pig. In: Forbes, J.M., Varley, M.A. and Lawrence, T.L.J. (eds) *The Voluntary Food Intake of Pigs*, Occasional Publication of the British Society of Animal Production, pp. 51–60.

Fowler, V.R., McWilliam, R. and Aitken, R. (1981) Voluntary feed intake of boars, castrates and gilts given diets of different nutrient density. *Animal Production* 32, 357.

Fowler, V.R., McWilliam, R., Pennie, K. and James, M. (1984) The effects of dietary novelty and frequency of feeding on the food intake and performance of growing pigs. *Animal Production* 38, 535–536.

Fox, D.G., Preston, R.L., Senft, B. and Johnson, R.R. (1974) Plasma growth hormone levels and thyroid secretion rates during compensatory growth in beef cattle. *Journal of Animal Science* 38, 437–441.

Fox, M.T., Jacobs, D.E., Campling, R.C., Pocknee, B.R., Clampitt, R. and Hart, I.C. (1985) Effect of thiabendazole treatment on feed intake, digestibility and selected blood values in lactating dairy cows. *Veterinary Record* 116, 257–260.

Fraser, A.F. (ed.) (1985) *Ethology of Farm Animals*. Elsevier, Amsterdam, 500pp.

Fraser, D. and Broom, D.M. (1990) *Farm Animal Behaviour and Welfare*. Bailliere Tindal, London, 437pp.

Fraser, D. and Rushen, J. (1992) Colostrum intake by newborn piglets. *Canadian Journal of Animal Science* 72, 1–14.

Fraser, D., Patience, J.F., Phillips, P.A. and McLeese, J.M. (1990) Water for piglets and lactating sows, quantity, quality and qaundaries. In: Haresign, W. and Cole, D.J.A. (eds) *Recent Advances in Animal Nutrition*, Butterworths, London, pp. 137–160.

Frederick, G., Forbes, J.M. and Johnson, C.L. (1988) Masking the taste of rapeseed meal in dairy compound food. *Animal Production* 46, 518.

Freer, M. (1966) The utilisation of irrigated pastures by dairy cows. 2. The effect of stocking rate. *Journal of Agricultural Science* 54, 243–256.

Freer, M. and Campling, R.C. (1963) Factors affecting the voluntary intake of food by cows. 5. The relationship between the voluntary intake of food, the amount of digesta in the reticulo-rumen and the rate of disappearance of digesta from the alimentary tract with diets of hay, dried grass or concentrates. *British Journal of Nutrition* 17, 79–88.

Friedman, M.I. and Sawchenko, P.E. (1984) Evidence for hepatic involvement in control of ad libitum food intake in rats. *American Journal of Physiology* 247, R106–113.

Friedman, M.I., Tordoff, M.G. and Ramirez, I. (1986) Integrated metabolic control of food intake. *Brain Research Bulletin*, 17, 855–859.

Friend, D.W. (1970) Self-selection of feeds and water by swine during pregnancy and lactation. *Journal of Animal Science* 32, 658–666.

Friend, D.W. (1973) Self-selection of feeds and water by unbred gilts. *Journal of Animal Science* 37, 1137–1141.

Friend, T.M., Polan, C.E. and McGilliard, M.L. (1977) Free stall and feed bunk requirements relative to behavior, production and individual feed intake in dairy cows. *Journal of Dairy Science* 60, 108–116.

Fuller, M.F. (1965) The effect of environmental temperature on the nitrogen metabolism and growth of the young pig. *British Journal of Nutrition* 19, 531–546.

Funk, E.M. (1932) Can the chick balance its ration? *Poultry Science* 11, 94–97.

Furuse, M., Yang, S.I., Choi, Y.H., Kawamura, N., Takahashi, A. and Okomura, J. (1991) A note on plasma cholecystokinin concentration in dairy cows. *Animal Production* 53, 123–125.

Galef, B.G. (1989) Enduring social enhancement of rats: preferences for the palatable and the piquant. *Appetite* 13, 81–92.

Gallouin, F. and Le Magnen, J. (1987) Evolution historique des concepts de faim, satiete et appetits. *Reproduction, Nutrition, Developpement* 27, 109–128.

Garnsworthy, P.C. and Huggett, C.D. (1992) The influence of the fat concentration of the diet on the response by dairy cows to body condition at calving. *Animal Production* 54, 7–13.

Garnsworthy, P.C. and Jones, G.P. (1987) The influence of body condition at calving and dietary protein supply on voluntary food intake and performance in dairy cows. *Animal Production* 44, 347–353.

Garnsworthy, P.C. and Topps, J.H. (1982) The effect of body condition of dairy cows at calving on their food intake and performance when given complete diets. *Animal Production* 35, 113–119.

Gatel, F. and Guion, P. (1990) Effects of monosodium 1 glutamate on diet palatability and piglet performance during the sucking and weaning periods. *Animal Production* 50, 365–372.

Gavin, M.L., Gray, J.M. and Johnson, P.R. (1984) Estrogen-induced effects on food intake and body weight in ovariectomised, partially lipectomised rats. *Physiology and Behavior* 32, 55–60.

Geary, N. (1979) Food intake and behavioural caloric compensation after protein repletion in the rat. *Physiology and Behavior*, 23, 1089.

Geiselman, P.J., Martin, J.R., Vanderweele, D.A. and Novin, D. (1980) Multivariate analysis of meal patterning in intact and vagotomised rabbits. *Journal of Comparative and Physiological Psychology* 94, 388–399.

Gengler, W.R., Martz, F.A., Johnson, H.D., Krause, G.F. and Hahn, L. (1970) Effect of temperature on food and water intake and rumen fermentation. *Journal of Dairy Science* 53, 434–437.

Gentle, M.J. (1971) Taste and its importance to the domestic chicken. *British Poultry Science* 12, 77–86.

Gentle, M.J. (1976) The effect of gold thioglucose on the central nervous system of chicks (*Gallus domesticus*). *Toxicology and Applied Pharmacology* 35, 223–228.

Gentle, M.J. and Richardson, A. (1972) Changes in the electro-encephalogram of the chicken produced by stimulation of the crop. *British Poultry Science* 13, 163–170.

Gentle, M.J., Dewar, W.A., Wight, P.A.L. and Dick, K.M. (1982) The effects of high dietary zinc on food intake in the domestic fowl. *Appetite* 3, 53–60.

Gherardi, S.G. and Black, J.L. (1991) Effect of palatability on voluntary feed intake by sheep. I. Identification of chemicals that alter the palatability of a forage. *Australian Journal of Agricultural Research* 42, 571–584.

Gherardi, S.C., Black, J.L. and Colebrook, W.F. (1991) Effect of palatability on voluntary feed intake by sheep. II. The effect of altering the palatability of wheaten hay on long-term intake and preference. *Australian Journal of Agricultural Research* 42, 585–598.

Gibbs, J., Young, R.C. and Smith, G.P. (1973) Cholecystokinin elicits satiety in rats with open gastric fistulas. *Nature* 245, 323–325.

Gidlewski, T., Cherry, J.A., Siegel, P.B. and Van Krey, H.P. (1982) Feed intake responses of four populations of chickens to calories in liquid form. *Archivs fur Geflugelkunde* 46, 136–142.

Giles, L.R., Murison, R.D. and Wilson, B.R. (1981) Backfat studies in growing pigs. 1. Influence of energy intake on growth and carcass measurements at varying liveweights. *Animal Production* 32, 39–46.

Gill, M.S. and Castle, M.E. (1983) The effects of the frequency of feeding concentrates on milk production and eating behaviour in Ayrshire dairy cows. *Animal Production* 36, 79–86.

Gill, M. and England, P. (1984) Effect of degradability of protein supplements on voluntary intake and nitrogen retention in young cattle fed grass silage. *Animal Production* 39, 31–36.

Gillette, K., Martin, G.M. and Bellingham, W.P. (1980) Differential use of food and water cues in the formation of conditioned aversions by domestic chicks (*Gallus gallus*). *Journal of Experimental Psychology: Animal Behavior Processes* 6, 99–111.

Gillingham, M.P. and Bunnel, F.L. (1989) Effects of learning on food selection and searching behaviour of deer. *Canadian Journal of Zoology* 67, 24–32.

Glick, Z. (1979) Intestinal satiety with and without upper intestinal factors. *American Journal of Physiology* 236, R142–R146.

Glimp, H.A. (1971) Effect of diet composition on diet preference by lambs. *Journal of Animal Science* 33, 861–864.

Goatcher, W.D. and Church, D.C. (1970) Review of some nutritional aspects of the sense of taste. *Journal of Animal Science* 31, 973–981.

Golian, A. and Polin, G. (1984) Passage rate of feed in very young chickens. *Poultry Science* 63, 1013–1019.

Gordon, C.H., Derbyshire, J.C., Wiseman, H.G. and Kane, E.A. (1961) Preservation and feeding value of alfalfa stored as hay, haylage, and direct cut silage. *Journal of Dairy Science* 44, 1299–1311.

Gordon, I.J. and Illius, A.W. (1992) Foraging strategy: from mosaic to monoculture. In: Speedy, A.W. (ed.) *Progress in Sheep and Goat Research*, CAB

International, Wallingford, pp. 153–177.

Gordon, J.G. (1964) Effect of time of year on the roughage intake of housed sheep. *Nature* 204, 798–799.

Gordon, J.G. (1965) The effect of water deprivation upon the rumination behaviour of housed sheep. *Journal of Agricultural Science* 64, 31–35.

Gordon, J.G. and Tribe, D.E. (1951) The self-selection of diet by pregnant ewes. *Journal of Agricultural Science* 41, 187–190.

Gordon, J.G., Tribe, D.E. and Graham, T.C. (1954) The feeding behaviour of phosphorus-deficient cattle and sheep. *British Journal of Animal Behaviour* 2, 72–74.

Gous, R.M. and DuPreez, J.J. (1975) The sequential feeding of growing chickens. *British Journal of Nutrition* 34, 113–117.

Graham, N.M. (1969) The influence of body weight (fatness) on the energetic efficiency of adult sheep. *Australian Journal of Agricultural Research* 20, 375–385.

Graham, N.M. and Searle, T.W. (1975) Studies of weaner sheep during and after a period of weight stasis. 1. Energy metabolism and nitrogen utilization. *Australian Journal of Agricultural Research* 26, 343–353.

Graham, N.M. and Williams, A.J. (1962) The effects of pregnancy on the passage of food through the digestive tract of sheep. *Australian Journal of Agricultural Research* 13, 894–900.

Graham, W.R. (1932) Can we learn anything from a free-choice of feeds as expressed by chicks? *Poultry Science* 11, 365–366.

Grant, S.A., Suckling, D.E., Smith, H.K., Torvell, L., Forbes, T.D.A. and Hodgson, J. (1985) Comparative studies of diet selection by sheep and cattle: the hill grasslands. *Journal of Ecology* 73, 987–1004.

Green, G.C., Elwin, R.L., Mottershead, B.E., Keogh, R.G. and Lynch, J.J. (1984) Long term effects of early experience to supplementary feeding in sheep. *Proceedings of the Australian Society of Animal Production* 15, 373–380.

Greenhalgh, J.F.D. (1982) An introduction to herbage intake measurements. In: Leaver, J.D. (ed.) *Herbage Intake Handbook*. British Grassland Society, Maidenhead, Berks, pp. 1–10.

Greenhalgh, J.F.D. and Reid, G.W. (1967) Separating the effects of digestibility and palatability on food intake in ruminant animals. *Nature* 214, 744.

Greenhalgh, J.F.D. and Reid, G.W. (1969) The effects of grazing intensity on herbage consumption and animal production. 3. Dairy cows grazed at two intensities on clean and contaminated pastures. *Journal of Agricultural Science* 72, 223–228.

Greenhalgh, J.F.D., Reid, G.W. and Aitken, J.N. (1966) The effects of grazing intensity on herbage consumption and animal production. 1. Short-term effects in strip-grazing dairy cows. *Journal of Agricultural Science* 67, 13–23.

Greenwood, G.B. and Demment, M.W. (1988) The effect of fasting on short-term cattle grazing behavior. *Grass and Forage Science* 43, 377–386.

Gregory, P.C. and Rayner, D.V. (1987) The influence of gastrointestinal infusion of fats on regulation of food intake in pigs. *Journal of Physiology* 385, 471–481.

Gregory, P.C., McFadyen, M. and Rayner, D.V. (1987) The influence of gastro-intestinal infusions of glucose on regulation of food intake in pigs.

*Quarterly Journal of Experimental Physiology* 72, 525–535.

Grill, H.J. (1986) Caudal brainstem contributions to the integrated neural control of energy homeostasis. In: Ritter, R.C., Ritter, S. and Barnes, C.D. (eds) *Feeding Behavior – Neural and Humoral Controls*. Academic Press, New York, pp. 103–129.

Grimmett, R.E. (1939) Arsenical soils of the Waiotopee Valley. *New Zealand Agriculture* 58, 383.

Grovum, W.L. (1979) Factors affecting the voluntary intake of food by sheep. 2. The role of distension and tactile input from compartments of the stomach. *British Journal of Nutrition* 42, 425–436.

Grovum, W.L. (1981) Cholecystokinin administered intravenously did not act directly on the central nervous system or on the liver to suppress food intake by sheep. *British Journal of Nutrition* 45, 183–201.

Grovum, W.L. (1987) A new look at what is controlling food intake. In: Owens, F.N., (ed.) *Symposium Proceedings, Feed Intake by Beef Cattle*. Oklahoma State University, Stillwater, Oklahoma, pp. 1–40.

Grovum, W.L. and Bignell, W.W.(1989) Results refuting volatile fatty acids per se as signals of satiety in ruminants. *Proceedings of the Nutrition Society* 48, 3A.

Grovum, W.L. and Chapman, H.W. (1988) Factors affecting the voluntary intake of food by sheep. 4. The effect of additives representing the primary tastes on sham intakes by oesophageal-fistulated sheep. *British Journal of Nutrition* 59, 63–72.

Grovum, W.L. and Phillips, G.D. (1978) Factors affecting the voluntary intake of food by sheep. 1. The role of distension, flow-rate of digesta and propulsive motility in the intestines. *British Journal of Nutrition* 40, 323–336.

Grovum, W.L., Brobeck, J.R. and Baile, C.A. (1974) Pentagastrin depressed feeding in sheep. *Journal of Dairy Science* 57, 608.

Gunn, R.G., Doney, J.M., Smith, W.F., Sim, D.A. and Hunter, E.A. (1991) A note on herbage intake by Greyface ewes on perennial ryegrass/white clover swards in the autumn. *Animal Production* 53, 257–260.

Hacker, J.B. (ed.) (1982) *Nutritional Limits to Animal Production from Pastures*. CAB, Farnham Royal, 536pp.

Hadjipieris, G. and Holmes, W. (1966) Studies on feed intake and feed utilisation by sheep. 1. The voluntary feed intake of dry, pregnant and lactating ewes. *Journal of Agricultural Science* 66, 217–223.

Hahn, G. (1981) Housing and management to reduce climatic impacts on livestock. *Journal of Animal Science* 52, 175–185.

Hancock, J. (1954) Studies in monozygotic cattle twins. *New Zealand Department of Agriculture Animal Research Division, Publication No. 63*.

Harb, M.Y. and Campling, R.C. (1983) Effects of the amount of barley and time of access to grass silage on the voluntary intake, eating behaviour and production of dairy cows. *Grass and Forage Science* 38, 115–119.

Harding, R. and Leek, B.F. (1972) Gastro-duodenal receptor responses to chemical and mechanical stimuli, investigated by a 'single fibre' technique. *Journal of Physiology* 222, 139P–140P.

Harding, R. and Leek, B.F. (1973) The effects of peripheral influences on gastric centre neuronal activity in sheep. *Journal of Physiology* 225, 309–338.

Harding, R., Sigger, J.N., Poore, E.R. and Johnson, P. (1984) Ingestion in fetal sheep and its relation to sleep states and breathing movements. *Quarterly Journal of Experimental Physiology* 69, 477–486.

Harper, A.E. (1974) Amino acids in nutrition. In: White, P.L. and Fletcher, D.C. (eds) *Processed Foods – Protein*, Publishing Science Group, Acton, MA. pp. 49–54.

Harper, A.E. and Kumata, U.S. (1970) Effects of ingestion of disproportionate amounts of amino acids. *Physiological Reviews* 50, 428–558.

Harris, C.E. and Raymond, W.F. (1964) The effect of ensiling on crop digestibility. *Journal of the British Grassland Society* 18, 204–212.

Hawkes, M.P.G. and George, J.C. (1975) Effects of hypothalamic lesions on levels of plasma free fatty acids in the Mallard duck. *International Archives of Physiology and Biochemistry* 83, 763–770.

Hawkins, C.D. and Morris, R.S. (1978) Depression of productivity in sheep infected with *Fasciola hepatica*. *Veterinary Parasitology* 4, 341–351.

Hayne, H., Rovee-Collier, C. and Gargano, D. (1986) Ambient temperature effects on energetic relations in growing chicks. *Physiology and Behavior* 37, 203–212.

Hays, V.W. (1979) Effectiveness of feed additive usage of antibacterial agents in swine and poultry production. In: Office of Technical Assessment (ed.) *Drugs in Livestock Feed. Vol. 1*, United States Congress, Washington DC.

Healy, W.J., Gill, B.P., English, P.R. and Davidson, F.M. (1993) The selection by young pigs of dietary cereal and protein fractions supplemented with amino acids to idealise protein contents. *Animal Production* 56, 468A.

Heaney, D.P. and Pigden, W.J. (1972) Effects of pre-conditioning on voluntary intake assay results using sheep. *Journal of Animal Science* 35, 619–623.

Heaney, D.P., Pigden, W.J., Minson, D.J. and Pritchard, G.I. (1963) Effect of pelleting on energy intake of sheep from forages cut at three stages of maturity. *Journal of Animal Science* 22, 752–757.

Heaney, D.P., Pritchard, G.I. and Pigden, W.J. (1968) Variability in ad libitum forage intakes by sheep. *Journal of Animal Science* 27, 159–164.

Heitman, H., Hahn, L., Kelly, C.F. and Bond, T.E. (1961) Space allotment and performance of growing finishing swine raised in confinement. *Journal of Animal Science* 20, 543–546.

Heitzman, R.J. and Walker, M.S. (1973) The antiketogenic action of an anabolic steroid administered to ketotic cows. *Research in Veterinary Science* 15, 70–77.

Hemsley, J.A. and Moir, R.J. (1963) The influence of higher volatile fatty acids on the intake of urea-supplemented low-quality cereal hay by sheep. *Australian Journal of Agricultural Science*, 14, 509–517.

Henning, P.H. (1987) The effect of increased energy demand through walking exercise on intake and ruminal characteristics on sheep fed a roughage diet. *Journal of Agricultural Science* 109, 53–59.

Henry, R.W., Pickard, D.W. and Hughes, P.E. (1985) Citric acid and fumaric acid as food additives for early-weaned piglets. *Animal Production* 40, 505–509.

Henry, Y. (1968) Libre consommation de principes inergetiques et azotes chez le rat and chez le porc selon la nature de la source azotee, sa concentration dans la regime et le modede presentation. [Choice intake of energy and nitrogen in the rat and pig, according to the source of nitrogen, its concentration and mode of presentation.] *Annales de Nutrition et Alimentation* 22, 141–154.

Henry, Y. (1985) Dietary factors involved in feed intake regulation in growing pigs: a review. *Livestock Production Science* 12, 339–354.

Henry, Y., Colleaux, Y. and Seve, B. (1992) Effects of dietary level of lysine and of level and source of protein on feed intake, growth performance, and plasma amino acid pattern in the finishing pig. *Journal of Animal Science* 70, 188–195.

Herpin, P., Bertin, R., Le Dividich, J. and Portet, R. (1987) Some regulatory aspects of thermogenesis in cold-exposed piglets. *Comparative Biochemistry and Physiology* 87, 1073–1081.

Hervey, G.R. (1959) The effects of lesions in the hypothalamus in parabiotic rats. *Journal of Physiology* 145, 336–352.

Hervey, G.R. and Tobin, G. (1983) Luxuskonsumption: diet-induced thermogenesis and brown fat: a critical review. *Clinical Science* 64, 7–18.

Hess, E.H. and Gogel, W.C. (1954) Natural preferences of the chick for objects of different colours. *Journal of Psychology* 38, 483–493.

Hidari, H. (1977) Diurnal changes of volatile fatty acid concentration in the rumen of sheep fed in free access. *Japanese Journal of Zootechnical Science* 48, 38–46.

Hidari, H. (1981) The relationships between rumen load and diurnal eating pattern of sheep fed in various times of access to feed. *Japanese Journal of Zootechnical Science* 52, 219–226.

Hijikuro, S. and Takewasa, M. (1981) Studies on the palatability and utilization of whole grains for finishing broilers. *Japanese Poultry Science* 18, 301.

Hill, F.W. and Dansky, L.M. (1954) Studies of the energy requirements of chickens. 1. The effect of dietary energy level on growth and feed consumption. *Poultry Science* 33, 112–119.

Hill, F.W., Carew, L.B. and van Tienhoven, A. (1958) Effect of diethylstilbesterol on utilization of energy by the growing chick. *American Journal of Physiology* 195, 654–658.

Hill, J.A. (1977) The relationship between food and water intake in the laying hen. PhD thesis, Huddersfield Polytechnic.

Hill, J.A., Powell, A.J. and Charles, D.R. (1979) Water intake. In: Boorman, K.N. and Freeman, B.M. (eds) *Food Intake Regulation in Poultry*. Longman, Edinburgh, pp. 231–257.

Hill, K.J. (1979) Physical effects of food in the digestive tract in relation to intake. In: Boorman, K.N. and Freeman, B.M. (eds) *Food Intake Regulation in Poultry*. Longman, Edinburgh, pp. 191–198.

Hill, R.W. (1976) *Comparative Physiology of Animals. An Environmental Approach*. Harper & Row, New York.

Hillman, D., Lassiter, C.A., Huffman, C.F. and Duncan, C.W. (1958) Effect of all-hay vs. all-silage rations on dry matter intake of lactating dairy cows; moisture and pH factors affecting appetite. *Journal of Dairy Science* 41, 720.

Hinch, G.N., Thwaites, C.J. and Lynch, J.J. (1982) A note on the grazing behaviour of young bulls and steers. *Animal Production* 35, 289–291.

Hinton, V., Rosofsky, M., Granger, J. and Geary, N. (1986) Combined injection potentiates the satiety effects of pancreatic glucagon, cholecystokinin, and bombesin. *Brain Research Bulletin* 17, 613–615.

Hinton, V., Esguerra, M., Farhoody, N., Granger, J. and Geary, N. (1987) Epinephrine inhibits feeding nonspecifically in the rat. *Physiology and Behavior* 40, 109–115.

Hocking, P.M. and Bernard, R. (1993) Evaluation of putative appetite suppressants in the domestic fowl (*Gallus domesticus*). *British Poultry Science* 34, 393–404.

Hodge, R.W.(1966) The relative pasture intake of grazing lambs at two levels of milk intake. *Australian Journal of Experimental Agriculture and Animal Husbandry* 6, 314–316.

Hodgkin, A.L. and Katz, B. (1949) The effect of sodium ions on the electrical activity of the giant axon of the squid. *Journal of Physiology* 225, 309–338.

Hodgkiss, J.P. (1981) Distension-sensitive receptors in the crop of the domestic fowl (*Gallus domesticus*). *Comparative Biochemistry and Physiology* 70A, 73–78.

Hodgkiss, J.P. (1984) Cholinergic neurones project orally in the intestinal nerve of the fowl. *Journal of Physiology* 349, 36P.

Hodgson, J. (1968) The relationship between the digestibility of a sward and the herbage consumption by grazing calves. *Journal of Agricultural Science* 70, 47–51.

Hodgson, J. (1971a) The development of solid food intake in calves. 1. The effect of previous experience of solid food, and the physical form of the diet, on the development of food intake after weaning. *Animal Production* 13, 15–24.

Hodgson, J. (1971b) The development of solid food intake in calves. 4. The effect of the addition of material to the rumen, or its removal from the rumen, on voluntary food intake. *Animal Production* 13, 581–592.

Hodgson, J. (1971c) The development of solid food intake in calves. 5. The relationship between liquid and solid food intake. *Animal Production* 13, 593–597.

Hodgson, J. (1973) The effect of the physical form of the diet on the consumption of solid food by calves, and the distribution of food residues in their alimentary tracts. *Animal Production* 17, 129–138.

Hodgson, J. (1982) Ingestive behaviour. In: Leaver, J.D. (ed.) *Herbage Intake Handbook*. British Grassland Society, Maidenhead, Berks, pp. 113–138.

Hodgson, J. (1985) The control of herbage intake in the grazing ruminant. *Proceedings of the Nutrition Society* 44, 339–346.

Hodgson, J. (1990) *Grazing Management: Science into Practice*. Longman Scientific and Technical, Harlow, Essex, 203pp.

Hodgson, J. and Maxwell, T.J. (1981) Grazing reearch and grazing management. In: *Hill Farming Research Organisation Biennial Report, 1979–91*, H.F.R.O., Edinburgh, pp. 169–187.

Hodgson, J. and Wilkinson, J.M. (1967) The relationship between live-weight and herbage intake in grazing cattle. *Animal Production* 9, 365–376.

Hodgson, J., Rodriguez Capriles, J.M. and Fenlon, J.S. (1977) The influence of sward characteristics on the herbage intake of grazing calves. *Journal of Agricultural Science* 89, 743–750.

Hogan, J.A. (1973) Development of food recognition in young chicks. 1. Maturation and nutrition. *Journal of Comparative and Physiological Psychology* 83, 355–366.

Holcombe, D.J., Roland, D.A. and Harms, R.H. (1975) The ability of hens to adjust calcium intake when given a choice of diets containing two levels of calcium. *Poultry Science* 54, 552–561.

Holcombe, D.J., Roland, D.A. and Harms, R.H. (1976a) The ability of hens to regulate phosphorus intake when offered diets containing different levels of phosphorus. *Poultry Science* 55, 308–317.

Holcombe, D.J., Roland, D.A. and Harms, R.H. (1976b) The ability of hens to regulate protein intake when offered a choice of diets containing different levels of protein. *Poultry Science* 55, 1731–1737.

Holcombe, D.W., Hallford, D.M. and Hoefler, W.C. (1988) Reproductive and lactational responses and serum growth hormone and insulin in fine-wooded ewes treated with ovine growth hormone. *Animal Production* 46, 195–202.

Holder, J.M. (1963) Chemostatic regulation of appetite in sheep. *Nature* 200, 1074–1075.

Holder, M.D. (1991) Conditioned preferences for the taste and odour components of flavors: blocking but not overshadowing. *Appetite* 17, 29–45.

Holme, D.W. and Coey, W.E. (1967) The effect of environmental temperature and method of feeding on the performance and carcass composition of bacon pigs. *Animal Production* 9, 209–218.

Holmes, E.G. and Fraser, F.J. (1965) An attempt to produce hyperphagia in sheep by electrical damage to the hypothalamus. *Australian Journal of Biological Science* 18, 345–352.

Holmes, P.H. (1993) Interactions between parasites and animal nutrition – the veterinary consequences. *Proceedings of the Nutrition Society* 52, 113–120.

Holmes, W. (ed.) (1989) *Grass, its Production and Utilisation, 2nd edn.* Blackwell Scientific, Oxford.

Holmes, W., Jones, J.G.W. and Drake-Brockman, R.M. (1961) The feed intake of grazing cattle. 2. The influence of size of animal on feed intake. *Animal Production* 3, 251–260.

Hopkins, J.R. (1985) Feeding the dairy cow by maximising forage and minimising concentrate input. Mimeograph, ADAS Regional Nutrition Chemist, Leeds, 12pp.

Horton, G.M.J., Malinowski, K. and Talbot, J.A. (1990) Effect of confinement on performance and physiological indicators of stress in lambs. *Journal of Animal Science* 68 Suppl 1, 260.

Hou, X.Z., Emmans, G.C., Anderson, D., Illius, A. and Oldham, J.D. (1991a) The effect of different pairs of feeds offered as a choice on food selection by sheep. *Proceedings of the Nutrition Society* 50, 94A.

Hou, X.Z., Lawrence, A.B., Illius, A., Anderson, D. and Oldham, J.D. (1991b) Operant studies on feed selection in sheep. *Proceedings of the Nutrition Society* 50, 95A.

Houpt, K.A. and Houpt, T.R. (1976) Comparative aspects of the ontogeny of taste. *Chemical Senses and Flavor* 2, 219–228.

Houpt, K.A. and Houpt, T.R. (1977) The neonatal pig, a biological model for the development of taste preferences and controls of ingestive behavior. In:

Weiffenbach, J.M. (ed.) *Taste and Development.* US Dept. Health, Education and Welfare, Bethesda, Maryland, pp. 86–98.

Houpt, K.A. and Wolski, T. (1982) *Domestic Animal Behavior for Veterinarians and Animal Scientists.* Iowa State University Press, Ames.

Houpt, K.A., Houpt, T.R. and Pond, W.G. (1977) Food intake controls in the suckling pig: glucoprivation and gastrointestinal factors. *American Journal of Physiology* 232, E510–E514.

Houpt, K.A., Houpt, T.R. and Pond, W.G. (1979) The pig as a model for the study of obesity and of control of food intake: a review. *Yale Journal of Biology and Medicine* 52, 307–329.

Houpt, T.R. (1974) Stimulation of food intake in ruminants by 2-deoxy-D-glucose and insulin. *American Journal of Physiology* 227, 161–167.

Houpt, T.R. (1983a) The controls of food intake in the pig. In: Laplace, J.P., Corring, T. and Rerat, A. (eds) *Physiologie Digestive Chez le Porc*, INRA, Paris, pp. 17–28.

Houpt, T.R. (1983b) The sites of action of cholecystokinin in decreasing meal size of pigs. *Physiology and Behavior* 31, 693–698.

Houpt, T.R. (1985) Control at the gut level. *Proceedings of the Nutrition Society* 44, 323–330.

Houpt, T.R., Baldwin, B.A. and Houpt, K.A. (1983) Effects of duodenal osmotic loads on spontaneous meals in pigs. *Physiology and Behavior* 30, 787–796.

Hovell, F.D.D. and Greenhalgh, J.F.D. (1978) The utilisation of diets containing acetate, propionate or butyrate salts by growing lambs. *British Journal of Nutrition* 40, 171–183.

Hovell, F.D.D., Ngambi, J.W.W., Barber, W.P. and Kyle, D.J. (1986) The voluntary intake of hay by sheep in relation to its degradability in the rumen as measured in nylon bags. *Animal Production* 42, 111–118.

Howes, G.A. and Forbes, J.M. (1987a) Food intake of domestic fowl injected with adrenergic agonists and antagonists into the hepatic portal vein. *Pharmacology, Biochemistry and Behavior* 26, 757–764.

Howes, G.A. and Forbes, J.M. (1987b) A role for the liver in the effects of glucagon on food intake in the domestic fowl. *Physiology and Behavior* 39, 587–592.

Hsia, L.C. and Wood-Gush, D.G.M. (1983) A note on social facilitation and competition in the feeding behaviour of pigs. *Animal Production* 37, 149–152.

Huber, J.T. and Soejono, M. (1976) Organic acid treatment of high dry matter corn silage fed lactating dairy cows. *Journal of Dairy Science* 59, 2063–2070.

Huffman, C.F. (1959) Summer feeding of dairy cattle. A review. *Journal of Dairy Science* 42, 1495–1551.

Hughes, B.O. (1971) Allelomimetic feeding in the domestic fowl. *British Poultry Science*, 13, 359–366.

Hughes, B.O. (1972) A circadian rhythm of calcium intake in the domestic fowl. *British Poultry Science* 13, 485–493.

Hughes, B.O. (1979) Appetites for specific nutrients. In: Boorman, K.N. and Freeman, B.M. (eds) *Food Intake Regulation in Poultry.* Longman, Edinburgh, pp. 141–169.

Hughes, B.O. and Black, A.J. (1976) Battery cage shape: its effect on diurnal feeding pattern, egg shell cracking and feather pecking. *British Poultry Science* 17, 327–336.

Hughes, B.O. and Dewar, W.A. (1971) A specific appetite for zinc in zinc-depleted domestic fowls. *British Poultry Science* 12, 255–258.

Hughes, B.O. and Wood-Gush, D.G.M. (1971a) Investigations into specific appetites for sodium and thiamine in domestic fowls. *Physiology and Behavior* 6, 331–339.

Hughes, B.O. and Wood-Gush, D.G.M. (1971b) A specific appetite for calcium in domestic chickens. *Animal Behaviour* 19, 490–499.

Hungate, R.E. (1966) *The Rumen and its Microbes*. Academic Press, New York, 533pp.

Hunter, E.J., Broom, D.M., Edwards, S.A. and Sibly, R.M. (1988) Social hierarchy and feeder access in a group of 20 sows using a computer-controlled feeder. *Animal Production* 47, 139–148.

Hurnik, J.F., Jerome, F.M., Reinhart, B.S. and Summers, J.D. (1971) Color as a stimulus for food consumption. *Poultry Science* 50, 944–949.

Hurnik, J.F., Piggins, D.J., Reinhart, B.S. and Summers, D.J. (1974) The effect of visual pattern complexity of feeders on food consumption of laying hens. *British Poultry Science* 15, 97–105.

Hurnik, J.F., King, G.J. and Robertson, H.A. (1975) Estrous and related behavior in postpartum Holstein cows. *Journal of Animal Science* 39, 968.

Hurwitz, S., Sklan, D. and Bartov, I. (1978) New formal approaches to the determination of energy and amino acid requirements of chicks. *Poultry Science* 57, 197–200.

Huston, J.E., Engdahl, B.S. and Bales, K.W. (1988) Intake and digestibility in sheep and goats fed three forages with different levels of supplemental protein. *Small Ruminant Research* 1, 81–92.

Hutchinson, K.J. and Wilkins, R.J. (1971) The voluntary intake of silage by sheep. 2. The effects of acetate on silage intake. *Journal of Agricultural Science* 77, 539–543.

Hutchinson, K.J., Wilkins, R.J. and Osbourn, D.F. (1971) The voluntary intake of silage by sheep. 3. The effects of post-ruminal infusions of casein on the intake and nitrogen retention of sheep given silage ad libitum. *Journal of Agricultural Science* 77, 545–547.

Hutson, G.D. (1991) A note on hunger in the pig: sows on restricted rations will sustain an energy deficit to gain additional food. *Animal Production* 52, 233–235.

Hutson, G.D. (1992) A comparison of operant responding by farrowing sows for food and nest-building material. *Applied Animal Behaviour Science* 34, 221–230.

Hutson, G.D. and Wilson, P.N. (1984) A note on the preference of sheep for whole or crushed grains and seeds. *Animal Production* 38, 145–146.

Hyde, R.J. and Witherly, S.A. (1993) Dynamic contrast: a sensory contribution to palatability. *Appetite* 21, 1–16.

Illius, A.W. and Gordon, I.J. (1987) The allometry of food intake in grazing ruminants. *Journal of Animal Ecology* 65, 989–999.

Illius, A.W. and Gordon, I.J. (1991) Prediction of intake and digestion in ruminants by a model of rumen kinetics integrating animal size and plant characterstics. *Journal of Agricultural Science* 116, 145–157.

Illius, A.W., Clark, D.A. and Hodgson, J. (1992) Discrimination and patch choice by sheep grazing grass-clover swards. *Journal of Animal Ecology* 61, 183–194.

Ingram, D.L. (1968) Effects of heating and cooling the hypothalamus on food intake in the pig. *Brain Research* 11, 714–716.

Ingram, D.L. and Legge, K.F. (1974) Effects of environmental temperature on food intake in growing pigs. *Comparative Physiology and Biochemistry* 48A, 573–581.

Ingvartsen, K.L., Andersen, H.R. and Foldager, J. (1992a) Effect of sex and pregnancy on feed intake capacity of growing cattle. *Acta Agriculturae Scandinavica, Section A, Animal Science* 42, 40–46.

Ingvartsen, K.L. Andersen, H.R. and Foldager, J. (1992b) Random variation in voluntary dry matter intake and the effect of day length on feed intake capacity in growing cattle. *Acta Agriculturae Scandinavica, Section A, Animal Science* 42, 121–126.

Injidi, M.H. (1981) The involvement of melatonin, thyroid hormones and glucose in the control of feed and growth of chickens. PhD thesis, University of Leeds, 280pp.

Injidi, M.H. and Forbes, J.M. (1983) Growth and food intake of intact and pinealectomised chickens treated with melatonin and triiodothyronine. *British Poultry Science* 24, 463–469.

Injidi, M.H. and Forbes, J.M. (1987) Stimulation of food intake and growth of chickens by cyproheptadine: lack of interaction with the effects of pinealectomy and melatonin. *British Poultry Science* 28, 139–145.

INRA (1979) *Alimentation des Ruminants*. Versailles, Institut National de la Recherche Agronomique, 597pp.

Ivy, R.E. and Gleaves, E.W. (1976) Effect of egg production level, dietary protein and energy on feed consumption and nutrient requirements of laying hens. *Poultry Science* 55, 2166–2171.

Jackson, D.A, Johnson, C.L. and Forbes, J.M. (1991) The effect of compound composition and silage characteristics on silage intake, feeding behaviour, production of milk and live weight change in lactating dairy cows. *Animal Production* 52, 11–20.

Jackson, H.M. and Robinson, D.W. (1971) Evidence for hypothalamic $\alpha$ and $\beta$ adrenergic receptors involved in the control of food intake in the pig. *British Veterinary Journal* 127, li–lii.

Jackson, P., Hodgson, J. and Rook, J.A.F. (1968) The voluntary intake of acetate by dairy cows given ammonium salts of short chain fatty acids in their drinking water. *Animal Production* 10, 473–481.

Jacobs, H.L. (1967) Sensory and metabolic regulation of food intake: thoughts on a dual system regulated by energy balance. *Proceedings of the 7th International Congress of Nutrition*. Pergamon, London, pp. 17–29.

Jacobs, H.L. and Scott, S. (1957) Factors mediating food and liquid intake in chickens. I. Studies on the preference for sucrose and saccharin solutions. *Poultry Science* 36, 8–15.

Janowitz, H.D. and Grossman, M.I. (1949) Some factors affecting the food intake of normal dogs and dogs with esophagotomy and gastric fistula. *American Journal of Physiology* 159, 143–148.

Janowitz, H.D. and Hollander, F. (1955) The time factor in the adjustment of food intake to varied caloric requirement in the dog: a study of the precision of appetite regulation. *Annals of the New York Academy of Sciences* 63, 56–67.

Jarrige, R., Demarquilly, C., Dulphy, J.P., Hoden, A. and Robelin, J. (1986) The INRA 'fill unit' system for predicting the voluntary intake of forage-based diets in ruminants: a review. *Journal of Animal Science* 63, 1737–1758.

Jen, K.L.C., Bodkin, N.L., Metzger, B.L. and Hansen, B.C. (1985) Nutrient composition: effects on appetite in monkeys with oral factors held constant. *Physiology and Behavior* 34, 655–660.

Jensen, A.H., Becker, D.E. and Harmon, B.G. (1969) Response of growing/ fattening swine to different housing environments during winter seasons. *Journal of Animal Science* 29, 451–456.

Jensen, M.B., Kyriazakis, I. and Lawrence, A.B. (1993) The activity and straw directed behaviour of pigs offered foods with different crude protein content. *Applied Animal Behaviour Science* (in press).

Johnson, J. and Reid, W.M. (1971) Pathogenicity of *Eimeria mivati* in light and heavy coccidial infections. *Poultry Science* 50, 1202–1205.

Johnson, J.E., Hindery, G.A., Hill, D.H. and Guidry, A. (1961) Factors concerned in hot weather effects on growth and feed efficiency of dairy heifers. *Journal of Dairy Science* 44, 976.

Johnson, K.G. (1987) Shading behaviour of sheep: preliminary studies of its relation to thermoregulation, feed and water intakes, and metabolic rate. *Australian Journal of Agricultural Research* 38, 587–596.

Johnson, M.H., Bolhuis, J. and Horn, G. (1985) Interaction between acquired preferences and developing predispositions in an imprinting situation. *Animal Behaviour* 33, 1000–1006.

Johnson, R.R. and McClure, K.E. (1973) High fat rations for ruminants. 2. Effects of fat added to corn plant material prior to ensiling on digestibility and voluntary intake. *Journal of Animal Science* 36, 397–406.

Johnson, W.L, Trimberger, G.W., Wright, M.J., Van Vleck, L.D. and Henderson, C.R. (1966) Voluntary intake of forage by Holstein cows as influenced by lactation, gestation, body weight and frequency of calving. *Journal of Dairy Science* 49, 856–864.

Johnsson, I.D., Hathorn, D.J., Wilde, R.M., Treacher, T.T. and Butler-Hogg, B.W. (1987) The effects of dose and method of administration of biosynthetic bovine somatotropin on live-weight gain, carcass composition and wool growth in young lambs. *Animal Production* 44, 405–414.

Jones, G.M. (1971) Volatile fatty acids in concentrate rations for lactating dairy cows. *Journal of Dairy Science* 54, 1142–1149.

Jones, G.P. and Garnsworthy, P.C. (1988) The effects of body condition at calving and dietary protein content on dry-matter intake and performance in lactating cows given diets of low energy content. *Animal Production* 47, 321–334.

Jones, G.P. and Garnsworthy, P.C. (1989) The effects of dietary energy content on the response of dairy cows to body condition at calving. *Animal Production* 49, 183–192.

Jones, J.E., Hughes, B.L. and Barnett, B.D. (1976) Effect of changing dietary energy and environmental temperatures on feed consumption and egg production of single comb White Leghorns. *Poultry Science* 55, 274–277.

Jones, R. and Forbes, J.M. (1984) A note on effects of glyphosate and quinine on the palatability of hay for sheep. *Animal Production* 38, 301–303.

Jordan, C.A., Waitt, W.P. and Scholz, N.E. (1965) Effects of orally-administered diethylstilbestrol and methyltestosterone on finishing barrows and gilts. *Journal of Animal Science* 24, 890.

Joshua, I.G. (1976) The development and regulation of a calcium appetite in growing chickens. *Dissertation Abstracts* 37, 2091–2092B.

Joshua, I.G. and Mueller, W.J. (1979) The development of a specific appetite for calcium in growing broiler chicks. *British Poultry Science* 20, 481–490.

Joubert, D.M. and Ueckerman, L. (1971) A note on the effect of docking on fat deposition in fat-tailed sheep. *Animal Production* 13, 191–192.

Kabuga, J.D. (1992a) Social interactions in N'dama cows during periods of idling and supplementary feeding post-grazing. *Applied Animal Behaviour Science* 34, 11–22.

Kabuga, J.D. (1992b) Social relationships in N'dama cattle during supplementary feeding. *Applied Animal Behaviour Science* 34, 285–290.

Kahn, H.E. and Spedding, C.R.W. (1984) A dynamic model for the simulation of cattle herd production systems. 2. An investigation of various factors influencing the voluntary intake of dry matter and the use of the model in their validation. *Agricultural Systems* 13, 63–82.

Kalat, J.W. and Rozin, P. (1971) Role of interference in taste-aversion learning. *Journal of Comparative and Physiological Psychology* 77, 53–58.

Kaminska, B. (1979) Evaluation of chickens ability to meet nutrient requirements in case of free choice of different protein-level mashes. *Instytut Zootechniki Prace Bad. Zakl. Hod. Drobiu* 8, 47–57.

Kang, H.S. and Leibholz, J. (1973) The roughage requirement of the early-weaned calf. *Animal Production* 16, 195–203.

Kanis, E. and de Vries, A.G. (1992) Optimization of selection for food intake capacity in pigs. *Animal Production* 55, 247–255.

Kare, M.R. and Maller, O. (1967) Taste and food intake in domestic and jungle fowl. *Journal of Nutrition* 92, 191–196.

Kare, M.R. and Pick, H.L. (1960) The influence of the sense of taste on feed and fluid consumption. *Poultry Science* 39, 697–706.

Kare, M.R., Pond, W.C. and Campbell, J. (1965) Observations on the taste reactions in pigs. *Animal Behaviour* 13, 265–269.

Karkeek, W.F. (1845) An essay on fat and muscle. *Journal of the Royal Agricultural Society* 5, 245–266.

Karue, C.N., Evans, J.L. and Tillman, A.D. (1973) Voluntary intake of dry matter by African zebu cattle. Quality of feed and the reference base. *Journal of Animal Science* 36, 1181–1185.

Katle, J. (1992a) Relationship between food consumption in growing chicks and their residual food consumption as adult laying hens. *Acta Agriculturae Scandinavica, Section A, Animal Science* 42, 14–19.

Katle, J. (1992b) Genetic and economic consequences of including residual food consumption in a multi-trait selection program for laying hens. *Acta*

*Agriculturae Scandinavica, Section A, Animal Science* 42, 63–70.

Katle, J. and Nordli, H. (1992) Variation in residual food consumption between cocks in a highly productive egg-laying strain. *Acta Agriculturae Scandinavica, Section A, Animal Science* 42, 20–26.

Kato, S., Sasaki, Y. and Tsuda, T. (1979) Food intake and rumen osmolality in the sheep. *Annales de Recherches Veterinaire* 10, 229–230.

Kaufman, L. and Collier, G. (1983) Meal-taking by domestic chickens (*Gallus gallus*). *Animal Behavior* 31, 397–404.

Kaufman, L.W., Collier, G. and Squibb, R.L. (1978) Selection of an adequate protein–carbohydrate ratio by domestic chicks. *Physiology and Behavior* 20, 339–344.

Kay, M., MacDearmid, A. and MacLeod, N.A. (1970) Intensive beef production. 10. Replacement of cereals with chopped straw. *Animal Production* 12, 261–266.

Kay, R.N.B. (1979) Seasonal changes of appetite in deer and sheep. *Agricultural Research Council Research Reviews* 5, 13–15.

Kay, R.N.B. and Suttie, J.M. (1980) Relationship of seasonal cycles of food intake and sexual activity in Soay rams. *Journal of Physiology* 310, 34–35P.

Kellerup, S.U., Parker, J.E. and Arscott, G.H. (1965) Effect of restricted water consumption on broiler chickens. *Poultry Science* 44, 78–83.

Kempster, H.L. (1916) Food selection by laying hens. *Journal of the American Association of Institutions and Investigators in Poultry Husbandry* 3, 26–28.

Kendrick, K.M. (1991) Cognition and learning in sheep. *AFRC Institute of Animal Physiology and Genetics Research Report for 1990–91*, p. 137.

Kendrick, K.M. (1992) Cognition. In: Phillips, C.J.C. and Piggins, D. (eds) *Farm Animals and the Environment.* CAB International, Wallingford, pp. 209–231.

Kennedy, G.C. (1953) The role of depot fat in the hypothalamic control of food intake in the rat. *Proceedings of the Royal Society B* 140, 578–592.

Kennedy, J.M. and Baldwin, B.A. (1972) Taste preferences in pigs for nutritive and non-nutritive sweet solutions. *Animal Behaviour* 20, 706–718.

Kennedy, P.M., Christopherson, R.J. and Milligan, L.P. (1985) Digestive responses to cold. In: Milligan, L.P., Grovum, W.L. and Dobson, A. (eds) *Control of Digestion and Metabolism in the Ruminant.* Prentice-Hall, New Jersey, pp. 285–306.

Kenney, P.A. and Black, J.L. (1984) Factors affecting diet selection by sheep. I. Potential intake rate and acceptability of feed. *Australian Journal of Agricultural Research* 35, 551–563.

Kennington, M.H., Perry, T.W. and Beeson, W.M. (1958) Effects of adding animal fat to swine rations. *Journal of Animal Science* 17, 1166.

Kenwright, A.D. and Forbes, J.M. (1993) Relationships between social dominance and feeding behaviour in lactating heifers during periods of heavy competition. *Animal Production* 56, 457A.

Ketelaars, J.J.M.H. and Tolkamp, B.J. (1992a) Toward a new theory of feed intake regulation in ruminants. 1. Causes of differences in voluntary feed intake, critique of current views. *Livestock Production Science* 30, 269–296.

Ketelaars, J.J.M.H. and Tolkamp, B.J. (1992b) Toward a new theory of feed intake regulation in ruminants. 3. Optimum feed intake, in search of a physiological background. *Livestock Production Science* 31, 235–258.

Khalaf, F. and Robinson, D.W. (1972a) Observations on the phagic response of the pig to infusions of dextrose and sodium pentobarbital into the ventromedial area of the brain. *Research in Veterinary Science* 13, 1–4.

Khalaf, F. and Robinson, D.W. (1972b) Aphagia and adipsia in pigs with induced hypothalamic lesions. *Research in Veterinary Science* 13, 5–7.

Khazaal, K., Dentinho, M.T., Ribeiro, J.M. and Orskov, E.R. (1993) A comparison of gas production during incubation with rumen contents in vitro and nylon bag degradability as predictors of the apparent digestibility in vivo and the voluntary intake of hays. *Animal Production* 57, 105–112.

Kibon, A. and Orskov, E.R. (1993) The use of degradation characteristics of browse plants to predict intake and digestibility by goats. *Animal Production* 57, 247–251.

Kidwell, J.F., Bohman, V.R. and Hunter, J.E. (1954) Individual and group feeding of experimental beef cattle as influenced by hay maturity. *Journal of Animal Science* 13, 543–547.

Kilgour, R. (1978) The application of animal behaviour and the humane care of farm animals. *Journal of Animal Science* 45, 1478–1486.

King, B., Stmoutsos, B.A. and Grossman, S.P. (1979) Delayed response to 2-deoxy-D-glucose in hypothalamic obese rats. *Pharmacology, Biochemistry and Behavior* 8, 259–262.

King, R.H. (1979) The effect of adding a feed flavour to the diets of young pigs before and after weaning. *Australian Journal of Experimental Agriculture and Animal Husbandry* 19, 695–697.

Kleiber, M. (1961) *Fire of Life*. Wiley, New York, 326pp.

Kiketsu, Y., Dial, G.D., March, W.E. and Pettigrew, J.E. (1992) Patterns of lactational feed intake and their influence on reproductive performance. *Minnesota Nutrition Conference, September 1992.*

Konggaard, S.P. and Krohn, C.C. (1978) [Investigation concerning feed intake and social behaviour among group fed cows under loose housing conditions. 3. Effects of isolating first lactation cows from older cows.] *Beretning fra Statens Husbyrbrugforsog* 469, 30pp.

Kornegay, E.T. and Notter, D.R. (1984) Effects of floor space and number of pigs per pen on performance. *Pig News and Information* 5, 523.

Kornegay, E.T., Tinsley, S.E. and Bryant, K.L. (1979) Evaluation of rearing systems and feed flavours for pigs weaned at two and three weeks of age. *Journal of Animal Science* 48, 999–1006.

Kostal, L., Savory, C.J. and Hughes, B.O. (1992) Diurnal and individual variation in behaviour of restricted fed broiler breeders. *Applied Animal Behaviour Science* 32, 361–374.

Kovalcik, K. and Kovalcik, M. (1986) Learning ability and memory testing in cattle of different ages. *Applied Animal Science* 15, 27–30.

Krabill, L.F., Wangsness, P.J. and Baile, C.A. (1978) Effects of Efazepam on digestibility and feeding behaviour in sheep. *Journal of Animal Science* 46, 1356–1359.

Krebs, H.A. (1966) Bovine ketosis. *Veterinary Record* 78, 187–191.

Kronfeld, D.S. (1970) Ketone body metabolism, its control, and its implications in pregnancy toxaemia, acetonaemia and feeding standards. In: Phillipson, A.T. (ed.) *Physiology of Digestion and Metabolism in the Ruminant.* Oriel

Press, Newcastle upon Tyne, pp. 566–583.

Krysl, L.J. and Hess, B.W. (1993) Influence of supplementation on behavior of grazing cattle. *Journal of Animal Science* 71, 2546–2555.

Kuenzel, W.J. (1982) Transient aphagia produced following bilateral destruction of the lateral hypothalamic area and quintofrontal tract of chicks. *Physiology and Behavior* 28, 237–244.

Kuenzel, W.J. (1989) Neuroanatomical substrates involved in the control of food intake. *Poultry Science* 68, 926–937.

Kuenzel, W.J. and McMurtry, J. (1988) Neuropeptide Y: brain localisation and central effects on plasma insulin. *Physiology and Behavior* 44, 669–678.

Kuenzel, W.J., Douglass, L.W. and Davidson, B.A. (1987) Robust feeding following central administration of neuropeptide Y or peptide YY in chicks, *Gallus domesticus. Peptides* 8, 823–828.

Kushner, L.R. and Mook, D.G. (1984) Behavioral correlates of oral and post-ingestive satiety in the rat. *Physiology and Behavior* 33, 713–718.

Kutlu, H.R. and Forbes, J.M. (1993a) Changes in growth and blood parameters in heat-stressed broiler chicks in response to dietary ascorbic acid. *Livestock Production Science* 36, 335–350.

Kutlu, H.R. and Forbes, J.M. (1993b) Self-selection of ascorbic acid in coloured foods by heat-stressed broiler chicks. *Physiology and Behaviour* 53, 103–110.

Kutlu, H.R. and Forbes, J.M.(1993c) Effect of changes in environmental temperature on self-selection of ascorbic acid in coloured feeds by broiler chicks. *Proceedings of the Nutrition Society* 52, 29A.

Kyriazakis, I. and Emmans, G.C. (1991) Diet selection in pigs: dietary choices made by growing pigs following a period of underfeeding with protein. *Animal Production* 52, 337–346.

Kyriazakis, I. and Emmans, G.C. (1992) The growth of mammals following a period of nutritional limitation. *Journal of Theoretical Biology* 156, 485–498.

Kyriazakis, I. and Emmans, G.C. (1993) The effect of protein source on the diets selected by pigs given a choice between a low and high protein food. *Physiology and Behavior* 53, 683–688.

Kyriazakis, I. and Oldham, J.D. (1993) Diet selection in sheep: the ability of growing lambs to select a diet that meets their crude protein (nitrogen × 6.25) requirements. *British Journal of Nutrition* 69, 617–629.

Kyriazakis, I., Emmans, G.C. and Whittemore, C.T. (1990) Diet selection in pigs: choices made by growing pigs given foods of different protein concentrations. *Animal Production* 51, 189–199.

Kyriazakis, I., Emmans, G.C. and Whittemore, C.T. (1991) The ability of pigs to control their protein intake when fed in three different ways. *Physiology and Behavior* 50, 1197–1203.

Kyriazakis, I., Anderson, D.H., Cooper, S.D.B., Oldham, J.D., Coop, R.L. and Jackson, F. (1993a) The effect of subclinical parasitism with *Trichostrongylus colubriformis* on the diet selection of growing sheep. *Proceedings of the Nutrition Society* 52, 353A.

Kyriazakis, I., Emmans, G.C. and Taylor, A.J. (1993b) A note on the diets selected by boars given a choice between two foods of different protein concentrations from 44 to 103 kg live weight. *Animal Production* 56, 151–154.

Kyriazakis, I., Leus, K., Emmans, G.C., Haley, C.S. and Oldham, J.D. (1993c) The effect of breed (Large White × Landrace v. purebred Meishan) on the diets selected by pigs given a choice between two foods that differ in their crude protein content. *Animal Production* 56, 121–128.

Lacy, M.P., Van Krey, H.P., Skewes, P.A. and Denbow, D.M. (1986a) Food intake in the domestic fowl: effects of intrahepatic lipid and amino acid infusion. *Physiology and Behavior* 36, 533–538.

Lacy, M.P., Van Krey, H.P., Skewes, P.A. and Denbow, D.M. (1986b) Intra-duodenal glucose infusions do not affect food intake in the fowl. *Poultry Science* 65, 565–569.

Lambert, R.J., Ellis, M., Smithard, R. and Davis, M. (1992a) Influence of variety and site of cultivation on the nutritive value of rapeseed meal for growing pigs. *Animal Production* 54, 482.

Lambert, R.J., Hawkins, C.G. and Ellis, M. (1992b) Time taken by growing pigs to consume meals from different varieties of rapeseed. *Animal Production* 54, 482–483A.

Lambourne, L.J. (1964) Stimulation of wool growth by thyroxine implantation. 2. Feed intake of grazing Merino wethers treated repeatedly with thyroxine. *Australian Journal of Agricultural Research* 15, 676–697.

Lamming, G.E., Swan, H. and Clarke, R.T. (1966) Studies on the nutrition of ruminants. 1. Substitution of maize by milled barley straw in a beef fattening diet and its effect on performance and carcass quality. *Animal Production* 8, 303–311.

Land, C. and Leaver, J.D. (1980) The effect of body condition at calving on the milk production and feed intake of dairy cows. *Animal Production* 30, 449.

Langhans, W. and Scharrer, E. (1986) Evidence for a vagally mediated satiety signal derived from hepatic fatty acid oxidation. *Journal of the Autonomic Nervous System* 18, 13–18.

Langhans, W. and Scharrer, E. (1987) Evidence for a role of the sodium pump of hepatocytes in the control of food intake. *Journal of the Autonomic Nervous system* 20, 199–205.

Langhans, W., Damaske, U. and Scharrer,E. (1984a) Subcutaneous glycerol injection fails to reduce food intake in rats fed on a high protein diet. *Physiology and Behavior* 32, 785–790.

Langhans, W., Pantel, K., Muller-Schell, W., Eggenberger, E. and Scharrer, E., (1984b) Hepatic handling of pancreatic glucagon and glucose during meals in rats. *American Journal of Physiology* 247, R827–R832.

Langhans, W., Egli, G. and Scharrer, E. (1985a) Regulation of food intake by hepatic oxidative metabolism. *Brain Research Bulletin* 15, 425–428.

Langhans, W., Egli, G. and Scharrer, E. (1985b) Selective hepatic vagotomy eliminates the hypophagic effect of different metabolites. *Journal of the Autonomic Nervous System* 13, 255–262.

Langhans, W., Pantel, K. and Scharrer, E. (1985c) Dissociation of epinephrine's hyperglycemic and anorectic effect. *Physiology and Behavior* 34, 457–464.

Langhans, W., Senn, M., Scharrer, E. and Eggenberger, E. (1988) Free-feeding pattern of pygmy goats eating a pelleted diet. *Journal of Animal Physiology and Animal Nutrition* 59, 160–166.

Langlands, J.P. (1969) Studies of the nutritive value of the diet selected by grazing sheep. *Animal Production* 11, 369–375.

Laplace, J.-P. (1970) Omaso-abomasal motility and feeding behaviour in sheep: a new concept. *Physiology and Behavior* 5, 61–65.

Larsson, S. (1954) On the hypothalamic organisation of the nervous mechanism regulating food intake. *Acta Physiologica Scandinavica* 32, Supplement 115.

Laswai, G.H., Close, W.H. and Keal, H.D. (1991) The voluntary intake of modern pig genotypes. *Animal Production* 52, 601.

Latshaw, J.D. (1993) Dietary lysine concentration from deficient to excessive and the effects on broiler chicks. *British Poultry Science* 34, 951–958.

Launchbaugh, K.L., Provenza, F.D. and Burritt, E.A. (1993) How herbivores track variable environments: responses to variability of toxins. *Journal of Chemical Ecology* 19, 1047–1056.

Lawrence, A.B. and Rushen, J. (eds) (1993) *Stereotypic Animal Behaviours: Fundamentals and Applications to Welfare*. CAB International, Wallingford, Oxon, 224pp.

Lawrence, A.B. and Wood-Gush, D.G.M. (1988) Influence of social behaviour on utilization of supplemental feedblocks by Scottish hill sheep. *Animal Production* 46, 203–212.

Lawrence, A.B., Appleby, M.C. and Macleod, H.A. (1988) Measuring hunger in the pig using operant conditioning: the effect of food restriction. *Animal Production* 47, 131–138.

Lawrence, A.B., Appleby, M.C., Illius, A.W. and MacLeod, H.A. (1989) Measuring hunger in the pig using operant conditioning, the effect of dietary bulk. *Animal Production* 48, 213–221.

Lawrence, A.B., Terlouw, E.M.C. and Kyriazakis, I. (1993) The behavioural effects of undernutrition in confined farm animals. *Proceedings of the Nutrition Society* 52, 219–229.

Leaver, J.D. (1973) Rearing of dairy cattle. 4. Effect of concentrate supplementation on the live-weight gain and feed intake of calves offered roughages ad libitum. *Animal Production* 17, 43–52.

Leaver, J.D. (1974) Rearing of dairy cattle. 5. The effect of stocking rate on animal and herbage production in a grazing system for calves and heifers. *Animal Production* 18, 273–284.

Leaver, J.D. and Yarrow, N.H. (1980) A preliminary study to compare individual feeding through Calan electronic feeding gates to group feeding. *Animal Production* 30, 303–306.

Leaver, J.D., Campling, R.C. and Holmes, W. (1968) The use of supplementary feeds for grazing cows. *Dairy Science Abstracts* 30, 355–361.

Leclercq, B. and Guy, G. (1991) Further investigations on protein requirement of genetically lean and fat chickens. *British Poulry Science* 32, 789–798.

Le Dividich, J. and Noblet, J. (1982) Growth rate and protein and fat gain in early-weaned piglets housed below thermoneutrality. *Livestock Production Science* 9, 717–729.

Le Du, Y.L.P. and Penning, P.D. (1982) Animal-based techniques for estimating herbage intake. In: Leaver, J.D. (ed.) *Herbage Intake Handbook*. British Grassland Society, Maidenhead, UK, pp. 37–75.

Le Du, Y.L.P., Baker, R.D. and Barker, J.M. (1976) The effect of length of milk feeding period and milk intake on herbage intake and performance of grazing calves. *Journal of Agricultural Science* 87, 197–204.

Lee, C.E., Scholes, J.C. and Herry, C.L. (1949) The effect of 'free choice', grain feeding on egg production and feed consumption. *Poultry Science* 28, 10–13.

Lee, K. (1978) The influence of Marek's disease vaccination with cell-free HVT vaccine and age of debeaking on food consumption, egg production and other traits in White Leghorns. *Poultry Science* 57, 1151.

Lee, P.A. and Hill, R. (1983) Voluntary food intake of growing pigs given diets containing rapeseed meal, from different types and varieties of rape, as the only protein supplement. *British Journal of Nutrition* 50, 661–672.

Lee, P.J.W., Gulliver, A.L. and Morris, T.R. (1971) A quantitative analysis of the literature concerning the restriction of growing pullets. *British Poultry Science* 12, 413–437.

Lee, R.F. (1974) Effect of physiological state upon voluntary intake of Ruminantia. PhD thesis, University of Cambridge.

Leek, B.F. (1969) Reticulo-ruminal mechanoreceptors in sheep. *Journal of Physiology* 202, 585–609.

Leek, B.F. (1977) Abdominal and pelvic visceral receptors. *British Medical Bulletin* 33, 163–168.

Leek, B.F. (1983) Clinical diseases of the rumen, a physiologist's view. *Veterinary Record*, 113, 10–15.

Leek, B.F. (1986) Sensory receptors in the ruminant alimentary tract. In: Milligan, L.P., Grovum, W.L. and Dobson, A. (eds) *Control of Digestion and Metabolism in the Ruminant.* Prentice-Hall, Englewood Cliffs, New Jersey, pp. 3–17.

Leek, B.F. (1987) The control of the motility of the reticulo-rumen. In: Ooms, L.A.A., Degryse, A.D. and van Miert, A.S.J.P.A.M. (eds) *Physiological and Pharmacological Aspects of the Reticulo-rumen.* Martinus Nijhoff, Dordrecht, pp. 1–20.

Leek, B.F. and Harding, R.H. (1975) Sensory nervous receptors in the ruminant stomach and the reflex control of reticulo-ruminal motility. In: McDonald, I.W. and Warner, A.C.I. (eds) *Digestion and Metabolism in the Ruminant.* University of New England, Armidale, pp. 60–76.

Leeson, S. and Summers, J.D. (1978a) Dietary selection of protein and energy by pullets and broilers. *British Poultry Science* 19, 425–430.

Leeson, S. and Summers, J.D. (1978b) Dietary self-selection by turkeys. *Poultry Science* 57, 1579–1585.

Leeson, S. and Summers, J.D. (1983) Performance of laying hens allowed self-selection of various nutrients. *Nutrition Reports International* 27, 837–843.

Leibowitz, S.F., Weiss, G.F., Yee, F. and Tretter, J.B. (1985) Noradrenergic innervation of the paraventricular nucleus: specific role in control of carbohydrate ingestion. *Brain Research Bulletin* 14, 561–567.

Leibowitz, S.F., Lucas, D.J., Leibowitz, K.L. and Jhanwar, Y.S. (1991) Developmental patterns of macronutrient intake in female and male rats from weaning to maturity. *Physiology and Behavior* 50, 1167–1174.

Le Magnen, J. (1976) Interactions of glucostatic and lipostatic mechanisms in the regulatory control of feeding. In: Novin, D., Wyrwicka, W. and Bray, G. (eds) *Hunger, Basic Mechanisms and Clinical Implications.* Raven Press, New York, pp. 89–101.

Le Magnen, J. (1992) *Neurobiology of Feeding and Nutrition.* Academic Press, San Diego.

Le Magnen, J. and Devos, M. (1980) Parameters of the meal pattern in rats: their assessment and physiological significance. *Neuroscience and Biobehavioral Reviews* 4 (Suppl.1), 1–11.

Le Magnen, J. and Devos, M. (1984) Meal to meal energy balance in rats. *Physiology and Behavior* 32, 39–44.

Le Magnen, J. and Tallon, S. (1966) Spontaneous periodicity of meal taking in the white rat. *Journal of Physiology (Paris)* 58, 323–349.

Lemenager, R.P., Owens, F.N., Lusby, K.S. and Totusek, R. (1978) Monensin, forage intake and lactation of beef cows. *Journal of Animal Science* 47, 247–254.

Lenkeit, W., Witt, M., Farries, E. and Djamai, R. (1966) [Studies of weight changes and feed intake at the end of pregnancy and the beginning of lactation.] *Nutrition Abstracts and Reviews* 37, 262–263.

Lepkovsky, S. and Furuta, F. (1971) The role of homeostasis in adipose tissues upon the regulation of food intake of White Leghorn cockerels. *Poultry Science* 50, 573–577.

Lepkovsky, S. and Yasuda, M. (1966) Hypothalamic lesions, growth and body composition of male chickens. *Poultry Science* 45, 582–588.

Lepkovsky, S., Dimick, M.K., Furuta, F., Snapir, N., Park, R., Narita, N. and Komatsu, K. (1967) Response of blood glucose and plasma free fatty acids to fasting and to injection of insulin and testosterone in chickens. *Endocrinology* 81, 1001–1006.

Levine, A.S. and Morley, J.E. (1981) Reduction of feeding in rats by calcitonin. *Brain Research* 222, 187–191.

Lewis, M. (1981) Equations for predicting silage intake by beef and dairy cattle. *Proceedings of the VI Silage Conference*, Edinburgh, pp. 35–36.

Liebelt, R.A., Ichinoe, S. and Nicholson, N. (1965) Regulatory influences of adipose tissue on food intake and body weight. *Annals of the New York Academy of Sciences*, 131, 559–582.

Lightfoot, A.L., Miller, B.G. and Spechter, H.H. (1987) The effect of pre-weaning diet on post-weaning health and performance of 3-week weaned pigs. *Animal Production* 44, 490.

Lin, L., York, D. and Bray, G. (1992) Acute effects of intracerebroventricular corticotropin-releasing hormone (CRH) on macronutrient selection. *International Journal of Obesity* Suppl 1, 52.

Lindvall, R.N. (1981) Effect of flooring material and number of pigs per pen on nursery pig performance. *Journal of Animal Science* 53, 863–868.

Little, W., Sansom, B.F., Manston, R. and Allen, W.M. (1976) Effects of restricting water intake of dairy cows upon their milk yield, body weight and blood composition. *Animal Production* 22, 329–339.

Little, W., Manston, R., Wilkinson, J.I.D. and Tarrant, M.E. (1991) Some factors related to the voluntary intake of silage by individual dairy cows housed as a group during two winter-feeding periods. *Animal Production* 53, 19–25.

Lobato, J.F.P., Pearce, G.R. and Beilharz, R.G. (1980) Effect of early familiarisation with dietary supplements on the subsequent ingestion of molasses–urea blocks by sheep. *Applied Animal Ethology* 6, 149–161.

Lodge, G.A., Fisher, L.J. and Lessard, J.R. (1975) Influence of prepartum feed intake on performance of cows fed ad libitum during pregnancy. *Journal of Dairy Science* 58, 696–702.

Lopez, S. and Hovell, F.D. de B.(1993) Effect of intraruminal infusions of volatile fatty acids on the intake of a low-digestibility straw by sheep. *Animal Production* 56, 446A.

Luiting, P. (1990) Genetic variation of energy partitioning in laying hens: causes of variation in residual feed consumption. *World's Poultry Science Journal* 46, 133–152.

Lunchick, C., Clawson, A.J., Armstrong, W.D. and Linnerud, A.C. (1978) Protein level, lysine level and source interaction in young pigs. *Journal of Animal Science* 47, 176–183.

Lynch, J.J. and Bell, A.K. (1987) The transmission from generation to generation in sheep of the learned behaviour of eating grain supplements. *Australian Veterinary Journal* 64, 291–292.

Lynch, J.J., Keogh, R.G., Elwin, R.L, Green, G.C. and Mottershead, B.E. (1983) Effects of early experience on the post-weaning acceptance of whole grain wheat by fine-woolled Merino lambs. *Animal Production* 36, 175–183.

Lynch, J.J., Hinch, G.N. and Adams, D.B. (1992) *The Behaviour of Sheep: Biological Principles and Implications for Production.* CAB International, Wallingford, 237pp.

Lynch, P.B. (1989) Voluntary intake of sows and gilts. In: Forbes, J.M., Varley, M.A. and Lawrence, T.L.J. (eds) *The Voluntary Food Intake of Pigs.* Occasional Publication of the British Society of Animal Production, pp. 71–77.

Lyons, T., Caffrey, P.J. and O'Connell, W.J. (1970) The effect of energy, protein and vitamin supplementation on the performance and voluntary intake of barley straw by cattle. *Animal Production* 12, 323–334.

Macari, M., Dauncey, M.J. and Ingram, D.L. (1983) Changes in food intake in response to alterations in the ambient temperature: modifications by previous thermal and nutritional experience. *Pflugers Archivs fur Physiologie* 396, 231–237.

Macari, M., Zuim, S.M.F., Secato, E.R. and Guerreiro, J.R. (1986) Effects of ambient temperature and thyroid hormones on food intake by pigs. *Physiology and Behavior* 36, 1035–1040.

MacDiarmid, B.N. and Watkin, B.R. (1972) The cattle dung patch. 3. Distribution and rate of decay of dung patches and their influence on grazing behaviour. *Journal of the British Grassland Society* 27, 48–54.

MacKenzie, D.D.S. (1967) Production and utilisation of lactic acid by the ruminant. A review. *Journal of Dairy Science* 50, 1772–1786.

Maddison, S. and Baldwin, B.A. (1983) Diencephalic neuronal activity during acquisition and ingestion of food in sheep. *Brain Research* 278, 195–206.

Mahan, D.C. and Fetter, A.W. (1982) Dietary calcium and phosphorus levels for reproducing sows. *Journal of Animal Science* 54, 285–291.

Mahan, D.C. and Gerber, D.B. (1984) Gilt and barrow performance responses from 130 to 300 pounds body weight. *Ohio Swine Research and Industry Report, Ohio State University Animal Science Series Publication No. 84,* Columbus, Ohio.

Mahan, D.C. and Mangan, L.T. (1975) Evaluation of various protein sequences on the nutritional carry-over from gestation to lactation with first-litter sows. *Journal of Nutrition* 105, 1291–1298.

Makela, A. (1956) Studies on the question of bulk in the nutrition of farm animals with special reference to cattle. *Annals of Agricultural Science, Fennica* 85, 1–130.

Maloiy, G.M.O. and Clemens, E.T. (1980) Gastrointestinal osmolality, electrolyte and organic acid composition in five species of East African herbivorous mammals. *Journal of Animal Science* 51, 917–924.

Mann, D.L., Goode, L. and Pond, K.R. (1987) Voluntary intake, gain, digestibility, rate of passage and gastrointestinal tract fill in tropical and temperate breeds of sheep. *Journal of Animal Science* 64, 880–886.

Manning, R., Alexander, G.I., Krueger, H.M. and Bogart, R. (1959) The effect of intravenous glucose injections on appetite in adult ewes. *American Journal of Veterinary Research* 20, 242–246.

March, B.E., Chu, S. and Macmillan, C. (1982) The effects of feed intake on adipocytes in the abdominal fat pad of mature broiler-type female chickens. *Poultry Science* 61, 1137–1146.

Margules, D.L. (1979) Beta-endorphin and endoloxone: hormones of the autonomic nervous system for the conservation or expenditure of bodily resources and energy in anticipation of famine or feast. *Neuroscience and Biobehavioral Reviews* 3, 155–162.

Markowitz, H. (1982) *Behavioural Enrichment in the Zoo*. Van Nostrand Reinhold, New York.

Marsden, D. and Wood-Gush, D.G.M. (1986) A note on the behaviour of individually-penned sheep regarding their use for research purposes. *Animal Production* 42, 157–159.

Marsh, R. (1979) The effects of wilting on fermentation in the silo and on the nutritive value of silage. *Grass and Forage Science* 34, 1–9.

Marsh, R., Campling, R.C. and Holmes, W. (1971) A further study of a rigid grazing management system for dairy cows. *Animal Production* 13, 441–448.

Martin, G.M., Bellingham, W.P. and Storlien, L.H. (1977) Effects of varied colour experience on chickens' formation of colour and texture aversions. *Physiology and Behavior* 8, 415–420.

Martin, H.F. and Baile, C.A. (1972) Feed intake of goats and sheep following acetate or propionate injections into rumen, ruminal pouches, and abomasum as affected by local anesthetics. *Journal of Dairy Science* 55, 606–613.

Martin, H.F., Seoane, J.R. and Baile, C.A. (1973) Feeding in satiated sheep elicited by intraventricular injections of CSF from fasted sheep. *Life Sciences* 13, 177–184.

Martz, F.A., Mishra, M., Campbell, J.R., Daniels, L.B. and Hilderbrand, E. (1971) Relation of ambient temperature and time postfeeding on ruminal, arterial and venous volatile fatty acids, and lactic acid in Holstein steers. *Journal of Dairy Science* 54, 520–525.

Masic, B., Wood-Gush, D.G.M., Duncan, I.J.H., McCorquodale, C. and Savory, C.J. (1974) A comparison of feeding behaviours of young broiler and layer males. *British Poultry Science* 15, 499–505.

Mason, S. and Shelford, J.A. (1990) A computerized forage feeding system allowing measurement of individual intakes, meal patterns and competitive feeding behavior. *Journal of Dairy Science* 73, Suppl. 1, 174.

Mastika, M. and Cumming, R.B. (1981) Performance of two strains of broiler chickens offered free choice from different ages. *Proceedings of the Fourth Australasian Poultry and Stock Feed Convention* (mimeograph).

Mastika, I.M. and Cumming, R.B. (1985) Effect of nutrition and environmental variations on choice feeding of broilers. In: Farrell, D.J. (ed.), *Recent Advances in Animal Nutrition in Australia 1985.* Armidale, NSW, University of New England, paper 19.

Mastika, M. and Cumming, R.B. (1987) Effect of previous experience and enviromental variations on the performance and pattern of feed intake of choice fed and complete fed broilers. *Recent Advances in Animal Nutrition in Australia 1987* pp. 260–282.

Matei-Valdescu, C., Apostol, G. and Popescu, V. (1977) Reduced food intake following cerebral intraventricular infusion of glucose in *Gallus domesticus. Physiology and Behavior* 19, 7–10.

Mateos, G.G., Sell, J.L. and Eastwood, J.A. (1982) Rate of food passage (transit time) as influenced by level of supplemental fat. *Poultry Science* 61, 94–100.

Matthewman, R.W., Oldham, J.D. and Horgan, G.W. (1993) A note on the effect of sustained exercise on straw intake and body weight in lactating cattle. *Animal Production* 57, 491–494.

Matthews, L.R. and Kilgour, R. (1980) Learning and associated factors in ruminant feeding behaviour. In: Ruckebusch, Y. and Thivend, P. (eds) *Digestive Physiology and Metabolism in Ruminants.* MTP Press, Lancaster, pp. 123–144.

Maurice, D.V., Whisehunt, J.E., Jones, J.E. and Smoak, K.D. (1983) Effect of lipectomy on control of feed intake and homeostasis of adipose tissue in chickens. *Poultry Science* 62, 1466.

Maust, L.E., McDowell, R.E. and Hooven, N.W. (1972) Effect of summer weather on performance of Holstein cows in three stages of lactation. *Journal of Dairy Science* 55, 1133–1139.

May, J.D. and Lott, B.D. (1992) Effect of periodic feeding and photoperiod on anticipation of feed withdrawal. *Poultry Science* 71, 951–958.

Mayer, J. (1953) Glucostatic regulation of food intake. *New England Journal of Medicine* 249, 13–16.

Maynard, L.A. and Loosli, J.K. (1962) *Animal Nutrition.* McGraw-Hill, New York, 182pp.

Mayne, C.S. (1990) An evaluation of an inoculant of *Lactobacillus plantarum* as an additive for grass silage for dairy cattle. *Animal Production* 51, 1–13.

Mayne, C.S. (1992) An evaluation of the concentrate sparing effect of four silage additives. *Animal Production* 54, 488.

Mayne, C.S. (1993) The effect of formic acid, sulphuric acid and a bacterial inoculation on silage fermentation and the food intake and milk production of lactating dairy cows. *Animal Production* 56, 29–42.

Mayne, C.S. and Wright, I.A. (1988) Factors affecting herbage intake and utilization by the grazing cow. In: Garnsworthy, P.C. (ed.) *Nutrition and*

*Lactation in the Dairy Cow.* Butterworths, London, pp. 280–293.

Mbanya, J.N. (1988) Effects of ruminal administration of acetate, propionate and distension on forage intake by dairy cows. PhD thesis, University of Leeds, 276pp.

Mbanya, J.N., Anil, M.H. and Forbes, J.M. (1993) The voluntary intake of hay and silage by lactating cows in response to ruminal infusion of acetate or propionate, or both, with and without distension of the rumen by a balloon. *British Journal of Nutrition* 69, 713–720.

McCann, J.P. and Reimers, T.J. (1985) Insulin response to glucose in estrous and diestrous obese and lean heifers. *Journal of Animal Science* 61, 619–624.

McCann, J.P., Bergmann, E.N. and Beerman, D.H. (1992) Dynamic and static phases of severe dietary obesity in sheep: food intakes, endocrinology and carcass and organ chemical composition. *Journal of Nutrition* 122, 496–505.

McCarthy, I.D., Houlihan, D.F., Carter, C.G. and Moutou, K. (1993) Variation in individual food consumption rates of fish and its implications for the study of fish nutrition and physiology. *Proceedings of the Nutrition Society* 52, 427–436.

McCoy, J.G. and Avery, D.D. (1990) Bombesin – potential integrative peptide for feeding and satiety. *Peptides* 11, 595–607.

McCulloch, T.A. (1969) A study of factors affecting the voluntary intake of food by cattle. *Animal Production* 11, 145–153.

McDonald, M.A. and Bell, J.M. (1958) Effects of low fluctuating temperatures on farm animals. 2. Influence of ambient air temperature on water intake of lactating Holstein–Friesian cows. *Canadian Journal of Animal Science* 38, 23–32.

McDonald, P. (1981) *The Biochemistry of Silage.* Wiley, Chichester, 226pp.

McDonald, P., Henderson, A.R. and Heron, S.J.E. (1991) *The Biochemistry of Silage* 2nd edn. Wiley, Chichester.

McDonald, R. and Emmans, G.C. (1980) Choice feeding of turkey breeder hens in single cages. *World's Poultry Science Journal* 36, 68–73.

McGlone, J.J., Stansbury, W.F. and Tribble, L.F. (1988) Management of lactating sows during heat stress: effects of water drip, snout coolers, floor type and a high energy-density diet. *Journal of Animal Science* 66, 885–891.

McKinley, M.J., Denton, D.A., Gellatly, D., Miselis, R.R., Simpson, J.B. and Weisinger, R.S. (1987) Water drinking caused by intracerebroventricular infusion of hypertonic solutions in cattle. *Physiology and Behavior* 39, 459–464.

McLaughlin, C.L., Baldwin, B.A. and Baile, C.A. (1974) Olfactory bulbectomy and feeding behavior. *Journal of Animal Science* 39, 136.

McLaughlin, C.L., Baile, C.A., Buckholtz, L.L. and Freeman, S.K. (1983) Preferred flavors and performance of weaning piglets. *Journal of Animal Science* 56, 1287–1293.

McLaughlin, C.L., Baile, C.A. and Buonomo, F.C. (1985) Effect of CCK antibodies on food intake and weight gain in Zucker rats. *Physiology and Behavior* 34, 277–282.

McLeod, D.S., Wilkins, R.J. and Raymond, W.F. (1970) The voluntary intake by sheep and cattle of silage differing in free-acid content. *Journal of Agricultural Science* 75, 311–319.

McPhee, C.P. (1981) Selection for efficient lean growth in a pig herd. *Australian Journal of Agricultural Research* 32, 681–690.

McSweeney, C.S. and Pass, M.A. (1983) The mechanism of ruminal stasis in lantana-poisoned sheep. *Quarterly Journal of Experimental Physiology* 68, 301–313.

Mears, G.J. and Mendel, V.E. (1974) Correlation of food intake in lambs with adipocyte glucose metablism and NEFA release. *Journal of Physiology* 240, 625–637.

Mehren, M.J. and Church, D.C. (1976) Influence of taste-modifiers on taste responses of pigmy goats. *Animal Production* 22, 255–260.

Mei, N. (1985) Intestinal chemosensitivity. *Physiological Reviews* 65, 211–237.

Meijs, J.A.C. (1986) Concentrate supplementation of grazing dairy cows. 2. Effect of concentrate composition on herbage intake and milk production. *Grassland and Forage Science* 41, 229–235.

Meijs, J.A.C. and Hoekstra, J.A. (1984) Concentrate supplementation of grazing dairy cows. 1. Effect of concentrate intake and herbage allowance on herbage intake. *Grass and Forage Science* 39, 59–66.

Meijs, J.A.C., Walters, R.J.K. and Keen, A. (1982) Sward methods. In: Leaver, J.D. (ed.) *Herbage Intake Handbook*. British Grassland Society, Maidenhead, pp. 11–36.

Mench, J.A. (1992) The welfare of poultry in modern production systems. *Poultry Science Reviews* 4, 107–128.

Mench, J.A., Van Tienhoven, A., Kaszovitz, B., Huber, A. and Cunningham, D.L. (1986) Behavioral effects of intraventricular dibutyryl cyclic AMP in domestic fowl. *Physiology and Behavior* 37, 483–488.

Mertens, D.R. (1973) Applications of theoretical mathematical models to cell wall digestion and forage intake in ruminants. PhD thesis, Cornell University.

Mertens, D.R. (1977) Dietary fiber components: relationship to the rate and extent of ruminal digestion. *Federation Proceedings* 36, 187–192.

Mertens, D.R. and Ely, L.O. (1979) A dynamic model of fiber digestion and passage in the ruminant for evaluating forage quality. *Journal of Animal Science* 49, 1085–1095.

Metz, J.H. (1975) Time patterns of feeding and rumination in domestic cattle. *Medededlingen Landbouwhhogeschool, Wageningen* 75, 1–66.

Metz, J.H.M. (1983) Food competition in cattle. In: Baxter, S.H., Baxter M.R., and MacCormack, J.A.C. (eds) *Farm Animal Housing and Welfare*. Martinus Nijhoff, Lancaster, pp. 164–170.

Meunier-Salaun, M.C., Monnier, M., Coileaux, Y., Seve, B. and Henry, Y. (1991) Impact of dietary tryptophan and behavioural type on behaviour, plasma cortisol and brain metabolites of young pigs. *Journal of Animal Science* 69, 3689–3698.

Meyer, A.H., Langhans, W. and Scharrer, E. (1989) Vasopressin reduces food intake in goats. *Quarterly Journal of Experimental Physiology* 74, 465–473.

Meyer, G.B., Babcock, S.W. and Sunde, M.L. (1970) Decreased feed consumption and increased calcium intake associated with pullet's first egg. *Poultry Science* 49, 1164–1169.

Meyer, J.H. and Hargus, W.A. (1959) Factors influencing food intake of rats fed low-protein rations. *American Journal of Physiology* 197, 1350–1352.

Mezzadra, C., Paciaroni, R., Vulich, S., Villareal, E. and Melucci, L. (1989) Estimation of milk consumption curve parameters for different genetic groups of bovine calves. *Animal Production* 49, 83–87.

Michell, A.R. and Moss, P. (1988) Salt appetites during pregnancy in sheep. *Physiology and Behavior* 42, 491–493.

Milford, R. and Minson, D.J. (1966) Intake of tropical pasture species. *Proceedings of the 9th International Grassland Congress* 1, 815–822.

Milk Marketing Board (1987) *Milk Costs 1986–87. Booklet 2. Feed Use and Grassland Production for the Dairy Herd.* MMB, Thames Ditton.

Miller, K. and Wood-Gush, D.G.M. (1991) Some effects of housing on the social behaviour of dairy cows. *Animal Production* 53, 271–278.

Miller, M.G. and Teates, J.F. (1986) The role of taste in dietary self-selection in rats. *Behavioral Neuroscience* 100, 399–409.

Miller, W.J., Clifton, C.M., Miller, J.K. and Fowler, P.R. (1965) Effects of feeding unlike forages, singly and in combination, on voluntary dry matter consumption and performance of lactating cows. *Journal of Dairy Science* 48, 1046–1052.

Miller, W.J., Blackmon, D.M., Powell, G.W., Gentry, R.P. and Hiers, J.M. (1966) Effects of zinc deficiency per se and of dietary zinc level on urinary and endogenous fecal excretion of 65-Zn from a single intravenous dose by ruminants. *Journal of Nutrition* 90, 335–341.

Milne, J.A., Macrae, J.C., Spence, A.M. and Wilson, S. (1978) A comparison of the voluntary intake and digestion of a range of forages at different times of the year by the sheep and the red deer (*Cervus elaphus*). *British Journal of Nutrition* 40, 347–357.

Milne, J.A., Maxwell, T.J. and Souter, W. (1981) Effect of supplementary feeding and herbage mass on the intake and performance of grazing ewes in early lactation. *Animal Production* 32, 185–195.

Miner, J.L., Della-Fera, M.A., Paterson, J.A. and Baile, C.A. (1990) Alpha2-adrenoceptor blockade does not block feeding induced by neuropeptide Y in sheep. *Physiology and Behavior* 48, 61–65.

Ministry of Agriculture, Fisheries and Food (MAFF) (1975) *Energy Allowances and Feeding Systems for Ruminants.* Technical Bulletin 33, HMSO, London, 79pp.

Minson, D.J. (1963) The effect of pelleting and wafering on the feeding value of roughages – a review. *Journal of the British Grassland Society* 18, 39–44.

Minson, D.J. (1982) Effects of chemical and physical composition of herbage eaten upon intake. In: Hacker, J.B. (ed.) *Nutritional Limits to Animal Production from Pasture.* Commonwealth Agricultural Bureaux, Farnham Royal, pp. 167–182.

Minson, D.J. and Ternouth, J.H. (1971) The expected and observed changes in the intake of three hays by sheep after shearing. *British Journal of Nutrition* 26, 31–39.

Mirza, S.N. and Provenza, F.D. (1992) Effects of age and conditions of exposure on maternally mediated food selection by lambs. *Applied Animal Behaviour Science* 33, 35–42.

Miselis, R.R. and Epstein, A.N. (1975) Feeding induced by intracerebro-ventricular 2-deoxy-D-glucose in the rat. *American Journal of Physiology* 229, 1438–1447.

Mongin, P. and Sauveur, B. (1979) The specific calcium appetite of the domestic fowl. In: Boorman, K.N. and Freeman, B.M. (eds) *Food Intake Regulation in Poultry.* Longman, Edinburgh, pp. 171–189.

Mongin, P., Jastrebebski, M. and van Teinhoven, A. (1978) Temporal patterns of ovulation, oviposition and feeding of laying hens under skeleton photo-periods. *British Poultry Science* 19, 747–753.

Monteiro, L.S. (1972) The control of appetite in lactating cows. *Animal Production* 14, 263–282.

Montgomery, M.J. and Baumgardt, B.R. (1965) Regulation of food intake in ruminants. 1. Pelletted rations varying in energy concentration. *Journal of Dairy Science* 48, 569–574.

Mook, D.G., Brane, J.A., Kushner, L.R. and Whitt, J.A. (1983) Glucose solution intake in the rat: the specificity of postingestive satiety. *Appetite* 4, 1–9.

Mook, D.G., Atkinson, B., Johnston, L. and Wagner, S. (1993) Persistence of sham feeding after intergastric meals in rats. *Appetite* 20, 167–179.

Moose, M.G., Ross, C.V. and Pfander, W.H. (1969) Nutritional and environmental relationships in lambs. *Journal of Animal Science* 29, 619–627.

Moran, J.B. (1976) Beef production as influenced by grazing and feeding management and by mature size. PhD thesis, Wye College, University of London.

Moran, J.B. and Holmes, W. (1978) The application of compensatory growth in grass/cereal production beef systems in the United Kingdom. *World Review of Animal Production* 14, 65–73.

Moran, J.B., Lemerle, C. and Trigg, T.E. (1988) The intake and digestion of maize silage-based diets by cows and sheep. *Animal Feed Science and Technology* 20, 299–312.

Morgan, D.J. and L'Estrange, J.L. (1977) Voluntary feed intake and metabolism of sheep when lactic acid is administered in the feed or intraruminally. *Journal of the British Grassland Society* 32, 217–224.

Morita, S. and Nishino, S. (1991) Distribution of eating bouts and inter-bout intervals in steers offered mixed ration ad libitum. *Journal of Rakuno Gakuen Universit* 16, 21–25.

Morley, F.H.W. (1986) *Grazing Animals.* Elsevier, Amsterdam, 459pp.

Morley, J.E. and Blundell, J.E. (1988) The neurobiological basis of eating disorders: some formulations. *Biological Psychiatry* 23, 53–78.

Morris, B.A. and Taylor, T.G. (1967) The daily food consumption of laying hens in relation to egg formation. *British Poultry Science* 8, 251–257.

Morris, T.R. (1968a) Light requirements of the fowl. In: Carter, T.C. (ed.), *Environmental Control in Poultry Production.* Oliver and Boyd, Edinburgh, pp. 15–39.

Morris, T.R. (1968b) The effect of dietary energy level on the voluntary caloric intake of laying birds. *British Poultry Science* 9, 285–295.

Morris, T.R. and Nurju, D.M. (1990) Protein requirement of fast and slow growing chicks. *British Poultry Science* 31, 803–809.

Morrison, S.R., Hintz, H.F. and Givens, R.L. (1968) A note on the effect of exercise on behaviour and performance of confined swine. *Animal Production* 10, 341–344.

Morrison, S.R., Heitman, H. and Bond, T.E. (1969) Effect of humidity on swine at temperatures above optimum. *International Journal of Biometeorology* 13, 135–139.

Morrison, S.R., Givens, R.L. and Heitman, H. (1976) A note on growth and feed conversion in pigs at different air temperatures and ventilation rates. *Animal Production* 23, 249–252.

Morrow, A.T.S. and Walker, N. (1991) The effect of number of single space feeders and the provision of an additional drinker or toy on the performance and feeding behaviour of growing pigs. *Animal Production* 52, 577.

Morrow, A.T.S. and Walker, N. (1992) The effect of increasing workload to obtain feed ad libitum on performance and behaviour of finishing pigs. *Animal Production* 54, 481A.

Moseley, G. and Jones, D.I.H. (1974) The effect of sodium chloride supplementation of a sodium adequate hay on digestion, production and mineral nutrition in sheep. *Journal of Agricultural Science* 83, 37–42.

Moser, R.L. (1985) Lactation feed intake management. *Pigs* (May), 26–29.

Mottershead, B.E., Lynch, J.J., Elwin, R.L. and Green, G.C. (1985) A note on the acceptance of several types of cereal grain by young sheep with and without prior experience of wheat. *Animal Production* 41, 257–259.

Mount, L.E. (1968) *The Climatic Physiology of the Pig*. Arnold, London, 271pp.

Mount, L.E., Holmes, C.W., Close, W.H., Morrison, S.R. and Start, C.B. (1971) A note on the consumption of water by the growing pig at several environmental temperatures and levels of feeding. *Animal Production* 13, 561–563.

Mowatt, D.N. (1963) Factors affecting rumen capacity and the physical inhibition of feed intake. PhD thesis, Cornell University, New York.

Moxon, A.L. and Rhian, M. (1943) Selenium poisoning. *Physiological Reviews* 23, 305–337.

Mrode, R.A. and Kennedy, B.W. (1993) Genetic variation in measures of food efficiency in pigs and their genetic relationships with growth rate and backfat. *Animal Production* 56, 225–232.

Muhikambele, V.R.M., Owen,E. and Owen, J.E. (1993) Vertical 'reach' capacity of sheep and goats fed through barriers. *Animal Production* 56, 456A.

Muinga, R.W., Thorpe, W. and Topps, J.H. (1992) Voluntary food intake, liveweight change and lactation performance of crossbred dairy cows given ad libitum *Pennisetum purpureum* (napier grass var. Bana) supplemented with leucaena forage in the lowland semi-humid tropics. *Animal Production* 55, 331–338.

Mullan, B.P. and Williams, I.H. (1989) The effect of body reserves at farrowing on the reproductive performance of first-litter sows. *Animal Production* 48, 449–458.

Muller, L.D. and Colenbrander, V.F. (1970) Effect of insulin administration on blood acetate and feed intake of sheep. *Journal of Animal Science* 31, 145–148.

Murdoch, J.C. (1965) The effect of length of silage on its voluntary intake by cattle. *Journal of the British Grassland Society* 20, 54–58.

Murdoch, J.C. and Rook, J.A.F. (1963) A comparison of hay and silage for milk production. *Journal of Dairy Research* 30, 391–397.

Murnane, D. (1934) Sarcophagia in herbivorous animals. *Journal of the Council for Scientific and Industrial Research of Australia* 7, 143–144.

Murphy, M.E. and King, J.R. (1989) Sparrows discriminate between diets differing in valine or lysine concentrations. *Physiology and Behavior* 45, 423–430.

Murphy, M.E. and Pearcy, S.D. (1993) Dietary amino acid complementation as a foraging strategy for wild birds. *Physiology and Behavior* 53, 689–698.

Mutsvangwa, T., Edwards, I.E., Topps, J.H. and Paterson, G.F.M. (1992) The effect of dietary inclusion of yeast culture (Yea-Sacc) on patterns of rumen fermentation, food intake and growth of intensively fed bulls. *Animal Production* 55, 35–40.

Myers, R.D. (1971) *Methods of Psychology: Laboratory Techniques in Neuropsychology and Neurobiology.* Academic Press, New York, 356pp.

Myers, R.D. and Veale, W.L. (1971) Spontaneous feeding in the satiated cat evoked by sodium or calcium ions perfused within the hypothalamus. *Physiology and Behavior* 6, 507–512.

Neal, H.D.S., Thomas, C. and Cobby, J.M. (1984) Comparison of equations for predicting voluntary intake by dairy cows. *Journal of Agricultural Science* 103, 1–10.

Neal, H.D.S., France, J., Orr, R.J. and Treacher, T.T. (1985) A model to maximize hay intake when formulating rations for pregnant ewes. *Animal Production* 40, 93–100.

Neal, H.D.S., Gill, M., France, J., Spedding, A. and Marsden, S. (1988) An evaluation of predictions equations incorporated in a computer program to ration beef cattle. *Animal Production* 46, 169–179.

Neilson, D.R., Whittemore, C.T., Lewis, M., Alliston, J.C., Roberts, D.J., Hodgson-Jones, L.S., Mills, J., Parkinson, H. and Prescott, J.H.D. (1983) Production characteristics of high-yielding dairy cows. *Animal Production* 36, 321–334.

Neumark, H. (1967) On the areas of the stomach of sheep that are sensitive to formic acid and histamine. *Journal of Agricultural Science* 69, 297–302.

Neumark, H., Bondi, A. and Volcani, R. (1964) Amines, aldehydes and keto-acids in silages and their effect on food intake by ruminants. *Journal of the Science of Food and Agriculture* 15, 487–492.

Newman, J.A., Parsons, A.J. and Harvey, A. (1992) Not all sheep prefer clover: diet selection revisited. *Journal of Agricultural Science* 119, 275–283.

Newman, J.A., Penning, P.D., Parsons, A.J., Harvey, J. and Orr, R.J. (1994) Fasting affects intake behaviour and diet preference of grazing sheep. *Animal Behaviour* 47, 185–193.

Newman, R.K. and Sands, D.C. (1983) Dietary selection for lysine by the chick. *Physiology and Behavior* 31, 13–20.

Newton, J.E. and Jackson, C. (1983) A note on the effect of dentition and age in sheep on the intake of herbage. *Animal Production* 37, 133–136.

Nicholson, J.W.G. (1984) Digestibility, nutritive value and feed intake. In: Sundstol, F. and Owen, E. (eds) *Straw and Other Fibrous By-products as Feed.* Elsevier, Amsterdam, pp. 340–372.

Nicolaidis, S. and Rowland, N. (1976) Metering of intravenous versus oral nutrients. *American Journal of Physiology* 231, 661–668.

Nielsen, B.L., Whittemore, C.T. and Lawrence, A.B. (1993) Effect of group size on the feeding behaviour of pigs using a computerized single-space feeding system. *Animal Production* 56, 420–521A.

Niijima, A. (1969) Afferent impulses from glucoreceptors in the liver of the guinea pig. *Annals of the New York Academy of Sciences* 157, 690.

Nir, I. and Levy, V. (1973) Response of blood plasma glucose, free fatty acids, triglycerides, insulin and food intake to bovine insulin in geese and cockerels. *Poultry Science* 52, 886–892.

Nir, I., Shapira, N., Nitsan, Z. and Dror, Y. (1974) Force-feeding effects on growth, carcass and blood composition in young chicks. *British Journal of Nutrition* 32, 229–239.

Noblet, J. and Henry, Y. (1977) [Consequences of a reduction in protein level of the feed on feed intake and growth of pigs according to amino acid balance and energy concentration.] *Annales de Zootechnie* 26, 379–394.

Nolte, D.L. and Provenza, F.D. (1992a) Food preference in lambs after exposure to flavors in solid foods. *Applied Animal Behavioural Science* 32, 337–347.

Nolte, D.L. and Provenza, F.D. (1992b) Food preferences in lambs after exposure to flavors in milk. *Applied Animal Behaviour Science* 32, 381–389.

Nolte, D.L., Provenza, F.D. and Balph, D.F. (1990) The establishment and persistence of food preferences in lambs exposed to selected foods. *Journal of Animal Science* 68, 998–1002.

Norman, M.J.T. and Green, J.O. (1958) The local influence of cattle dung and urine upon the yield and botanical composition of permanent pasture. *Journal of the British Grassland Society* 13, 39–45.

Novin, D. (1976) Visceral mechanisms in the control of food intake. In: Novin, D., Wyrwicka, W. and Bray, G. (eds) *Hunger, Basic Mechanisms and Clinical Implications.* Raven Press, New York, pp. 357–367.

Novin, D. (1983) The integration of visceral information in the control of feeding. *Journal of the Autonomic Nervous System* 9, 233–246.

Novin, D., Sanderson, J.D. and Vanderweele, D.A. (1974) The effect of isotonic glucose on eating as a function of feeding condition and infusion site. *Physiology and Behavior* 13, 3–7.

NRC (1957) *Nutrient Requirements of Domestic Animals. Nutrient Requirements of Sheep.* National Research Council, Washington DC, Publication 5047, No. V.

NRC (1963) *Nutrient Requirements of Domestic Animals. Nutrient Requirements of Cattle.* National Research Council, Washington DC, Publication 1137, No. IV.

NRC (1981) *Effect of Environment on Nutrient Requirements of Domestic Animals.* National Research Council, Washington DC, National Academy Press, 152pp.

NRC (1984a) *Nurient Requirements of Beef Cattle, 6th revised edn.* National Academy Press, Washington DC.

NRC (1984b) *Nutrient Requirements of Poultry, 8th revised edn.* National Academy Press, Washington DC.

NRC (1987) *Predicting Feed Intake of Food-Producing Animals.* National Academy Press, Washington DC, 85pp.

Nys, Y., Sauveur, B., Lacarsagne, L. and Mongin, P. (1976) Food, calcium and water intakes by hens lit continuously from hatching. *British Poultry Science* 17, 351–358.

Odoi, F.N.A. and Owen, E. (1992) Offering barley straw to lambs near weaning as a means of increasing their subsequent readiness to eat straw. *Australian Journal of Agricultural Research* 54, 492–493A.

Odoi, F.N.A. and Owen, E. (1993) Encouraging store lambs to eat barley straw at housing: influence on intake of pen to pen visibility and number of lambs per pen. *Animal Production* 56, 455.

Odwongo, W.O. and Conrad, H.R. (1983) Prediction of digestible net energy intake in lactating dairy cows. *Journal of Dairy Science* 66 (Suppl 1), 166.

Oetting, R.L. and Vanderweele, D.A. (1985) Insulin suppresses intake without inducing illness in sham feeding rats. *Physiology and Behavior* 34, 557–562.

O'Grady, J.F. and Lynch, P.B. (1978) Voluntary feed intake by lactating sows: influence of system of feeding and nutrient density of the diet. *Irish Journal of Agricultural Research* 17, 1–5.

O'Grady, J.F., Lynch, P.B. and Kearney, P.A. (1985) Voluntary feed intake by lactating sows. *Livestock Production Science* 12, 355–365.

Ollivier, L. (1978) [The unfavourable effect of mixing sexes in fattening pigs in groups.] *Annales de Zootechnie* 26, 615–619.

Olsson, K. (1969) Effects of slow infusions of KC1 into the 3rd brain ventricle. *Acta Physiologica Scandinavica* 77, 358–364.

Olsson, K. and McKinley, M.J. (1980) Central control of water and salt intake in goats and sheep. In: Ruckebusch, Y. and Thivend, P. (eds) *Digestive Physiology and Metabolism in Ruminants*, MTP Press, Lancaster, pp. 161–175.

Oltjen, R.R., Davies, R.E. and Hiner, R.L. (1965) Factors affecting performance and carcass characteristics of cattle fed all-concentrate rations. *Journal of Animal Science* 24, 192–197.

O'Mary, C.C., Pope, A.L., Wilson, G.D., Bray, R.W. and Casida, L.E. (1952) The effects of diethylstilbestrol, testosterone and progesterone on growth and fattening and certain carcass characteristics of Western lambs. *Journal of Animal Science* 11, 656–673.

Onibi, G.E., Gill, P.B. and English, P.R. (1992) Feed ingredient selection in growing and finishing pigs: effects on performance and carcass quality. *Animal Production* 54, 451–452A.

Oomura, Y. (1976) Significance of glucose, insulin and free fatty acids on the hypothalamic feeding and satiety neurones. In: Novin, D.A., Wyyrwicka, W. and Bray, G. (eds), *Hunger Basic Mechanisms and Clinical Implications*. Raven Press, New York, pp. 145–158.

Orr, R.M. (1977) A study on the role of body fatness in the control of voluntary feed intake in sheep. PhD thesis, University of Edinburgh.

Orr, R.J. and Treacher, T.T. (1984) The effect of concentrate level on the intake of hays by ewes in late pregnancy. *Animal Production* 39, 89–98.

Orr, R.J. and Treacher, T.T. (1989) The effect of concentrate level and the intake of grass silage by ewes in late pregnancy. *Animal Production* 48, 109–120.

Orr, R.J. and Treacher, T.T. (1994) The effect of concentrate level on the intakes of silages or hays by ewes in the 1st month of lactation. *Animal Production* 58, 109–116.

Orsini, J.P.G. (1990) 'SummerPack', a user-friendly simulation software for the management of sheep grazing dry pastures or stubbles. *Agricultural Systems* 33, 361–376.

Orskov, E.R. and McDonald, I. (1979) The estimation of protein degradability in the rumen from incubation measurements weighted according to rate of passage. *Journal of Agricultural Science, Cambridge* 92, 499–503.

Orskov, E.R., Fraser, C. and Corse, E.L. (1971) The effect of protein supplementation via the abomasum on the voluntary intake of concentrate by young growing sheep. *Proceedings of the Nutrition Society* 30, 25–26A.

Orskov, E.R., Reid, G.W. and Kay, M. (1991) Influence of straw quality and level of concentrate in a completely mixed diet on intake and growth rate in steers. *Animal Production* 52, 461–464.

Ortega-Reyes, L. and Provenza, F.D. (1993) Amount of experience and age affect the development of foraging skills of goats browsing blackbrush (*Coleogyne ramosissima*). *Applied Animal Behaviour Science* 36, 169–183.

Osbourn, D.F. (1967) The intake of conserved forages. In: *Fodder Conservation*. Occasional Symposium of the British Grassland Society, No. 3, pp. 20–28.

Osbourn, D.F. and Wilson, P.N. (1960) Effects of different patterns of allocation of a restricted quantity of food upon the growth and development of cockerels. *Journal of Agricultural Science* 54, 278–289.

Ostergaard, V. (1979) *Strategies for Concentrate Feeding to Attain Optimum Feeding Level in High Yielding Dairy Cows*. National Institute of Agricultural Science, Copenhagen, 138pp.

Osuji, P.O., (1974) The physiology of eating and the energy expenditure of the ruminant at pasture. *Journal of Range Management* 27, 437–443.

Ott, E.A., Smith, W.H., Harrington, R.B. and Beeson, W.M. (1966) Zinc toxicity in ruminants. 1. Effect of high levels of dietary zinc on gains, feed consumption and feed efficiency of lambs. *Journal of Animal Science* 25, 414–418.

Owen, J.B. (1979) *Complete Diets for Cattle and Sheep*. Farming Press, Ipswich, 159pp.

Owen, J.B. and Ingleton, J.W. (1963) A study of food intake and production in grazing ewes. 2. The interrelationships between food intake and grazing output. *Journal of Agricultural Science* 61, 329–340.

Owen, J.B. and Ridgman, W.J. (1967) The effect of dietary energy content on the voluntary feed intake of pigs. *Animal Production* 9, 107–113.

Owen, J.B. and Ridgman, W.J. (1968) Further studies of the effect of dietary energy content on the voluntary intake of pigs. *Animal Production* 10, 85–91.

Owen, J.B., Miller, E.L. and Bridge, P.S. (1968) A study of the voluntary intake of food and water and the lactation performance of cows given diets of varying roughage content ad libitum. *Journal of Agricultural Science* 70, 223–235.

Owen, J.B., Miller, E,.L. and Bridge, P.S. (1969) Complete diets given ad libitum to dairy cows – the effect of the level of inclusion of milled straw. *Journal of Agricultural Science* 72, 351–357.

Ozanne, P.G. and Howes, K.M.W. (1971) Preference of grazing sheep for pasture of high phosphate content. *Australian Journal of Agricultural Research* 22, 941–950.

Pain, B.F., Leaver, J.D. and Broom, D.M. (1974) Effects of cow slurry on herbage production, intake by cattle and grazing behaviour. *Journal of the British Grassland Society* 29, 85–91.

Pajor, E.A., Fraser, D. and Kramer, D.L. (1991) Consumption of solid food by suckling pigs: individual variation and relation to weight gain. *Applied Animal Behaviour Science* 32, 139–155.

Pamp, D.E., Goodrich, R.D. and Meiske, J.C. (1976) A review of the practice of feeding minerals free choice. *World Review of Animal Production* 12, 13–18.

Panksepp, J. (1978) Analysis of feeding patterns: data reduction and theoretical implications. In: Booth, D.A. (ed.) *Hunger Models: Computable Theory of Feeding Control*. Academic Press, London, pp. 143–166.

Paquay, R. and Vernaillen, F. (1984) Effects of oleic acid esters on food intake in sheep. *Canadian Journal of Animal Science* 64 (Supplement), 316–317.

Parrott, R.F. and Baldwin, B.A. (1978) Effects of intracerebroventricular injections of 2-deoxy-D-glucose, D-glucose and xylose on operant feeding in pigs. *Physiology and Behavior* 21, 329–331.

Parrott, R.F. and Baldwin, B.A. (1981) Operant feeding and drinking in pigs following intracerebroventricular injection of synthetic cholecystokinin octapeptide. *Physiology and Behavior* 26, 419–422.

Parrott, R.F. and Baldwin, B.A. (1982) Centrally-administered bombesin produces effects unlike short-term satiety in operant feeding pigs. *Physiology and Behavior* 28, 521–524.

Parrott, R.F., Heavens, R.P. and Baldwin, B.A. (1986) Stimulation of feeding in the satiated pig by intracerebroventricular injection of neuropeptide Y. *Physiology and Behavior* 36, 523–525.

Parsons, A.J., Newman, J.A., Penning, P.D., Harvey, A. and Orr, R.J. (1994) Diet preference by sheep: effects of recent diet, physiological state and species abundance. *Journal of Animal Ecology* 63, 465–478.

Partridge, G.G., Fisher, J., Gregory, H. and Prior, S.G. (1992) Automated wet feeding of weaner pigs versus conventional dry feeding – effects on growth rate and feed consumption. *Animal Production* 54, 484A.

Patrick, H. and Ferrise, A. (1962) Water requirements of broilers. *Poultry Science* 41, 1363–1367.

Patterson, I.W. and Coleman, D.D. (1982) Activity patterns of seaweed-eating sheep on North Ronaldsay, Orkney. *Applied Animal Ethology* 8, 137–146.

Patterson, T.L. (1927) Gastric movements in the pigeon with economy of animal material – Comparative studies 5. *Journal of Laboratory Clinical Medicine* 12, 1003–1008.

Pearson, R.A. and Lawrence, P.R. (1992) Intake, digestion, gastro-intestinal transit time and nitrogen balance in working oxen, studied in Costa Rica and Nepal. *Animal Production* 55, 361–370.

Peel, C.J., Bauman, D.E., Gorewit, R.C. and Sniffen, C.J. (1981) Effect of exogenous growth hormone on lactational performance high yielding dairy cows. *Journal of Nutrition* 111, 1662–1671.

Peel, C.J., Sandles, L.D., Quelch, K.J. and Herington, A.C. (1985) The effects of long-term administration of bovine growth hormone on the lactational performance of identical-twin dairy cows. *Animal Production* 41, 135–142.

Pekas, J.C. (1983) A method for direct gastric feeding and the effect on voluntary ingestion in young swine. *Appetite* 4, 23–30.

Pekas, J.C. and Trout, W.E. (1993) Cholecystokinin octapeptide immunization: effect on growth of barrows and gilts. *Journal of Animal Science* 71, 2499–2505.

Penning, P.D. and Hooper,G.E. (1985) An evaluation of the use of short-term weight changes in grazing sheep for estimating herbage intake. *Grass and Forage Science* 40, 109–116.

Penning, P.D., Corcura, P. and Treacher, T.T. (1980) Effect of dry matter concentration of milk substitute and method of feeding on intake and performance by lambs. *Animal Feed Science and Technology* 5, 321–336.

Penning, P.D., Steel, G.L. and Johnson, R.H. (1984) Further development and use of an automatic recording system in sheep grazing studies. *Grass and Forage Science* 39, 345–351.

Penning, P.D., Hooper, G.E. and Treacher, T.T. (1986) The effect of herbage allowance on intake and performance of ewes suckling twin lambs. *Grass and Forage Science* 41, 199–351.

Penning, P.D., Orr, R.J. and Treacher, T.T. (1988) Responses of lactating ewes, offered fresh herbage indoors and when grazing, to supplements containing differing protein concentrations. *Animal Production* 46, 403–415.

Penning, P.D., Parsons, A.J., Orr, R.J. and Treacher, T.T. (1991a) Intake and behaviour responses by sheep to changes in sward characteristics under continuous stocking. *Grass and Forage Science* 46, 15–28.

Penning, P.D., Rook, A.J. and Orr, R.J. (1991b) Patterns of ingestive behaviour of sheep continuously stocked on monocultures of ryegrass or white clover. *Applied Animal Behaviour Science* 31, 403–415.

Penning, P.F., Parsons, A.J., Newman, J.A., Orr, R. and Harvey, A. (1993) The effects of group size on time budgets in grazing sheep. *Applied Animal Behaviour Science* 37, 101–109.

Penzhorn, E.J. and Meintjes, J.P. (1972) Influence of pregnancy and lactation on the voluntary feed intake of Afrikaner heifers and cows. *Agroanimalia* 4, 83–92.

Perez, C. and Sclafani, A. (1991) Cholecystokinin conditions flavor preferences in rats. *American Journal of Physiology* 260, R179–R185.

Perry, G.C. (1992) Olfaction and taste. In: Phillips, C.J.C. and Piggins, D. (eds) *Farm Animals and the Environment*, CAB International, Wallingford, pp. 185–199.

Persaud, P. and Simm, G. (1991) Genetic and phenotypic parameters for yield, food intake and efficiency of dairy cows fed ad libitum. 2. Estimates for part lactation measures and their relationship with 'total' lactation measures. *Animal Production* 52, 445–450.

Petchey, A.M. and Abdulkader, J. (1991) Intake and behaviour of cattle at different food barriers. *Animal Production* 52, 576–577.

Petchey, A.M. and Broadbent, P.J. (1980) The performance of fattening cattle offered barley and grass silage in various proportions either as discrete feeds or as a complete diet. *Animal Production* 31, 251–257.

Peters, J.P., Bergman, E.N. and Elliot, J.M. (1983) Changes of glucose, insulin and glucagon associated with propionate infusion and vitamin B-12 status in sheep. *Journal of Nutrition* 113, 1229–1240.

Peters, R.R., Chapin, L.T., Emery, R.S. and Tucker, H.A. (1980) Growth and hormonal response of heifers to various photoperiods. *Journal of Animal Science* 51, 1148–1153.

Peters, R.R., Chapin, L.T., Emery, R.S. and Tucker, H.A. (1981) Milk yield, feed intake, prolactin, growth hormone and glucocorticoid response of cows to supplemental light. *Journal of Dairy Science* 64, 1671–1678.

Peterson, A.D., Baile, C.A. and Baumgardt, B.R. (1972) Cerebral ventricle injections of pentobarbital, glucose and sodium chloride into sheep and calves, and feeding. *Journal of Dairy Science* 55, 822–828.

Petherick, J.C. and Rutter, S.M. (1990) Quantifying motivation using a computer-controlled push-door. *Applied Animal Behaviour Science* 27, 159–167.

Petherick, J.C. and Waddington, D. (1991) Can domestic fowl (*Gallus domesticus*) anticipate a period of food deprivation? *Applied Animal Behaviour Science* 32, 219–226.

Petherick, J.C., Beattie, A.W. and Bodero, D.A.V. (1989) The effect of group size on the performance of growing pigs. *Animal Production* 49, 497–502.

Petherick, J.C., Sutherland, R.H., Waddington, D. and Rutter, S.M. (1992) Measuring the motivation of domestic fowl in response to a positive and negative reinforcer. *Applied Animal Behaviour Science* 33, 357–366.

Pettyjohn, J.D., Everett, J.P. and Mochrie, R.D. (1963) Responses of dairy calves to milk replacer fed at various concentrations. *Journal of Dairy Science* 46, 710–714.

Pfister, J.A., Muller-Schwarze, D. and Balph, D.F. (1990) Effects of predator fecal odors on feed selection by sheep and cattle. *Journal of Chemical Ecology* 16, 323–329.

Phillip, L.E., Buchanan-Smith, J.G. and Grovum, W.L. (1981a) Effects of infusing the rumen with acetic acid and nitrogenous constituents in maize silage extracts on food intake, ruminal osmolality and blood acid–base balance in sheep. *Journal of Agricultural Science* 96, 429–438.

Phillip, L.E., Buchanan-Smith, J.G. and Grovum, W.L. (1981b) Food intake and ruminal osmolality in sheep: differentiation of the effect of osmolality from that of the products of maize silage fermentation. *Journal of Agricultural Science* 96, 439–445.

Phillips, C.J.C. and Schofield, S.A. (1989) The effect of supplementary lighting on the production and behaviour of dairy cows. *Animal Production* 48, 293–304.

Phipps, R.H., Bines, J.A. and Cooper, A. (1983) A preliminary study to compare individual feeding through Calan electronic feeding gates to group feeding. *Animal Production* 36, 544.

Phipps, R.H., Sutton, J.D., Jones, B.A., Allen, D. and Fisher, W.J. (1993) The effect of mixed forage diets on feed intake and milk production of dairy cows. *Animal Production* 56, 424A.

Pickard, D.W., Swan, H. and Lamming, G.E. (1969) Studies on the nutrition of ruminants. 4. The use of ground straw of different particle sizes for cattle from twelve weeks of age. *Animal Production* 11, 543–550.

Pickard, D.W., Hedley, W.G. and Skilbeck, S. (1977) Calcium appetite in growing pigs. *Proceedings of the Nutrition Society* 36, 87A.

Pickard, D.W., Beevors, J.A., Hughes, G. and Knibb, H.F. (1978) The voluntary intake of calcium by dairy cows at the end of pregnancy and its effect on plasma calcium at parturition. *Animal Production* 26, 365.

Pierce, A.W. (1962) Studies on salt tolerance of sheep. 4. The tolerance of sheep for mixtures of sodium chloride and calcium chloride in the drinking water. *Australian Journal of Agricultural Research* 13, 479–486.

Piggins, D. (1992) Visual perception. In: Phillips, C.J.C. and Piggins, D. (eds) *Farm Animals and the Environment*, CAB International, Wallingford, pp. 131–158.

Pilbrow, P.J. and Morris, T.R. (1974) Comparison of lysine requirements amongst eight stocks of laying fowl. *British Poultry Science* 15, 51–73.

Plegge, S.D., Godrich, R.D., Hanson, S.A. and Kirick, M.A. (1984) Predicting dry matter intake of feedlot cattle. *Proceedings of the Minnesota Nutrition Conference*, p. 56.

Plotka, E.D., Morley, J.E., Levine, A.S. and Seal, U.S. (1986) Effects of opiate antagonists on feeding and spontaneous locomotion in deer. *Physiology and Behavior* 35, 965–970.

Polin, D. and Wolford, J.H. (1973) Factors influencing food intake and calorific balance in chickens. *Federation Proceedings* 32, 1720–1726.

Polin, D. and Wolford, J.H. (1977) Role of estrogen as a cause of fatty liver syndrome. *Journal of Nutrition* 107, 873–886.

Poppi, D.P., Gill, M. and France, J. (1994) Quantification of theories of intake regulation in growing ruminants. *Journal of Theoretical Biology* 167, 129–145.

Powell, T.S., Douglas, C.R., Stonerock, R.H. and Harms, R.H. (1972) Feed intake of hens fed various levels of energy from feed and/or sucrose-water. *Poultry Science* 51, 1851.

Prasad, B.M., Horton, G.M.J. and Blethen, D.B. (1990) Effect of garlic (*Allium sativum*) on the voluntary feed consumption of horses, sheep and pigs. *Journal of Animal Science* 68, Suppl 1, 257.

Prescott, N.J., Waithes, C.M., Kirkwood, J.K. and Perry, G.C. (1985) Growth, food intake and development in broiler cockerels raised to maturity. *Animal Production* 41, 239–246.

Provenza, F.D., Pfister, J.A. and Cheney, C.D. (1992) Mechanisms of learning in diet selection with reference to phytotoxicosis in herbivores. *Journal of Range Management* 45, 36–45.

Provenza, F.D., Lynch, J.J. and Nolan, J.V. (1993) The relative importance of mother and toxicosis in the selection of foods by lambs. *Journal of Chemical Ecology* 19, 313–323.

Provenza, F.D., Lynch, J.J. and Cheney, C.D. (1994) An experimental analysis of the effects of a salient flavor and food deprivation on the response of sheep to novel foods. *Applied Animal Behavioural Science* Submitted.

Provenza, F.D., Lynch, J.J. and Nolan, J.V. (1994a) Food aversion conditioned in anaesthetized sheep. *Physiology and Behavior* 55, 429–432.

Provenza, F.D., Ortega-Reyes, C.B., Scott, C.B., Lynch, J.J. and Burritt, E.A. (1994b) Antiemetic drugs attenuate food aversions in sheep. *Journal of Animal Science* 72, 1989–1994.

Pulina, G., Rossi, G., Cannas, A., Brandano, P., Rassu, S.P.G. and Serra, A. (1992) The use of a pelleted feed as stimulator of chewing activity in dairy sheep.

Proceedings of the 43rd Annual Meeting of the European Association of Animal Production, Madrid, p. 376.

Purser, D.B. and Moir, R.J. (1966) Rumen volume as a factor involved in individual sheep differences. Journal of Animal Science 25, 509–515.

Putnam, P.A. and Bond, J. (1971) Drylot feeding patterns for the reproducing beef cow. Journal of Animal Science 33, 1086–1090.

Putnam, P.A., Lehmann, R. and Davis, R.E. (1965) Effect of electric lighting on drylot-feeding behavior of cattle. Proceedings of the Conference on Electromagnetic Radiation in Agriculture, pp. 16–19.

Pym, R.A.E. and Nichols, R.J. (1979) Selection for food conversion in broilers: direct and correlated responses to selection for body weight gain, food consumption, and food conversion ration. British Poultry Science 20, 73–86.

Ralphs, M.H. and Olsen, J.D. (1990) Adverse influence of social facilitation and learning context in training cattle to avoid eating larkspur. Journal of Animal Science 68, 1944–1952.

Ralston, S.L. and Baile, C.A. (1982) Gastrointestinal stimuli in the control of feed intake in ponies. Journal of Animal Science 55, 243–253.

Ramirez, I. (1992) Chemoreception for fat: do rats sense triglycerides directly? Appetite 18, 193–206.

Ramos, A. and Tennessen, T. (1992) Effect of previous grazing experience on the grazing behaviour of lambs. Applied Animal Behaviour Science 33, 43–52.

Ramos, A. and Tennessen, T. (1993) A note on the effect of dietary variety on food intake of cattle. Animal Production 57, 323–325.

Raun, A.P., Cooley, C.O., Potter, E.L., Rathmacher, R.P. and Richardson L.F. (1976) Effect of monensin on feed efficiency of feedlot cattle. Journal of Animal Science 43, 670–677.

Rawson, R.O. and Quick, K.P. (1971) Unilateral splanchnotomy: its effect on the response to intra-abdominal heating in the ewe. Pflugers Archiv. 330, 362–365.

Rayburn, E.B.(1986) Quantitative aspects of pasture management. Seneca Trail RC&D Technical Manual, Seneca Trail RC&D, Franklinville, New York.

Raymond, F., Redman, P. and Waltham, R. (1986) Forage Conservation and Feeding. Farming Press, Ipswich, 188pp.

Rayner, D.V. (1992) Gastrointestinal satiety in animals other than man. Proceedings of the Nutrition Society 51, 1–6.

Rayner, D.V. and Gregory, P.C. (1985) Gastrointestinal influences on short-term regulation of food intake in pigs. Proceedings of the Nutrition Society 44, 56.

Rayner, D.V. and Gregory, P.C. (1989) The role of the gastrointestinal tract in the control of voluntary food intake. In: Forbes, J.M., Varley, M.A. and Lawrence, T.L.J. (eds) The Voluntary Food Intake of Pigs. Occasional Publication of the British Society of Animal Production, Edinburgh, BSAP, pp. 27–39.

Rayner, D.V., Miller, S. and Lopez, S. (1991) MK-329, L-365,260 and the inhibition of food intake, gastric emptying, volume and pressure to duodenal emulsified fat infusion in the pig. Regulatory Peptides 35, 255.

Read, N.W. (1992) Gastrointestinal satiety in man. Proceedings of the Nutrition Society, 51, 7–11.

Reed, D.R., Friedman, M.I. and Tordoff, M.G. (1992) Experience with a macronutrient source influences subsequent macronutrient selection. *Appetite* 18, 223–232.

Reid, C.S.W. (1963) Diet and the motility of the forestomachs of the sheep. *Proceedings of the New Zealand Society of Animal Production* 23, 169–188.

Reid, G.W., Greenhalgh, J.F.D. and Aitken, J.N. (1972) The effects of grazing intensity on herbage consumption and animal production. IV. An evaluation of two methods of avoiding the rejection of fouled herbage by dairy cows. *Journal of Agricultural Science* 78, 491–496.

Reid, R.L. aand Hinks, N.J. (1962) Studies on the carbohydrate metabolism of sheep. 17. Feed requirements and voluntary feed intake in late pregnancy, with particular reference to prevention of hypoglycaemia and hyperketonaemia. *Australian Journal of Agricultural Research* 13, 1092–1111.

Reid, R.L., Hinks, N.T. and Mills, S.C. (1963) Alloxan diabetes in pregnant ewes. *Journal of Endocrinology* 27, 1–19.

Reiner, R.J., Bryant, F.C., Farfan, R.D. and Craddock, B.F. (1987) Forage intake of alpacas grazing Andean rangeland in Peru. *Journal of Animal Science* 4, 868–871.

Renner, R. and Hill, F.W. (1961) Utilization of fatty acids by the chicken. *Journal of Nutrition* 74, 259–264.

Rezek, M., Schneider, K. and Novin, D. (1975) Regulation of food intake following vagotomy, coeliectomy and a combination of both procedures. *Physiology and Behavior* 15, 517–522.

Rice, R.W., Morris, J.G., Maeda, B.T. and Baldwin, R.L. (1974) Simulation of animal functions in models of production systems: ruminants on the range. *Federation Proceedings* 33, 188–195.

Richard, P. (1967) *Atlas Stereotaxique du Cerveau de Brebis.* INRA, Paris, 76pp.

Richardson, A.J. (1970a) Blood glucose levels and food intake in the domestic chicken. *British Poultry Science* 11, 501–504.

Richardson, A.J. (1970b) The role of the crop in the feeding behaviour of the domestic chicken. *Animal Behaviour* 18, 633–639.

Richardson, A.J. (1972) The effect of duodenal constriction on food and water intake of the Brown Leghorn cockerel. *British Poultry Science* 13, 175–177.

Richter, C.P. and Eckert, J.F. (1937) Mineral appetite of parathyroidectomised rats. *Endocrinology* 21, 50–54.

Ricks, C.A., Dalrymple, R.H., Baker, P.K. and Ingle, D.L. (1984) Use of a β-agonist to alter fat and muscle deposition in steers. *Journal of Animal Science* 59, 1247–1255.

Rijpkema, Y.S., van Reeuwijk, L., Peel, C.J. and Mol, E.P. (1987) Responses of dairy cows to long-term treatment with somatotropin in a prolonged release formulation. *Proceedings of the 38th Annual Meeting of the European Association of Animal Production*, Lisbon.

Riley, J.E. (1989) Recent trends in pig production: the importance of intake. In: Forbes, J.M., Varley, M.A. and Lawrence, T.L.J. (eds) *The Voluntary Intake of Pigs*. Occasional Publication of the British Society of Animal Production, No. 13, 1–5.

Rinaldo, D. and Le Dividich, J. (1991) Assessment of optimal temperature for performance and chemical body composition. *Livestock Production Science* 29, 61–75.

Rinaldo, D., Salaun, M.C. and Le Dividich, J. (1989) [Effect of a reduction in environmental temperature or a nighttime decrease in ambient temperature on the performance of weaned pigs.] *Journées Recherche Porcine en France* 21, 239–244.

Ritter, R.C. and Edwards, G.I. (1986) Dorsomedial hindbrain participation in control of food intake. In: Ritter, R.C., Ritter, S. and Barnes, C.D. (eds) *Feeding Behavior – Neural and Humoral Controls*. Academic Press, New York, pp. 131–161.

Ritter, S. (1986) Glucoprivation and the glucoprivic control of food intake. In: Ritter, R.C., Ritter, S. and Barnes, C.D. (eds) *Feeding Behavior – Neural and Humoral Controls*, New York, Academic Press, pp. 271–313.

Riviere, P. and Bueno, L. (1987) Influence of regimen and insulaemia on orexigenic effects of GRF 1-44 in sheep. *Physiology and Behavior* 39, 347–350.

Robert, S., Matte, J.J. and Girard, C.L. (1991) Effect of feeding regimen on behaviour of growing-finishing pigs supplemented or not supplemented with folic acid. *Journal of Animal Science* 69, 4428–4436.

Robert, S., Matte, J.J., Farmer, C., Girard, C.L. and Martineau, G.P. (1993) High-fibre diets for sows: effects on stereotypies and adjunctive drinking. *Applied Animal Behaviour Science* 37, 297–309.

Roberts, R.E. (1934) Methods of feeding ducks. *Poultry Science* 13, 338–342.

Robinson, D. (1985) Performance of laying hens as affected by split time and split composition dietary regimens using ground and unground cereals. *British Poultry Science* 26, 299–399.

Robinson, D.W. (1974) Food intake regulation in pigs. 3. Voluntary food selection between protein-free and protein-rich diets. *British Veterinary Journal* 130, 522–527.

Robinson, D.W. (1975a) Food intake regulation in pigs. 5. The influence of dietary amino acid pattern on free choice food selection. *British Veterinary Journal* 131, 707–715.

Robinson, D.W. (1975b) Food intake regulation in pigs. 4. The influence of dietary threonine imbalance on food intake, dietary choice and plasma amino acid patterns. *British Veterinary Journal* 131, 595–600.

Robinson, D.W., Holmes, J.H.G. and Bayley, H.S. (1974) Food intake regulation in pigs. 1. The relationship between dietary protein concentration, food intake and plasma amino acids. *British Veterinary Journal* 130, 361–365.

Robinzon, B. and Snapir, N. (1983) Intraventricular glucose administration inhibits feeding in satiated but not in 24 hours food deprived cocks. *Pharmacology, Biochemistry and Behavior* 19, 929–932.

Robinzon, B., Snapir, N. and Perek, N. (1977) Removal of olfactory bulbs in chickens: consequent changes in food intake and thyroid activity. *Brain Research Bulletin* 2, 263–272.

Robinzon, B., Snapir, N. and Perek, M. (1978) Hyperphagia without obesity in septal lesioned cocks. *Physiology and Behavior* 20, 1–6.

Robinzon, B., Snapir, N. and Lepkovsky, S. (1982) Hypothalamic hyperphagia, obesity and gonadal disfunction. Absence of consistent relationship between lesion site and physiological consequences. In: Scanes, C.G., Ottinger, M.A., Kenny, A.D., Balthazer, J., Crowther, J. and Chester-Jones,

I. (eds) *Aspects of Avian Endocrinology: Practical and Theoretical Implications*, Texas Tech University Press, Lubbock Texas, pp. 201–210.

Roe, R. and Mottershead, B.E. (1962) Palatability of *Phalaris arundinacea,*L. *Nature* 193, 255–256.

Roffler, R.E. and Thacker, D.L. (1983) Influence of reducing dietary crude protein from 17 to 13.5 percent on early lactation. *Journal of Dairy Science* 66, 51–58.

Rogers, L.J. (1986) Organisation of brain and behaviour in the chicken, the influence of nutrition on it and its effects on learning and feeding. *Poultry Husbandry Research Foundation Symposium Proceedings*, University of Sydney, pp. 64–73.

Rogers, L.J. (1989) Some factors determining the food intake of young chicks. *Recent Advances in Animal Nutrition in Australia* 322–342.

Rogers, Q.R. and Egan, A.R. (1975) Amino acid imbalance in the milk-fed lamb. *Australian Journal of Agricultural Science* 28, 169–182.

Rogers, Q.R. and Leung, P.M.B. (1973) The influence of amino acids on the neuroregulation of food intake. *Federation Proceedings* 32, 1709–1718.

Rogerson, A., Ledger, H.P. and Freeman, G.H. (1968) Food intake and live-weight gain comparisons of *Bos indicus* and *Bos taurus* steers on a high plane of nutrition. *Animal Production* 10, 373–380.

Rolls, B.J. (1986) Sensory-specific satiety. *Nutrition Reviews* 44, 93–101.

Rolls, B.J. and Rolls, E.T. (1982) *Thirst*. Cambridge University Press, Cambridge, 194pp.

Ronning, M. and Laben, R.C. (1966) Response of lactating cows to free-choice feeding of milled diets containing from 10 to 100% concentrates. *Journal of Dairy Science*, 49, 1080–1085.

Rook, A.J. and Gill, M. (1990) Prediction of the voluntary intake of grass silages by beef cattle. 1. Linear regression analysis. *Animal Production* 50, 425–438.

Rook, A.J., Dhanoa, M.S. and Gill, M. (1990a) Prediction of the voluntary intake of grass silages by beef cattle. 2. Principal component and ridge regression analysis. *Animal Production* 50, 439–454.

Rook, A.J., Dhanoa, M.S. and Gill, M. (1990b) Prediction of the voluntary intake of grass silages by beef cattle. 3. Precision of alternative prediction models. *Animal Production* 50, 455–466.

Rook, A.J., Gill, M., Wilkins, R.D. and Lister, S.J. (1991) Prediction of voluntary intake of grass silages by lactating cows offered concentrates at a flat rate. *Animal Production* 52, 407–420.

Rook, J.A.F. and Thomas, P.C. (eds) (1983) *Nutritional Physiology of Farm Animals*. Longman, London, 704pp.

Rook, J.A.F., Balch, C.C. and Johnson, V.W. (1965) Further observations on the effects of intraruminal infusions of volatile fatty acids and of lactic acid on the yield and composition of milk of the cow. *British Journal of Nutrition* 19, 93–99.

Rose, S.P. and Abbas, G. (1993) Diet selection of cockerels and the feeding value of wheat. *Animal Production* 56, 469.

Rose, S.P. and Kyriazakis, I. (1991) Diet selection of pigs and poultry. *Proceedings of the Nutrition Society* 50, 87–98.

Rose, S.P. and Lambie, I.T.M. (1986) Comparison of a choice-feeding regimen for broilers under continuous and intermittent lighting programmes. *Proceedings of the 7th European Poultry Conference*, Paris, Tours, France, World's Poultry Science Association, pp. 903–906.

Rose, S.P. and Michie, W. (1986) Effect of temperature and diet during rearing of layer strain pullets. In: Fischer, C. and Boorman, K.N. (eds) *Nutrient Requirements of Poultry and Poultry Research*. Butterworths, London, pp. 214–216.

Rose, S.P. and Njeru, F.N. (1989) Effect of enzyme supplementation of cereals on the diet selection of choice-fed broilers. *British Poultry Science* 27, 975–976.

Rose, S.P., Burnett, A. and Elmajeed, R.A. (1986) Factors affecting the diet selection of choice-fed broilers. *British Poultry Science* 27, 215–224.

Rose, S.P., Fielden, M. and Gardin, P. (1993) Sequential feeding of whole grain wheat to broiler chickens. *Animal Production* 56, 435.

Ross, P.A. and Hurnik, J.F. (1983) Drinking behaviour of broiler chickens. *Applied Animal Ethology* 11, 25–31.

Rovee-Collier, C.K., Clapp, B.A. and Collier, G.H. (1982) The economics of food choice in chicks. *Physiology and Behavior* 28, 1097–1102.

Roy, J.H.B. (1980) *The Calf*, 4th edn. Butterworths, London, 442pp.

Rugg, W.C. (1925) Feeding experiments, free choice of feeds. *Victoria, Australia, Department of Agriculture Bulletin* 54, 36–56.

Rusby, A.A. and Forbes, J.M. (1985) The effect of portal vein infusion of 2-deoxy-glucose and 3-methyl-glucose on the food intake of cockerels. *Proceedings of the Nutrition Society* 44, 59A.

Rusby, A.A. and Forbes, J.M. (1987) Effects of infusions of lysine, leucine and ammonium chloride into the hepatic portal vein of chickens on voluntary food intake. *British Journal of Nutrition* 58, 325–331.

Rusby, A.A., Anil, M.H., Chatterjee, P. and Forbes, J.M. (1987) The effects of intraportal infusion of glucose and lysine on the food intake of intact and hepatic vagotomised chickens. *Appetite* 9, 65–72.

Rushen, J., De Passille, A.M.B. and Schouten, W. (1990) Stereotypic behavior, endogenous opioids, and postfeeding hypoalgesia in pigs. *Physiology and Behavior* 48, 91–96.

Russek, M. (1963) Participation of hepatic glucoreceptors in the control of food intake. *Nature* 197, 79–80.

Russek, M. (1976) A 'conceptual' equation of intake control. In: Novin, D., Wyrwicka, W. and Bray, G. (eds) *Hunger: Basic Mechanisms and Clinical Implications*. Raven Press, New York, pp. 128–147.

Russek, M. (1981) Reply to commentary on 'Current status of the hepatostatic theory of food intake control'. *Appetite* 2, 157–162.

Rutter, S.M., Jackson, D.A., Johnson, C.L. and Forbes, J.M. (1987) Automatically recorded competitive feeding behaviour as a measure of social dominance in dairy cows. *Applied Animal Ethology* 17, 41–50.

Saghier, O.A.S. and Campling, R.C. (1991) Energy and protein supplements to straw-based diets for yearling cattle: effects on straw intake and digestibility. *Animal Production* 52, 83–92.

Salmon-Legagneur, E. and Rerat, A. (1962) Nutrition of sows during pregnancy. In: Morgan, J.J. and Lewis, D. (eds) *Nutrition of Pigs and Poultry*. Butterworths, London, pp. 207–223.

Sanderson, R., Thomas, C. and McAllan, A.B. (1992) Fish-meal supplementation of grass silage given to young growing steers: effect on intake, apparent digestibility and live-weight gains. *Animal Production* 55, 389–396.

Savory, C.J. (1975) Effects of group size on the feeding behaviour and growth of chicks. *British Poultry Science* 16, 343–350.

Savory, C.J. (1976) Effects of different lighting regimes on diurnal feeding patterns of the domestic fowl. *British Poultry Science* 17, 341–350.

Savory, C.J. (1977) Effects of egg production on the patterns of food intake of broiler hens kept in continuous light. *British Poultry Science* 18, 331–337.

Savory, C.J. (1979) Feeding behaviour. In: Boorman, K.N. and Freeman, B.M. (eds) *Food Intake Regulation in Poultry.* Longman, Edinburgh, pp. 277–323.

Savory, C.J. (1984) Regulation of food intake by brown leghorn cockerels in response to dietary dilution with kaolin. *British Poultry Science* 25, 253–258.

Savory, C.J. (1985) An investigation into the role of the crop in control of feeding in Japanese quail and domestic fowls. *Physiology and Behavior* 35, 917–928.

Savory, C.J. (1987) An alternative explanation for apparent satiating properties of peripherally administered bombesin and cholecystokinin in domestic fowl. *Physiology and Behavior* 39, 191–202.

Savory, C.J. (1988) Rate of eating by domestic fowls in relation to changing food deficits. *Appetite* 10, 57–65.

Savory, C.J. (1989) Responses of fowls to an operant feeding procedure and its potential use for reducing randomness in meal occurrence. *Physiology and Behavior* 45, 373–379.

Savory, C.J. and Fisher, R.D.A. (1992) Influence of a period of 'freeze-feeding' on behaviour of growing layer pullets. *Applied Animal Behaviour Science* 35, 55–66.

Savory, C.J. and Gentle, M.J. (1980) Intravenous injections of cholecystokinin and cerulin suppress food intake in domestic fowl. *Experientia* 36, 1191–1192.

Savory, C.J. and Gentle, M.J. (1983) Brain cholecystokinin and satiety in fowls. *Appetite* 4, 223.

Savory, C.J. and Gentle, M.J. (1984) Effects of food deprivation, strain, diet and age on feeding responses to intravenous injections of cholecystokinin. *Appetite* 4, 165–177.

Savory, C.J. and Hodgkiss, J.P. (1984) Influence of vagotomy in domestic fowls on feeding activity, food passage, and satiety effects of two peptides. *Physiology and Behavior* 33, 937–944.

Savory, C.J. and Smith, C.J.V. (1987) Are there hunger and satiety factors in the blood of domestic fowls? *Appetite* 8, 101–110.

Savory, C.J., Wood-Gush, D.G.M. and Duncan, I.J.H. (1978) Feeding behaviour in a population of domestic fowls in the wild. *Applied Animal Ethology* 4, 13–27.

Savory, C.J., Duke, G.E. and Bertoy, R.W. (1981) Influence of intravenous injections of cholecystokinin on gastrointestinal motility in turkeys and domestic fowls. *Comparative Biochemistry and Physiology* 70A, 179–189.

Savory, C.J., Gentle, M.J. and Yeomans, M.R. (1989) Opioid modulation of feeding and drinking in fowls. *British Poultry Science* 30, 379–392.

Savory, C.J., Maros, K. and Rutter, S.M. (1993) Assessment of hunger in growing broiler breeders in relation to a commercial restricted feeding programme. *Animal Welfare* 2, 131–152.

Scallett, A.C., Della-Fera, M.A. and Baile, C.A. (1985) Satiety, hunger and regional brain content of cholecystokinin and met-enkephalin in sheep. *Peptides* 6, 937.

Schanbacher, B.D. and Crouse, J.D. (1980) Growth and performance of growing-finishing lambs exposed to long and short photoperiods. *Journal of Animal Science* 51, 943–948.

Schanbacher, B.D. and Crouse, J.D. (1981) Photoperiodic regulation of growth. A photosensitive phase during the light dark cycle. *American Journal of Physiology* 241, E1–E5.

Scharrer, E. and Langhans, W. (1986) Control of food intake by fatty acid oxidation. *American Journal of Physiology* 250, R1003–R1006.

Scharrer, E. and Langhans, W. (1990) Mechanisms for the effect of body fat on food intake. In: Forbes, J.M. and Hervey, G.R. (eds) *The Control of Body Fat Content.* Smith-Gordon, London, pp. 63–86.

Schelling, G.T. and Hatfield, E.E. (1968) Effect of abomasally infused nitrogen sources on nitrogen retention of growing lambs. *Journal of Nutrition* 96, 319–326.

Schmitt, M. (1973) Influences of hepatic portal receptors on hypothalamic feeding and satiety centres. *American Journal of Physiology* 225, 1089–1095.

Schutze, J.V., Jensen, L.S., Carver, J S. and Matson, W.E. (1960) Influence of various lighting regimes on the performance of growing chickens. *Washington Agricultural Experimental Station Bulletin* 36.

Scott, T.A. and Balnave, D. (1989) Responses of sexually-maturing pullets to self-selection feeding under different temperature and lighting regimes. *British Poultry Science* 30, 135–150.

Scott, T.R. (1992) Taste, the neural basis of body wisdom. In: Simopoulos, A.P. (ed.) *Nutritional Triggers for Health and Disease.* World Reviews of Nutrition and Dietetics, Basel, Karger, pp. 67.

Scottish Agricultural College (SAC) (1992) *Langhill 92.* SAC, Edinburgh, 89pp.

Seebeck, R.M., Springell, P.H. and O'Kelly, J.C. (1971) Alterations in host metabolism by the specific and anorectic effects of the cattle tick (*Boophilus microplus*). 1. Food intake and body weight growth. *Australian Journal of Biological Science* 24, 373–380.

Seidenglanz, J., Golder, J. and Sramek, J. (1974) The effect of the physical form of concentrate feeds on the rate of their intake my milch-cows. *Zivocisna Vyroba (Praha)* 19, 243–251.

Seigel, P.B., Cherry, J.A. and Dunnington, E.A. (1984) Feeding behaviour and feed consumption in chickens selected for body weight. *Annales Agriculturae Fenniae* 23, 247–252.

Seoane, J.R. (1982) Relationships between the physico-chemical characteristics of hays and their nutritive value. *Journal of Animal Science* 55, 422–431.

Seoane, J.R. and Baile, C.A. (1972a) Effects of intraventricular (III ventricle) injections of 2-deoxy-d-glucose, glucose and xylose on feeding behavior of sheep. *Physiology and Behavior* 9, 423–428.

Seoane, J.R. and Baile, C.A. (1972b) Ionic changes in cerebrospinal fluid and feeding, drinking and temperature of sheep. *Physiology and Behavior* 10, 915–923.

Seoane, J.R. and Baile, C.A. (1973) Feeding elicited by injections of $Ca^{2+}$ and $Mg^{2+}$ into the third ventricle of sheep. *Experientia* 29, 61–62.

Seoane, J.R., Baile, C.A. and Martin, H.F. (1972a) Humoral factors modifying feeding behavior of sheep. *Physiology and Behavior* 8, 993–995.

Seoane, J.R., Warner, R.G. and Seoane, N.A. (1972b) Heparin-induced lipolysis and feeding behavior in sheep. *Physiology and Behavior* 9, 419–422.

Seoane, J.R., McLaughlin, C.L. and Baile, C.A. (1975) Feeding following intra-hypothalamic injections of calcium and magnesium ions in sheep. *Journal of Dairy Science* 58, 349–361.

Seoane, J.R., Bedard, L. and Caron, N. (1988) Comparison between pentobarbital- and muscimol-induced feeding in satiated sheep. *Canadian Journal of Physiology and Pharmacology* 66, 703–706.

Shaobi, T.S. and Forbes, J.M. (1985) Do chickens consider a glucose solution to be food or water? *Proceedings of the Nutrition Society* 44, 57A.

Shaobi, T.S. and Forbes, J.M. (1987) Feeding responses to infusions of glucose solutions into the duodenum of chickens, and the influences of pre-fasting or vagotomy. *British Poultry Science* 28, 407–413.

Share, I., Martyniuk, E. and Grossman, M.I. (1952) Effect of prolonged intra-gastric feeding on oral food intake in dogs. *American Journal of Physiology* 169, 229–235.

Shariatmadari, F. and Forbes, J.M. (1990a) Growth and food intake responses of broiler and layer chickens to diets of different protein contents, and a choice of protein content. *Proceedings of the Nutrition Society* 49, 217A.

Shariatmadari, F. and Forbes, J.M. (1990b) The influences of meal composition on subsequent food selection in broiler and layer chickens. *Proceedings of the Nutrition Society* 49, 219A.

Shariatmadari, F. and Forbes, J.M. (1991) A comparison of a split diet system and choice feeding on food intake and growth of broilers. *Proceedings of the Nutrition Society* 50, 96A.

Shariatmadari, F. and Forbes, J.M. (1992a) Diurnal food intake patterns of broiler chickens offered a choice of feed varying in protein content. *Animal Production* 54, 470A.

Shariatmadari, F. and Forbes, J.M. (1992b) The effect of force-feeding various levels of protein on diet selection and growth of broiler chickens. *Proceedings of the Nutrition Society* 51, 56A.

Shariatmadari, F. and Forbes, J.M. (1993) Growth and food intake responses to diets of different protein contents and a choice between diets containing two levels of protein in broiler and layer strains of chicken. *British Poultry Science* 34, 959–970.

Sherrit, G.W., Graves, H.B., Gobble, J.L. and Hazlett, V.E. (1974) Effects of mixing pigs during the growing-finishing period. *Journal of Animal Science* 39, 834–837.

Sherwin, C.M., Alvey, D.M. and Williamson, J.D. (1993) Effects of cage-front design on the feeding behaviour of laying hens. *Applied Animal Behaviour Science* 38, 291–299.

*References*

Sherwood, D.H., Caskey, C.D., Krautmann, B.A., Van Wormer, M.C., Smith, S.B. and Ward, R.F. (1964) Management and feeding of meat-type broiler chicks. *Poultry Science* 43, 1272–1278.

Shimizu, N., Oomura, Y., Novin, D., Grijalva, C.V. and Cooper, P.H. (1983) Functional correlations between lateral hypothalamic glucose-sensitive neurons and hepatic portal glucose-sensitive units in rat. *Brain Research* 265, 49–54.

Shurlock, T.G.H. and Forbes, J.M. (1981a) Factors affecting food intake in the domestic chicken: the effect of infusions of nutritive and non-nutritive substances into the crop and duodenum. *British Poultry Science* 22, 323–331.

Shurlock, T.G.H. and Forbes, J.M. (1981b) Evidence for hepatic glucostatic regulation of food intake in the domestic chicken and its interaction with gastrointestinal control. *British Poultry Science* 22, 333–346.

Shurlock, T.G.H. and Forbes, J.M. (1984) Effects on voluntary intake of infusions of glucose and amino acids into the hepatic portal vein of chickens. *British Poultry Science* 25, 303–308.

Sibbald, A.R., Maxwell, T.J. and Eadie, J. (1979) A conceptual approach to the modelling of herbage intake by hill sheep. *Agricultural Systems* 4, 119–134.

Siebrits, F.K. and Kemm, E.H. (1982) Body composition and energetic efficiency of lean and obese pigs. *Proceedings of the European Association of Animal Production.* Lillehammer, Norway, p. 237.

Silankove, N. (1987) Impact of shelter in hot Mediterranean climate on feed intake, feed utilization and body fluid distribution in sheep. *Appetite* 9, 207–215.

Silankove, N. (1989) Interrelationship between water, food and digestible energy intake in desert and temperate goats. *Appetite* 12, 163–170.

Silankove, N. and Gutman, M. (1992) Interrelationships between lack of shading, shelter and poultry litter supplementation: food intake, live weight, water metabolism and embryo loss in beef cows grazing dry Mediterranean pasture. *Animal Production* 55, 371–376.

Silverman, H.J. and Zucker, I. (1976) Absence of post-fast food compensation in the golden hamster (*Mesocricetus auratus*). *Physiology and Behavior* 17, 271–283.

Simkins, K.L., Suttie, J.M. and Baumgardt, B.R. (1965) Regulation of food intake by ruminants. 4. Effect of acetate, propionate, butyrate and glucose on voluntary food intake in dairy cattle. *Journal of Dairy Science* 48, 1635–1642.

Simm, G., Persaud, P., Neilson, D.R., Parkinson, H. and McGuirk, B.J. (1991) Predicting food intake in dairy heifers from early lactation records. *Animal Production* 52, 421–434.

Simpson, A.D.F. and Raine, H. (1981) The prediction of feed intake – the primary step in the modelling of broiler growth. *Computers in Animal Production.* British Society of Animal Production Occasional Publication No. 5, pp. 152–153.

Simpson, C.W., Baile, C.A. and Krabill, L.F. (1975) Neurochemical coding for feeding in sheep and steers. *Journal of Comparative and Physiological Psychology* 88, 176–182.

Simpson, S.J., James, S., Simmonds, M.S.J. and Blaney, W.M. (1991) Variation in chemosensitivity and the control of dietary selection behaviour in the locust. *Appetite* 17, 141–154.

Sinurat, A.P. and Balnave, D. (1986) Free-choice feeding of broilers at high temperature. *British Poultry Science* 29, 577–584.

Smith, A.J. (1972) Some nutritional problems associated with egg production at high environmental temperatures. 3. The effect of environmental temperature on water intake and calcium utilisation by pullets and on certain aspects of carcass composition. *Rhodesian Journal of Agricultural Research* 10, 31–40.

Smith, C.J.V. (1969) Alterations in the food intake of chickens as a result of hypothalamic lesions. *Poultry Science* 48, 475–477.

Smith, C.J.V. and Baranowski-Kish, L.L. (1976) The response of chickens to D-mannoheptulose: feeding behavior and blood glucose. *Poultry Science* 55, 444–447.

Smith, C.J.V. and Baranowski-Kish, L.L. (1979) Mechanisms of regulation of energy intake in poultry. In: Boorman, K.N. and Freeman, B.M. (eds) *Food Intake Regulation in Poultry*. Longman, Edinburgh, pp. 63–76.

Smith, C.J.V. and Bright-Taylor, B. (1974) Does a glucostatic mechanism for feed intake control exist in chickens? *Poultry Science* 53, 1720–1724.

Smith, C.J.V. and Pilz, D.R. (1970) Feeding behaviour of chickens: effects of cropectomy. *Poultry Science* 49, 226.

Smith, C.J.V. and Szper, I. (1976) The influence of direct implantation of gold thioglucose into the brain of chickens on food consumption and weight gain. *Poultry Science* 55, 2421–2423.

Smith, C.J.V., Hatfield, J., Fowler, S. and Bright-Taylor, B. (1975) Changes in food consumption and blood glucose levels in the domestic chicken, *Gallus domesticus* in response to the administration of 2 deoxy-glucose. *Comparative Biochemistry and Physiology* 51, 811–814.

Smith, E.J. and Clapperton, J.L. (1981) The voluntary food intake fo sheep when silage juice is infused into the rumen. *Proceedings of the Nutrition Society* 40, 22A.

Smith, G.P., Jerome, C., Cushing, B.J., Eterno, R. and Simansky, K.J. (1981) Abdominal vagotomy blocks the satiety effect of cholecystokinin in the rat. *Science* 213, 1036–1037.

Smith, W.C., Ellis, M., Chadwick, J.P. and Laird, R. (1991) The influence of index selection for improved growth and carcass characteristics on appetite in a population of large white pigs. *Animal Production* 52, 193–199.

Snapir, N. and Robinzon, B. (1989) Role of the basomedial hypothalamus in regulation of adiposity, food intake and reproductive traits in the domestic fowl. *Poultry Science* 68, 948–957.

Snapir, N., Ravona, H. and Perek, M. (1973a) Effect of electrolytic lesions in various regions of the basal hypothalamus in White Leghorn cockerels upon food intake, blood plasma triglycerides and proteins. *Poultry Science* 52, 629–636.

Snapir, N., Robinzon, B., Godschalk, M., Heller, E.D. and Perek, M. (1973b) The effect of intrahypothalamic administration of sodium pentobarbital on eating behavior and feed intake in chickens. *Physiology and Behavior* 10, 97–100.

Snapir, N., Yaakobi, M., Robinzon, B., Ravona, H. and Perek, M. (1976) Involvement of the medial hypothalamus and the septal area in the control of food intake and body weight in geese. *Pharmacology, Biochemistry and Behavior* 5, 609–615.

Sonoda, T., Kisanuki, K., Fujimoto, Y. and Yoshioka, Z. (1974) *Bulletin of the Faculty of Agriculture, Miyazaki University* 21, 389–392.

Spahlinger, D.E. and Hobbs, N.T. (1992) Mechanisms of foraging in mammalian herbivores: new models of functional response. *American Naturalist* 140, 325–348.

Sparkes, G.H., Cole, D.J.A. and Lewis, D. (1981) The effect of dietary protein level on voluntary food intake in the pig. *Animal Production* 32, 356–357.

Spurlock, G.M. and Clegg, M.T. (1962) Effect of cortisone acetate on carcass composition and wool characteristics of weaned lambs. *Journal of Animal Science* 21, 494–500.

Squires, V.R. (1981) *Livestock Management in the Arid Zone.* Inkata Press, Melbourne.

Squires, V.R. and Wilson, A.D. (1971) Distance between food and water supply and its effect on drinking frequency, and food and water intake of Merino and Border Leicester sheep. *Australian Journal of Agricultural Research* 22, 283–290.

Standing Committee on Agriculture; Ruminant Subcommittee (1990) Prediction of feed intake. *Feeding Standards for Australian Livesotck. Ruminants,* Chapter 6, CSIRO, pp. 209–224.

Stansbury, W.F., McGlone, J.J. and Tribble, L.F. (1987) Effects of season, floor type, air temperature and snout odours on sow and litter performance. *Journal of Animal Science* 65, 1507–1513.

Stedman, J.A. and Hill, R. (1987) Voluntary food intake in a limited time of lambs and calves given diets containing rapeseed meal from different types and varieties of rape, and rapeseed meal treated to reduce the glucosinolate concentration. *Animal Production* 44, 75–82.

Steen, R.W.J. (1991) The effect of level of protein supplementation on the performance and carcass composition of young bulls given grass silage ad libitum. *Animal Production* 52, 465–476.

Steen, R.W.J. (1992) A comparison of soya-bean meal, fish meal and maize gluten feed as protein sources for calves offered grass silage ad libitum. *Animal Production* 54, 333–339.

Steffens, A.B., Van der Gugten, J., Godeke, J., Luiten, P.G.M. and Strubbe, J.H. (1986) Meal-induced increases in parasympathetic and sympathetic activity elicit simultaneous rises in plasma insulin and free fatty acids. *Physiology and Behavior* 37, 119–122.

Steinacker, G., Devlin, T.J. and Ingalls, J.R. (1970) Effect of methionine supplementation posterior to the rumen on nitrogen utilisation and sulphur balance of steers on a high roughage ration. *Canaadian Journal of Animal Science* 50, 319–324.

Steinruck, U. and Kirchgessner, M. (1992) [Regulation of protein intake of hens with high laying performance by self-selecting diets with different protein levels.] *Archivs fur Geflugelkunde* 56, 163–171.

Steinruck, U., Kirchgessner, M. and Roth, F.X. (1990a) [Selective methionine intake of broilers by changing the position of the diets.] *Archivs fur Geflugelkunde* 54: 245–250.

Steinruck, U., Roth, F.X. and Kirchgessner, M. (1990b) [Selective feed intake of broilers during methionine deficiency.] *Archivs fur Geflugelkunde* 54: 173–183.

Steinruck, U., Roth, F.X. and Kirchgessner, M. (1991) [Selective vitamin B6 intake of broilers.] *Journal of Animal Physiology and Animal Nutrition,* 65: 110–119.

Stephens, D.B. (1980) The effects of alimentary infusions of glucose, amino acids, or neutral fat on meal size in hungry pigs. *Journal of Physiology* 299, 453–463.

Stephens, D.B. (1985) Influence of intraduodenal glucose on meal size and its modification by 2-deoxy-d-glucose or vagotomy in hungry pigs. *Quarterly Journal of Experimental Physiology* 70, 129–135.

Stephens, D.B. and Baldwin, B.A. (1974) The lack of effect of intrajugular or intraportal injections of glucose or amino-acids on food intake of pigs. *Physiology and Behavior* 12, 923–929.

Stephens, D.B., Ingram, D.L. and Sharman, D.F. (1983) An investigation into some cerebral mechanisms involved in schedule-induced drinking in the pig. *Quarterly Journal of Experimental Physiology* 68, 653–660.

Stephens, D.W. and Krebs, J.R. (1986) *Foraging Theory.* Princeton University Press, Princeton, 247pp.

Stevenson, J.S., Pollman, D.S., Davis, D.L. and Murphy, J.P. (1983) Influence of supplemental light on sow performance during and after lactation. *Journal of Animal Science* 56, 1282–1286.

Stewart, A.H., Edwards, S.A., Brouns, F. and English, P.R. (1993) An assessmsent of the effect of feeding system on the production and social organisation of group housed gilts. *Animal Production* 56, 422.

Stobbs, T.H. (1973) The effect of plant structure on the intake of tropical pastures. 1. Variation in the bite size of grazing cattle. *Australian Journal of Agricultural Research* 24, 809–819.

Stock, M.J. and Rothwell, N.J. (1982) Evidence for diet-induced thermogenesis in hyperphagic cafeteria-fed rats. *Proceedings of the Nutrition Society* 41, 133–135.

Stolba, A. and Wood-Gush, D.G.M. (1989) The behaviour of pigs in a semi-natural environment. *Animal Production* 48, 419–426.

Stolz, S.B. and Lott, D.F. (1964) Establishment in rats of a persistent response producing a net loss of reinforcement. *Journal of Comparative and Physiological Psychology* 57, 147–153.

Stone, C.C., Brown, M.S. and Waring, G.H. (1974) An ethological means to improve swine production. *Journal of Animal Science* 39, 137.

Stone, R.L. (1975) The requirements for metabolizable energy and nitrogen for maintenance in parenterally fed sheep. PhD thesis, Ohio State University, Columbus.

Stricker, E.M. and McCann, M.J. (1985) Visceral factors in the control of food intake. *Brain Research Bulletin* 14, 687–692.

Stricker, E.M., Rowland, N., Saller, C.F. and Friedman, M.I. (1977) Homeostasis during hypoglycemia: central control of adrenal secretion and peripheral control of feeding. *Science* 196, 79–81.

Stricklin, W.R. (1988) Influence of photoperiod on eating patterns of beef cattle. In: Phillips, C.J.C. and Forbes, J.M. (eds) *Photoperiodic Manipulation of Dairy Cattle.* University of Wales Dairy Research Unit Technical Report No. 4, 8–15.

Stricklin, W.R. and Gonyou, H.W. (1981) Dominance and eating behaviour of cattle fed from a single stall. *Applied Animal Ethology* 7, 135–140.

Strubbe, J.H., Steffens, A.B. and De Ruiter, L. (1977) Plasma insulin and the time pattern of feeding in the rat. *Physiology and Behavior* 18, 81–86.

Sturkie, P.D. (1976) *Avian Physiology.* Springer-Verlag, New York, 400pp.

Sturkie, P.D. and Joiner, W.P. (1959) Effects of foreign bodies in cloaca and rectum of the chicken of food consumption. *American Journal of Physiology* 197, 1337–1338.

Sugahara, M., Baker, D.H. and Scott, H.M. (1969) Effect of different patterns of excess amino acids on performance of chicks fed amino acid deficient diets. *Journal of Nutrition* 97, 29.

Sugahara, M., Baker, D.H., Harman, B.G. and Jensen, A.H. (1970) Effect of ambient temperature on performance and carcass development in young swine. *Journal of Animal Science* 31, 59–62.

Summers, J.D. (1974) Factors influencing food intake in practice – broilers. In: Swan, H. and Lewis, D. (eds) *Nutrition Conference for Feed Manufacturers, 7,* Butterworths, London, pp. 127–140.

Summers, J.D. and Leeson, S. (1979) Diet presentation and feeding. In: Boorman, K.N. and Freeman, B.M. (eds) *Food Intake Regulation in Poultry.* Longman, Edinburgh, pp. 445–469.

Summers, J.D., Moran, E.T. and Pepper, W.T. (1967) A chloride deficiency in a practical diet encountered as a result of using a common sodium sulfate antibiotic potentiating procedure. *Poultry Sicence* 46, 1557–1560.

Sunde, M.L. (1956) Effect of fats and fatty acids in chick rations. *Poultry Science* 35, 362–370.

Susmel,P., Spanghero, M., Stefanon, B., Mills, C.R. and Cargnelutti, C. (1991) Effect of NDF concentration and physical form of fescue hay on rumen degradability, intake and rumen turnover of cows. *Animal Production* 53, 305–313.

Sutton, J.D., Aston, K., Beever, D.E. and Fisher, W.J. (1992) Body composition and performance of autumn-calving Holstein–Friesian dairy cows during lactation: food intake, milk constituent output and live weight. *Animal Production* 54, 473A.

Suzuki, S., Fujita, H. and Shinde, Y. (1969) Change in the rate of eating during a meal and the effect of the interval between meals on the rate at which cows eat roughages. *Animal Production* 11, 29–41.

Sykes, A.H. (1983) Food intake and its control. In: Freeman, B.M. (ed.) *Physiology and Biochemistry of the Domestic Fowl, vol. 4.* Academic Press, London, pp. 1–29.

Sykes, A.R. and Coop, R.L. (1976) Intake and utilisation of food by growing lambs with parasitic damage to the small intestine caused by daily dosing with *Trichostrongylus colubriformis* larvae. *Journal of Agricultural Science* 86, 507–515.

Sykes, A.R. and Coop, R.L. (1977) Intake and utilisation of food by growing lambs with parasitic damage to the small intestine caused by daily dosing with *Ostertagia circumcincta* larvae. *Journal of Agricultural Science* 88, 671–677.

Sykes, A.R., Coop, R.L. and Rushton, B. (1980) Chronic subclinical fascioliasis in sheep: effects on food intake, food utilisation and blood constituents. *Research in Veterinary Science* 28, 63–70.

Syme, G.J. and Syme, L.A. (1979) *Social Structure in Farm Animals*. Elsevier, Amsterdam, 200pp.

Symons, L.E.A. (1985) Anorexia. *Advances in Parasitology* 24, 103–133.

Symons, L.E.A. and Hennessy, D.R. (1981) Cholecystokinin and anorexia in sheep infected by the intestinal nematode *T. colubriformis*. *International Journal of Parasitology* 11, 55–58.

Tadtiyanant, C., Lyons, J.J. and Vandepopuliere, J.M. (1988) The influence of wet and dry feed on production under heat stress. *Poultry Science* 67, 164.

Tadtiyanant, C., Lyons, J.J. and Vandepopuliere, J.M. (1991) Influence of wet and dry feed on laying hens under heat stress. *Poultry Science* 70, 44–52.

Talbot, C. (1993) Some aspects of the biology of feeding and growth in fish. *Proceedings of the Nutrition Society* 52, 403–416.

Tanner, J.C., Owen, E., Winugroho, M. and Gill, M. (1993) Cut-and-carry feeding of indigenous grasses in Indonesian smallholder sheep production: effect of amount offered on intake and growth, and on output of compost made from refusals and excreta. *Animal Production* 56, 449A.

Tarttelin, M.F. (1968) Cyclical variations in food and water intakes in ewes. *Journal of Physiology* 195, 29P–31P.

Tarttelin, M.F. (1969) The physiology of the ventromedial hypothalamus of the sheep with special reference to food and water intake. PhD thesis, University of London.

Tauson, R. and Elwinger, K. (1986) Prototypes for application of choice feeding in caged laying hens using flat chain feeders. *Acta Agralia Scandinavica* 36, 129–146.

Tauson, R., Jansson, L. and Elwinger, K. (1991) Whole grain/crushed peas and a concentrate in mechanised choice feeding for caged laying hens. *Acta Agralia Scandinavica* 41, 75–83.

Tayler, J.C. (1959) A relationship between weight of internal fat, 'fill', and the herbage intake of grazing cattle. *Nature* 184, 2021–2022.

Tayler, J.C. and Aston, K. (1972) Feed factors in milk production. *Annual Report of the Grassland Research Institute, 1971*.

Tayler, J.C. and Gibbs, B.G. (1975) Evaluation of the conserved products of grasses and legumes and their use with other feeds for beef production. *Annual Report of the Grassland Research Institute, 1974*, 72–73.

Tayler, J.C. and Wilkins, R.J. (1976) Conserved forage – complement or competitor to concentrates. In: Swan, H. and Broster, W.H. (eds) *Principles of Cattle Production*, Butterworths, London, pp. 343–364.

Taylor, G.C. and Forbes, J.M. (1988) Food intake and growth of broiler chickens following removal of the abdominal fat pad. *Proceedings of the Nutrition Society* 47, 90A.

Taylor, St C.S., Moore, A.J. and Thiessen, R.B. (1986) Voluntary food intake in relation to body weight among British breeds of cattle. *Animal Production* 42, 11–18.

Taylor, W. and Leaver, J.D. (1984) Systems of concentrate allocation for dairy cattle. 1. A comparison of three patterns of allocation for autumn-calving cows offered grass silage ad libitum. *Animal Production* 39, 315–324.

Telle, P.P., Preston, R.L., Kintner, L.D. and Pfander, W.H. (1964) Definition of the ovine potassium requirement. *Journal of Animal Science* 23, 59–66.

Ternouth, J.H. and Beattie, A.W. (1970) A note on the voluntary food consumption and the sodium–potassium ratio of sheep after shearing. *Animal Production* 12, 343–346.

Ternouth, J.H. and Beattie, A.W. (1971) Studies of the food intake of sheep at a single meal. *British Journal of Nutrition* 25, 153–164.

Ternouth, J.H., Stobo, I.J.F. and Roy, J.H.B. (1978a) The effect of dry matter concentration on milk substitute intake by the calf. *Proceedings of the Nutrition Society* 37, 57A.

Ternouth, J.H., Stobo, I.J.F. and Roy, J.H.B. (1978b) The effect of milk substitute concentration on the intake of milk, dry feed and water by the calf. *Proceedings of the Nutrition Society* 37, 85A.

Tetlow, R.M. and Wilkins, R.J. (1977) The effect of density on the intake of dried forage pellets by young ruminants. *Animal Production* 25, 61–70,

Thiago, L.R.L., Gill, M. and Sissons, J.S. (1992) Studies of methods of conserving grass herbage and frequency of feeding in cattle. 2. Eating behaviour, rumen motility and rumen fill. *British Journal of Nutrition* 67, 319–336.

Thikey, H.M. (1985) The use of conditioned reflexes to enhance feed intake in the growing pig. PhD thesis, University of Aberdeen.

Thomas, C. (1987) Factors affecting substitution rates in dairy cows on silage based rations. In: Haresign, W. and Cole, D.J.A. (eds) *Recent Advances in Animal Nutrition – 1987*, pp. 205–218.

Thomas, C., Gill, M. and Austin, A.R. (1980a) The effect of supplements of fish meal and lactic acid on voluntary intake of silage by calves. *Grass and Forage Science* 35, 275–279.

Thomas, C., Gill, M. and Austin, A.R. (1980b) The effect of supplements of fish meal and lactic acid on voluntary intake of silage by calves. *Grass and Forage Science* 35, 275–279.

Thomas, C., Aston, K., Bass, J., Daley, S.R. and Hughes, M. (1984) The effect of composition of concentrate on the voluntary intake of silage and milk output. *Animal Production* 38, 519.

Thomas, C., Aston, K. and Daley, S.R. (1985) Milk production from silage, a comparison of red clover with grass silage. *Animal Production* 41, 23–31.

Thomas, C.K. and Pearson, R.A. (1986) Effect of ambient temperature and head cooling on energy expenditure, food intake and heat tolerance of Brahman and Brahman × Friesan cattle working on treadmills. *Animal Production* 43, 83–90.

Thomas, J.W., Moore, L.A. and Sykes, J.F. (1961a) Further comparisons of alfalfa hay and alfalfa silage for growing dairy heifers. *Journal of Dairy Science* 44, 862–973.

Thomas, J.W., Moore, L.A., Okamoto, M. and Sykes, J.F. (1961b) A study of factors affecting rate of intake of heifers fed silage. *Journal of Dairy Science* 44, 1471–1483.

Thomas, P.C. and Chamberlain, D.G. (1983) Silage as a feedstuff. In: *Silage for*

*Milk Production*. Technical Bulletin No. 2, NIRD, HRI, pp. 63–102.

Thompson, J.M. and Parks, J.R. (1983) Food intake, growth and mature size in Australian Merino and Dorset Horn sheep. *Animal Production* 36, 471–479.

Thompson, J.M., Parks, J.R. and Perry, D. (1985) Food intake, growth and body composition in Australian Merino sheep selected for high and low weaning weight. 1. Food intake, food efficiency and growth. *Animal Production* 40, 55–70.

Thonney, M.L., Touchberry, R.W., Goodrich, R.D. and Meiske, J.C. (1976) Intraspecies relationship between fasting heat production and body weight, a re-evaluation of $W^{0.75}$. *Journal of Animal Science* 43, 692–703.

Thorhallsdottir, A.G., Provenza, F.D. and Ralph, D.F. (1987) Food aversion learning in lambs with or without a mother: discrimination, novelty and persistence. *Applied Animal Behaviour Science* 18, 327–340.

Thorne, D.H.M., Vandepopuliere, J.M. and Lyons, J.J. (1989) Automated high moisture diet feeding system for laying hens. *Poultry Science* 68, 1114–1117.

Thornley, J.H.M., Parsons, A.J., Newman, J.A. and Penning, P.D. (1994) A cost–benefit model of grazing intake and diet selection in a two-species temperate grassland sward. *Functional Ecology* 8, 5–16.

Thornton, R.F. and Minson, D.J. (1973) The relationship between apparent retention time in the rumen, voluntary intake, and apparent digestibility of legume and grass diets in sheep. *Australian Journal of Agricultural Research* 24, 889–898.

Thrasher, G.W., Shively, J.E. and Askelton, C.E. (1970) Effects of Carbadox on performance and carcass traits of growing swine. *Journal of Animal Science* 31, 333–338.

Thye, F.W, Warner, R.G. and Miller, P.D. (1970) Relationship of various blood metabolites to voluntary feed intake in lactating ewes. *Journal of Nutrition* 100, 565–572.

Tindal, J.S., Knaggs, G.S., Hart, I.C. and Blake, L.S. (1978) Release of growth hormone in lactating and non-lactating goats in relation to behaviour, stages of sleep, electroencephalograms, environmental stimuli and levels of prolactin, insulin, glucose and free fatty acids in the circulation. *Journal of Endocrinology* 76, 333–346.

Titchen, D.A., Reid, C.S.W. and Vlieg, P. (1966) Effects of intra-duodenal infusions of fat on the food intake of sheep. *Proceedings of the New Zealand Society of Animal Production* 26, 36–51.

Toates, F.M. and Booth, D.A. (1974) Control of food intake by energy supply. *Nature* 251, 710–711.

Tobin, G. and Boorman, K.N. (1979) Carotid artery or jugular amino acid infusions and food intake in the cockerel. *British Journal of Nutrition* 41, 157–167.

Tolkamp, B.J. and Ketelaars, J.J.M.H. (1992) Toward a new theory of feed intake regulation in ruminants. 2. Costs and benefits of feed consumption: an optimization approach. *Livestock Production Science* 30, 297–317.

Tordoff, M.G. and Friedman, M.I. (1986) Hepatic portal glucose infusions decrease food intake and increase food preference. *American Journal of Physiology* 251, R192–R196.

Tordoff, M.G. and Novin, D. (1982) Coeliac vagotomy attenuates the ingestive responses to epinephrine and hypertonic saline but not insulin, 2 deoxy-D-glucose or polyethylene glycol. *Physiology and Behavior* 29, 605–613.

Tordoff, M.G., Tepper, B.J. and Friedman, M.I. (1987) Food flavor preferences produced by drinking glucose and oil in normal and diabetic rats: evidence for conditioning based on fuel oxidation. *Physiology and Behavior* 41, 481–487.

Toutain, P.L., Toutain, C., Webster, A.J.F. and McDonald, J.D. (1977) Sleep and activity, age and fatness, and the energy expenditure in confined sheep. *British Journal of Nutrition* 38, 445–454.

Tribe, D.E. (1949) The importance of the sense of smell to the grazing sheep. *Journal of Agricultural Science* 39, 309–312.

Tribe, D.E. and Gordon, J.G. (1949) The importance of colour vision to the grazing sheep. *Journal of Agricultural Science* 39, 313–314.

Troelson, J.E. and Bigsby, F.W. (1964) Artificial mastication – a new approach for predicting voluntary forage consumption by ruminants. *Journal of Animal Science* 23, 1139–1142.

Tsiagbe, V.K., Straub, R.J., Cok, M.E., Harper, A.E. and Sunde, M.L. (1987) Formulating wet alfalfa juice protein concentrate diets for chicks. *Poultry Science* 66, 1023–1027.

Tulloh, N.M. (1966) Physical studies of the alimentary tract of grazing cattle. 3. Seasonal changes of the alimentary tract of grazing cattle. *New Zealand Journal of Agricultural Research* 9, 252–260.

Tweeton, J.R., Phillips, R.E. and Peek, F.W. (1973) Feeding behaviour elicited by electrical stimulation of the brain in chickens. *Poultry Science* 52, 165–172.

Ulyatt, M.J., Blaxter, K.L. and McDonald, I. (1967) The relations between the apparent digestibility of roughages in the rumen and lower gut of sheep, the volume of fluid in the rumen and voluntary feed intake. *Animal Production* 9, 463–470.

Vadiveloo, J. and Holmes, W. (1979) The prediction of the voluntary feed intake of dairy cows. *Journal of Agricultural Science* 93, 553–562.

Valentine, J.F.(1990) *Grazing Management*. Academic Press, San Diego.

Van Choubroek, F., Coucke, L. and Van Spaendonk, R. (1971) The quantitative effect of pelleting feed on the performance of piglets and fattening pigs. *Nutrition Abstracts and Reviews* 41, 1–9.

Van den Broek, G.W., Robertson, J., Keim, D.A. and Baile, C.A. (1979) Feeding and depression of abomasal secretion in sheep elicited by elfazepam and 9-aza-cannabinal. *Pharmacology, Biochemistry and Behavior* 11, 51–56.

Vandepopuliere, J.M. and Lyons, J.J. (1983) Methane digester effluent provided to caged laying hens via feed and water. In: *Proceedings of the 3rd Annual Solar Biomass Workshop*, USDA Agriculture Research Service, Crop System Research Unit, Coastal Plains Experimental Station, Tifton, GA, pp. 94–97.

Vandermeerschen-Doize, F. and Paquay, R. (1984) Effects of continuous long-term intravenous infusion of long-chain fatty acids on feeding behaviour and blood components of adult sheep. *Appetite* 5, 137–146.

Vandermeerschen-Doize, F., Bouckoms-Vandermeier, M. and Paquay, R. (1982) Effects of long-term ad libitum feeding on the voluntary food intake, body weight, body composition and adipose tissue morphology of lean adult sheep. *Reproduction, Nutrition, Developpement* 22, 1049–1061.

van Houtert, M.F.J. and Leng, R.A. (1991) A note on the effects of high levels of dietary calcium, phosphorus and sodium on nutrient utilization by sheep offered a roughage-based diet. *Animal Production* 53, 249–252.

Van Miert, A.S.J.P.A.M. and Van Duin, C.T.M. (1991) Feed intake and rumen motility in dwarf goats. Effects of some $\alpha_2$-adrenergic agonists, prostaglandins and posterior pituitary hormones. *Veterinary Research Communications* 15, 57–67.

Van Niekerk, A.I., Greenhalgh, J.F.D. and Reid, G.W. (1973) Importance of palatability in determining the feed intake of sheep offered chopped and pelleted hay. *British Journal of Nutrition* 30, 95–105.

Van Soest, P.J. (1967) Development of a comprehensive system of feed analysis and its application to forages. *Journal of Animal Science* 26, 119–128.

Van Soest, P.J. (1982) *Nutritional Ecology of the Ruminant.* O and B Books, Corvallis,Oregon, 374pp.

Vasilatos, R. and Wangsness, P.J. (1980) Changes in concentrations of insulin, growth hormone and metabolites in plasma with spontaneous feeding in lactating dairy cows. *Journal of Nutrition* 110, 1479–1489.

Vera, R.R., Morris, J.G. and Koong, L.J. (1977) A quantitative model of energy intake and partition in grazing sheep in various physiological states. *Animal Production* 25, 133–153.

Verstegen, J.W.A., Brascamp, E.W. and van der Hel, W. (1978) Growing and fattening of pigs in relation to temperature of housing and feeding level. *Canadian Journal of Animal Science* 58, 1–13.

Vetter, R.L. and Von Glan, K.N. (1978) Abnormal silages and silage related disease problems. In: McCullough, M.E. (ed.) *Fermentation of Silage – A Review,* West Des Moines, National Feed Ingredients Association, pp. 281–332.

Vidal, J.M., Edwards, S.A., McPherson, O., English, P.R. and Taylor, A.G. (1991) Effect of environmental temperature on dietary selection in lactating sows. *Animal Production* 52, 597.

Vidal, J.M., Brouns, F., Edwards, S.A., English, P.R., MacPherson, O., Taylor, A.G. and Haley, C.S. (1992) Dietary protein selection by Chinese and European growing pigs given free choice feeding. *Animal Production* 54, 483.

Vipond, J.E., King, M.E., Inglis, D.M. and Hunter, E.A. (1987) The effect of winter shearing of housed pregnant ewes on food intake and animal performance. *Animal Production* 45, 211–222.

Vo, K.Y., Boone, M.A. and Johnstone, W.E. (1978) Effect of three life ambient temperatures on growth, feed and water consumption and various blood components in male and female Leghorn chickens. *Poultry Science* 57, 798–803.

Wade, G.N. and Gray, J.M. (1979) Gonadal effects on food intake and adiposity: a metabolic hypothesis. *Physiology and Behavior* 22, 583–593.

Wade, G.N. and Zucker, I. (1970) Modulation of food intake and locomotor activity in female rats by diencephalic hormone implants. *Journal of Comparative Physiology and Psychology* 72, 328–336.

Wagnon, K.A. (1965) Social dominance in range cows and its effects on supplemental feeding. *California Agricultural Experiment Station Bulletin* 819, 31pp.

Wahed, R.A., Owen, E., Naate, M. and Hosking, B.J. (1990) Feeding straw to small ruminants: effect of amount offered on intake and selection of barley straw by goats and sheep. *Animal Production* 51, 283–289.

Waite, R., McDonald, W.B. and Holmes, W. (1951) Studies in grazing management. 3. The behaviour of dairy cows grazed under the close-folding and rotational systems of management. *Journal of Agricultural Science* 41, 163–173.

Waldern, D.E. (1972) Effects of supplemental hay on consumption of low and medium dry matter corn silage by high-producing dairy cows. *Canadian Journal of Animal Science* 52, 491–496.

Waldern, D.E. and Van Dyk, R.D. (1971) Effect of monosodium glutamate in starter rations on feed consumption of early weaned calves. *Journal of Dairy Science* 54, 262–265.

Waldo, D.R., Miller, R.W., Okamoto, M. and Moore, L.A. (1965a) Ruminant utilisation of silage in relation to hay, pellets and hay plus grain. 1. Composition, digestion, nitrogen balance, intake and growth. *Journal of Dairy Science* 48, 910–916.

Waldo, D.R., Miller, R.W., Okamoto, M. and Moore, L.A. (1965b) Ruminant utilisation of silage in relation to hay, pellets and hay plus grain. 2. Rumen content, dry matter passage and water intake. *Journal of Dairy Science* 48, 1473–1480.

Walker, P.S., van Krey, H.P., Cherry, J.A. and Siegal, P.B. (1981) The effect of gold thioglucose on feed consumption in domestic fowl. *Poultry Science* 60, 1325–1332.

Wallace, M., Fraser, C.D., Clements, J.A. and Funder, J.W. (1981) Naloxone, adrenalectomy and steroid replacement: evidence against a role for circulting β-endorphin in food intake. *Endocrinology* 108, 189–192.

Wangsness, P.J. and Muller, L.D. (1981) Maximum forage for dairy cows: review. *Journal of Dairy Science* 64, 1–13.

Wangsness, P.J. and Soroka, G.H. (1978) Effect of energy concentration of milk on voluntary intake of lean and obese piglets. *Journal of Nutrition* 108, 595–600.

Wangsness, P.J., Chase, L.E., Peterson, A.D., Hartstock, T.G., Kellmel, D.J. and Baumgardt, B.R. (1976) System for monitoring feeding behavior of sheep. *Journal of Animal Science* 42, 1544–1549.

Wanyoike, M.M. and Holmes, W. (1981) A comparison of indirect methods of estimating feed intake on pasture. *Grass and Forage Science* 36, 221–225.

Waran, N.K. and Broom, D.M. (1992) The influence of a barrier on the behaviour and growth of early-weaned piglets. *Animal Production* 56, 115–119.

Wardrop, I.D. (1960) The post-natal growth of the visceral organs of the lamb. 2. The effect of diet on growth rate, with particular reference to the parts of the alimentary canal. *Journal of Agricultural Science* 55, 127–132.

Warner, A.C.I. and Stacy, B.D. (1965) Solutes in the rumen of the sheep. *Quarterly Journal of Experimental Physiology* 50, 169–184.

Warner, A.C.I. and Stacy, B.D. (1968) The fate of water in the rumen. 2. Water balances throughout the feeding cycle in sheep. *British Journal of Nutrition* 22, 389–410.

Warner, A.C.I. and Stacy, B.D. (1977) Influence of ruminal and plasma osmotic pressure on salivary secretion in sheep. *Quarterly Journal of Experimental Physiology* 62, 133–142.

Warnick, V.D., Arave, C.W. and Mickelsen, C.H. (1977) Effects of group, individual and isolated rearing of calves on weight gain and behavior. *Journal of Dairy Science* 60, 947–953.

Weatherford, S.C. and Ritter, S. (1986) Glucagon satiety, diurnal variation after hepatic branch vagotomy or intraportal alloxan. *Brain Research Bulletin* 17, 545–550.

Webb, A.J. (1989) Genetics of food intake in the pig. In: Forbes, J.M., Varley, M.A. and Lawrence, T.L.J. (eds) *The Voluntary Food Intake of Pigs*. Occasional Publication of the British Society of Animal Production, pp. 1–50.

Webster, A.J.F., Smith, J.S. and Brockway, J.M. (1972) Effects of isolation, confinement and competition for feed on the energy exchanges of growing lambs. *Animal Production* 15, 189–201.

Weddell, J.R. (1992) The effects of Maxgrass treatment of bale silage on the performance of beef cattle. *Animal Production* 54: 487.

Weeth, H.J., Sawhney, D.S. and Lesperance, A.L. (1967) Changes in body fluids, excreta and kidney function of cattle deprived of water. *Journal of Animal Science* 26: 418–423.

Weingarten, H.P. (1993) How do we measure palatability in animals? *Appetite,* 22: 216.

Welch, J.D. (1967) Appetite control in sheep by indigestible fibres. *Journal of Animal Science* 26, 849–854.

Welch, J.G. (1982) Rumination, particle size and passage from the rumen. *Journal of Animal Science* 54, 885–894.

Weller, R.F. and Phipps, R.H. (1985a) Milk production from grass and maize silages. *Animal Production* 40, 560–561.

Weller, R.F. and Phipps, R.H. (1985b) The effect of silage preference on the performance of dairy cows. *Animal Production* 42, 435.

Weller, R.F. and Phipps, R.H. (1989) Preliminary studies on the effect of flavouring agents on the dry-matter intake of silage by lactating dairy cows. *Journal of Agricultural Science* 112, 67–71.

Wernli, C.G. and Wilkins, R.J. (1971) The voluntary intake of grass silage supplemented with dried grass or barley. *Animal Production* 13, 397.

Westoby, M. (1974) An analysis of diet selection by large generalist herbivores. *American Naturalist* 108, 290–304.

Wheeler, J.L., Reardon, T.F. and Lambourne, L.J. (1963) The effect of pasture availability and shearing stress on herbage intake of grazing sheep. *Australian Journal of Agricultural Research* 14, 364–372.

Widdowson, E. and McCance, R.A. (1960) Some effects of accelerating growth. 1. General somatic development. *Proceedings of the Royal Society, B* 152, 188–206.

Wierenga, H.K. and Hopster, H. (1986) Behavioural research to improve systems for automatic concentrate feeding. *Proceedings of the International Symposium on Applied Ethology in Farm Animals*, Balatonfured, Hungary.

Wiese, A.C., Johnson, B.C., Mitchell, H.H. and Nevens, W.B. (1947) Riboflavin deficiency in the dairy calf. *Journal of Nutrition* 33, 263–270.

Wilcoxon, H.C., Dragoin, W.B. and Kral, O.A. (1971) Illness-induced aversions in rat and quail: relative salience of visual and gustatory cues. *Science* 171, 826–828.

Wilkins, R.J. (1974) The nutritive value of silages. In: Swan, H. and Lewis, D. (eds) *Nutrition Conference for Feed Manufacturers, 8.* Butterworths, London, pp. 167–189.

Wilkins, R.J., Hutchinson, K.J., Wilson, R.F. and Harris, C.E. (1971) The voluntary intake of silage by sheep. 1. Interrelationships between silage composition and intake. *Journal of Agricultural Science* 77, 531–537.

Wilkins, R.J., Lonsdale, C.R., Tetlow, R.M. and Forrest, T.J. (1972) The voluntary intake and digestibility by cattle and sheep of dried grass wafers containing particles of different size. *Animal Production* 14, 177–188.

Wilkinson, J.M., Penning, I.M. and Osbourn, D.F. (1978) Effect of stage of harvest and fineness of chopping on the voluntary intake and digestibility of maize silage by young beef cattle. *Animal Production* 26, 143–150.

Wilkinson, S.C. and Chestnutt, D.M.B. (1988) Effect of level of food intake in mid and late pregnancy on the performance of breeding ewes. *Animal Production* 47, 411–420.

Williams, A.J. (1964) The effect of daily photoperiod on wool growth of Merino rams subjected to unrestricted and restricted feeding regimes. *Australian Journal of Experimental Agriculture and Animal Husbandry* 4, 124–128.

Williams, G., McKibbin, P.E. and McCarthy, H.D. (1991) Hypothalamic regulatory peptides and the regulation of food intake and energy balance: signals or noise? *Proceedings of the Nutrition Society* 50, 527–544.

Wilson, A.D. (1966) The tolerance of sheep to sodium chloride in food and drinking water. *Australian Journal of Agricultural Research* 17, 503–514.

Wilson, B.J. and Emmans, G.C. (1979) The animal's relationship to its food. In: Boorman, K.N. and Freeman, B.M. (eds) *Food Intake Regulation in Poultry.* Longman, Edinburgh, pp. 3–10.

Wilson, P.N. and Osbourn, D.F. (1960) Comensatory growth after undernutrition in mammals and birds. *Biological Reviews* 35, 324–363.

Wilson, R.K. and Flynn, A.V. (1974) Observations of the eating behaviour of individually fed beef cattle offered grass silage ad libitum. *Irish Journal of Agricultural Research* 13, 347–349.

Winchester, C.F. and Morris, M.J. (1956) Water intake of cattle. *Journal of Animal Science* 15, 722–740.

Winfield, C.G., Brown, W. and Lucas, I.A.M. (1968) Some effects of compulsory exposure over winter on in-lamb Welsh Mountains ewes. *Animal Production* 10, 451–463.

Wirtshafter, D. and Davis, J.D. (1977a) Set points, settling points, and the control of body weight. *Physiology and Behavior* 19, 75–78.

Wiseman, J. and Cole, D.J.A. (1987) The digestible and metabolisable energy of two fat blends for growing pigs as influenced by level of inclusion. *Animal Production* 45, 117–122.

Wodzika, M. (1963) The effect of shearing on the appetite of sheep. *New Zealand Journal of Agricultural Research* 6, 440–447.

Wodzika, M. (1964) The effect of shearing on the appetite of two-tooth ewes. *New Zealand Journal of Agricultural Research* 7, 654–662.

Wood, J.D. (1989) Meat quality, carcass composition and intake. In: Forbes, J.M., Varley, M.A. and Lawrence, T.L.J. (eds) *The Voluntary Food Intake of Pigs*. Occasional Publication of the British Society of Animal Production, pp. 79–86.

Wood, P.D.P. (1969) Factors affecting the shape of the lactation curve in cattle. *Animal Production* 11, 307–316.

Wood-Gush, D.G.M. and Gower, D.M. (1968) Studies on motivation in the feeding behaviour of the domestic cock. *Animal Behaviour* 16, 101–107.

Wood-Gush, D.G.M. and Horne, A.R. (1971) The effect of egg formation and laying on the food and water intake of Brown Leghorn hens. *British Poultry Science* 11, 459–466.

Wood-Gush, D.G.M. and Kare, M.R. (1966) The behaviour of calcium deficient chickens. *British Poultry Science* 7, 285–290.

Woods, S.C., Lotter, E.C., McKay, D. and Porte, D. (1979) Chronic intra-cerebroventricular infusion of insulin reduces food intake and body weight of baboons. *Nature* 282, 503–505.

Woods, S.C., Stein, L.J., McKay, L.D. and Porte, D. (1984) Suppression of food intake by intravenous nutrients and insulin in the baboon. *American Journal of Physiology* 247, R393–401.

Woods, S.C., Porte, D., Strubbe, J.H. and Steffens, A.B. (1986) The relationships among body fat, feeding, and insulin. In: Ritter, R.C., Ritter, S. and Barnes, C.D. (eds) *Feeding Behavior: Neural and Humoral Controls*. Academic Press, Orlando, pp. 315–327.

Wright, I.A., Rhind, S.M, Whyte, T.K., Smith, A.J., McMillen, S.R. and Prado, R. (1990) Circulating concentrations of LH and FSH and pituitary responsiveness to GnRH in intact and ovariectomized suckled beef cows in two levels of body condition. *Animal Production* 51, 93–101.

Wright, P. (1976) The neural substrate of feeding behaviour in birds. In: Wright, P. and Caryl, P.G. (eds) *Neural and Endocrine Aspects of Behaviour in Birds*. Elsevier, Amsterdam, pp. 319–349.

Wyburn, R.S. (1980) The mixing and propulsion of the stomach contents of ruminants. In: Ruckebusch, Y. and Thivend, P. (eds) *Digestive Physiology and Metabolism in Ruminants*. MTP, Lancaster, pp. 35–51.

Wylie, A.R.G. and Chestnutt, A.M.B. (1992) The effect of silage quality and frequency of feeding of supplementary concentrates on serum metabolite and insulin-like growth factor 1 (IGF-1) concentrations in the late pregnant ewe. *Animal Production* 54, 455–456A.

Wyrwicka, W. and Dobrzecka, C. (1960) Relationship between feeding and satiation centers of the hypothalamus. *Science* 132, 805–806.

Yalda, A.Y. and Forbes, J.M. (1990) Effect of energy restriction on the relationship between body fat and food intake in broilers. *Proceedings of the Nutrition Society* 49, 215A.

Yalda, A.Y. and Forbes, J.M. (1991) The effect of force-feeding on the relationship between body fat and food intake in broilers. *Proceedings of the Nutrition Society* 50, 99A.

Yang, T.S., Howard, B. and McFarlane, W.V. (1981) Effects of food on drinking behaviour of growing pigs. *Applied Animal Ethology* 7, 259–270.

Yeomans, M.R. and Savory, C.J. (1989) Altered spontaneous and osmotically induced drinking for fowls with permanent access to quinine. *Physiology and Behavior* 46, 917–922.

Young, R.J. and Lawrence, A.B. (1994) Feeding behaviour of pigs in groups monitored by a computerized feeding system. *Animal Production* 58, 145–152.

Young, R.J., Lawrence, A.B. and Carruthers, J. (1993) The effects of food level and a foraging device on the behaviour of sows. *Animal Production* 56, 440A.

Zahorik, D.M. and Houpt, K.A. (1981) Species differences in feeding strategies, food hazards and the ability to learn food aversions. In: Kamil, A.C. and Sargent, T.D. (eds) *Foraging Behavior.* Garland Press, New York, pp. 289–310.

Zainuri, A.S., Hoskinson, R.M. and Kellaway, R.C. (1991) Production responses of lambs immunized against somatostatin. *Animal Production* 53, 339–344.

Zamel, L.N., Colenbrander, V.F., Callahan, C.J., Chew, B.P., Erb, R.E. and Moeller, N.J. (1979) Variables associated with peripartum traits in dairy cows. 1. Effect of dietary forages and disorders on voluntary intake of feed, body weight and milk yield. *Theriogenology* 11, 229–244.

Zeigler, H.P. (1975) Trigeminal deafferentiation and hunger in the pigeon. *Journal of Comparative and Physiological Psychology* 89, 827–844.

Zoiopoulous, P.E., English, P.R. and Topps, J.H. (1983) A note on intake and digestibility of a fibrous diet self fed to primiparous sows. *Animal Production* 37, 153–156.

# Index